THE ROLE OF THE TRYPANOSOMIASES
IN AFRICAN ECOLOGY

THE ROLE OF THE
TRYPANOSOMIASES
IN AFRICAN ECOLOGY

———

A STUDY OF THE TSETSE FLY PROBLEM

———

BY

JOHN FORD

CLARENDON PRESS · OXFORD

1971

Oxford University Press, Ely House, London W.1

GLASGOW   NEW YORK   TORONTO   MELBOURNE   WELLINGTON
CAPE TOWN   SALISBURY   IBADAN   DAR ES SALAAM   LUSAKA   ADDIS ABABA
BOMBAY   CALCUTTA   MADRAS   KARACHI   LAHORE   DACCA
KUALA LUMPUR   SINGAPORE   HONG KONG   TOKYO

PRINTED IN GREAT BRITAIN
BY BUTLER AND TANNER LTD
FROME AND LONDON

PREFACE

MANY years ago I began to have doubts about official colonial doctrine concerning the importance of the tsetse in tropical Africa. I have attributed this doctrine, in Chapter 1, to Sir Richard Burton, although it had earlier beginnings. These insects and the diseases they transmit do, of course, present very serious problems of health, both human and animal, but Burton was quite wrong in supposing that the African tropics would become an agricultural paradise if they could be removed.

It seems to me that the applied scientist ought to want to understand why he is employed. If, as a consequence of his curiosity, he comes to the conclusion that his successes or failures will not have the results his employers expect from them, he should try to find a basis for alternative strategies for dealing with what is still a very serious and difficult problem.

This book presents, in narrative form, the story of the trypanosomiases in five different areas in which I have worked. These narratives are preceded by five chapters which contain the minimum of technical background necessary for their understanding. The concluding two chapters contain what seem the main lessons to be drawn from the study.

ACKNOWLEDGEMENTS

FIRST it is a pleasure and a duty to thank the Wellcome Trustees for their munificent generosity, which has enabled me to write this book. Without that support it could not have been written.

On an earlier occasion, I collected material during a travelling fellowship granted by the Food and Agricultural Organization. Dr. N. Ansari invited me to visit Geneva, where I was able to use the World Health Organization library. Professor P. G. Janssens allowed me to work at the Prince Leopold Institute of Tropical Medicine in Antwerp, and I am also indebted to him for permission to reproduce the graph on page 473. Dr. R. J. Onyango has been unfailingly generous with the resources of the East African Trypanosomiasis Research Organization at Sukulu, and Mr. T. M. Leach, on three occasions, allowed me to work in the laboratories of the Nigerian Institute for Trypanosomiasis Research at Kaduna and Vom. Mr. K. J. R. Maclennan, of the Ministry of Forest and Animal Resources, Kaduna, not only supplied me with abundant information but also gave up much time to taking me around Nigeria. I am most grateful to Mallam Bukar Shaib, Permanent Secretary of that Ministry, for facilitating my Nigerian field work. Professor Desmond Hill arranged for me to work in the library of Ibadan University. Mr. H. R. Binns, of the East African Veterinary Research Organization, arranged for use of the library at Muguga. Among the many who have given time to taking me around Africa, I have to thank especially Mr. D. B. Turner and Mr. G. Clausen in Tanzania, Dr. P. E. Glover and Mr. J. le Roux in Kenya, and Mr. J. Bernacca, Dr. W. R. Wooff, and Mr. H. R. Clifford in Uganda. Dr. P. Finelle at Bouar and Dr. J. Gruvel at Fort Lamy were most generous and hospitable in demonstrating situations in the Central African and Chad Republics, and I am grateful to Dr. M. Graber, Directeur de la Région de Récherches Veterinaire et Zootechniques de l'Afrique Centrale, and Dr. J. Desrotour, Directeur de l'Elevage, for hospitality in those two countries.

Dr. A. de Barros Machado, Dr. M. Thomé, Dr. T. A. M. Nash, Professor E. Bursell, Mr. W. P. Boyt, Mr. J. A. K. Farrell, Dr. J. Weir, Dr. G. R. Scott, Mr. A. G. Robertson, and Mr. P. M. Mwambu have been generous in answering letters and sending unpublished material. I am grateful to Messrs Baillière, Tindall, and Cassell for permission to quote at length from the 16th edition of Manson's *Tropical Diseases*.

I am greatly indebted to Dr. F. I. C. Apted, Mr. D. A. T. Baldry, Dr. G. F. Cockbill, Mr. J. M. B. Harley, Mr. T. M. Leach, Mr. K. J. R. Maclennan, Mr. W. H. Potts, Dr. K. D. B. Thomson, Professor D. J. B. Wijers, and Dr. Guy Yeoman, who, between them, have ready nearly all of the book and given valuable criticism, correction, and information.

Miss Mary Potter has been most careful in drawing many of the maps, and I am indebted to Dr. David Rogers for a similar service. The staff of the Clarendon Press have been unfailingly patient and helpful, and I thank them.

In making these acknowledgements I am conscious of many other people who have given freely of their skills and knowledge to assist me. I must, however, mention especially Professor W. E. Kershaw, Dr. F. C. Hawking, Professor B. Weitz, and Mr. W. H. Potts of the Trypanosomiasis Panel of the Ministry of Overseas Development for their continuing encouragement. I also owe a large debt of gratitude to Professor G. C. Varley for giving me room to write in one of the oldest homes of glossinology, the Hope Department of Zoology at Oxford.

Finally my debt to my wife is immeasurable. She has typed all the book once and most of it many times. Without her, it would never have been written.

J. F.

Oxford, 19th August 1970

CONTENTS

CONTENTS

LIST OF FIGURES

LIST OF MAPS

LIST OF TABLES

I

ORGANISMS INVOLVED IN THE AFRICAN TRYPANOSOMIASIS PROBLEM AND THEIR INTERRELATIONSHIPS

THE colonial period in tropical Africa may be taken as beginning in 1885 with the Congress of Berlin and as ending about 1960, three-quarters of a century later. During its last sixty years the European powers chiefly involved, Britain, France, Belgium, and Portugal, maintained organizations to investigate and attempt to solve the problems created by the presence of tsetse flies (*Glossina*) and the diseases of man and domestic animals transmitted by them. For sixty years a large number of scientists, some of them of great distinction, worked on 'the tsetse problem' and an appreciable portion of African colonial budgets was devoted to the upkeep of research and control services. There grew up a large body of knowledge about tsetse flies and about trypanosomes, the causative organisms of human sleeping sickness and of animal trypanosomiasis. P. A. Buxton, one of the leaders in this research, said of the study of tsetse flies that, 'The work of the entomologist has been so full and well planned, that it is of general biological interest. *Glossina* is indeed one of the classical organisms on which certain methods of field survey and of estimating population have been developed' (Buxton 1955).

One of the first to make up his mind on tsetse flies was Richard Burton who wrote, 'It is difficult to conceive the purpose for which this plague was placed in a land so eminently fitted for breeding cattle and for agriculture, which without animals cannot be greatly extended, except as an exercise for human ingenuity to remove. Possibly at some future date, when the country becomes valuable, the tsetse may be exterminated by the introduction of some insectivorous bird, which will be the greatest benefactor that Central Africa ever knew' (Burton 1860). This study is a commentary upon the explorer's text. It was not until about 1930 that his assessment of the problem began to be challenged. When, forty years after him, the appalling mortality of the Uganda sleeping sickness epidemic and Bruce's discovery of the role of *Glossina* in its transmission drew widespread attention to the tsetse fly, everything seemed to reinforce Burton's opinion. The official view was clearly stated by the East Africa Commission in 1925. 'The ravages of the tsetse-fly are the greatest menace to the development of tropical Africa, and constitute one of its most serious problems' (Ormsby-Gore 1925).

Although the search for an insectivorous bird soon became a minor side-line, British research was almost entirely confined to problems of tsetse elimination until well after the Second World War. It was pursued in complete confidence that the achievement of that objective would indeed be the greatest of all benefactions that a colonial power could bestow upon Africa. By that time, however, biologists in other disciplines had put forward another view, that the expulsion of *Glossina* might be a disaster. Today neither opinion seems right.

A variety of methods for tsetse extermination now exist. In addition, the doctor or veterinarian whose task is to treat human or animal trypano-somiasis has available a whole battery of drugs for treatment and temporary prophylaxis. Yet it is certain that the area infested with tsetse in Africa is larger than it was in 1900 after the passage of the rinderpest (Chapters 8, 11, 17, and elsewhere) and it is likely that the overall incidence of sleeping sickness is greater than it was a century ago. There is a need, therefore, to re-examine the premises for investigation and treatment of the problem.

The organisms

The trypanosomes (*Trypanosoma*) are flagellated Protozoa belonging to the class Zoomastigophorea, order Kinetoplastida. Characteristically they possess a kinetoplast, a body of deeply staining nucleoprotein (DNA) situated near the base of the flagellum. There are many trypanosomes beside those associated with tsetses, some of them causing diseases and some harmless. All are haemoflagellates, parasites in the blood, and some-times other tissues, of various vertebrates. Their transmission from one vertebrate host to another is performed by an intermediate invertebrate host, the vector. *Trypanosoma equiperdum*, the cause of a venereal disease of horses, is the sole exception to this rule. It plays no part in the African disease complex within the tsetse belts.

Infection by one or other of the trypanosomes is known as trypano-somiasis. This infection in man gives rise to a disease that takes a variety of forms, one of which may correctly be called sleeping sickness because the patient, at one stage, is unable to keep awake. The cattle trypanosomiases are sometimes called by the Zulu name *nagana*. The causal trypanosomes of these diseases in tropical Africa are essentially blood parasites of larger wild animals, and transmission from one host to another is performed by tsetse flies. We may follow Weitz (1964) in speaking of these animals as the *natural* hosts of the trypanosomes. Sometimes the insect vector will bite and transmit the flagellates to man or his domestic animals, which then perform the role of *adventitious* hosts. However, there are circumstances in which the flies come to depend entirely upon man or domestic livestock for their blood meals, and in this case the adventitious hosts may take over the role of the natural hosts of the trypanosomes. But this is a secondary development and the tsetse-borne trypanosomiases, in general, may be grouped together as zoonoses; that is, as diseases caused by parasites of animals which accidentally become established in man or, in this case, man's own domestic symbionts, cattle, sheep, goats, horses, pigs, and dogs. The transmission of trypanosomes from one host to another by tsetse flies (*Glossina*) is cyclical and obligatory, for they undergo a part of their life-cycle in these insects.

The genus *Glossina* belongs to the insect order of Diptera, family Muscidae, subfamily Stomoxydinae. Other Diptera, especially perhaps species of *Stomoxys* and the Tabanidae, that live by blood sucking, can participate in the transmission of trypanosomes from one host to another. This may happen when one of these insects is interrupted in a meal from an infected host and immediately transfers its attention to another in the same herd. The proboscis is then full of blood containing trypanosomes, and by piercing the skin and injecting saliva into the circulation of the second animal, infective trypanosomes are transferred. Possibly tsetse flies themselves may function in this way when similarly interrupted. Such transmission is called 'mechanical' or 'acyclical' transmission and may play an important part in some epidemics and epizootics. It is a difficult subject to investigate. At present it seems a safe assumption that extermination of the genus *Glossina* in Africa would eliminate the diseases with which this study is concerned, but it is not certain.

There are 34 species, subspecies, and races of *Glossina* now recognized. At least half of them have little more than academic interest to people concerned with the control of trypanosomiasis. Among the trypanosomes four, in a broad sense, cause diseases of domestic livestock, and one of these has developed 'races' that cause trypanosomiasis in man.

Weitz (1963) lists 51 species or genera of wild mammals as having been fed upon by one or other of the 15 species of tsetse flies that he has investigated, plus the ostrich and other birds, as well as reptiles which include crocodiles and the large lizard *Varanus* and perhaps some tortoises. Trypanosomes pathogenic to domestic livestock have been identified in over 30 species of wild mammals.

The purpose of this study is to inquire what are the effects of this complex of parasites, hosts, and vectors upon the distribution and numbers and habits of men and their domestic animals in Africa. Of the latter, camels, horses, sheep, goats, and dogs can be regarded as such, without any further subdivision; but it will be necessary to take account of four apparently basic races of cattle and numerous types into which they may be divided.

Finally, there is man. One of the more stupid generalizations that have warped judgement on many African problems, including the problems of trypanosomiasis, is that nearly all Africans have the same habits, culture, and character. There are four races of indigenous peoples in tropical Africa, and one authority lists over 700 major tribal groups (Murdock 1959). Of these this study will concern over thirty. Between them they inhabit a wide range of environments and use a dozen or so types of social organization and culture to gain their livings as communities. Appreciable numbers of peoples of seven European countries have come to tropical Africa as merchants and would-be colonizers, as well as many Indians, Pakistanis, and Levantines. In the past Persians and Arabs have colonized its eastern Coast, and the Arabs and Berbers have made their impact from the Sahara. Individuals of any of these groups might die of sleeping sickness if infected with an appropriate trypanosome; but their reactions when considered as societies, to the ecological complexes in which tsetse flies and trypanosomes are involved, have often been very different.

It seems necessary to give some account of the behaviour of tsetse flies and trypanosomes before turning to their distribution in Africa, and this is done in Chapters 2 and 4. One would like to refer to authoritative sources of information on the ecology of the wild hosts of these insects and their common parasites, but it is only recently that study of the larger African fauna has begun to be put upon a sound basis and it is seldom possible to point to features in wild animal behaviour (save in general terms) that are relevant to the epidemiology and epizootiology of trypanosomiasis. As to the human inhabitants, they too are only now beginning to receive objective study and, perhaps more important, are themselves communicating with the world outside Africa in ways of which notice must be taken. The large mammals, human and other, must therefore be described separately in the areas chosen for detailed examination.

Rates of change

We shall shortly consider the nature of the inquiry to be made into the relationships of these various organisms, and at this point it is worth noting that both ecology and epidemiology, in some of their aspects, are concerned with the analysis of systems which are made up of and acquire their nature from the rates of change in biological processes and interactions. Basic among these are the rates of reproduction which can be measured by the length of interval between generations. Trypanosomes, at least in the blood of the mammal host, have generation intervals that are specific, and vary from about 5 to about 7 hours (Muhlpfordt 1964). At 25°C there is an interval of 57 days between the emergence of a young female tsetse fly from her puparium and the emergence of her first offspring from its puparium. At 30°C the time is 44 days, and at 20°C it is 90 days. The natural hosts of trypanosomes and tsetse flies vary considerably in their generation intervals. The rhinoceros on which, according to Weitz (1963), *Glossina longipennis* mostly feeds in Kenya, probably matures at about 20 years and pregnancy lasts 7 months, but the corresponding figures for the warthog, the principal host of *G. morsitans* and *G. swynnertoni*, are 2 years and 25 weeks. African cattle generally do not reproduce until they are 4–5 years old and carry their unborn calves for 9–10 months. In Sukumaland, in Central Tanzania,

Laurie, Brass, and Trant (n.d.) found that 28 years was the mean of specific fertility distribution for local women. Clark (1967) gives a corresponding figure of somewhat under 25 years for mothers of the Ivory Coast and Guinea.

Perhaps on some future occasion another student of the trypanosomiases may be able to describe them and their effects in terms of this kind; indeed, Glasgow (1963a) was able to bring together enough quantitative data to construct a life table with age-specific fecundity and net reproduction rates for *Glossina* at 26°C. Work of this kind has since been greatly extended by Saunders (1967).

Vegetation, climates, and ecological systems

The four chapters following describe what seem to be the relevant features of the biology and geographical distribution of tsetse flies and trypanosomes. Then follow accounts of the trypanosomiases and their relationships with societies living in five separate sample areas. Between them these sample areas cover a wide range of climates and ecological systems. Two are situated near the geographical and ecological limits of *Glossina*: one, in Nigeria, where high temperature appears to be the critical factor preventing northward expansion; another, in Rhodesia, where cold is probably the main obstacle to spread southward. The other three are placed centrally in Africa, around Lake Victoria. These also cover a wide variety of climates and vegetation that varies from tropical rain forest to semi-arid grass steppe, so that in addition to the numerous animals that have to be considered, there is also a wide spectrum of plant life which provides their energy and gives them shelter.

Had this study been attempted ten years ago it is likely that this chapter would have included a fifth category of relevant organisms, the plant species, or at any rate, the major vegetation communities and their dominant trees. Until about 1960 it was an accepted dogma that different species of tsetse flies lived in obligatory association with certain plant communities, and that the 'structure' of the latter provided the key to the understanding of a corresponding 'structure' in the distribution of tsetse-fly populations. This was not a completely erroneous notion, but it now seems a more fruitful line of approach merely to look upon vegetation as providing the visible framework within which tsetse carry out cycles of behaviour that are still by no means fully understood. Certainly, in no study of any species of *Glossina* has the point yet been reached at which one would have to name a particular plant as an essential component of an observed behaviour pattern. It is useful to add precision to description by using botanical nomenclature; but the plants do not interact, in the phenomena to be described in this book, in the same way as do the trypanosomes, the tsetse flies, the wild fauna, and man and his domestic animals.

Nevertheless, having thus rejected both botany and the concepts of tsetse fly behaviour in which the writer was educated along with other glossinologists, it is necessary to affirm the belief that understanding is not fully to be achieved except within the framework of the evolution of ecosystems (Tansley 1949). In them the plant world is the intermediary that transforms the energy that operates the biological systems to be studied. These include man and his works, but the plant world is also the principal obstacle to man's solution of the problems posed for him by the existence of trypanosomes.

Earlier ideas of the role of the trypanosomes in African ecology

Ecological problems can only finally be solved when they are stated quantitatively. But first it is necessary to decide what problems need to be solved. A British Government committee, set up in 1911, decided that the way to remove the burden of the tsetse-borne diseases from tropical Africa was to eliminate tsetses (Desart 1914). French and Belgian authorities took a different view and made their target the elimination of trypanosomes by medical methods. If this could be done the tsetses would become harmless. The French and Belgians had to deal with successive epidemics of sleeping sickness among people living, for the most part, in or on the borders of the Congo basin. In this environment domestic animals were few and of little importance economically or, it was thought, as integral components of the epidemiological situation it was desired to change. When, in the 1920s, British West African countries began to suffer epidemics of sleeping sickness, French methods were adopted. It was not until after the Second World War that the trypanosomiases began to assume much importance among the diseases of domestic livestock in West Africa.

In East Africa, once the Uganda epidemic had been brought under control, the 'tsetse problem' came to be seen as very largely a veterinary matter. An epidemic spread of sleeping sickness through Tanzania in the 1920s and 1930s, although alarming enough in the communities it affected, did not infect large populations and caused relatively little social disorganization. One disquieting feature of the East African problem at that time was that everywhere it seemed that the tsetses were spreading or 'advancing' and driving the stricken peasantry before them. Tsetses suddenly appeared or began to 'advance', cattle began to die, and their owners, seeing their wealth disappear, abandoned their homes and moved to other areas where there were no flies.

To explain these 'advances' the theory was propounded that the African was an incompetent farmer, too idle to rotate his crops and conserve soil fertility or, by correct tilling, to prevent soil erosion. Driven by their self-inflicted poverty families had to move or starve. When they left, the bush grew up and formed an environment for the tsetses, the first few of which infected cattle belonging to people still in the area. They also moved, leaving more room for the bush to grow. The wild animals, natural hosts of the flies, now began to invade the abandoned lands and soon all reverted once more to savanna or woodland, inhabited only by the wild game and *Glossina*. The next step in the process came when people who had fled from the infection found that there was no room in the tsetse-free lands, which had become overcrowded so that their inhabitants were now forced back to the bush. Here their activities in felling trees, cultivating, and hunting wild animals destroyed the habitat of the flies and killed off their natural hosts. So the process went on in a never-ending and unbreakable cycle, for before long soil exhaustion followed again upon incompetent farming and another 'advance' of tsetse intervened. The process was not thought of as being entirely the fault of the African peasantry. The presence of the tsetses had prevented them from developing a proper animal husbandry. They had been unable to use such things as wheels and ploughs (and therefore had failed to invent them) and, because of the tsetses, did not understand the art of manuring. As the cattle populations of East Africa nearly all live out of contact with tsetses, much of this hypothesis does not bear critical examination. However, the idea was developed that if tsetses were eliminated, cattle would flourish and their owners would take to eating them instead of using them as purely pecuniary assets. This would give them the energy needed to overcome the fatal cycle of soil exhaustion, semi-starvation, land abandonment, overcrowding, bush felling for more cultivation, and again more soil exhaustion. This sort of concept was widely held and formed the basis for official policies.

This book had its origin in a conversation between its author and some Africans in Western Uganda in 1945. Tsetses, *Glossina morsitans*, had been 'advancing' in Ankole from the south since 1907, and the local people asserted that until the Europeans had arrived in that part of the continent, just west of Lake Victoria, there had been no tsetses in their country. This assertion would have been dismissed as absurd had it not been discovered shortly afterwards and quite by chance that it was certainly true, and that for some hundreds of years there can have been at least no *G. morsitans* there, whatever may have been the case with other species of tsetse. Moreover bush was spreading rapidly in country that clearly had not been exhausted by bad husbandry. The theories that were then current obviously did not apply in Ankole. This disillusioning experience led to further investigation of the histories of other areas and it soon became evident that the 'advances' of tsetse which had been in progress throughout Tanzania in the 1930s and were in progress over most of Uganda during the 1940s could not possibly be explained by the theory of bush invasion of soils exhausted by misuse. Having reached this conclusion, one began to ask whether eliminating tsetses would have the beneficial effects that were predicted.

One of the earlier results of this historical approach to the problem of the spread of tsetse in Ankole was to show that a movement of another species,

G. pallidipes, into the north of Ankole had been initiated by the evacuation of people from densely populated regions in the Rift Valley below Mount Ruwenzori, as a preventive measure against the spread of sleeping sickness. This disease had assumed epidemic proportions as a result of administrative measures taken by the Belgians in the Semliki river valley, west of the mountain, when they first occupied it at the end of the nineteenth century. Thus, in 1945, I found myself trying to deal with a problem that had its origin half a century before my time and over sixty miles away from the place in which I was working (Ford 1950). It seemed that my efforts and those of my colleagues were, perhaps, very misdirected. We were feebly scratching at the surface of events that we hardly knew existed, and if we achieved anything at all, it was often to exacerbate the ills of the societies we imagined ourselves to be helping. Some years later Varley (1957) elaborated similar ideas in general terms in relation to tropical ecology, and mentioned anti-tsetse operations, among other similar exercises, as having initiated changes that had taken place without subsequent ecological observation. We had failed to learn the ecological lessons that might have been taught.

In so far as these remarks imply criticism of the methods of people confronted with practical problems, whether in Africa or elsewhere, it is possible to answer that, having assumed their imperial roles, the colonial powers had no choice but to deal with the problems they encountered. They had to make what use they could of scientific knowledge as it existed at the time. Unfortunately, with very few exceptions, it was psychologically impossible for men and women concerned in imperial expansion in Africa to believe that their own actions were more often than not responsible for the manifold disasters in which they found themselves caught up. The scientists they called in to help them were as ignorant as they of the problems they had to tackle. Above all, they were compelled to act. When, in 1907, Sir H. Hesketh Bell, first governor of Uganda, made his own interpretation of the findings of the Royal Society Commission on Sleeping Sickness in that country and ordered the evacuation of populations from infected areas, 200 000 people had already died of the disease. The Governor then initiated a chain of events that are still in progress and have led, among other things, to an epidemic of the same disease at Alego in the Central Nyanza province of Kenya in 1964. By 1912 Fiske, the Uganda government's medical entomologist, had begun to doubt if evacuation had been either right or necessary (Fiske 1920). One cannot now perform experiments to answer the problem.

In eastern Africa it took thirty-five years to change the research policies initiated by the Desart committee, and another decade to implement the change. But by the time of political independence, research, at least in the laboratories, had been placed upon a proper foundation, able to support biological approaches to the trypanosomiasis problem from any direction. But emergencies will continue to occur. Governments and international agencies will have to take action to save life. They will also take action in the interests of commerce and economic development. It may be of use to describe the history of some major ecological events associated with trypano-some infection in the hope that some remnants of Professor Varley's lost lessons of ecology may be salvaged.

The confrontation of ecosystems and natural foci of infection

The circumstances in which vast ecological experiments have been initiated in Africa are seldom clear. To people brought up in an environ-ment almost entirely conditioned by a long history of human exploitation of nature, as in Europe, the special problems associated with the confronta-tion between relatively highly organized human societies and natural, undisturbed, ecosystems are not always apparent. In the history of western Europe it is clear that civilization could not have developed in the way it did—indeed, perhaps, could not have developed at all—had not the forests that once clothed it, from the Urals to Land's End, been felled and replaced by managed vegetations. This was the great work of the Dark Ages. It gained in momentum for hundreds of years until, from 1050 onwards for 200 years or so, the heroic period of European reclamation, *l'age des grands défrichements*, provided the economic foundation for the Renaissance and the scientific revolution (Darby 1956, 1957). In an earlier epoch similar centuries of work had preceded the emergence of the Mediterranean, Chinese, and other civilizations. It is a process that still continues, and those involved with it have always been exposed to risk of serious infection from the parasites that escape from their natural environments and invade the tissues of men who create new ecosystems to supplant the old. Apollo Smintheus loosing his arrows on the beaches of Troy; the succession of plague pandemics in Europe of the Middle Ages; the recent outbreak of a new and very fatal haemorrhagic fever in Colombia when insecticides poisoned the village cats, and rats invaded the unprotected homes (Woodall 1968), are only three of a long series of diseases that have affected man in the course of the confrontation of his artificial ecosystems with those of nature. It is a curious comment to make upon the efforts of colonial scien-tists to control the trypanosomiases, that they almost entirely overlooked the very considerable achievements of the indigenous peoples in over-coming the obstacle of trypanosomiasis to tame and exploit the natural ecosystem of tropical Africa by cultural and physiological adjustment both in themselves and their domestic animals.

These aspects of zoonotic diseases were neglected as a basis for control policies in colonial dependencies in Africa. Western science continues to make a piecemeal approach to disease whenever and wherever it breaks out. A basis for a systematic approach to the epidemiological consequences of ecosystem confrontation emerged in the 1930s in Russia, where Pav-lowsky and his associates began to analyse the patterns of disease caused by the tick-borne virus of spring–summer encephalitis among people trying to invade and exploit the great forests of the taiga. From their work has emerged the concept of natural foci of infection or, as it is sometimes called, the nidality of disease, as a separate scientific discipline (Pavlowsky 1963). The essence of this is that epidemic conditions arise where the various organisms involved interact together so that there is continual circulation of the pathogenic agent, via the vector, between the natural and the adventitious hosts. Such a biocenosis can only occur where the environment is such that all its components can meet in favourable conditions of time and space.

The ideas of the Pavlowsky school are now familiar. From the practical viewpoint they were superior to the somewhat similar notions that had a partial development among workers on trypanosomiasis, in their insistence on the complex nature of the processes involved in a natural focus of infection, and therefore of the need for joint investigation by zoologists, ecologists, and parasitologists. The colonial governments in Africa were only beginning to come around to this sort of team work when independence came. They left to the new countries a legacy of ideas that had little relevance to the biological processes with which they had unwittingly interfered.

Much highly sophisticated research is now being done on the trypanosomiases in the laboratories of Europe and America. The knowledge gained is intended for use in Africa and it is important to understand the circumstances in which it will be used. The problem with which the following chapters deal may be stated thus: To define the factors leading to the infection of a man (or a cow, pig, horse) A, by the trypanosome B, at the place C, and time D. This definition will not be achieved, but some new paths towards it may be a little illuminated.

The practical uses of an epidemiology of trypanosomiasis

It is not irrelevant to inquire why such a study should be valuable. If it were possible to assert that this or that technique could be applied at a calculable rate and cost, in confidence that at the end of the operation African trypanosomiasis would be eliminated, the study of circumstantial epidemiology would be of academic interest only. An informed estimate made in 1957, for ridding the continent of *Glossina* (and therefore very probably, but not certainly, of trypanosomiasis) was given at £1000 million sterling to be spent over fifty to seventy-five years (Phillips 1959). If there were any sense in arguing about such figures this estimate should now be doubled or trebled. The geographical magnitude of the problem is such that a policy based upon elimination is not a practical one. There are a few countries in which the area of infestation by *Glossina* is small enough to contemplate removal of the tsetse from within their borders, but in nearly every case they adjoin other countries where there is a prospect of infestation prolonging itself indefinitely. Further, where large-scale programmes have been promulgated to eliminate either the tsetse or the trypanosomcs and have achieved a high degree of success, when the attempt was made voluntarily or involuntarily to put an end to the work, disasters of the most catastrophic kind intervened.

We shall find that in the underdeveloped countries of tropical Africa there may be advantages in preserving some degree of trypanosome infection as an aid to attaining, as soon as is possible, a growing economy based upon balanced ecology. The real problem is not how to get rid of tsetse flies or how to cure sleeping sickness and the infections of domestic animals, but how to apply techniques of control in such a way that an expanding economy is not hampered by their mishandling. We must understand the advantages of infection in an underdeveloped world, just as much as we must understand the disasters that can follow upon loss of control. To achieve the levels of control that seem desirable it is essential to understand the interplay of factors which lead to infection. To do this we must first try to list what these factors are. That is the principal contribution that this book is intended to make towards the problem defined at the end of the last section.

Some of the factors will emerge in the brief accounts of tsetse and trypanosome biology that follow. Other factors, perhaps less familiar to students of these organisms, may emerge from the histories of sample areas given in the second section of the book. They are histories in two senses. Firstly they display what seem to be the historical contexts in which the series of epidemics and epizootics observed since the end of the nineteenth century have developed. Secondly they are also histories of the efforts made to control these events and of the ideas that prompted them. No attempt has been made at a comprehensive presentation of data, but wherever possible the selected fragments have been given a quantitative basis. The selection of data has been made to illustrate the argument put forward in the third section of the book. This looks forward, perhaps too optimistically, to a policy for dealing with trypanosomiasis and, by implication, other zoonotic infections, which will allow the peoples of the continent to resume their proper task of developing their own environment, within the world society; and to do this in ways that will ensure, in their confrontation with natural ecosystems, a minimum of unnecessary disease and death and the maximum conservation of natural resources.

The book is not a textbook. Much important research is scarcely touched upon because although of great intrinsic worth it is not yet assimilable at the mainly historical and geographical levels of the narratives presented in Chapters 6 to 24. Readers who wish to follow up subjects referred to briefly can consult the volume recently edited by Mulligan (1970). A useful but much briefer conspectus of the subject of African trypanosomiasis as a whole is that of Lumsden (1965). Glasgow's (1963a) study of tsetse populations provides a good introduction to glossinology. Another valuable review is found in the collection of papers by several authors published as Part 5–6 of volume 28 of the Bulletin of the World Health Organization in 1963. This Organization maintains an information service on the trypanosomiases and, periodically, in conjunction with the Food and Agriculture Organization of the United Nations, convenes meetings of experts to review the contemporary situation. The International Scientific Committee for Trypanosomiasis Research, which operated to 1960 under the auspices of the Committee for Technical Cooperation in Africa (CCTA), continues to meet, every two years, as an adjunct of the Organization for African Unity (OAU). Its proceedings provide another useful means for coordination of research and control.

2

RESPONSES OF TSETSES TO THEIR HOSTS

WHEN Buxton's great *Natural history of tsetse flies* (1955) was written, most of the research on these insects had been directed towards the two problems of measurement of the densities of their populations and of describing their biology by investigating where they lived, especially in relation to vegetation communities. From about 1920 to 1950 very little attention was given to the relationships of tsetses to the animals on which they fed. Research was directed towards eliminating them rather than to understanding their role as vectors of disease. This was, however, an important subject to Fiske whose unorthodox views about the Uganda epidemic have already been noted. He was one of the earliest students of *Glossina* in the field. His work provides a convenient starting point for what is seen by the observer who attempts to study tsetse behaviour in the African bush.

Fiske's study of *Glossina fuscipes fuscipes*

W. F. Fiske was an American entomologist who went to Uganda shortly after the great epidemic of sleeping sickness of 1900–8 to study the vector of the disease, *Glossina fuscipes fuscipes*, then included in the species *G. palpalis*. He had already been a partner in writing one of the classical papers of mathematical ecology (Howard and Fiske 1911). He came to the conclusion that the methods being taken by the Uganda Protectorate government for the control of human sleeping sickness were faulty, and one cannot help wondering what might have happened had his views prevailed. They will be discussed in Chapter 14.

Like other glossinologists of that time Fiske was interested in the disparity in numbers of male and female tsetses that were caught by a man walking through the bush. He went to a small island called Lula on Lake Victoria; its area is scarcely more than 10 000 yd². Employing a team of ten assistants he began systematically catching out the tsetse population of the island on the afternoon of 18 November 1913. On the first afternoon males were caught at a rate of 14·0 per catcher per hour, but the female rate was only 0·9, and females formed only 6 per cent of the catch. By the afternoon of the 20th, males were being caught at the rate of only 1·7 per hour, but females, which now formed 72 per cent of the catch, were being caught at a rate of 4·4 per hour. They continued to form about two-thirds of the catch until the end of the experiment on the 27th, when flies, of both sexes together, were still being caught at a rate of 2·2 per catcher per hour.

The most plausible explanation was that male flies are active and easily caught at all times during good weather, whether they are hungry or not, but that the females are normally inactive and not to be caught except when hungry or seeking food. It had been noticed that the presence of so many persons on the small island had temporarily banished from it several crocodiles and monitor lizards, *Varanus*. The experiment was followed by another on the island of Lugazi. Here on 19 and 20 December, 197 flies were caught and, after sex had been determined, were liberated, so that heavy initial catching of males should not affect the sex ratio, which turned out to be 166 : 31, or 15·5 per cent females. From the 22nd to the 27th all host animals, consisting of several *Varanus* and crocodiles were systematically hunted from the islet. On 26 and 27 December, 208 flies were caught, in the ratio of 89 : 119, or 57·2 per cent females.

Fiske concluded that (1) if the female percentage is low, food must be plentiful and man less liable to attack; (2) there must be a conspicuous correlation between variations in female percentage and the persistence with which tsetse flies press their attacks on man. The conclusion that man was not a favoured host does not seem to have been drawn, and Fiske believed that the low female percentage under normal conditions was due to females only coming to man to feed, while males chiefly appeared 'merely to seek the females'. Lloyd (1912) and Lamborn (1915) who had been studying *Glossina morsitans* in Zambia and Malawi respectively, reached the same conclusion.

This behaviour on the part of the male tsetse led to the formation of 'following swarms' which accompanied the observer or, it was to be supposed, any moving animal of sufficient size along the path he, or it, was using. When he stopped the following swarm also stopped, and the flies settled on the leaves of shrubs or the grasses on either side of the path. This mechanism led to the aggregation of males around stationary and complacent hosts. So little observation has been made on the behaviour of tsetse in the presence of their hosts that it is worth while to quote some of Fiske's notes in full.

Kitobo Island, 3rd December 1913

Varanus observed excavating burrow in sandy soil some distance from shelter [i.e. from the forest edge]. On approaching it made off rapidly, and on reaching the spot I was assailed by a great number of tsetse, which swept back and forth and around me like angry bees, 'buzzing' in their flight in a manner never before noted. After a few minutes they all dispersed, without any sign of them alighting upon me.

Bugalla Island, 23 November 1914

A large male situtunga was approached as it was feeding with its head concealed in a dense thicket. With glasses (Zeiss prismatic ×12) it was possible to make out that a peculiar dark colour of foreleg, lower shoulder and thorax, which were plainly seen through an opening in the bushes, was due to an unprecedented number of tsetse, which literally blackened its coat. It seemed entirely unmoved and phlegmatic under attack.

On being shot, the animal plunged directly through the thicket; ran a few yards at great speed and fell. On proceeding to the spot where it was feeding, I found a 'following swarm' of fly of unprecedented size (probably not less than 200 flies) buzzing like a great swarm of angry bees. They surrounded me, but hardly any alighted on me or followed me to where the antelope lay.

Damba Island, 13 September 1915

A large male situtunga was shot in an opening in the forest in the dusk of evening. It ran into the thickly shaded forest and fell. On reaching it I was amazed to find a considerable swarm of flies, partly outside, but judging by the noise they made, more inside than outside the forest (it was so dark they could not be seen). Is it possible that a swarm will follow an animal into the night, and perhaps remain on its body all night?

Bugalla Island, December 1914

[Original note lost.] On entering an open space in the jungle where formerly were plantations, a small herd of two female and two half-grown male situtunga was seen, with other animals feeding in the edge of the jungle out of sight. Those in sight did not immediately see me, who stood motionless watching them, nor upon seeing me did they betray alarm or more than mild curiosity. The whole herd moved in my direction and one female approached within three yards. Each animal was followed by a small swarm of tsetse—perhaps 15 or 20 flies—few of them on the animal itself, but principally on the vegetation close at hand, or hovering about. Not one of the flies was seen to feed, nor did the animals show signs of annoyance at their presence. On becoming alarmed the antelopes made off without undue haste, the flies following.

Fiske's paper is long and discursive. Some of his interpretations were wrong but the detailed observation of behaviour has scarcely since been matched. He noted, for example, that flies that had just fed rested on nearby vegetation:

Crocodile was never actually approached, for there are few animals more quick to take alarm at the sound of an intruder, and at the first alarm a crocodile —unlike many other animals—is sure to make off. But on several occasions when they have been seen to slip quietly into the water, the vegetation near the spot where they were resting has been found covered with engorged flies; on one occasion in such numbers that the bushes nearest at hand seemed thick with berries.

Later students of tsetse behaviour have found it convenient to commence at the moment when the tsetse leaves the animal on which it has been feeding, and begins the cycle of behaviour that accompanies its metabolism of the blood meal.

The relative attractiveness of different animals to *G. f. fuscipes* was measured by tethering various animals, and counting the number of bites they received per unit of time. It is not clear how the counting was done although 'the animals were exposed as equally as possible along a bit of beach'. On the animals only those flies that became engorged with blood were counted as having bitten, since some probed the skin without engorging. However, flies that bit man were not allowed to feed. Table 2.1 displays the results of three experiments. The monitor lizard and the crocodile were clearly more attractive or possibly, as Fiske maintained, were more complacent than any other host. He drew special attention to the different responses to three bulls in a fourth experiment. The Indian bull was immune to attack in comparison with the others.

This was entirely due to his very excitable temperament. He was intractable, and perhaps a bit dangerous, and became almost as excited under attack by *Glossina* as the sheep, which were even more intolerant of fly than the goats used

TABLE 2.1

The relative attractiveness of Varanus, *goat, pig, and man to* G. fuscipes†

Host	No. of hours exposed	No. of bites inflicted	No. of bites per hour
Varanus . . .	24	60	2·50
Pig	32·25	1	0·03
Goat	76	0	0·00
Man, African . .	38	1	0·03
Man, European . .	202	5	0·02

† From Fiske (1920).

in previous experiments. The Ankole, on the other extreme, was absolutely tractable and docile, and refused to become annoyed at the attack of either *Glossina* or *Stomoxys*, and the half breed was not much different.

There is a confusion in Fiske's thought. Although he had defined the following swarm as a male activity that ensured encounter with females, he did not distinguish clearly between this sexual behaviour and behaviour associated with feeding. Commenting on the low rate of biting observed on the tethered pig, he remarked that this result was untrustworthy for on one occasion he discovered a following swarm of fly about a pig that was shot, and so proved 'conclusively enough that this animal was a favoured host'.

This confusion was to remain for many years although the distinction between male sexual behaviour and feeding behaviour was also made, as noted above, by workers on *Glossina morsitans*. One of them, indeed, observed that if he caught only those flies that bit him, instead of catching at random all that approached, the sex ratio tended to reach equality (Lloyd

1912). The flies that fed and the flies that followed were not the same. The moving object behind which a following swarm congregated was not necessarily a favoured source of food. A favoured food host, moreover, could attract a following swarm that made no attempt to feed. On Bugalla Island on 23 November 1914, Fiske had seen so many tsetse feeding on a situtunga that they 'literally blackened its coat'. On the same island in December, however, he saw a small herd of the same antelopes, each followed by perhaps 15–20 flies, 'not one of which was seen to feed'.

Fiske thought that a complacent temperament, whether possessed by a man, a domestic animal, a monitor lizard, or a situtunga, was the essential quality in a preferred host. The idea has since commended itself to other workers such as Glasgow (1963a), and recently it has received support from Rhodesian entomologists. At Sengwa in the Zambezi tsetse belt, during 3 hours and 20 minutes observation on an impala and an ox kraaled together, no tsetse alighted on the impala, but they were seen to alight on the ox on 143 occasions. In another experiment totalling $15\frac{1}{4}$ hours, no tsetse alighted on the impala, but 77 were caught from the ox. It was particularly noticed that the impala was very irritable under attack by other biting flies, mainly Stomoxydinae, reacting with kicks, skin rippling, and head shaking (Cockbill 1966). The impala (*Aepyceros melampus*) is one of the commonest and certainly one of the most conspicuous of African antelopes, but in over 13 000 analyses of blood meals from tsetse of the *morsitans* group (see Chapter 17) its blood appeared in only 0·27 per cent. Langley (1968) has shown that *G. morsitans* can be maintained in the laboratory on impala blood as well as on any other. Complacency under tsetse attack may indeed be part of the explanation for host preference.

Behaviour towards 'hosts' in *G. morsitans* and *G. swynnertoni*

The study of tsetse behaviour has been rejuvenated in the last decade by Bursell and his colleagues, first at Shinyanga in Tanzania and later in the University College in Rhodesia. It cannot be claimed that the whole story is elucidated. The following is an account of the day-to-day life of *G. morsitans* as it appears to the writer when he applies Bursell's ideas to his own and other people's field observations. Bursell began with the tsetse full of fresh blood and looking to Fiske like a berry or, to Carpenter (1920), Fiske's medical colleague in Uganda, like a ripe redcurrant.

In this state, having taken up two to three times its own weight of blood, it flies, with some difficulty, for it may be unable to maintain height, to the nearest perch. There is an urgent need for the fully fed tsetse to reduce its weight and become fully mobile again and, perhaps, less visible.† It

† And therefore less subject to predation. 'The first *Bembex* that I ever saw at work was *B. capensis* which I found at Jinja in 1910. One was seen going into the burrow carrying a full fed tsetse, whose shining red, bloated abdomen full of blood was quite unmistakeable' (Carpenter 1920). *Bembex* is a large predatory wasp.

may begin to get rid of the excess water from the blood meal before feeding is finished. It is voided in small clear droplets from the anus and the process of dehydration of the blood meal continues for several hours.

Bursell (1961) who worked on *G. swynnertoni* and *G. morsitans* referred to the period in which the newly fed fly digests its blood meal as *Phase 1*. During this phase the fly is at rest, perched upon a tree or bush, and does not respond to the presence of moving objects or the scent of favoured food hosts. Possibly it moves about the tree on which it is resting to avoid unfavourable microclimates such as would be created by direct insolation, or to escape from predators. A specimen of *G. morsitans* was allowed to feed and was then marked with a conspicuous spot of red paint on the thorax. Having fed, it flew to the trunk of a large *Brachystegia* tree and settled while it extruded a globule of fluid. Then it moved by short upward flights on the tree trunk until lost to sight in the foliage of the crown. Recently Pilson and Pilson (1967) have located marked *G. morsitans* in tree canopies at heights of 40 ft. But on other occasions freshly fed tsetse have been seen to rest for several hours on the same place on a shrub only 5–6 ft from the ground. During this resting phase lipids are built up from the blood meal and stored in the fat bodies that occupy much of the abdominal cavity. At the same time various amino-acids become concentrated in the haemolymph, among them especially proline which provides the immediate source of energy for flight (Bursell 1963). Before the blood meal is fully digested *Phase 2* intervenes, perhaps when a threshold level of proline and other associated amino-acids is reached.

In Phase 2, male tsetses fly towards any sufficiently large moving object; or perhaps it need not be moving, but is merely an object that is new in the fly's accustomed field of vision. If the object that stimulated activity is moving at a speed not greater than about 15 mile/h the male in Phase 2 will follow it. When *G. morsitans* males are following a party of men along a path, they fly in a zigzag flight close to the ground and as soon as the men stop they stop too, and alight on the ground or low herbage. (*G. fuscipes* fly at a greater height above ground and come to rest at waist to shoulder height on shrubs and tall grasses.) In some conditions, perhaps of high temperature, Phase 2 males alight on the object they are following (a man walking or cycling or a slowly moving motor car) and may be carried long distances. In this state they do not attempt to feed.

Male tsetse are not capable of more than twenty minutes' activity daily. If no moving object stimulates participation in a following swarm, orthokinetic flights may also occur in Phase 2. During flight the available proline is consumed and other amino-acids, among which alanine is the most conspicuous, replace it in the haemolymph as waste products (Bursell 1965).

Phase 2 activity towards the same object by a number of mature males results in a 'following swarm'. Moving objects may also attract teneral females or very 'hungry' mature females. When this happens, the following swarm males begin a nuptial flight around the female and mating occurs (at any rate with young females).

After participating in the following swarm for a time, perhaps only a few minutes, during which the available proline is used up and replaced by alanine, *Phase 3* intervenes. This is also an active phase, but activity is now a response to a food stimulus. If none is perceptible at the end of Phase 2 the male tsetse comes to rest. During this rest metabolism continues and excretion of waste products leads to defaecation. Defaecation also happens quite often during feeding, perhaps under the stimulus of pressures developed by the distending crop. Conversion of the residual blood meal continues and Phase 2 activity may be again resumed without a meal having been taken. However, if the object followed during Phase 2 is a favoured host, the fly may alight on it and begin feeding at once, although high temperature or high light intensity may have an inhibiting effect. If the object followed is either not favoured or, perhaps, is repellent, flies at the end of Phase 2 will alight on nearby vegetation.

If the fly begins feeding at once then, after engorging itself, it will return to the immobile Phase 1. Its gut may now contain undigested blood from two different host species; the residual blood meal from the first host and the newly ingested meal. Double feeds are not unknown (Weitz and Jackson 1955) and must be more frequent than is shown by blood meal analysis since two meals from the same species of host will not be serologically separable (see Chapter 3).

If the fly after participating in a following swarm stays at rest for lack of the stimulus of a favoured food host, the residuum of the first blood meal will be digested, fat will build up and convertible amino-acids be replenished in the haemolymph. A physiological state may then be restored in which Phase 2 behaviour is resumed and the male responds again to a moving object rather than to a food host.

Eventually a condition will be reached at which no residual blood meal remains to be metabolized into fat, and beyond that only sufficient proline can be formed for a limited flight response to a favoured host. Feeding will again lead to repetition of the above processes.

These routines may fail to bring the fly into contact with a source of food. It enters Bursell's *Phase 4*. The fat bodies are exhausted, or nearly so, and now there can be no orthokinetic flight or participation in following swarms. Any moving object is at once attacked and probed for blood, even if it is inanimate, like the warm surface of a motor car tyre or an animal usually rejected as a food host, like a zebra or an impala. This is an assumption. Zebra have never and impala only rarely been demonstrated in blood meals (Weitz 1963), but they do become infected with trypanosomes in nature. This might be due to mechanical transmission (p. 3). Both *G. morsitans* and *G. swynnertoni* have been found on recently shot zebra

(Weitz and Jackson 1955), but perhaps these were flies that had been in a following swarm attracted to a moving object, not to a food source.

The 'hunger cycle', the mean interval between feeds, varies in length with season. In hot weather, *G. swynnertoni* feeds at a mean interval of rather less than three days, *G. morsitans* rather more (Jackson 1954). In the wet season the interval is longer. Glasgow (1961*a*) obtained rather longer mean hunger cycles for *G. swynnertoni* but produced histograms that suggested that the majority of flies feed at intervals of two or three days.

So far this account has dealt only with mature male flies. Nothing has been said about the females or about teneral and 'young' flies. The story is also incomplete in that it has not yet described two other cycles that control the cycles of metabolism and behaviour. One is the cycle of changing climate, especially of temperature and humidity associated with the alternation of day and night. The other is the cycle of activity displayed by the animals on which the tsetse feed and behind which, when they move, the mature male flies form their sexually appetitive swarms. It is convenient to consider the animals first.

Behaviour of the natural hosts

Lack of knowledge of wild host behaviour now becomes an obstacle. 'In Africa ... practically nothing is known of the game populations which existed in the past, still exist, or could exist in any area. ... Unfortunately data on the vital statistics of wild animals in Africa are almost completely lacking' (Vesey-Fitzgerald 1960). Since 1960 much research has begun but it is still only in general terms that one may think about how behaviour routines of *Glossina* fit those of their hosts.

About 40 per cent of *Glossina morsitans* meals are taken from warthog, *Phacochoerus aethiopicus*, and evidently much of the observed behaviour of this tsetse is regulated by successive stages in its metabolism of warthog blood. But although the warthog is one of the most familiar of African animals we know far less about it than we know about tsetse. One aspect of its behaviour that must favour it as a food source is its relative immobility. Many of the antelopes and other bovids seem to be as attractive to *G. morsitans* as are the pigs, but for the most part they move over fairly wide ranges. Together they may supply as much blood to *G. morsitans* as do warthogs, but they comprise many species and only rarely does one of these approach the contribution of that animal. Vesey-Fitzgerald (1960) suggests that the distribution of warthogs may be conditioned by the availability of aardvark (*Orycteropus*) holes in which they shelter and, although he was referring specifically to the fauna of the Lake Rukwa plains in Tanzania, this may well be true of warthogs in much of the African savanna vegetation. Although warthogs like to wallow in mud, and presumably to drink, they can do without water in the dry season, using only the moisture in the rhizomes of perennial grasses and bulbils of Cyperaceae. Such an animal is obviously an ideal host for an insect living in comparatively open woodland.

Weir and Davison (1965) recorded the drinking habits, in the dry season, of ten herbivores and four carnivores in the Wankie national park in Rhodesia. They divided the herbivores into four groups:

(1) Buffalo, zebra, and giraffe are evening and night drinkers. While they may be seen at a pan drinking at any time in the twenty-four hours, they show a distinct peak for drinking between 16.00 and 20.00 h.

(2) Wildebeest and eland are night and morning drinkers, mostly between 05.00 and 09.00 h.

(3) Kudu, sable, roan, and warthog are daytime drinkers. They rarely go to water at night, especially the warthog which shows two peak periods for drinking, one between 05.00 and 10.00 h, the other between 14.00 and 17.00 h.

(4) Elephants drink chiefly between 16.00 and 02.00 h.

Weir and Davison point out that their data were obtained from one area, at one time of year, and at one period of the month (full moon). Some animals rearranged their routines to avoid tourists; others did not. Elephants remain at pans often for hours at a time, other species tend to leave them rapidly after drinking. 'Often two or three hundred animals can arrive, drink and leave a pan within one hour, individuals remaining at the pan only for about five to ten minutes.'

Several of the animals mentioned by Weir and Davison are migratory. Elephants, in particular, must move over large territories if they are not to consume or kill off all the plant life of their environments. Other animals, like the wildebeest and the buffaloes that at some seasons form large herds, must move to new pastures. The bloodsucking arthropods that depend upon them must either travel with them (ticks, fleas, *Hippobosca*) or they must remain in an inactive pupal stage except in the seasons when the animals are available in their neighbourhood (Tabanidae). Insects like the tsetse that do not live like ticks, do not spend most of the year as pupae, have only sufficient energy reserves for very limited periods of daily activity, and must fit their behaviour patterns to those of animals that are found in the same locality throughout the year. The daily routines of host animals and of tsetse are both, in some degree, controlled by the diurnal rhythms of light, temperature, and humidity. The activity peaks observed by Weir and Davison around the Wankie pans occurred, for the most part, in the early morning or late afternoon, and correlate fairly well with the dry season activity peaks of *G. morsitans* in the same latitudes.

Animals drink at water-holes, rivers, or on lake shores, and most of them then return to the woodlands or tree savanna where they spend most of the day grazing or browsing or, especially in the heat of the afternoon, at rest in shady and concealed places. There is much evidence to suggest that most feeding by tsetse takes place in these sheltered spots.

The catch from the standing ox

The feeding habits of *Glossina morsitans* and of *G. pallidipes* have been much studied recently in the Zambezi valley. A distinguishing feature of the work has been that observation has been confined to those flies that actually visited a bait animal to feed. Only those seen to gorge themselves with blood were recorded and their subsequent movements observed.

The Zambezi studies (Pilson and Pilson 1967, and earlier papers by Pilson and Leggate) were begun partly to obtain a measure of the risk of infection suffered by an animal in tsetse-infested bush. Tsetse that approached an animal but went away without feeding obviously did not contribute to that risk. Another motive was to devise a measure of apparent density of the *Glossina* population that was not subject to variation due to differences in behaviour of tsetse at different times of day, at different seasons, and in different weathers. Such behaviour was not fully understood; but at least it was certain that all flies had to feed. By confining observations to the feeding element in the tsetse population and by recording throughout a whole day (beginning observation before there was any pre-sunrise activity and continuing until no more flies came to the bait after sundown) much of the variation that made other forms of observation difficult to interpret would be avoided. Another objective was to find out where flies went after feeding.

The first studies were made on a population of *Glossina pallidipes* inhabiting riverine forest in the floor of the Zambezi valley. Flies were allowed to feed, and when gorged with blood were caught, recorded, marked by a system that allowed each individual fly to be identified when recaptured, and then released. A team of assistants was employed to search all vegetation in an area of about one acre around the bait, so that the resting sites could be classified and their characteristics determined. Some of the results from this side of the work are described in Chapter 17.

Feeding is confined to periods of the day when temperature is above 18°C and below 32°C. When temperature is high and humidity low in the hot dry season (November) some flies come to feed at sunrise, but by 07.30 h only a few (about 5 per hour) are feeding and this low rate of attack continues through the day until after 16.00 h when it begins to increase rapidly, and by 17.30 h over 100 flies per hour are feeding. These are mean figures and sometimes many more than this are to be seen on the animal, so that at peak hours for feeding its legs seem to be clothed in black stockings, recalling the blackened coat of Fiske's situtunga. In the earlier part of the dry season when nights are cold, there is no morning peak of feeding which only begins after the temperature has risen to 18°C at about 07.30 h, and feeding frequency rises throughout the day, the females attacking earlier in the day than the males. Again there is a late afternoon peak, brought to an abrupt end at sunset.

The rains break in late November or December and continue until April or May. Feeding is now spread more evenly through the day, though still building up towards a late afternoon peak. In the middle of the rainy season far fewer flies come to the bait ox than at any other time. This is because the tsetse population is more widely dispersed throughout the bush and is not confined to the denser riverine thickets. At this time of the year the flies are not exposed to climatic stresses either of temperature or humidity, for shade is abundant and, above all, the host animals themselves are not restricted in their choice of pasture or browse, and do not seek the more heavily shaded parts of their habitat to escape the heat. There is little concentration either of host animals or of the tsetse that live on their blood.

Pilson and Pilson (1967) carried out a more extended survey of *G. morsitans* using the same technique, and demonstrated that this species showed similar patterns of behaviour throughout the seasons. However, variations in their general seasonal patterns were discernible when observations were made in different vegetation communities. In their work on *G. pallidipes*, females had accounted for 63·4 per cent of the total catch of 8106 flies in 1959 and 1960 (Pilson and Leggate 1962a). A possible explanation for the excess of females was given by the work of Jackson (1937, 1940) which indicated that they have a greater expectation of life than males, so that although they emerge in equal numbers from the puparia, they predominate as the population grows older. In Pilson and Pilson's study of *G. morsitans* we are not given all the data in the original form, but from one table we find that of 5968 *G. morsitans* marked and released at four intensively studied sites, only 42·4 per cent were females. For the most part it was not possible to detect significant departures from the 1 : 1 sex ratio. Data for 32 site-months were tested statistically. In 10 there was a significant excess of males over females, in 1 only were females more numerous, but in the other 21 there was no significant departure from equality.

One important conclusion was that in the area in which the Pilsons were working no concentration of flies took place in any specific vegetation at any time of the year, except in riverine vegetation in the hot dry season, and this concentration was confined to males only. This is in contrast with the conclusions drawn about *G. pallidipes* and also differs from the views of other workers about *G. morsitans* in other parts of Africa and, indeed, of Rhodesia, but there is no reason to dispute it and it may perhaps throw light on what is observed by men walking through the bush or resting in it, for this is the chief object of this study.

The nutritional state of *Glossina morsitans* caught by different sorts of bait

The various phases through which a tsetse passes during a hunger cycle, and the behavioural changes characteristic of each phase have been described above. These ideas were elaborated by Bursell (1961) as a result of comparing the nutrition reserves of flies caught at different baits. He extended this work in conjunction with the Pilsons (Bursell 1966), and compared the nutritional state of male *Glossina morsitans* caught at their stationary bait oxen with those caught by a 'standard catching party' on a fly-round. A fly-round (Potts 1930, Ford, Glasgow, Johns, and Welch 1959) is a means of sampling a tsetse population in which a party of people walk through the bush and stop at intervals to catch tsetse that have approached them. The resultant catch is usually expressed as numbers of flies per ten thousand yards. For our present purposes, the catch of feeding flies at the stationary bait animal is compared with the catch taken by moving men (who stop periodically to catch). In Bursell's observations, the Pilsons' method of catching engorged flies only was changed slightly. Flies were caught when they were observed to lower the proboscis to probe the skin of the ox; they were not given time to suck up blood.

We need not examine Bursell's results in detail. He included in his estimate of their nutrition reserves not only the amount of fat (chloroform extract from dried flies) but also the amount of undigested blood. This was assessed by colorimetric estimation of haematin. One microgram of haematin was equivalent to an amount of blood that would metabolize to 0·0375 mg of fat. Observations were made in the hot dry season (October) and the rainy season (February). Both the fat and the haematin estimates indicated that whether caught on the stationary bait ox or by the moving party of men, flies in *Brachystegia* or *Colophospermum mopane* woodlands were in a better nutritional state than flies caught in riverine bush or in *Combretum* savanna. The size of the flies was measured and although collecting sites were only a few miles apart, significant differences could be demonstrated between the mean sizes of local samples. This was in line with the work of Jackson (1940 and other papers) who showed that the average rate of dispersal is only about 200 yd a week, which seems small in an insect that can fly between 15 and 20 mile/h. It is of some interest that not only were the tsetse caught in the *Brachystegia* woodlands the best nourished, but they were also the largest, an observation that seems to support the view expressed in Chapter 3, that the evolution of the *morsitans* group of tsetse has run *pari passu* with the evolution of the *miombo* ecosystems.

Since our object is to compare responses to various baits, the feature of Bursell's work that is of most interest here is the difference observed between the nutrition state of flies caught at the stationary animal and those caught on the fly-round (i.e. by moving men). The nutrition reserves of *G. morsitans* males caught while following moving men are significantly greater than those of males caught when about to feed from the stationary ox. This would be expected if the former were exhibiting sexually appetitive behaviour, while the latter were responding to a food source. In the earlier terminology, the flies following the men were in Phase 2, those coming to the ox in Phase 3 or Phase 4.

In his earlier work, Bursell (1961) had thought that the behaviour change, from one phase to the next, was initiated when food reserves fell below a certain threshold. However, although in his Zambezi valley studies the flies following the moving men had larger nutrition reserves than those that fed on the stationary ox, there was a very wide overlap in the distributions of individual values. It seemed that some flies were as likely to be attracted to a moving party of men as to a stationary bait ox. However, one may be bitten by tsetse flies when walking through the bush, sometimes quite severely, so that it is perhaps wrong to think of all the flies caught on a fly-round as sexually appetitive. Most of them are, but to some of them the moving men act as a food host. On the stationary bait ox only those flies seen to be about to feed were caught. Any others that may have approached but which did not adopt a feeding posture were neglected. The comparison between flies caught off the stationary ox and those caught while following the moving men is not entirely valid. Moreover, there is considerable evidence that an ox is much more attractive as a source of food than is a man. Bursell (unpublished) found that the nutrition reserves of flies caught when just about to feed from an ox were very much greater than were those of flies caught (in the same locality) when just about to feed off a human being.†

Moving men and moving oxen as baits

Some of the difficulties of interpretation of Bursell's (1966) study might be resolved if one were to compare tsetse caught from moving men and from moving animals (or stationary men and stationary animals) and, at the same time, to sort the catch into as many behavioural categories as can be observed. This was done in two different areas in Nigeria (Ford 1969*b*). Five sorts of behaviour were recorded, all of them familiar to field workers on *Glossina morsitans*.

(1) Flies caught on the ground. A man walking along a path through woodlands infested with *G. morsitans* may not notice them at all unless he stops to look behind him, when he will find perhaps half a dozen flies sitting on the path within a yard or two of his feet. When he moves on they will follow, flying in zigzag flight about six inches above the ground. If he is pushing a way through tall grass the movement will be more difficult to see. Virtually all these flies are males.

† I am greatly indebted to Professor Bursell for allowing me to refer to this observation.

(2) At rare intervals he may notice that the flies are buzzing frantically about one another, usually three or four feet above the ground. If he contrives to catch them all he will discover that there may be up to a dozen males and in their midst a single female. This is the nuptial flight.

(3) It may also be found that some tsetse are sitting on the man's back, and closer observation will show that some are perched vertically with the proboscis pointing upwards towards the man's head and others, which we include in this third category, are perched with the proboscis pointing generally towards the ground, or sometimes they are at an angle to the vertical. These are recorded as 'head-down' flies.

(4) This category comprises the 'head-up' flies at rest on man.

(5) Finally there are those tsetses that actually bite the man and, if he does not notice, gorge themselves with his blood.

In the work to be described flies were not allowed to feed but were caught as soon as they were seen to lower the proboscis to do so. Every fly caught was assigned to one or other of these categories. The sex and species were noted (for some *Glossina tachinoides* were encountered near streams), as well as whether or not the flies were tenerals† and therefore had not had their first meal. Each fly was given a number and put in its own small glass tube and killed with ethyl acetate vapour. Measurements of size (using a section of the fourth longitudinal wing vein as an index) and of relative age, by assessing the amount of wing-fray (Jackson 1946), were made on return to the laboratory before drying the flies, weighing them, and then extracting the fat and again weighing to find the fatless weight (*residual dry weight*, or rdw).

The same procedures were followed when the catching party took with it a bait ox, but it was not possible to distinguish the two categories (3) and (4) when flies settled on the animal but did not feed. They were recorded as at rest on the ox when they stood lightly on the animal's coat and did not burrow down into it in order to insert the proboscis. When they did this they were caught, if possible, before any blood had been taken up.

The results of the fat extraction analysis of collections made during the dry season (March) in the Yankari game reserve in the Sudan zone of northern Nigeria are given in Table 2.2. From this it is seen that the various behaviour patterns described above tend to sort themselves out in the order given. Of the flies caught when the bait consisted of moving men, those in category (1), caught while following along the ground, have the heaviest residual dry weight and the greatest fat content; those in categories (4) and (5) are lightest in rdw and have the least fat. It is not possible to demonstrate that the weights or fat contents of the flies in the first three categories

† Glasgow (1963*a*) writes, 'Until they have had their first meal tsetse have a characteristic soft feel, and they are called "teneral". This word is not used in this sense of any other group of insects, but a special term is justified as the condition is an unusual one not known in any other group of insects.'

are significantly different, and we can include them all in the sexually appetitive swarm. Similarly there is no significant difference in the weights and fat proportions of flies that perch 'head-up' and those actually seen to begin to feed. Perhaps the 'head-up' flies would feed if watched long enough, but Glasgow (1961a) and Pilson and Pilson (1967) believe that high light intensity inhibits feeding. Possibly some flies approach moving

TABLE 2.2

The residual dry weight (rdw), and percentage fat content of male G. mor-sitans *caught at Yankari, Nigeria, in the dry season of 1967 by moving parties of men alone or accompanied by an ox*

Category	No. in sample	rdw with standard error (mg)	Mean of fat with standard error (%)
	Catches with men only		
(1) From ground . .	39	6·86 ± 0·236	34·78 ± 4·741
(2) Nuptial flight . .	11	6·83 ± 0·271	30·32 ± 1·716
(3) 'Head-down' on men	31	6·74 ± 0·062	28·12 ± 2·014
Following swarm totals .	81	6·81 ± 0·071	31·63 ± 1·105
(4) 'Head-up' on men .	26	6·22 ± 0·189	19·58 ± 2·043
(5) Probing . . .	31	6·38 ± 0·182	18·03 ± 1·596
Feeding totals . .	57	6·31 ± 0·130	18·74 ± 1·266
	Catches with ox		
(1) From ground . .	11	6·36 ± 0·291	38·82 ± 2·738
(2)	Not observed		
(3) Perched on ox . .	11	6·58 ± 0·269	30·29 ± 3·118
Following swarm totals .	22	6·48 ± 0·195	34·56 ± 2·229
(4)	Not distinguished on ox		
(5) Probing . . .	38	6·55 ± 0·263	23·99 ± 2·447

parties of men to feed and perch on them but are inhibited from feeding while the men are moving along unshaded paths.

Flies caught on an ox led by the men show a similar ranking of the fat contents. No nuptial flight occurred, so that category (2) is missing. It has already been noted that it is not possible to distinguish categories (3) and (4) on the ox. Fewer flies were taken from the ox simply because this bait was used on fewer occasions.

A number of comparisons can be made between the catch made by men alone and the catch when they were accompanied by the ox. The first point to note was that on no occasion when the ox was present was any fly caught off a man. All were from the ground or from the ox. Clearly the presence of the animal changed the response of the tsetse to man. Next it may be observed that the size of the following swarm in relation to the intensity of attack by flies coming to feed is smaller when the ox is used. To make the comparison we sum categories (1), (2), and (3) to give a total of 81 following flies, and (4) and (5) to give 57 feeding (or 'hungry' or 'head-up') flies coming to the party of men alone. When the ox is present the following swarm total includes those perched on the animal but not seen to feed, in all 22, as against 38 feeders. Comparing these proportions by χ^2, a value of 7·250 indicates that the proportions of followers to feeders differs significantly ($P < 0·01$) between the two baits. Evidently connected with this difference in observed behaviour is the difference in nutrition state between flies that fed from the ox and those that came to feed from man. The former had a mean of fat weights that was 23·99 ± 2·447 per cent of the residual dry weights. The latter, combining feeding and 'head-up' flies, gave a value of 18·74 ± 1·266 per cent fat. The difference of 5·25 per cent is significant ($P < 0·05$).

One explanation for these observations is that Phase 2 flies are all in the same state when they begin following either bait, but that when man alone is present they continue following longer. This will augment the size of the following swarm, and result in greater consumption of nutrition reserves. This suggests two propositions: that man is less attractive as a food host than the ox, and is only attacked by the more hungry flies, which, had a favoured host been present, would have fed earlier; and that flies leave the swarm to feed on the bait they are following if it is acceptable. Bursell's comparison of the hunger state of *G. morsitans* caught when about to feed from man with that when about to feed on an ox is evidence for the first proposition. Is there evidence for the second?

Similar observations were also made at Ilorin in Central Nigeria, where, as will be shown in Chapter 21, man is much less favoured as a food host by several species of *Glossina* than he is at Yankari. In the wet season of 1966 three men traversed a route on which they caught from the following swarm and released 53 male *G. morsitans* and (which was unusual) 1 female. Three males and 1 female attempted to feed and were captured but not released. Fifteen minutes later a second party followed with the ox. This party caught only 7 following flies, one of which had been marked. But they also caught 21 males and 5 females all feeding from the ox. Five of these feeding males and 1 of the females had been marked by the first party. The 5 males had a mean fat content of 24·15 per cent, but the 3 that attempted to feed from the men in the first party only showed a mean of 14·9 per cent fat. It looked very much as though it needed the presence of the favoured host, the ox, to induce the better-nourished flies to leave the swarm to feed.

Confirmation of the idea that the following swarm is in a sexually appetitive condition is found in the proportions of teneral flies. The teneral fly has only a limited amount of fat left over from its life as a larva and pupa to supply energy to seek its first meal. The amount of fat and therefore the time available for the search varies according to seasonal climate and to the size of the fly (which depends upon the nutritional condition of its mother). It is therefore important that this first meal be obtained quickly, and to ensure this the teneral fly is less selective in its food choice. It is as ready to feed from a man as from an ox. Of the flies seen to probe man at Yankari, 21·7 per cent were tenerals, but of those that attacked the ox there were only 11·6 per cent. At Ilorin where man was much less favoured as a food host, only 9·1 per cent of flies probing the ox were tenerals, but of the few that probed man, 50 per cent were taking their first meal (Ford 1969b).

This observation, then, goes some way towards explaining the greater fat content of flies that feed on the ox; for the tenerals are, by definition, likely to have depleted nutrient reserves. The data in Table 2.2 include all flies caught. To determine if the flies that feed on man really are 'hungrier' than those that feed on the ox, it is necessary to exclude the teneral flies. There is another source of error. When catching flies that are about to feed, especially from the ox, it is difficult sometimes to net them before they have taken up any blood. Any fly that showed any signs of having sucked up fresh blood was specially recorded. The blood ingested would raise the residual dry weight and hence depress the percentage weight of fat. Among the 38 flies that probed the ox at Yankari were 5 tenerals, and 6 that had taken up a little blood. This left 27 flies, which gave a mean fat content of $27·3 \pm 3·154$ per cent. Among the 31 flies that probed man there were 4 tenerals, but none that showed fresh blood. These 27 gave $18·77 \pm 1·759$ per cent fat, and they are therefore significantly less well provided with fat than those that fed on the ox $(t = 7·5387, P < 0·001)$. Thus there seems little doubt that the physiological condition of flies that attack man is different from that of those that feed on an ox. This is not necessarily incompatible with Fiske's notion, so strongly supported by the recent comparisons between the attack on ox and on impala, that the favoured hosts are the more complacent.

'Feeding grounds'

Enough has been said about the behaviour of some of the commoner tsetses to allow some discussion of the role they play as vectors of trypanosomes between the wild animals, and man and his domestic livestock. Nothing has been said about development of infection in *Glossina*. No reference has yet been made to species other than *Glossina morsitans*, *G. swynnertoni*, and *G. pallidipes*, the most widely encountered savanna tsetses, and the lacustrine and riverine *G. fuscipes*. So far as is known, Fiske's observations around Lake Victoria on the last-mentioned species would apply with equal validity to the other subspecies of *G. fuscipes* and *G. palpalis*. In the next chapter the relationships of the latter two species will be discussed, as well as the distribution and habits, so far as they are known, of other tsetses. Finally, in the context of the present chapter, nothing has been said about 'feeding grounds'. This concept is so frequently encountered in papers about the savanna tsetses from 1930 onwards that it must be examined briefly. It was developed by members of the Tanganyika Tsetse Research department, especially Jackson (1930, 1933, 1949, 1955) and Nash (1930, 1933). It has been disposed of by Glasgow (1963a), but it is useful to see how the sort of observations already described in this chapter led to its formulation.

It was supposed that the 'home' (Jackson 1933) or the 'true habitat' (Nash 1933) of *G. morsitans* was the *Brachystegia–Julbernardia* woodland. Here the females rested when not feeding or depositing their larvae under fallen trees, in rot holes in tree boles, under rocks, or in other suitably protected places. These are the classical breeding sites where puparia may usually be found. When flies of either sex became 'hungry' they were supposed to move out of the woodland into open glades, usually associated with drainage lines or water courses and variously called, in different countries, *mbugas*, *dambos*, *vleis*, etc.

Both Jackson and Nash (working at the same time but in different parts of Tanzania) had recognized that in some places the proportion of females and teneral flies in the catch was higher than in others. These they first spoke of as female and male areas, and both came to the same conclusion as had Fiske (1920), working on *G. fuscipes*, that a high proportion of females indicated a 'hungry' population. They also noted that the female areas, where flies were hungry, were usually open glades. The idea that flies were hungry in these areas, now designated 'feeding grounds', was much strengthened by the use of 'hunger staging' (Jackson 1933) in which the appearance of the male flies was used as an index of the amount of their nutrient reserves. The catch of males in the 'female areas' tended to include a high proportion of 'Stage IV' flies. These have concave, translucent abdomens indicating much reduced fat bodies. In the male areas these emaciated males were rare and better-fed flies were common and, of course, there were fewer females. Jackson marked flies in the woodland and caught them in the 'feeding grounds', and vice versa. He 'naturally supposed, since some flies make such movements, that most flies do so. The truth may be that most flies find food animals resting under trees without having to fly very far looking for them, but that some are less fortunate and that such unlucky ones in due course arrive at the "feeding grounds" in an advanced state of hunger' (Glasgow 1963a). It is, of course, in these open glades, where there are few trees, that the human observer most often sees wild animals. In Chapter 17, the blood meal analyses of Weitz (1963) are reproduced. On the whole one finds that antelopes neglected by tsetse are grazing species which naturally favour open, grassy places, and those that are favoured as food hosts are browsers.

Nash came nearest to understanding the nature of 'feeding grounds'. They 'are areas to which hungry fly resort solely for the purpose of feeding. Probably these fly have failed to find food in the habitat and so have been forced to look for it elsewhere' (Nash 1933). One must remember that in nearly all field work up to about 1955 the bait was man himself, and we have seen that the nutrient reserves of *G. morsitans* that feed from man are smaller than those of flies feeding from the ox. Man is not a preferred host, though he is more attractive than zebra or impala.

It now seems that the phrase 'feeding ground' is a misnomer. Tsetse do not normally feed in them, although flies in Bursell's Phase 4, which are near to death by starvation and make a feeding attack on any object that provides a suitable stimulus, tend to accumulate where such objects (such as an entomologist) are most visible. As well as Phase 4 males, females in the same starved state and tenerals whose most urgent need is to get their first meal respond in the same way. Enhanced visibility must also assist formation of sexually appetitive swarms. Males approach and follow animals that leave the shelter of the bush to drink at water-holes. They also follow on the return journey and will eventually form an aggregation around the animals when they halt in the shade of the bush as postulated by Fiske (1920). The work of Weir and Davison (1965) showed that the activity cycles of some of the larger mammals approximately fit the times of maximum activity of tsetse in a nearby area. That *G. morsitans* will accumulate into a swarm around a moving object that emerges from the bush edge into an area of greater visibility was demonstrated in south-west Uganda. The peak build-up of the swarm, which occurred at different places on a path according to the direction in which the observers were walking, suggested that the flies had responded from distances of 150–400 yd (Ford 1958a). This fits the observation of Napier Bax (1937) that the closely related *G. swynnertoni* was visually activated at a distance of 150 yd (although not at 200) and with the recent deductions of Bursell and Slack (1968) that the distance flown by the average fly caught by a party of men is about 200 yd.

Males in following swarms may move straight from the swarm to the animal being followed, and begin to feed. If the animal is an unacceptable source of blood (such as man) following persists longer than if it is a preferred source (such as ox). In places where normally unacceptable animals (especially grazers like zebra) are particularly conspicuous, hunger induced by following for more than the normal interval will be more frequent. Moreover, in treeless glades high light intensity may inhibit feeding so that even when following an acceptable host animal, males may lose more than the normal quantity of their nutrient reserve and a condition of extreme hunger may result. If one wishes to experience a really savage attack by tsetse the best way is to drive along a bush road at about 15 mile/h and, while crossing a stream bed, which will usually have involved a prior traverse of the associated *mbuga* or *vlei*, stop with the windows open. The flies that have hitherto been prevented by the motion of the car from locating its passengers now respond to the scent of the human animal and attack with a quite intolerable voracity.

'Feeding grounds' therefore are not places where flies habitually feed. They are places where flies tend to become starved more quickly than in the 'true habitat', the bush or woodland, and where, therefore, they lose their customary discrimination and attack animals normally ignored, including man. Glossinologists, being men who for many years did not appreciate that they were less acceptable as sources of blood than warthogs, were misled into supposing that because they were mostly attacked in these places, so were all other animals. This was not so.

There is one more point to note about 'feeding grounds'. Essentially they are open spaces where moving objects are especially visible. In his attack on wildlife ecosystems, man becomes vulnerable to tsetse bite when, in making roads or clearing ground to build huts or to cultivate, he creates artificial 'feeding grounds'. It is an activity more or less balanced by its effect in destroying the habitats of the animal reservoirs of trypanosomes.

Other aspects of female behaviour

The early conclusions of Lloyd, Lamborn, and Fiske on the significance of the female ratio in catches by moving parties of men are supported by recent research. In order to clarify future references to female *Glossina*, a very brief note on the processes of reproduction must conclude this chapter.

The female need only mate once. This usually happens before she takes her first meal and is still in the teneral state. The sperm is stored in two spermathecae and suffices for fertilization of all eggs produced during her life. Tsetses are larviparous. The female does not lay eggs but gives birth, at intervals, to a single larva. When this happens she is about three weeks old. Other larvae are born at more or less regular intervals. The intervals before the first larva is born, and between subsequent births are regulated by temperature. At 24°C larvae of *Glossina fuscipes* appear every 10 days, *G. morsitans* every 11 days. At 18°C and 30°C females of the latter species larviposit at intervals of 25 and 8 days respectively (Jack 1939).

The larva, which at birth attains a weight greater than that of its mother, quickly burrows beneath the soil on which it has been deposited. The pregnant female chooses sites for larviposition which vary according to season, but ensure that her offspring are protected, during their further development, from extremes of climate. Birth takes place during the third larval instar. When burrowing is completed, usually at a half to one inch below the soil surface, the larval skin hardens to form the puparium.

Within this shell the insect undergoes a fourth larval instar and then pupates and metamorphoses to become a pharate adult which in due course emerges to the open air and, as a teneral insect, begins within a few hours the cycles of behaviour already described. The interval between larviposition and emergence is 31 days at 24°C, and at other temperatures can be calculated by the formula $1/0.0323 - 0.0028(t - 24)$, t being the mean temperature of maintenance (Jackson 1949, Glasgow 1963a).

Here one aspect of this process may be noted very briefly. It has been shown that teneral flies and fully adult non-tenerals respond somewhat differently to potential food hosts. It can also be shown that male tsetses, as they grow older, participate less frequently in sexually appetitive swarms (Ford 1969a). Age in males is assessed by measuring the amount of fraying of the posterior edge of the wings by a method devised by Jackson (1946). The older the fly the greater the amount of wing-fray. The method could be used for females, except for the difficulty of catching large enough numbers to achieve accurate calibration of the amount of fray. An entirely different technique was first developed by Russian entomologists on mosquitoes and other bloodsucking flies. It was applied to *Glossina* by Saunders (1960) and extended by Challier (1965). Female tsetses possess two ovaries, right and left, each containing two ovarioles. The eggs develop from follicles in the four ovarioles in a definite sequence, the first and third from the right pair of ovarioles, the second and fourth from the left. The fifth egg appears in a second follicle in the first ovariole of the right ovary, and so on. After ovulation, when the egg has descended into the uterus, the remains of its follicle can still be seen. It is thus possible to see, by dissection, how often and in what order ovulation has taken place and, knowing the interval of production of eggs, to assess the age of the fly. The Saunders–Challier technique has many uses (for example in the study of age-specific fecundity rates and net reproduction rates as in Saunders 1967). Here it is mentioned because, in Chapter 4, it will become necessary to describe the factors affecting the frequency of infection of tsetses by trypanosomes. One of these factors is the mean age of the tsetse population.

3

PATTERNS OF TSETSE DISTRIBUTION AND EVOLUTION

The evolution of *Glossina*

IT is impossible to explain the epidemiological relationships of trypanosomes, tsetses, and their natural hosts unless we look upon them as
having evolved together and as having influenced each other's evolution.
Three authors have concerned themselves with the evolutionary phylogeny
of the genus *Glossina*. Their views are briefly discussed in the first sections
of this chapter. A fourth system of possible phylogenetic influences is then
examined. It will be seen that the various factors supposed to have influenced the evolution of *Glossina* are not mutually exclusive.

Insects are rare among fossils and no fossil tsetse has been found in
Africa; but four fossil species from the Oligocene shales at Florissant in
Colorado, U.S.A., are generally accepted as *Glossina*. If they are then it
may be that the genus still survives in the New World (Glasgow 1967), for
forest species with habits like the most recently discovered African species,
G. nashi Potts 1955, are difficult to find. If they exist then they do not
transmit trypanosomes to Central American livestock.

The Florissant fossils must fit into the same evolutionary and geographical scheme as the modern tsetse of tropical Africa. That a dispersal
of the genus leading to its separation into a number of phylogenetic groups
took place in the remote past cannot be disputed. The three extant *fusca*,
morsitans, and *palpalis* groups (sometimes given subgeneric status as
Austenina, *Glossina*, and *Nemorhina*) are the survivors of this process. A
scheme for their evolution that takes account of present-day geography as
well as of the Florissant fossils was suggested by Evens (1953) following the
ideas of Jeannel (1942). The latter found in the continental drift hypothesis
of Wegener a suitable basis for explanation of the geographical distribution
of certain groups of Coleoptera. For long disputed by geophysicists, though
generally supported by biologists, the hypothesis of continental drift has
now found wide acceptance.

Evens excuses his speculations on the pardonable grounds that 'on ne
saurait étudier la dispersion des Tsé-tsés au Congo Belge, le pays le plus
riches en espèces, sans avoir l'esprit ouvert à l'évolution historique de
cette famille de Muscidae, dont la triste renommée a conquis le monde'.
Machado (1954, 1959) who in some essentials does not agree with Evens,
also evokes the orogenies and climatic fluctuations of the distant past
to explain phylogeny. The major epidemiological patterns of the African

trypanosomiases are founded upon the geographical distinctions between the distributions of the three subgeneric groups of tsetse. The speculations of Evens and Machado are valuable not only as starting points for zoogeographical discussion, but also because they provide a background to the long evolutionary history of tsetse-borne disease.

Flight in insects may have begun in the Upper Carboniferous in response to the development of abundant vertically growing large plants. The Diptera emerged much later, in the Permian. When some insects abandoned plant juices as food and adopted a bloodsucking habit, they introduced their own flagellate parasites to the circulation of vertebrates. This stage may already have been reached during the Mesozoic with the appearance of an *Ur-Glossina* that fed on giant terrestrial reptiles in that portion of Wegener's early world that later formed the great mass of Eurasia. The transmission of a Stercorarian trypanosome, *Trypanosoma grayi* Novy (see Chapter 4), a parasite of *Crocodilus niloticus*, by *Glossina fuscipes* is, perhaps, a survival from this era. The equator then passed through the area in which the Mediterranean sea was later to appear, so that the *Ur-Glossina* already inhabited a warm or sub-tropical climate.

Evens thinks that expansion of the genus took place in two directions. A westward movement took it north of a much larger Aralo-Caspian sea into Laurentia, the continental forerunner of North America, Greenland, and western Europe. A second area of expansion was the area later to become Asia Minor (Mesogaea). With the movement of the equator, tsetse disappeared from the main Eurasian mass and followed the progress of the tropics southward. One branch moved west and south towards the American tropics and West Africa, not yet separated by the formation of the Atlantic trough. The eastern branch, skirting the eastern shores of the Tethys sea and later of a Saharan sea, invaded East Africa (Gondwana) and then spread westwards. The formation of the African rift valleys and the volcanic mountain chains, that lasted from the Miocene into the Pleistocene, then produced another division in the eastern branch of *Glossina*. Finally during part of the Miocene, a vast lake in what later became the basin of the Congo river created another isolating factor contributing to speciation in the original western line (*Austenina*) and also in the western fork of the eastern line (*Nemorhina*).

This two-pronged invasion of Gondwana, of which the future African continent formed the central mass, led to the appearance of three dispersal centres: (1) that of the *fusca* group around the Bay of Biafra; (2) that of the *palpalis* group, also around the Bay of Biafra; (3) that of the *morsitans* group in Africa east of the Central Rift.

A classification of *Glossina* species is given in Table 3.1 on p. 42, and the main outlines of their modern distributions are shown in Maps 3.1, 3.2, and 3.3. Eight of fourteen species or sub-species of the *fusca* group are to be found within a comparatively small area adjoining the Bay of Biafra. Six of

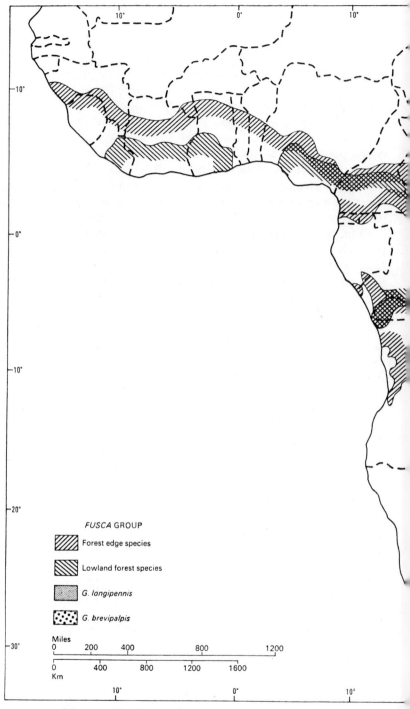

MAP 3.1. Distribution of lowland forest, forest–savanna mosaic or fores
G. brevipalp

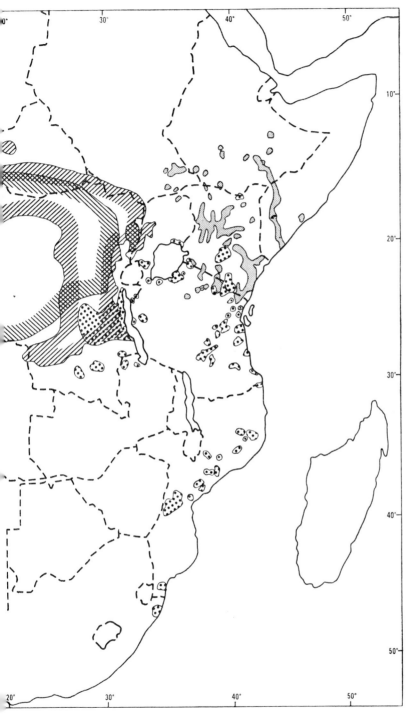

of *fusca* group tsetses, and the relict species in woodland and savanna,
ipennis.

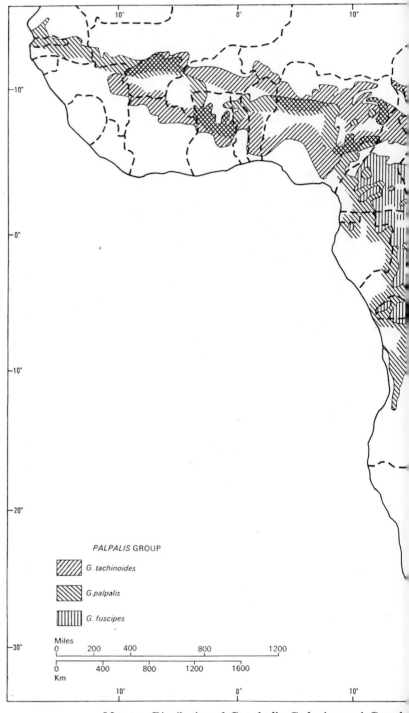

MAP 3.2. Distribution of *G. palpalis*, *G. fuscipes*, and *G. tach*

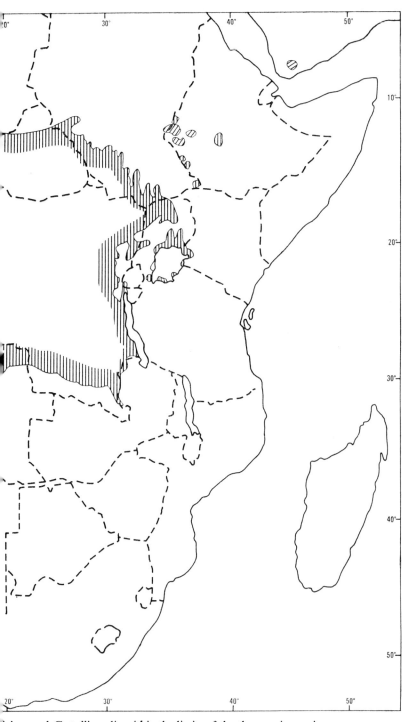

ginea and *G. pallicera* lie within the limits of the three main species.

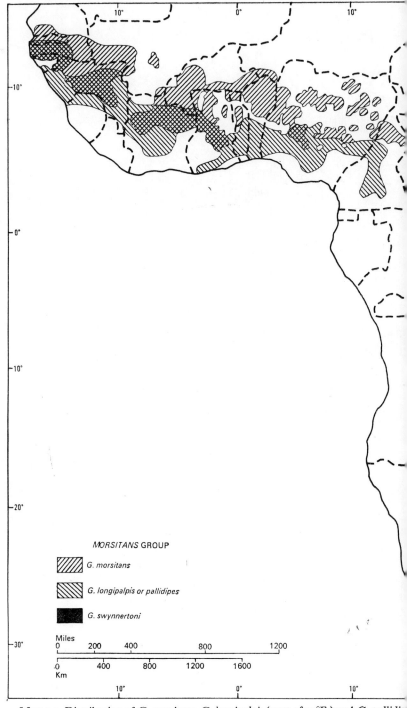

MAP 3.3. Distribution of *G. morsitans*, *G. longipalpis* (west of 25°E.) and *G. pallidip*
miles of the East

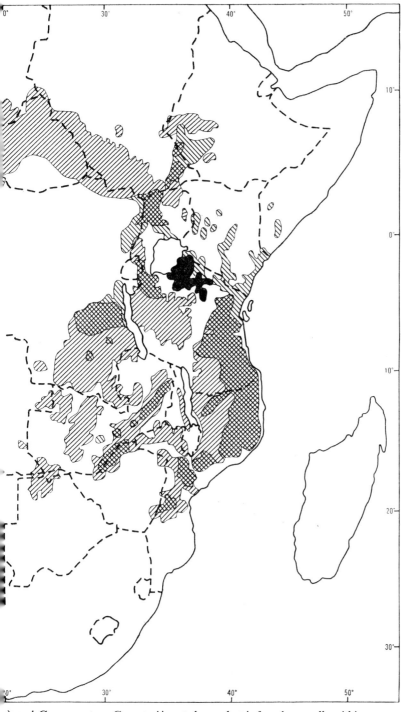

.), and *G. swynnertoni*. *G. austeni* is not shown, but is found generally within 150
:tween 2°N. and 27°S.

TABLE 3.1

Classification of Glossina

Order: INSECTA
Order: Diptera
Family: Muscidae
Subfamily: Stomoxydinae
Genus: *Glossina* Wiedemann 1830

Fusca group	*Palpalis* group	*Morsitans* group
Glossina fusca fusca Walker 1849	*Glossina palpalis palpalis* Robineau-Desvoidy 1830	*Glossina morsitans morsitans* Westwood 1850
G. fusca congolensis Newstead and Evans 1921	*G. palpalis gambiensis* Vanderplank 1949	*G. morsitans submorsitans* Newstead 1910
G. tabaniformis Westwood 1850	*G. fuscipes fuscipes* Newstead 1910	*G. morsitans centralis* Machado 1970
G. longipennis Corti 1895	*G. fuscipes martinii* Zumpt 1933	*G. swynnertoni* Austen 1923
G. brevipalpis Newstead 1910	*G. fuscipes quanzensis* Pires 1948	*G. longipalpis* Wiedemann 1830
G. nigrofusca nigrofusca Newstead 1910	*G. caliginea* Austen 1911	*G. pallidipes* Austen 1903
G. nigrofusca hopkinsi Van Emden 1944	*G. pallicera pallicera* Bigot 1891	*G. austeni* Newstead 1912
G. fuscipleuris Austen 1911	*G. pallicera newsteadi* Austen 1929	
G. medicorum Austen 1911	*G. tachinoides* Westwood 1850	
G. severini Newstead 1913		
G. schwetzi Newstead and Evans 1921		
G. haningtoni Newstead and Evans 1922		
G. vanhoofi Henrard 1952		
G. nashi Potts 1955		

the nine species or sub-species of the *palpalis* group are also found in the same region. Whether or not Evens' hypothesis as to the formation of these two centres is correct, modern geography supports his view of the importance of this zone as a centre of relatively intense speciation. No such focus is to be found among the *morsitans* group.

Evens regards the Rift Valley as a major isolating influence, but it seems clear that speciation has also been influenced by the more or less concentric pattern of drier climates and associated biota around the central high rainfall forests.

The fusca *group*

Two factors chiefly influenced evolution of the *fusca* group in Africa. The eastward and southward spread from the dispersal centre around the epicontinental sea in what later became the Congo basin (or alternatively the appearance, in another epoch, of very dry conditions in the centre of the basin) led to the isolation and speciation of *G. severini*, *G. vanhoofi*, *G. schwetzi*, and *G. fuscipleuris*, species now found around the edge of the Congo basin. Its spread further eastward throughout or around the periphery of a great East African plcistoccnc forcst isolated the two East African species, *G. brevipalpis* and *G. longipennis*. Relict belts of *G. fuscipleuris* east of Lake Victoria, in Central Tanzania (Buxton 1955) and in the Limpopo basin (Santos Dias 1962) may be survivals from the same process. Evens (1953) believes that the Western Rift Valley was the principal isolating agent in the origin of *G. longipennis* and *G. brevipalpis*. He regards the presence of the latter in the south-eastern Congo, west of Lake Tanganyika, as a secondary migration westwards through or around the Rift. In the same way *G. fusca*, *G. fuscipleuris*, and *G. nigrofusca hopkinsi* have invaded the country east of the Rift by various suitable routes. This seems unnecessary. A reduction of an East African forest that had, at one time, extensive links with the Congo forest would provide an appropriate means of isolation.

It is often assumed that the evolution of the *palpalis* and *morsitans* groups was a process in which an ancestral line of *fusca*-like species, living in a wet climate, branched off from the parent stock and adapted itself to drier conditions. To what extent the present pattern of distribution of the three groups with regard to climate is an indication of this trend is not easy to say. Evens, in company with most glossinologists, supposes that the two East African species *G. longipennis* and *G. brevipalpis* have adapted themselves to a dry climate, but Machado (1959) cannot accept this. He holds that *G. longipennis*, the most xerophilous of all *Glossina*, is, morphologically, the most primitive. He quotes floristic evidence to show that the Florissant fossils were laid down under a semi-arid climate. He believes there is no sound evidence to show that the ancestral *Glossina* was an insect living in humid conditions.

The Florissant fossil tsetse were not all large insects. *Glossina oligocena* indeed had wings 16 mm long, some 3 mm longer than the largest modern tsetse, *G. brevipalpis*. On the other hand *G. osborni* had wings only 7 mm long, about the size of those of an average *G. tachinoides* or a small *G. austeni*. *G. armatipes* (perhaps, according to Buxton 1955, not a *Glossina*) was also very small (Cockerell 1918). Doubtless the Florissant shales were laid down over a long time and one need not assert that all four fossil species (*G. veterna* is the fourth) lived under the same climate or in the same general habitat. But there is no reason why they should not have done so. Machado makes the point that the Florissant climate was in respect of temperature probably very close to, if not outside, the cold climate limits of modern tsetse distribution. The case is paralleled in the Sitatonga Hills in Mozambique where *G. brevipalpis* and *G. austeni* (representing modern extremes of size) may be found with *G. pallidipes* and *G. morsitans* (Pires, Marques da Silva, and Teles e Cunha 1950). Here these species are indeed approaching close to their climatic limits, but they may be found together in various localities nearly all the way north to Mombasa. Just short of latitude 4°S., *G. morsitans* disappears, but the three other species are soon joined by *G. longipennis*, the example *par excellence* of adaptation to arid, almost desert conditions. In West Africa similar assemblages could be found and among them *G. tachinoides*, usually thought of as a dry climate fly, sometimes lives in very wet climates. We must therefore agree with Machado that the Florissant fossils do not reveal anything about the environment of the *Ur-Glossina*. We do know, however, that during the Oligocene, the Colorado area was infested by a number of species of tsetse fly, as distinct from one another as, for example, the modern *G. fusca*, *G. longipalpis*, and *G. tachinoides*, to name three members of an assemblage to be found in the same area in Ghana.

The palpalis *group*

Machado's (1954) revision of the *palpalis* group has now found general acceptance. It collects together three subspecies for long thought to belong to the original *G. palpalis* Robineau-Desvoidy 1830, namely *G. palpalis fuscipes* Newstead, *G. p. martinii* Zumpt, and *G. p. quanzensis* Pires, to restore *Glossina fuscipes* Newstead 1910. The isolating factor that led to the geographically separate evolution of these three subspecies, as well as their separation as a whole from *G. palpalis*, was drought and not the presence of a central sea in the middle of the Congo basin.

In general one may say that *G. palpalis* inhabits the rivers along the Congo and West African coasts that drain directly into the sea. *G. fuscipes* infests the Congo river and its tributaries and, in the east, the subspecies *G. fuscipes fuscipes* overflows into the basin of the Nile. It also occupies the northern half of the Congo basin, i.e. the Congo river itself, the Ubangi and the Uele rivers, the Aruwimi, the Lomami, and the Lower Lualaba. The headwaters of the Lualaba and, through their connection via the Lukuga river, the shores of Lake Tanganyika, provide the habitat of *G. fuscipes martinii*. The third subspecies, *G. fuscipes quanzensis*, occupies the rivers of the south-western quarter of the Congo basin, the Sankara, Kasai, Kwilu, and Kwango, and along their courses penetrates into Angola.

There is some overlapping. On the Lualaba near Kasongo (4° 30′S.) all three subspecies have been recorded as well as some intermediate forms. Near the Congo mouth *G. f. fuscipes*, *G. f. quanzensis*, and *G. palpalis palpalis* are found in the same general area, and there is overlapping of *G. f. fuscipes* and *G. p. palpalis* in southern Cameroun, the Central African Republic, and the Congo Republic. In general, however, the distribution in the Congo basin and its neighbouring areas is distinct.

Machado supposes that *G. palpalis* and *G. fuscipes* derive from a common ancestor and that the present geographical division between them, i.e. between *G. palpalis* on the coastal rivers and *G. fuscipes* in the drainage system of the *cuvette congolaise*, reflects their origin. The elevation of the rim and the sinking of the centre of the Congo basin took place at the beginning of the Miocene. A new watershed was formed that separated the short rivers running down to the Atlantic from Gabon to northern Angola from the great central Congo basin. This divided the distribution area of the common *palpalis/fuscipes* ancestor. The basin formed by the sinking of the central part of the Congo captured the Upper Lualaba and Upper Kasai rivers, already in existence as part of the hydrological system of an earlier epoch. The basin filled and formed a great lake that persisted until its western rim was breached at Stanley Falls and the modern Congo began to flow into the Atlantic.

G. *fuscipes* was thus isolated from G. *palpalis* and evolved in the forests around the shores of the Miocene lake. Machado believes that the present subspecies G. *fuscipes fuscipes*, which occupies a far greater area than either G. *f. martinii* or G. *f. quanzensis*, is closest to the ancestral form. The two latter species became isolated as a result of later climatic desiccation.

A large part of the Congo forests is rooted in Kalahari sands redistributed by winds in the middle Pleistocene. There was an arid period 75 000–52 000 years B.P. and perhaps another about 10 000 B.P. Sands were blowing in north-east Angola from 13 000 to 11 000 B.P. These dry epochs that followed the gradual emptying of the Miocene lake may have reduced peripheral lacustrine forests to mere gallery forests. Such a process could have segregated the G. *fuscipes* populations of the Kasai and Lukeni rivers from the northern portions of the Congo system, leading to the appearance of the *quanzensis* subspecies.

G. *f. martinii* evolved around the shores of Lake Tanganyika at a time when its effluent, the Lukuga, was closed. Lake Tanganyika for a long time after its final formation during the middle Pliocene was completely isolated from other hydrological systems, and during this period it developed its own unique endemic fauna. It is supposed that during this period of isolation the shores of Lake Tanganyika were free of G. *fuscipes*, which invaded when the Lukuga gap appeared. Later, perhaps during the same dry period responsible for the segregation of G. *f. quanzensis*, this connection ceased to exist. G. *f. martinii* then evolved independently on the shores of Tanganyika and finally, in a more recent humid epoch, re-invaded the Congo basin by the same route.

If geographical isolation in the past was the principal factor leading to the speciation of the three forms of G. *fuscipes*, their subsequent differentiation may have been assisted by the ecological distinctions between the ecosystems in which eventually they found themselves. G. *f. fuscipes* belongs to the great rain forest of the central Congo (although capable in the north and north-east of surviving in gallery forests in a savanna climate), G. *f. quanzensis* is a gallery forest tsetse in derived savanna or forest mosaic vegetation, while G. *f. martinii* is a gallery forest fly in country now occupied by *Brachystegia-Julbernardia* woodland.

Machado (1954) has commented upon the paucity of intermediate forms

in zones where different species and subspecies meet. 'Une seule explic-
ation parait valable: il y a une barrière, non de nature géographique ou
écologique, mais biocènotique, à l'étalement de *palpalis* vers l'hinterland et
de *fuscipes* vers la région cotière; cette barrière est constituée, pour chaque
espèce, par la présence de l'autre. L'absence d'une zone d'intergradation
et l'existence d'une bande de superposition entre les aires des deux
espèces favorisè l'idée de la competition, de preference à celle de l'hybrid-
ation.' However, he rightly remarks that 'La pauvreté de nos connaissances
actuelles sur l'écologie comparée des deux formes et sur leurs rapports
reproductifs naturels ... nous empêches toutefois d'être plus affirmatifs'.

Mouchet, Gariou, and Rateau (1958) studied areas of overlap between
G. f. fuscipes and G. palpalis and were unable to find intermediate forms
which would have been expected had abundant hybridization taken place;
nor were they able to distinguish habitat differences although, in the area
studied, the two species occupied distinct stretches of the same rivers.

Vanderplank (1949b) crossed G. palpalis from Nigeria with G. fuscipes
fuscipes from Uganda. Table 3.2 is taken from his paper. Of his controls, the

TABLE 3.2

Results of hybridization of G. palpalis *and* G. fuscipes†

Male	Female	Pairs	Inseminated	Alive at 21 days	No. that produced puparia	Total pupae produced
G. p. × G. p.		44	32	24	22	130
G. f. × G. f.		41	30	22	22	51
G. p. × G. f.		64	61	45	2	3
G. f. × G. p.		29	28	24	6	12

† From Vanderplank (1949b).

palpalis × *palpalis* puparia gave 98 per cent emergence and the *fuscipes*
× *fuscipes* 100 per cent. Only one of the three *palpalis* male × *fuscipes*
female puparia emerged successfully and of the *fuscipes* male × *palpalis*
female cross only four of the twelve. Twenty-seven per cent of female G.
fuscipes died from injuries received in mating with G. *palpalis* males. To
achieve successful mating the females had to be protected either by cutting
off the points of the male claspers or by coating their abdomens with
cellulose acetate paint. It is clear that if these experiments reproduce what
happens in nature, the failure of Mouchet and his colleagues to find hybrids
in the *palpalis–fuscipes* overlap zones was to be expected. Random mating
between the two species, followed by failures of various sorts, including
high mortality among G. *fuscipes* females, is the basis of the separation observed in nature.

Little is known of *Glossina pallicera* or of *G. caliginea*, but *G. tachinoides* is a species of great interest, both for the light it throws upon the geography of *Glossina* and in its role as a vector of sleeping sickness. It has a greater environmental range (at least in terms of the physical and biotic characteristics of the places in which it is found) than any other species of tsetse. It is also the only living species that has been found outside the African continent, although that part of Southern Arabia in which it was collected by Carter (1906) is included by zoogeographers in the Ethiopian region and was linked to the African continent by a land bridge during the Pliocene. *G. tachinoides* occurs together with *G. fuscipes fuscipes* in south-west Ethiopia (Ovazza 1956, Balis and Bergeon 1968). This provides a geographical link with its main area of dispersion, from the Central African Republic to the Republic of Guinea.

Machado (1954) regards *G. tachinoides* as perhaps having derived from *G. fuscipes* from which it became isolated in the basin of the Upper Niger or of Lake Chad. The latter reached its maximum (Mega-Chad), with a shore line 400 miles north of its present limits 22 000 years ago, and it was still the same size as late as 8500 B.P. By 4500 B.P. it was much shrunk. Further east, the Sudd in the southern Sudan is the relic of a great lake. These events, however, cannot account for Carter's South Arabian tsetse if the Bab-el-Mandeb was flooded by the Indian Ocean during the Pliocene (Furon 1963). But whatever the date of its origin, its distribution from southern Arabia westwards implies an earlier continuity and, moreover, a continuity associated with permanent riverine or lacustrine vegetation. It seems easiest to think of *G. tachinoides* as a species derived from the common ancestor of *G. fuscipes* and *G. palpalis* rather than from the former only.

If the west to east range of *G. tachinoides* is remarkable, its north to south distribution in West Africa is no less so. In Northern Nigeria it lives along streams running through country with as little as 15 inches mean yearly rainfall. In the south, in the Cross river area of Eastern Nigeria it lives under a rainfall of 130 inches a year. This remarkable ecological variability is reflected in the feeding habits of the species, and hence influences its role as a vector of trypanosomiasis (see Chapter 21).

The morsitans group

Bursell (1958) also has discussed the phylogeny of *Glossina*. He has seen the evolution of the three subgenera primarily as a process of development of water-proofing mechanisms. He supposes that the *fusca* group are the nearest in structure to the ancestral tsetse and that the latter was, like most of its modern representatives, a dweller in forests with humid climates. The evolution of the *palpalis* and *morsitans* groups was, at least in part, the evolution of water-proofing mechanisms and drought avoidance behaviour patterns. The puparia of *G. brevipalpis* and *G. fuscipleuris*, species living in residual forest or relatively humid secondary forest communities in eastern Africa, cannot tolerate environments with humidity less than 70 per cent; on the other hand *G. swynnertoni* and *G. morsitans centralis* can complete their development in an atmosphere of 10 per cent relative humidity. *G. morsitans submorsitans* needs a relative humidity of 30 per cent while *G. pallidipes*, *G. tachinoides*, *G. fuscipes fuscipes*, and *G. austeni* have tolerance levels between 40 and 50 per cent relative humidity. The *palpalis* group flies living in habitats associated with lake edges or rivers, avoid the climate extremes of the areas in which they are found.

There are two anomalies in Bursell's phylogenetic scheme. *G. austeni*, a member of the *morsitans* group, lives in evergreen thickets along the east coast of Africa often in company with *G. brevipalpis*. It is assumed that *G. austeni* developed a puparial shell with high water-proofing efficiency in a dry climate, along with other members of its group, although it is not confined to the more humid climate of the East African coast. The other anomaly is presented by *G. longipennis*, a member of the *fusca* group that is better adapted than any other tsetse to life in an arid environment. Large puparia (as in all the *fusca* group) are at an advantage in resisting desiccation because their surface area is small in relation to weight. *G. longipennis* is confined to the semi-arid regions of Tanzania, Kenya, and Somalia and has a puparium larger than *G. brevipalpis*, its puparial shell and pupal skin are both less permeable to water, and it can tolerate a greater loss of weight through water loss. It can complete its development in completely dry air. There seems no doubt that by and large puparial water-proofing efficiency is related to the climatic stresses that the puparium must endure; but there are difficulties in the way of full acceptance of Bursell's theory. Thus although *G. austeni* is supposed to have adjusted itself to a wetter climate, much of the East African coast in the distribution range of this species has a dry climate, for example, in Somalia and parts of Kenya. This in itself would not be a difficulty were it not for the fact that *G. brevipalpis*, taken as an example of a dweller in the ancestral wet climate, lives in the same area as not only *G. austeni*, but also with the powerfully drought-resistant *G. longipennis*. The bush along the Tana river or the arid country of the Tsavo game park in Kenya supports both *G. brevipalpis* and *G. longipennis* (the wet and dry extremes of Bursell's phylogenetic tree) as well as the intermediate species, *G. pallidipes* and *G. austeni*. A study of the microclimates of larviposition sites of these four species would be interesting, for they seem likely to differ very much.

Whatever may be the true phylogenetic relationships of the three groups of tsetse flies, it is certain today that the *fusca* group as a whole live in humid environments, the *palpalis* group is generally confined to waterside habitats, and the third, or *morsitans* group, is associated with more arid 'savanna' type vegetation.

It will have become evident that Bursell's phylogeny must be unacceptable to Machado, whose interpretation of the Florissant fossils has been discussed. Machado believes that *G. longipennis*, far from being a species that has undergone specialized adaptation to a dry climate, is actually the most primitive and simple of all modern tsetse. It is also unacceptable to him that the morphological distinctions upon which taxonomy is based are, as it were, incidental phenotypic manifestations of an evolutionary process that was chiefly a response to the need to invade drier climates. The view is supported by Bursell's own data for *G. m. centralis* and those of Buxton and Lewis (1934) for *G. m. submorsitans*. Both are certainly of the same species and both belong to the same ecosystem, the *Brachystegia–Isoberlinia* woodlands, or *miombo*. The former can tolerate a relative humidity as low as 10 per cent, but *G. m. submorsitans* has a much higher tolerance level, between 30 and 50 per cent r.h. The development of a hyper-efficient water-proofing mechanism in the one subspecies, or its loss in the other, may have accompanied but seems unlikely to have controlled the morphological characters upon which the two are separated. Glasgow (1963a) thinks that its phylogenetic significance presents a problem that must be left unsolved, but that pupal water balance is a limiting factor in controlling the distribution of the various species of tsetse seems an unavoidable conclusion. In support of this he refers to Jackson (1945) who introduced two exotic species of tsetse, *G. morsitans morsitans* and *G. fuscipes fuscipes*, into the habitat of *G. swynnertoni*. There are places in Tanzania where the latter species and *G. morsitans* meet and produce sterile cross matings. It was therefore to be supposed that *G. morsitans* would survive, at least for a time, in the *swynnertoni* habitat. It did so on a scale large enough to produce a second generation. *G. fuscipes* failed in this. They fed and mated, for gravid females were captured which, taken into the laboratory, larviposited. From the puparia produced by these larvae second-generation adults emerged. But in the bush there was no sign of a second generation. It was supposed that the female *G. fuscipes* were unable to find sites for larviposition with humidities high enough for puparial life to be completed. But another view is possible. Swynnerton (1923b) recorded two examples of larviposition, by *G. morsitans* and *G. pallidipes*, in completely unshaded open ground. Most of them were dead and it might well be thought that death was due to overheating rather than to desiccation. Failure of inherent behaviour routines to achieve necessary end results may occur in environments entirely different from that in which genetic selection had led to their development. The *G. fuscipes* in the Shinyanga bush might not have been able to find sufficiently humid sites; on the other hand they could equally well have been unable to begin the processes which, in normal circumstances, would lead to them. It will be necessary to look again at the climatic controls on tsetse behaviour and distribution, especially in Chapters 17 and 21.

Feeding and speciation

So far speciation has been considered as a response to geographical isolation and to isolation produced by climatic change. No thought has been given to isolation due to adaptation to new hosts. If we accept a late Palaeozoic or early Mesozoic origin for *Glossina* (and this seems necessary to account for the Florissant fossils) then we must also postulate an original dependence on large reptiles. The great terrestrial reptiles flourished during the Cretaceous and then abruptly became extinct. By the Eocene only snakes, lizards, and some tortoises were living on land. The crocodiles and turtles remained in aquatic habitats. At the beginning of the Tertiary, *Glossina* could either remain committed to the crocodiles and large lizards in riverine or lacustrine environments, and some of them did, or attach themselves, as did others, to the new rapidly evolving mammals. If the habits of ancestral forms were similar to those of their modern descendants, one would look to the forest and the thicket pigs (ancestral forest hogs and bushpigs) and to large animals like elephant, buffalo, rhinoceros, or hippopotamus ancestors in these habitats to provide the most easily available alternatives to large reptiles. Transfer of preference to such species would enable tsetse to move further away from the aquatic reptile habitats into the forests, and eventually to the savannas.

It seems possible that tsetse which had adopted a predominantly forest or thicket pig diet could, in appropriate situations, transfer their preference to warthog ancestors with little alteration in their feeding responses. Support for this view is found in the ideas of Baker (1963). He believes that many Trypanosomatidae began as gut parasites of annelids, and thence adapted themselves to vertebrate hosts (fishes, amphibia, reptiles) via the leeches. In the latter they developed in the 'anterior station' (see Chapter 4). Insect trypanosomes originally developed in the 'posterior station', and used the stercorarian mechanism (as in *G. palpalis* and *Trypanosoma grayi*) to transfer to the vertebrate host. The pathogenic African trypanosomes were thus first acquired by the mammal hosts from leeches and then found in *Glossina*, already carrying trypanosomes in the posterior station, a new vector with a vacant anterior station.

This change in habitat of the trypanosomes can only have occurred in humid environments where leeches were common. The forest pigs seem to fit these requirements. Knowledge about trypanosome infections in wild animals, and there is not a lot, is summarized in Chapter 4. Wild Suidae, among the susceptible animals, are better adapted than are most other species, save perhaps buffaloes, to trypanosome infection. When they are artificially infected, parasitaemia is transitory, while it is unusual to obtain positive blood smears from wild pigs. Antelopes are much more productive of positive blood smears, while some, at least in captivity, are easily killed by trypanosome infection. It is tentatively suggested that anterior station trypanosomes were acquired by *Glossina* from forest pigs and that from them tsetse turned their attentions to warthogs. The priority thus given to the Suidae has enabled them to achieve a degree of adjustment to trypanosome infection greater than is found in the antelopes. These essentially open-country animals became 'secondary' hosts of tsetse of the

TABLE 3.3

Rearrangement and summary of blood meal analysis tables of Weitz (1963) excluding man and domestic animals as well as blood meals not fully identified

	Host	%
Lacustrine and riverine feeders		
Palpalis group tsetse	Reptiles	55·6
	Bushbuck	22·3
	Remainder	22·1
Forest, thicket, or forest-edge feeders		
Group (A) *G. tabaniformis,*	Bushpig and forest	
G. fuscipleuris, G. austeni	hog	74·4
	Remainder	25·6
Group (B) *G. fusca, G. pallidipes*	Bushbuck	61·1
G. longipalpis	Bushpig	11·9
	Remainder	27·0
Savanna feeders		
G. m. morsitans, G. m. submorsitans	Warthog	57·2
G. swynnertoni	Buffalo	20·6
	Giraffe and kudu ⎱ Remainder ⎰	22·2
Specialized East African *fusca* group flies		
G. brevipalpis, G. longipennis	Elephant ⎱ Rhinoceros Hippopotamus and ⎰ buffalo	70·9
	Bushpig	17·6
	Remainder	11·5

morsitans group, after *Glossina* had invaded the savannas in the wake of the warthogs.

The feeding patterns of the commoner tsetse have been analysed by Weitz (1963). After some rearrangement his five tables are summarized in Table 3.3. (See also Chapter 17 for another rearrangement.) All blood meals attributed to man or cattle are excluded. We are concerned with events that occurred before man developed habits that permitted him or his livestock to act as hosts (Lambrecht 1964, Ford 1965).

Infections of trypanosomes in wild animals are discussed at greater length in Chapter 4. Among those which are preferred hosts of tsetse the pigs seldom display infections (10 per cent). Among the bovids, bushbuck and situtunga are outstanding both as tsetse hosts and as carriers of trypanosomes in the peripheral circulation. Among the forest or thicket feeders, Group (B), bovids other than bushbuck only supply 1·5 per cent of all blood meals. Among the Savanna feeders only four bovids make a relatively large contribution to tsetse diet and of these only the giraffe (37 per cent), kudu (45 per cent), and eland (29 per cent) show frequent infections. Nine other bovid genera listed by Weitz as supplying blood meals to the savanna tsetse together contribute only 4·0 per cent of all blood meals. Of these, some like the waterbuck and reedbuck frequently show trypanosome infections but they are seldom bitten by tsetse. They are not well adjusted to infection because their habits are such that contact with *Glossina* is infrequent. Other bovids, such as impala, perhaps display few parasitaemias because they are not attractive as food hosts to *Glossina*. Feeding patterns and trypanosome infections both suggest that the bovids, in general, are less well adjusted to trypanosome infection than are the pigs. Indeed there is a third group of bovids which, at least in captivity, may be unable to withstand infection (by *T. brucei*) and die of trypanosomiasis. These include Thomson's gazelle, duiker, and dik-dik.

To recapitulate: tsetse were originally reptile feeders and, as such, became involved with the transmission of *Trypanosoma grayi*, which persists between the *palpalis* group and the crocodiles. The anterior station trypanosomes entered the African Artiodactyla via leech attack on forest mammals, particularly Suidae (and, perhaps, the buffaloes). This prior acquisition of trypanosomes has produced a high degree of adjustment to infection (revealed by the relatively infrequent peripheral parasitaemias) in the pigs and buffaloes. The savanna-dwelling warthogs enabled *Glossina* to enter the savanna ecosystems, in which the *morsitans* group evolved as a separate entity. During the process, the Bovidae and Giraffidae also became hosts to the trypanosomes, but as yet they are less well adjusted than the Suids.

Support for the view that Suidae were earlier hosts of tsetse other than Artiodactyla comes from the fossil record. Non-ruminants of this order, which today include pigs, peccaries, and hippopotami, greatly predominated during the Eocene and Oligocene. The ruminants, which now include the antelopes, giraffe, and buffalo, only assumed their present importance during the Pliocene (Simpson 1950).

Group (B) of the forest, thicket, or forest-edge tsetses in Table 3.3 feed mainly on an antelope, the bushbuck. This group includes *G. pallidipes* and *G. longipalpis*, two very closely related species of the *morsitans* group, and *G. fusca*, type species of the *fusca* group, which is also a very widespread forest-edge or seral forest species. May one, perhaps, regard the first two of these as savanna species that have reverted to forest or seral forest habitats, and *G. fusca* as a forest fly that has taken to thicket and to the forest edge, for here also is the habitat of their principal food host.

G. longipennis and *G. brevipalpis* are aberrant species. The most peculiar feature in their feeding is their reliance upon very large animals to provide blood. Elephants, rhinoceros, and buffalo are fed on when sheltering in the thickets or secondary forest patches with which these flies are associated. *G. brevipalpis* is not invariably found beside hippopotamus infested rivers, but when it is, the precision with which the male flies appear at sunset on the paths made by these animals as they leave the water forcibly strikes anyone who has observed it (for example, as described by Van den Berghe and Lambrecht 1954). It is evidently a specialized manifestation of the sexual appetitive swarm. A key factor in the survival of *fusca* group flies after the recession of the Pleistocene forests in eastern Africa was the use made of relic forest islands or thickets as refuges by the very large mammals.

There remains *G. austeni*, a species which, like *G. brevipalpis*, recently extended its range within the East African coastal plain when abolition of slavery forced Arab farmers to abandon their plantations and turn to commerce. Weitz groups this tsetse with other mainly Suid feeders but in Table 3.3 it has been grouped with *G. tabaniformis* and *G. fuscipleuris* as a forest or thicket feeder on pigs. If Bursell (1958) was correct in supposing that *G. austeni* was a savanna species that had reverted to a thicket or forest life, then obviously it had to revert also to a thicket or forest animal diet and there is nothing odd in finding it grouped with two species seemingly phylogenetically remote from it.

Tsetse flies and vegetation

The correlations between the distribution of various species of *Glossina* and the different major vegetation communities of Africa which attracted so much attention in earlier research on the genus now seems to be an unprofitable line of study. These correlations, in so far as they exist, are fundamentally with the distributions of the tsetse hosts. When, in the past, successes in tsetse control were achieved by partial clearing of the bush, they resulted from the destruction of the habitat of the natural hosts rather than from destruction of the habitat of the tsetse. When all woody vegetation is felled then, perhaps, it may be said that the tsetse disappear because of exposure of the puparia to extremes of climate; but where there is appropriate shelter the flies have shown remarkable powers of adapting themselves to artificial environments provided the latter also shelter acceptable host animals.

By some earlier workers the control of trypanosomiasis was thought to be theoretically possible by either of two methods: the method of Koch was directed towards the elimination of the pathogen by essentially medical methods; the entomological method of Ross, by eliminating the insect vector, broke the cycle of development of the trypanosomes and so led to its extinction at the same time. However, on at least two occasions tsetse-borne trypanosomes have succeeded in adapting themselves to a life which does not involve cyclical development in *Glossina*,† while one might well suppose that elimination of trypanosomes would permit tsetses to establish themselves as successful domestic parasites of man.‡ It is therefore erroneous to suppose that an obligatory association exists between *Glossina* and the vegetation communities in which the various species are commonly found. Nevertheless the climate, the natural vegetation, and the topography of Africa do provide bases for geographical classification of these insects which is not without its practical uses.

The modern vegetation map of Africa (e.g. that of Keay, Aubréville, Duvigneaud, Hoyle, Mendonca, and Pichi-Sermolli 1958, and also in Ady 1965) may be looked upon as a map that displays the areas of potential distribution of the three subgenera of *Glossina*, except where adverse climates overlap the distribution of vegetation. Thus *Glossina morsitans* is associated over most of its range with *Brachystegia* or *Isoberlinia* woodlands; but in parts of Rhodesia and Angola these woodlands occupy country which is too cold to support tsetse during the winter months (see Chapter 17). In latitudes not far south of these areas the same tsetse is, in places, associated with *Colophospermum mopane* woodland, but much of this vegetation is free of tsetse, perhaps because it is found in country too dry to support a suitable population of mammal hosts.

Broadly speaking the *fusca* group can be divided into three environmental categories as follows:

(1) In tropical moist forest at low and medium altitudes: *G. tabaniformis, G. haningtoni, G. nashi, G. nigrofusca,* and possibly *G. vanhoofi* and *G. severini.*

(2) In forest–savanna mosaic or the edges of the tropical moist forests: *G. fusca, G. medicorum, G. fuscipleuris, G. schwetzi,* and locally *G. nigrofusca.*

(3) In relict secondary forest patches or thickets, in woodlands and savannas, *G. brevipalpis,* or in wooded steppe, *G. longipennis.*

The *morsitans* group can be arranged as follows:

(1) *G. morsitans morsitans* in the *Brachystegia–Julbernardia* woodlands of Mozambique and Rhodesia below 4000 ft above sea level; in Tanzania

† *Trypanosoma viennei,* a parasite of cattle in Central America transmitted mechanically by Tabanidae, is a strain of *T. vivax* imported from Africa in infected animals in the nineteenth century. *T. evansi,* the cause of surra in horses and camels, is a strain of *T. brucei,* also mechanically transmitted by Tabanidae, which, like syringe-passaged strains of the same species, has become monomorphic.

‡ *G. morsitans submorsitans* adapted itself to a diet of cattle blood in the Koalib hills of Kordofan (Ruttledge 1928). The peri-domestic habits of *G. tachinoides,* studied by Baldry (1964), are described in Chapters 21 and 22.

east of the central highlands as far north as the Kenya border just west of Mombasa; in the south the species is also found in *Colophospermum mopane* woodlands in the Zambezi valley. It formerly infested the same vegetation in the valley of the Limpopo.

(2) *G. morsitans centralis* in *Brachystegia–Julbernardia* woodlands west of Lusaka–Broken Hill–Mbeya and Iringa highlands in Zambia and Western Tanzania and in Katanga and Angola. Also in the Okovango swamps of Botswana, and in the north in *Acacia gerardii* wooded grassland west of Lake Victoria.

(3) *G. morsitans submorsitans* from Northern Uganda and the Southern Sudan Republic westwards to the Republic of Guinea in *Isoberlinia doka* and *I. dalzielli* woodlands, but overlapping north and south of this zone with, respectively, dry wooded savanna of the Sudan zone and the relatively more moist vegetation of the Southern Guinea zone. Relict isolated fly-belts survive in the valleys of western Ethiopia.

(4) Throughout these areas and sometimes overlapping with *G. brevipalpis* and *G. longipennis* (but intermediately between the two in its capacity to withstand drought) is *G. pallidipes*. It always inhabits thicket or forest-edge areas. Until eliminated by insecticides from Zululand (du Toit 1959) it extended further south in Africa than any other species. It occurs in the north-east of the Congo basin, but west of about 17°E. is replaced by the very similar *G. longipalpis*.

(5) *G. swynnertoni* was at first not distinguished from *G. morsitans* (with which, however, it does not form fertile hybrids). It is considered to be recently evolved from *G. morsitans* (Potts 1951). It occupies a relatively small area in north Central Tanzania, east of Lake Victoria in *Acacia–Commiphora* wooded steppe, a more xerophytic vegetation than that inhabited by the neighbouring *G. morsitans* (see Chapter 12).

(6) *G. austeni* is confined to the coastal plains of East Africa, only in a few places being found at altitudes of over 500 ft above sea level or more than 150 miles inland. During the last century it spread greatly when the suppression of slavery caused Arab land owners to abandon their farms, and cultivation was replaced by secondary thicket inhabited by bushpigs.

Finally there is the *palpalis* group. The whole group is, with minor exceptions, confined to the shores and banks of lakes and rivers that drain either into the Atlantic Ocean or into the Mediterranean. One exception is found where *G. fuscipes* infests the banks of the Omo river flowing into the internal drainage basin of Lake Rudolf. The second exception is found in the already-noted discovery by Carter (1906) of *G. tachinoides* in the Hadramaut in Southern Arabia. If, as one presumes, the flies were taken on a drainage system that had an oceanic outflow, then it must have entered the Indian Ocean.

Several countries have published atlases to show the distribution of

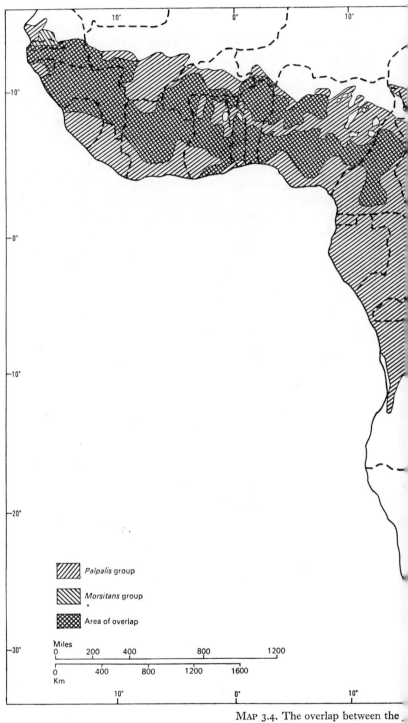

Palpalis group

Morsitans group

Area of overlap

Miles
0   200   400   800   1200

0   400   800   1200   1600
Km

MAP 3.4. The overlap between the

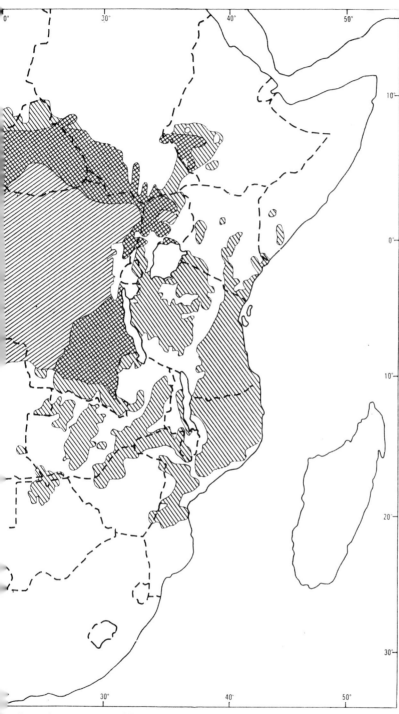

...nd *morsitans* groups of *Glossina*.

their tsetse belts, and the whole subject was last reviewed by Ford in 1963. There is no need to discuss details here, but it is important to draw attention to the zones in which the distributions of the subgeneric groups overlap, especially the *morsitans* group and the *palpalis* group (Map 3.4). It will appear in the course of the following narratives, that these areas of overlap, which are the areas in which trypanosomes are most liable to be transferred from wild animals to man and his livestock, are of profound epidemiological and epizootiological significance.

A note on *Glossina morsitans*

Marked differences are found between the epidemiological histories of human trypanosomiasis in the *G. morsitans* belts of eastern and central Tanzania (Ford 1965). In this chapter an unfamiliar nomenclature has been used to distinguish the races or subspecies which inhabit them. Westwood's (1850) type specimen was collected in the Limpopo river valley below the Zoutpansberg in the north-west Transvaal (see Map 17.1 on p. 286 and also Austen 1903). Vanderplank (1949*a*) was wrong in supposing that the *G. morsitans* belts of western Tanzania, western Zambia and south-eastern Congo were occupied by the type subspecies and therefore also wrong in giving the now familiar name *orientalis* to the flies of the Zambezi river valley, eastern Zambia, Mozambique and eastern Tanzania. The disentangling of these and other confusions now reconciles taxonomy with history and geography and has been described at greater length in Mulligan (1970). *G. morsitans morsitans* Westwood in Machado's (1970) revision now has its correct provenance and the flies of the western group of east and central African belts now become *G. morsitans centralis*.

4

TRYPANOSOMES AND TRYPANOSOMIASIS IN ANIMALS AND IN MEN

Classification

HOARE'S (1964) classification of the genus *Trypanosoma* is abridged in Table 4.1. Trypanosomes that are the causal agents of the African tsetse-borne trypanosomiases belong to the section Salivaria. They are placed here because when their development in the insect is completed they are transmitted by inoculation in its saliva when it sucks the blood of its vertebrate host. They are said to develop in the anterior station. There is one other tsetse-borne trypanosome, *Trypanosoma grayi* Novy 1906, which develops in the posterior station, the hind gut of the tsetse, whence it is ejected with the insect's faeces and thence, if they are suitably placed, enters the circulation of its vertebrate host, the crocodile, through the mucous membrane of the mouth (Hoare 1931). It is not pathogenic and its life-cycle and morphology place it in the section Stercoraria which includes the very numerous and mostly harmless trypanosomes that are voided by the invertebrate host when defaecating.

Nearly all literature on human trypanosomiasis speaks of two diseases, Gambian or West African sleeping sickness and Rhodesian sleeping sickness, and attributes them to infection by *Trypanosoma gambiense* Dutton 1902 or to *T. rhodesiense* Stephens and Fantham 1910. Recent opinion regards these 'species' as 'strains', 'demes', or 'clones' of *Trypanosoma* (*Trypanozoon*) *brucei* Plimmer and Bradford 1899 (Ormerod 1967). It is likely that this view will be generally accepted·and an end reached in an argument concerning their relationship, which is now nearly half a century old.

Had veterinary trypanosomiasis first been encountered on a large scale by teams of specialist parasitologists and clinicians, as were the human infections, similar classificatory difficulties might have beset the discussion of *T. vivax* and perhaps also of *T. congolense*. Both produce strains that give a wide range of pathogenic response and, like the *T. brucei* infections in man, display geographical relationships. It was once an accepted notion that *T. vivax* was the chief destroyer of cattle in West Africa, while in eastern Africa this role was held by *T. congolense*. Some of the connotations of these geographical distributions will be examined in the next chapter, but solutions to the problems posed await the exploration of trypanosome biology by modern techniques.

Other systems of classification may develop from the study of the

TABLE 4.1

The classification of trypanosomes†

PROTOZOA
Class: Zoomastigophorea
Order: Kinetoplastida
Genus: *Trypanosoma* Gruby 1843

Section: STERCORARIA
(1) Subgenus: *Megatrypanum*
   Type: *Trypanosoma (Megatrypanum) theileri* Laveran 1902
(2) Subgenus: *Herpetosoma*
   Type: *Trypanosoma (Herpetosoma) lewisi* (Kent 1880) Laveran and Mesnil 1901
(3) Subgenus: *Schizotrypanum*
   Type: *Trypanosoma (Schizotrypanum) cruzi* Chagas 1909
(4) Subgenus: *Endotrypanum*
   Type: *Trypanosoma (Endotrypanum) schaudinni* Mesnil and Brimont 1908

Section: SALIVARIA
(5) Subgenus: *Duttonella*
   Type: *Trypanosoma (Duttonella) vivax* Ziemann 1905
(6) Subgenus: *Nannomonas*
   Type: *Trypanosoma (Nannomonas) congolense* Broden 1904
(7) Subgenus: *Pycnomonas*
   Type: *Trypanosoma (Pycnomonas) suis* Ochmann 1905
(8) Subgenus: *Trypanozoon*
   Type: *Trypanosoma (Trypanozoon) brucei* Plimmer and Bradford 1899

---

† After Hoare (1964) and Baker (1969a).

immunology of the trypanosomiases. Different strains or even clones from the same strain of a single species may produce different immunological reponses in host animals (p. 87). The growth of trypanosomes in artificial culture media may perhaps be regarded as a special case of the immunological method. The relationship now beginning to be explored between the immunological and other physiological processes in trypanosomes and their ultrastructure offers yet another approach.

With few exceptions contemporary laboratory work on the trypanosomes finds little place in the following pages. It is not indeed irrelevant, but in its present stage it is conducted at a level that does not allow it to influence control policy although it has already led to improvement in diagnostic technique, or to influence epidemiological or epizootiological understanding, except in quite general terms.

Lumsden and his colleagues have applied to the study of trypanosomes some of the methods used in virology. If parasites that are morphologically indistinguishable and bear the same name cause different diseases in hosts also bearing identical specific names but endowed with different genetic ancestries, then the results of isolated research workers become difficult to reconcile and co-ordinate. Lumsden's method permits trypanosomes used in research to be given a more precise definition than can be provided, as yet, by taxonomic nomenclature alone. He has also attempted to standardize and define methods of measurement of parasitological phenomena (Lumsden 1963).

Another approach is being developed by Ormerod (1960, 1967, and other papers) who has used newer microscopical techniques allied with biochemistry to define geographical variants in trypanosome species. Here is an example of recent research which was related, at an early stage of its development, to the geographical pattern of human trypanosomiasis and at once seemed to fit, in an illuminating manner, with the work of entomologists and epidemiologists.

Trypanosomes and trypanosomiases in domestic animals

The more obvious and superficial aspects of trypanosome infections will be described in domestic livestock, in man, in wild animals, and finally, in tsetse flies. With livestock the intention will be to show the diseases as seen by African farmers and by field veterinarians and government livestock inspectors. In man, interest is in the disease as seen by relatives and neighbours of the sufferers or by doctors and field staffs who have to prevent epidemics and control them when they break out. The descriptions given are borrowed from well-known standard texts. The important subjects of the pathology, detailed diagnosis, and treatment of these diseases fall outside the scope of the study and the inquiring reader can refer to Mulligan (1970) or follow up the references given in the text.

Duttonella

Trypanosoma (D.) vivax *Ziemann 1905*. *T. vivax* (*T. cazalboui* in earlier French literature) was so named because of its habit, in fresh blood films, of swimming with great rapidity across the field of the microscope. It is a relatively large trypanosome 20–26 μm in length, with a free flagellum 3–6 μm long. There is a large kinetoplast situated close to the posterior end. (The kinetoplast, a deeply staining more or less rounded body, considerably smaller than the nucleus, was at one time thought to be concerned with agitating the flagellum. It is present in most trypanosomes. Its size and position in the protozoan body are of diagnostic significance.) Small laboratory animals are not easily infected with *T. vivax* but it infects all larger domestic animals except dogs and pigs. On one or two occasions it has produced a transient infection in man (Hoare 1949). In sheep and goats it tends to be of low virulence and in horses it produces a chronic disease from which there is usually a spontaneous recovery. *T. vivax* is therefore chiefly important as the cause of disease in cattle.

Trypanosoma (D.) uniforme *Bruce* et al. *1911*. *T. uniforme* is like a small *T. vivax* in appearance and causes similar infections. For practical purposes it is treated as *T. vivax*.

Nannomonas

Trypanosoma (N.) congolense *Broden 1904*. *T. congolense* was frequently referred to in early literature by the synonyms *T. pecorum* and *T. nanum*. It is a small trypanosome, less than half the length of *T. vivax* (9–18 μm). It lacks a free flagellum and possesses a medium-sized kinetoplast. In fresh blood films it is active but does not travel rapidly across the microscope field, tending rather to remain as a focus of turbulence among neighbouring blood corpuscles. The blood forms in *Nannomonas* are pleomorphic. They vary in form and size, with complete continuity of intermediate forms, but with extremes that are morphologically quite distinct (Godfrey 1960). Because of this *T. congolense* was once thought to include a second species, *T. dimorphon*. As their subgeneric name implies, they are small trypanosomes; some may have a free flagellum, others not, and the undulating membrane may be inconspicuous.

T. vivax *and* T. congolense *infections of cattle*

It is not possible to distinguish these two infections clinically. The experienced stockman will confidently diagnose trypanosomiasis on the appearance and the history of an ox, but without microscopical examination of blood smears will not know the causal trypanosome. Hornby (1952) described infections in several individual animals. His experimental ox No. 2785 suffered a sub-acute infection of *T. congolense*. This animal was put on a good ration of hay and artificially infected. Six days later he showed trypanosomes in the blood and continued to yield positive blood in every smear taken twice weekly for twenty-seven weeks. A gradual anaemia developed, but was never marked and there was a mild intermittent fever. His weight fell from 584 to 462 lb during the first sixteen weeks. His general condition deteriorated and he became lazy and dejected with drooping extremities and staring coat. He became weaker until he could not keep pace with the herd. His hair tended to fall out, but 'the condition was never pitiable'.

There was no marked crisis, but from week 26 onwards weight ceased to fall, there was some return of appetite, and the anaemia showed slight improvement. Trypanosomes now began to be occasionally absent from blood smears and eventually were only seen rarely. This condition continued for nineteen weeks but there was little obvious progress towards recovery.

The hay ration was now supplemented by an addition of cotton seed and a mineral supplement. Weight picked up rapidly and no trypanosomes were to be seen in the blood after the eleventh month. Sixteen months after the ox was infected, 150 ml of his blood were injected into a goat and failed to infect. He was judged to have recovered. This might have happened more quickly had he been given at the start a better diet than was provided by the ration. 'One sees the same thing in native herds, where mortality from trypanosomiasis is bound up with the severity of the period of poor nutrition before and just after the commencement of each rainy season' (Hornby 1952).

The symptoms of trypanosomiasis in cattle vary from area to area. In part this may be due to the different responses of genetically varying types of African cattle; in part it is associated with variation in the nutrition values of different pastures; in part reaction to infection is affected by climate; and finally, local customs in the use of cattle may subject them to different stresses. In his account of ox No. 2785, Hornby mentioned that no geophagism was seen and he added that earth-eating was a symptom more commonly seen in West than in East Africa. However, in the high rainfall climate of Zanzibar, with its poor pastures on soils derived from decayed coral, cattle trypanosomiasis is sometimes known as the earth-eating disease (*maradhi ya kula ardhi*).

In another of Hornby's oxen, an acute *T. congolense* infection ended with the animal's death ten weeks after inoculation. Another strain of the same species of trypanosome produced a mild disease which, judged by the appearance of parasites in the blood, although very scanty and infrequent, lasted for three years. During all this time it was impossible, from mere observation, to tell that the ox had any infection at all and only at the time of crisis was he slightly off colour for about a week. In *T. vivax* infections there is a similar variability in virulence of different strains.

Infection by either *T. congolense* or *T. vivax* may produce fulminating parasitaemia followed by death within fifteen days of the first appearance of trypanosomes in the circulation. On the other hand some strains scarcely give rise to any clinical disease, or the symptoms may be so generalized that they can hardly be distinguished from the effects of under-feeding or of overwork (Richardson and Kendall 1963).

T. congolense *and* T. vivax *in other domestic animals*

T. congolense causes disease in horses, donkeys, sheep, and goats which may be fatal, but may, as in the ox, show varying degrees of virulence. Pigs, on the other hand, are never more than slightly affected by *T. congolense* and the same may be said of indigenous African dogs. Exotic breeds of dogs, however, are unable to resist infection and generally die in a few weeks if not treated. *T. vivax* infections of dogs are very rare, but with other animals there is considerable variation in virulence, though the tendency to produce a mild, more chronic disease is more pronounced than with *T. congolense*.

Trypanosoma (N.) simiae *Bruce* et al. *1912*

T. simiae causes a very acute and rapidly fatal disease of domestic pigs. It is larger (12–24 μm) than *T. congolense*. Its rarity in diagnostic records of veterinary services is perhaps an indication of the rarity of pigs in the African domestic economy as compared with cattle, sheep, and goats.

Pycnomonas

Trypanosoma (P.) suis *Ochmann 1905*. This trypanosome, a cause of severe infections in domestic pigs, was forgotten after its description by Ochmann but was rediscovered by the Belgian parasitologists Peel and Chardome (1954) in the Eastern Congo.

Trypanozoon

Trypanosoma (T.) brucei *Plimmer and Bradford 1899*. *T. brucei* is a pleomorphic trypanosome. The blood infection typically shows 'slender', 'stumpy', and 'intermediate' forms. The slender forms are thin and long, averaging 35 μm, with a long free flagellum. Stumpy forms average about 18 μm and are broader than the slender forms as well as lacking a free flagellum. Intermediate forms have, as their name implies, measurements between these extremes and always have a free flagellum of medium length. There is a conspicuous undulating membrane and the kinetoplast is small. Most students believe that the intermediate forms are also intermediate in that they are stages in the transformation of slender to stumpy forms. The pleomorphism does not only consist in the simultaneous appearance of the three forms in the blood, but also in the presence of posteronuclear forms. These are stumpy forms in which the nucleus is displaced towards the posterior end of the body of the trypanosome, even to beyond the kinetoplast.

T. brucei *infections of domestic animals*

Hornby was veterinary surgeon with the Allied Forces in the East African Campaign of 1914–18. This gave him a unique opportunity of observing *T. brucei* infection in horses.

I had the humiliating experience of dealing with thousands of animals which after all attempts to cure the disease had failed, had to be regarded as incurable and destroyed. [In the infected horse] the ears tend to droop. The eyeballs are sunken. The coat is harsh. The penis is frequently extruded from the sheath. The whole appearance is dejected. As the disease progresses, evidences of oedema appear. . . . When riding a horse in the early stages of illness one of the first symptoms is that it stumbles. It sways when trotted. It tends to fall if turned sharply or pushed or has a leg raised. In advanced cases the weakness may amount to paraplegia (Hornby 1952).

Fever is intermittent and shows some correlation with the intensity of parasitaemia. The heart rate is increased. The disease may be chronic and trypanosomes may be difficult to detect in the bloodstream. Several months may pass before death intervenes. Acute cases, however, terminate fatally in two to four weeks after the onset of symptoms.

Perhaps *T. brucei* more than any other trypanosome has protected African people from invasion and African wildlife from destruction. The Allied armies in 1914–18 were not the first that had to go on foot because their horses died. Lugard's mounted infantry suffered heavy losses in Nigeria in 1903 (Griffiths 1937) and it was not the rifle so much as the horse that allowed the Afrikaners to destroy most of the South African fauna. When they had to hunt on their own feet the wild game survived (Tabler 1955).

T. brucei infections of dogs are usually acute and, if not treated, nearly always fatal. Partial paralysis and uncoordinated movements demonstrate, as in the horse and human, that the central nervous system has been invaded.

Cattle tolerate infection with *T. brucei* and throw it off usually with only a very slight reaction. Pigs, too, are easily infected but seldom show clinical symptoms. This tolerance of infection by *T. brucei* may be of great importance in the epidemiology of human trypanosomiasis (Chapters 16 and 22).

Sheep and goats die of infection with *T. brucei* within two or three months, but to gambian strains they react (like small laboratory animals and to some extent like man) less severely and tend to throw off an infection in a few months.

Nomenclature

In this book the data used are, for the most part, those collected by doctors, veterinarians, and field entomologists directly concerned with the control of the trypanosomiases in man and his domestic livestock. These men are not equipped with, nor do they need, in the present state of knowledge, the means of diagnostic precision already available to protozoologists. To the field veterinarian *T. (Duttonella) vivax* and *T. (D.) uniforme* are both *T. vivax* and even if the distinction were to be made between them, the treatment of the infection would still be the same. It would be more accurate, in the following pages, when results based upon field observation are discussed, to refer to *Duttonella* rather than *T. vivax*, for this includes both *T. (D.) vivax* and *T. (D.) uniforme*; and to *Nannomonas* rather than *T. congolense*. But on the grounds chiefly of familiarity and therefore of convenience the names *T. vivax* and *T. congolense* are retained, thus following the usages of the men who have had the task of controlling the infections and whose reports describe what they have seen in nature.

Trypanozoon **infections in man**

'There are as many trypanosomiases as there are specific trypanosomes. There may even be more, for every species of pathogenic trypanosome is capable of causing disease in several species of mammals, and the syndrome is not always the same' (Hornby 1952). Evidence is accumulating that strain behaviour is very constant (Gray 1966) and Hornby's remark ought, perhaps, to be modified to the effect that there can be as many trypanosomiases for a single host species as there are separate strains of trypanosomes.

In Hoare's classification of the tsetse-borne trypanosomes of the subgenus *Trypanozoon*, *Trypanosoma (Trypanozoon) brucei*, *T. (T.) rhodesiense*, and *T. (T.) gambiense* are given equal status although he has often expressed the opinion (e.g. Hoare 1965) that they are all variants of *T. (T.) brucei*. The terms '*rhodesiense*' and '*gambiense*' or rhodesian and gambian refer to variation in the clinical picture of the disease to which some strains of *T. (T.) brucei* give rise in man, and the geographical connotations with which they were formerly endowed can no longer be sustained. Ormerod's (1967) Zambezi strains, distinguishable by the form of certain cytoplasmic inclusions, are, he believes, geographically confined to the Zambezi basin.

In this book the view is taken that *T. (T.) brucei* is a parasite of wild mammals for which man and domestic livestock are, essentially, adventitious hosts to some, but not all, of its variant forms. Doctors continue to refer to *T. rhodesiense* and *T. gambiense*, but because it is desired to emphasize the connection with wild hosts the device is used here of using these terms as if they were subspecific, i.e. *T. brucei rhodesiense* and *T. brucei gambiense* or, on occasion, *T. 'rhodesiense'* or *T. 'gambiense'*. It would have been more accurate to use Hoare's subgeneric name of *Trypanozoon* on all save a few occasions, but it seems desirable to retain familiar terms and also to indicate what names were, in fact, used by the authors whose work is described.

These ideas long ago found expression in the views of the German parasitologist, Kleine. Before the First World War he had had experience of the rhodesian infection in the Rovuma river basin in Southern Tanzania and of the gambian disease on the shores of Lake Victoria. After the war he was a member of an international commission sent out to study human trypanosomiasis by the League of Nations and, having first been involved with the gambian disease in the Congo and on the shore of Lake Tanganyika, went across Lake Victoria to see the first rhodesian epidemic (the Maswa epidemic in Tanzania described in Chapter 12). Afterwards he wrote: 'Considered as a *whole*, the cases are without any doubt clinically distinct from those I had the opportunity of observing previously.' However, 'Not one of our patients (in Maswa) would, in the *palpalis* regions on Lake Tanganyika, the Congo, etc. be considered as presenting any unusual symptoms, but would merely be regarded as a case in which the disease was running a particularly severe course' (Kleine 1928).

The gambian disease or sleeping sickness

Classical gambian sleeping sickness is transmitted by tsetse of the *palpalis* group. The infection in man has a long history. Slave traders were well aware of it and knew its commoner symptoms. It failed to establish itself in Central America, although in the West Indies it was recognized that recently imported slaves might die of the 'negro lethargy'.

The following is a textbook account of gambian trypanosomiasis. In Chapter 23 the views will be quoted of the physician who, forty years ago, began to build up the special service instituted to control the growing epidemic in Nigeria. 'My experience . . . led me to regard the text book story as representing a state of things that only happens occasionally' (Lester 1939).

The incubation period after the infected fly-bite is 5–20 days but rarely is prolonged to months or even years. Commonly, but not always, such a bite develops into a 'trypanosome chancre', seen in Europeans as a hard red nodule surrounded by a paler periphery. Trypanosomes may be seen very briefly in the chancre before they appear in the general bloodstream (Gordon and Willett 1958). The chancre gradually disappears. The patient develops a fever which may be the first indication of infection, and his heart beat accelerates. He may develop a characteristic temporary rash. The fever fluctuates and the patient suffers from severe headaches. Glands become swollen and tender, especially the cervical glands towards the back of the neck. In the early stages of the infection these glands are soft and may continue enlarging until they seem like discrete tumours. In prolonged infections they become small and fibrous. The swelling of the cervical glands, Winterbottom's sign, was well known to slave traders. Its possession might save a slave from transportation to the Americas, but was also recognized by himself and his fellows as a prelude to sleeping sickness and probably death. Many tribes excised the swollen glands in an attempt to arrest progress of the disease.

The untreated patient may continue for months or years in this condition of irregular fever, accompanied by general debility and insomnia. The typically swollen glands will be evident as well as localized oedema, usually of the eyelids, the hands, feet, and ankles. The degree of illness may vary from time to time, and different patients may respond in different ways. Men may become impotent; pregnant women tend to abort. Some may remain infected and yet enjoy long periods of good health; some may throw off the infection and undergo a spontaneous cure; others may die comparatively quickly at the stage so far described, often with epileptic type convulsions or by falling into a coma.

The name 'sleeping sickness' is descriptive of the later stages of the disease. Trypanosomes appear in the circulation soon after infection though usually in about the third week, but as the disease continues may become very scanty and impossible to find in the blood. Puncture of the swollen cervical glands may show trypanosomes in the gland juice when blood examination is negative. Both blood and glands may fail to yield trypanosomes although the patient is still infected. Meanwhile there is a more or less continuous invasion by trypanosomes of the central nervous system. This is the beginning of 'sleeping sickness'.

Generally its first indications are

merely an accentuation of the debility and languor usually associated with trypanosome infection. There is a disinclination to exertion; slow, shuffling gait;

T A E—F

morose, mask-like expression; relaxation of features; hanging of the lower lip; puffiness and drooping of the eyelids; tendency to lapse into sleep or a condition simulating sleep, somnolence or 'near coma' during the day-time, contrasting with restlessness at night; slowness in answering questions; shirking of the day's task. Dull headache is generally present. He will walk, if forced to do so, with unsteady and swaying gait. Later there may be fibrillary twitching of muscles, especially of the tongue, and tremor of the hands, more rarely of the legs, indicating involvement of the motor centres. His speech is difficult to follow, becoming indistinct and staccato. By this time the patient has taken to bed, or he lies in the corner of his hut, indifferent to everything going on around him, but still able to speak and take food if brought to him. He never spontaneously engages in conversation, or even asks for food. As torpor deepens he forgets even to chew his food, falling asleep perhaps in the act of conveying it to his mouth, or with the half-masticated bolus still in his cheek. Nevertheless, such food as he can be persuaded to take is digested and assimilated. Consequently, if he is properly nursed, there may be no general wasting. So far the striking features are the mental and personal changes with a paucity of neurological signs. As time goes on, he begins to lose flesh, tremor of hands and tongue becomes more marked, and convulsive or choreic movements may occur in the limbs or in limited muscular areas. Sometimes, too, rigidity of the cervical muscles and retraction of the head occur. There is usually an intolerable pruritis of the skin; bedsores tend to form; the lips become swollen and saliva dribbles from the mouth. Gradually the lethargy deepens; the body wastes; the bedsores extend; the sphincters relax; and finally the patient dies comatose, or sinks from slowly advancing asthenia (Manson-Bahr 1966).

There are considerable variations in the course taken by the disease.

Mania is not uncommon: delusions may present themselves, or psychical and physical symptoms not unlike those of general paralysis of the insane are developed. In the European, death is frequently due to convulsions, probably from the presence of trypanosomes in the brain. Deep hyperaesthesia of the muscles is also quite common. The habits usually become bestial and he becomes a drooling, dribbling and drowsy idiot (Manson-Bahr 1966).

Death in persons infected with gambian *T. brucei* is often not due to the direct effects of trypanosomiasis, but to intercurrent diseases such as pneumonia or dysentery.

The rhodesian disease

Just as it had been supposed for many years that *Glossina palpalis*, in the older broad sense inclusive of *G. fuscipes*, was the vector of gambian sleeping sickness, so for an equally long time it was thought that human strains of *T. brucei* (*T. rhodesiense*) were transmitted by *G. morsitans* or its near relative, *G. swynnertoni*. Some authors supposed that the vector was specific for the disease. As late as 1938 Belgian epidemiologists held that in spite of reports of *rhodesiense*-like cases in Katanga, it was impossible that the disease should be present because human trypanosomiasis in that province was clearly transmitted by the riverine *G. fuscipes* (Van Hoof, Henrard, and Peel 1938). In an early review of human trypanosomiasis, Kleine and Fischer (1912) expressed the view that every species of trypanosome could, given the right conditions of climate, develop in any species of *Glossina*, and it is now accepted that not only is it impossible to draw a hard and fast line between the gambian and rhodesian forms of the disease, but that strains of trypanosomes productive of one or other diseases may be transmitted by *morsitans* group as well as *palpalis* group tsetse and vice versa. However, it remains the case that in general, trypanosomiasis of man displaying a relatively slow development of the disease towards a 'sleeping' condition is more common within the limits of *palpalis* group distribution, while the more rapidly fatal rhodesian infection tends to be associated with the presence of *G. morsitans* and *swynnertoni* and, locally, of *G. pallidipes*.

Essentially the rhodesian infection develops in the same way as the gambian, but because the development is more rapid some of the symptons of the latter are, as it were, telescoped and become less obvious. The reaction at the site of the bite is usually more severe. The incubation of the disease is more rapid and it may begin with a more severe fever and rigor. The lymph glands are less obviously swollen than in the gambian disease. Trypanosomes in the blood are usually more numerous and may appear earlier. The heart is soon affected and the pulse-rate is fast and remains so. The central nervous system is involved early and mental symptoms are commonly observed. It is usual, however, for death to intervene before the sleeping condition develops. This may often be caused by the effects of a more rapid infection on the heart, leading to severe inflammation of the myocardium. Untreated cases die in three to nine months after infection as against two to three or several years for the gambian infection. The cause of death may be heart failure, toxaemia due to the abundance of the parasite in the circulation or, as in the gambian type of infection, intercurrent disease.

Distinction between rhodesian and gambian infections

The sort of problem that greatly exercised epidemiologists until quite recent years is well displayed in a classical paper by Van Hoof (1947) who for many years was in charge of sleeping sickness services in the Belgian Congo. He recognized three types of gambian infection.

The first consisted of strains that were easily transmitted by tsetse, but produced a slowly developing infection. Lymph gland enlargement was late in appearing as was the involvement of the central nervous system. The infection responded well to treatment with the drug tryparsamide. Trypanosomes were rarely found in the blood, although tsetse fed on the patients became infected. Guinea pigs generally suffered a mild disease and showed few parasites in the blood. They usually survived for at least a year. In humans spontaneous cure sometimes occurred. These strains seemed to be adapted, both by their relatively chronic effect on the human host and the ease with which they could infect tsetse, to rapid and widespread extension.

Secondly, more virulent strains were recognized which would kill guinea pigs in three to four months and showed a heavy parasitaemia, especially in later weeks. In the human there were frequent relapses after treatment, although tryparsamide was generally effective. The cerebro-spinal fluid underwent alteration within six to twelve months after the flybite.

Thirdly, there were very virulent strains that turned up sporadically in all endemic areas. These, both in man and the guinea pig, tended to behave like *T. 'rhodesiense'*. Parasitaemia was pronounced and the clinical progress of the disease was very rapid. Guinea pigs died within the month, and in man the nervous stage began to develop in two or three months. The trypanosomes resisted treatment with tryparsamide and it was difficult to infect tsetse flies, especially from relapse cases.

Variations of this kind, as indicated by the observations of Kleine already noted, are to be found in most outbreaks, but the more chronic form, the slowly developing disease ending in 'sleep' preponderates in *'gambiense'*, the more acute in *'rhodesiense'* areas. To this it must be added that symptomless carriers of infection may also be found anywhere, though more frequently in old endemic foci of the gambian type of infection or, on the other side of the continent, in the Zambezi basin. Most doctors take the view that these 'healthy carriers' will, eventually, become sick and succumb; but this is not proven. As well as these symptomless persons there are, especially in *'gambiense'* areas, sufferers from a mild form of the disease which manifests itself in periods of slight illness with fever and headache. Such persons are unaware that they are suffering from anything different from the usual run of intermittent sickness from the great variety of infections that beset the African peasant. They may live thus for several years before the disease begins to develop its more severe symptoms leading, often quite rapidly, to death.

It was at one time supposed that '*T. gambiense*' infection was distinguished in five ways from '*T. rhodesiense*'. The disease was chronic in one and acute in the other. *T. 'gambiense'* responded favourably to treatment with the drug tryparsamide, but *T. 'rhodesiense'* did not. The former was transmitted by *palpalis* group tsetse, the latter by *G. morsitans*. In laboratory animals (guinea pigs or rats) *T. 'gambiense'* could only be established with some difficulty, trypanosomes were sparse, and there was a long interval to death. *T. 'rhodesiense'* rapidly produced a heavy parasitaemia and killed quickly. Finally, in these animals, posteronuclear forms were frequently observed in the *'rhodesiense'* infection, but were rare or absent in *'gambiense'* infections. But here, too, all gradations of every character have been observed.

The debate on the relationships of *T. brucei*, regarded as a species not infective to man, and *T. 'gambiense'* and *T. 'rhodesiense'* has been prolonged and not very productive. It has been well summarized by Ashcroft (1959*a*).

The Zambezi infection

Rhodesian sleeping sickness was so called because *T. rhodesiense* was described from a European who became infected in Northern Rhodesia (Zambia). Eventually the disease was recognized in many parts of eastern Africa and gave rise to a number of epidemics. Recently, however, the infection in the Zambezi basin has been given a separate identity by Ormerod (1967), partly on the basis of morphological differences in certain cell inclusions and partly on the epidemiological and clinical grounds. No epidemic has yet been observed in the Zambezi basin, but a persistent low endemic, with little variation in case incidence, has continued since the infections were first identified (as *T. rhodesiense*) in 1910. Moreover among the inhabitants of the Zambezi fly-belt, although acute cases predominate, an unusually high proportion of healthy symptomless 'carriers' has been found, again from early days up to the present. In contrast, strangers, and notably Europeans, acquire acute infections and form an unusually high proportion of recorded cases (see Chapter 20).

Infections of wild animals

Ashcroft (1959*b*) combined in a single table the results of eight parasitological surveys of wild animals beginning with Kinghorn, Yorke, and Lloyd (1913) and ending with his own attempt to isolate a human-infective strain of *T. brucei* from game animals (Ashcroft 1958). This feat was successfully accomplished at about the same time by Heisch, McMahon, and Manson-Bahr (1958) who obtained one from a bushbuck shot in the *G. pallidipes* bush in the endemic sleeping sickness area of the Lake Victoria coast north of the Kavirondo gulf (Chapter 16).

Ashcroft's summary shows that of 1242 animals examined over a long period of time in a variety of places, all by blood slides and some as well by inoculation of blood into experimental animals, 242 or 19·5 per cent were infected with trypanosomes. Fifty-three (4·2 per cent) were infected with *T. brucei*, 131 (10·4 per cent) with *T. congolense*, and 79 (6·3 per cent) with *T. vivax*. It will be seen in the next chapter that different methods of parasitological examination give different results when used to diagnose trypanosome infections in cattle. These records of infections in wild animals are certainly distorted in the same way. Ashcroft himself, when examining blood from 74 animals shot in Tanzania, found 7 infections by blood film and 4, different, infections by inoculating blood from the same animals into rats (Ashcroft 1958).

Lumsden (1962) made another review of earlier work and demonstrated

TABLE 4.2

Infections in game animals expressed as percentages of animals examined†

Order	Family	Subfamily	Genus	No. examined	T. v.	T. c.	T. b.	All
Artiodactyla	Hippopotamidae		Hippopotamus	655	0	0·5	0	0·5
	Suidae	Suinae	Phacochoerus	154	1	6	2	10
			Potamochoerus	26	12	0	0	12
				180	2	5	2	10
	Giraffidae		Giraffa	68	16	28	1	37
	Bovidae	Alcelophinae	Alcelophus	76	1	3	9	13
			Connochaetes	38	0	0	0	0
			Damaliscus	30	3	3	3	13
				144	1	2	6	10
		Cephalophinae	Sylvicapra	41	2	7	2	15
		Neotraginae	Ourebia	30	3	3	3	13
			Raphicerus	20	0	20	0	20
				50	2	10	2	14
		Madoquinae	Rhynchotragus	34	0	3	0	3
		Reduncinae	Adenota	70	3	0	1	4
			Kobus	110	33	9	24	52
			Redunca	39	25	15	8	43
				220	22	7	14	35
		Aepycerotinae	Aepyceros	151	1	9	1	11
		Antilopinae	Gazella	20	0	10	0	10
		Oryginae	Hippotragus	62	5	10	0	15
			Oryx	1	0	0	0	0
				63	5	10	0	14
		Tragelaphinae	Strepsiceros	40	3	45	0	45
			Taurotragus	63	5	21	5	29
			Tragelaphus	55	2	25	5	31
				158	3	28	4	34
		Bovinae	Syncerus	87	0	3	3	7
Perissodactyla	Rhinocerotidae		Diceros	8	0	0	0	0
	Equidae		Equus	109	2	3	0	6

T. v., T. vivax   T. c., T. congolense   T. b., T. brucei

† From Lumsden (1962).

that the Giraffidae and two subfamilies of the Bovidae, the Reduncinae and the Tragelaphinae, stood out as having a higher proportion (34–37 per cent) of parasitaemic individuals than others, none of which exceeded 16 per cent infected. The high incidence in the Reduncinae is mainly contributed by *T. vivax* and in the Tragelaphinae by *T. congolense*. Species yielding 5 per cent or more of *T. brucei* infections are the hartebeests (*Alcelophus*), the waterbucks (*Kobus*), the reedbucks (*Redunca*), the eland (*Taurotragus*), and the bushbuck (*Tragelaphus*). Lumsden's summary is reproduced in Table 4.2. A rearrangement of his data, omitting the Hippopotamidae, shows that of the 1333 animals examined, 4·42 per cent were infected with *T. brucei*, 9·53 per cent with *T. congolense*, and 5·77 per cent with *T. vivax*; much the same values as were obtained by Ashcroft. But in the tsetse these groups of trypanosomes are found in very different proportions.

Some of the *T. brucei* infections must have been also infective to man. Bruce himself believed that the morphological identity of the various strains of this trypanosome implied that all were dangerous to man, and he advocated the extermination of wild game should be vigorously undertaken in endemic areas. 'It would be as reasonable to allow mad dogs to live and be protected by law in our English towns and villages. Not only should all game laws restricting their destruction in fly country be removed, but active measures should, if feasible, be taken for their early and complete blotting out' (Bruce 1915). It would be interesting to record the details of the violent arguments and heroic experiments made to decide whether or not the wild game of Africa were the true source of these fatal infections. Dr. Taute and his veterinary colleague Huber were convinced that *T. brucei* and *T. 'rhodesiense'* were different. They inoculated themselves and 129 Africans with blood from horses naturally infected in a known sleeping sickness area. At that time infection meant almost certain death, but no ill effects resulted (Taute and Huber 1919). One suggestion was that infection with *T. brucei* might occur in rare, susceptible persons, or in people in poor health from other causes, and that once the trypanosome was established, it became adapted to the human environment and could be transmitted to other men. Much evidence exists to show that man-to-man transmission, via *Glossina* or perhaps other bloodsucking arthropods, is important in maintaining epidemics (e.g. Dye 1927). The theory was extended to include the hypothesis that once restored to a wild animal reservoir, the trypanosomes lost their infectivity to man. In order to settle this point an experiment was begun in Tanzania by Corson and continued by several successors at the Tinde Sleeping Sickness Laboratory. Here, for over twenty years, a *'rhodesiense'* strain of *T. brucei* was transmitted by tsetse-bite from sheep to sheep, with occasional extensions into various captured wild animals and with regular trials of its infectivity to man made by inoculation into human volunteers (Corson 1935, Fairbairn and Burtt 1946, Ashcroft

1959c, Willett and Fairbairn 1955). There was no doubt that the trypanosome kept its virulence to man when maintained in other mammals, provided that the passage was made by cyclical transmission through tsetse. It was shown, however, that when a human infective 'rhodesiense' strain was inoculated into rats simultaneously with a *T. brucei* morphologically indistinguishable but infective only to other animals, the second strain persisted and the infection, after a few transmissions, lost its ability to establish itself in man (Culwick, Fairbairn, and Culwick 1951; but see Vaucel and Jonchère 1954, and Vaucel and Fromentin 1958 for a more acceptable explanation of how this happened). Laboratory experiments with single strains of trypanosomes may not yield results that are directly applicable to the condition in nature where other trypanosomes must compete for survival in the same hosts and vectors. Another point established by the Tinde team was that the cyclical transmission through *Glossina* was essential if the trypanosome were to retain its characteristic features. If transmission from one animal to another was effected by syringe passage the trypanosomes not only lost their power to infect man, but also their pleomorphism.

The attempts to absolve the African wildlife of responsibility for harbouring the fatal 'rhodesiense' infection failed, and the argument has now reduced itself to the problem of whether the bushbuck alone is especially important as a reservoir or whether other animals are equally or more important. In the absence of experiment it is a futile debate. *Gambiense*-type strains can also be maintained in a variety of domestic animals (Chapter 24; see also Fairbairn 1954).

In recent years much attention has been given to conserving the African fauna and weighty arguments have been advanced in favour of ranching or farming the wild game instead of cattle. One argument less sound than others is that wild animals are not affected by trypanosome infection. As a generalization this is not true.

The effects of infection in wild animals

Ashcroft, Burtt, and Fairbairn (1959) analysed the results of infecting various animals with *T. brucei* (usually a 'rhodesiense' strain) at the Tinde Laboratory. They recognized two main groups, the second of which fell into three sub-groups.

(1) Animals that were usually killed by the infection and displayed parasites in the blood until death: Thomson's gazelle (*Gazella thomsonii*), dik-dik (*Rhynchotragus kirki*), blue forest duiker (*Philantomba monticola*), jackal (*Canis* sp.), 'fox' (probably *Otocyon* sp.), antbear (*Orycteropus afer*), hyrax (*Procavia* sp.), serval (*Leptailurus serval*), and monkey (probably *Cercopithecus aethiops*). None of these animals is commonly fed on by tsetse except the aardvark, but the very abnormal conditions of

laboratory captivity for such an animal might have predisposed it to a fatal infection.

(2) Animals tolerant of or resistant to infection:

(a) In this sub-group all were infectible and showed positive blood for a considerable time. This included: common duiker (*Sylvicapra grimmia*), eland (*Taurotragus oryx*), Bohor reedbuck (*Redunca redunca*), spotted hyaena (*Crocuta crocuta*), oribi (*Ourebia cottoni*), bushbuck (*Tragelaphus scriptus*), and impala (*Aepyceros melampus*).

(b) The following could usually be infected but exhibited very scanty parasitaemia: warthog (*Phacochoerus aethiopicus*), bushpig (*Potamochoerus koiropotamus*), and porcupine (*Hystrix africae-australis*).

(c) The uninfectible baboon (*Papio* spp.).

Lumsden (1962) preferred to recognize two states: (1) insusceptibility due to refractoriness, as in the baboon for all trypanosomes or as in man for all save some strains of *T. brucei*; (2) susceptibility, or the state of an animal which permits trypanosomes to multiply in it. Some animals achieve a state of adjustment in which, probably, they produce a succession of antibodies in response to a succession of antigens produced by the trypanosome population of the blood.

Desowitz (1960) studied infections of *T. brucei* and of *T. vivax* in two gazelles (*Gazella rufifrons*), a reedbuck (*Redunca redunca*), and two duikers (*Sylvicapra grimmia*). One of the gazelles died of the *T. brucei* infection. One duiker was refractory to another strain of *T. brucei* and did not develop a parasitaemia. A reedbuck similarly resisted infection with a strain of *T. vivax* which caused a mild disease in a duiker and a gazelle.

When she died, the famous lioness, Elsa, had trypanosomes (*T. brucei*) in her blood (Adamson 1965) but it was another protozoan blood parasite, a piroplasm, that killed her. Her son, Boy, became sick in his youth and was also found to have a trypanosome infection. He was treated and recovered. The drug used was a cure for both trypanosome and piroplasm infections. Hornby's observations on the effects of the nutrition upon the course of infection may apply with equal force to wild animals. In years of abundance adjustment may be easily achieved; but in dearth this may not be so, especially when two or more infections must be dealt with simultaneously.

Sachs, Schaller, and Baker (1967) found a *T. brucei* type infection in a young lion that was obviously ill, but could not say if the trypanosome was the cause of its disease. McCulloch (1967) saw two zebras in the Serengeti national park in Tanzania that were obviously sick. He shot them, and established that both were infected with *T. brucei* and noted symptoms that recalled Hornby's (1952) description of trypanosomiasis in horses. While the evidence is still slight it suggests that wild animals do suffer from trypanosomiasis, and in endemic areas it is probable that a proportion die of the infection and that the survivors acquire a natural immunity (Cunningham in Beaton 1968).

An interesting sideline of recent surveys has been the demonstration that carnivores in nature tend frequently to show trypanosomes in their blood. Baker (1969b) gives details of three hyaenas shot all showing infections of the *T. congolense* type. Out of 11 lions killed, 7 had *T. brucei* and 2 had *T. congolense*-type infections. In laboratories, on more than one occasion, cats have eaten infected rats or mice and have themselves acquired the infection. This, and not by tsetse-bite, may be the way in which carnivores usually become infected.

Trypanosomes in the insect vector

Tsetses become infected with trypanosomes when they feed on a vertebrate host that has trypanosomes in its circulation. This statement needs qualification: if a number of previously uninfected tsetse feed on an animal from which blood slides showing trypanosomes can be obtained, not all will become infected. In those that do, the trypanosomes undergo a definite cycle of development. The trypanosomes ingested with the blood meal (so-called 'blood forms') pass into the gut but are not digested. They undergo morphological changes and eventually assume a *crithidial* form. They now look like members of another genus belonging to the Kinetoplastida called *Crithidia*. In them the kinetoplast, the small deeply staining body near the root of the flagellum, is placed in front of the nucleus whereas in all other stages of the cycle it lies behind the nucleus.

Metamorphosis continues and the crithidial forms give rise to meta-cyclic trypanosomes. These are the infective forms which, if injected into the bloodstream of a vertebrate host while the tsetse is feeding, may establish themselves and complete the cycle by becoming 'blood forms'.

Development of the trypanosomes in the tsetse differs in the different subgenera. The *Duttonella* trypanosomes (*T. vivax*, *T. uniforme*) are the simplest. Ingested blood forms attach themselves to the proboscis wall and continue there while they turn into crithidial forms. The latter invade the hypopharynx where they become metacyclics and are then ready for inoculation into the vertebrate host. Blood forms of *T. vivax* that are carried beyond the proboscis when taken up in the fly's blood meal are digested.

This does not happen with the trypanosomes of the *Nannomonas* (*T. congolense*) subgenus. The blood forms begin their transformation in the mid-gut, where they become elongated and move forward to the proventriculus and thence to the proboscis where they attach themselves to its walls and pass through the crithidial stage. Later they migrate again into the hypopharynx where they become metacyclics and are ready for inoculation into the vertebrate host.

The cycle of development of *T. brucei* in the insect vector is more complicated than that of other trypanosomes. It starts, of course, with the ingestion of blood forms from the mammal host and their passage down the intestine to the mid-gut. *Glossina*, like many other insects, grows an internal protective lining for its mid-gut, the peritrophic membrane, a thin chitinous sheath or tube formed by secretion from a ring of glandular cells in the wall of the proventriculus. As secretion progresses, the cylindrical tube is pushed backwards down the gut, its anterior end remaining attached to the gut wall. Its lumen is continuous with that of the oesophagus. Its distal end, when it is fully developed, opens into the posterior portion of the mid-gut.

The peritrophic membrane may have an important role in the epidemiology of human trypanosomiasis, for it is impenetrable by trypanosomes. Nevertheless, *T. brucei* may appear in the ectoperitrophic space about four days after the infective blood meal and then multiply as elongated forms in both the ectoperitrophic and endoperitrophic spaces. One route into the ectoperitrophic space might be via the open distal end of the peritrophic membrane. Alternatively the parasites may pass through the membrane itself close to the glandular ring of cells from which it is secreted while it is still fluid.

Van Hoof, Henrard, and Peel (1937) fed *G. palpalis* on various laboratory animals and obtained a greater number of infected flies when the first meal was the infective one, but fewer when the infective meal was preceded by one or more feeds from uninfected animals. This suggested that the younger the fly the more easily it was infected. The problem was clarified by Wijers (1958) who demonstrated that flies feeding from an infective host on their first day of adult life are more likely themselves to develop an infection than if this first meal is taken on the second or third days. It is the age of the fly at the time of taking the infective meal which is important. Wijers concluded that for *G. palpalis* to become injected with *T. brucei gambiense* five conditions had to be fulfilled. The fly had to be ready to feed within 24 hours of its emergence from the puparium; its first host had to be a human being; that person had to be suffering from sleeping sickness; the disease had to be in an early stage with sufficient trypanosomes circulating in the peripheral blood, and finally, the fly had to live at least 18 days so that the trypanosomes could undergo the cycle of development which would end with them as metacyclics in the salivary glands.

With the proviso that on occasion infection may occur from an infected animal other than man, this account is entirely acceptable. It almost certainly applies also to the acquisition of all *brucei* type infections by all species of tsetse from any animal.

Having reached the ectoperitrophic space (and perhaps occasionally they move round the posterior open end of the membrane in older flies) the elongated trypanosomes move forward from the mid-gut into the proventriculus.

This must involve them once more in boring through the young cells of the anterior portion of the membrane at its point of origin. They arrive in the proventriculus between the 10th and 20th day after the blood meal and then make their way to the salivary glands where first crithidial forms and then metacyclics are produced. This whole cycle may be completed in 17 days, but its speed is controlled, in part, by environmental factors. High temperature in the environment of the pupa ensures that the emergent fly may be more easily and more rapidly infected than if it had undergone its pupal stage at a lower temperature (Burtt 1946a, Fairbairn and Culwick 1950). With a low temperature of the pupal environment it may be difficult or impossible to obtain infections in laboratory flies.

The species of mammal host on which the fly feeds may also affect its chances of developing an infection. This appeared from the studies, already mentioned, of Van Hoof, Henrard, and Peel (1937). In two experiments in which the infected hosts were guinea pigs, when the infective meal was preceded by several uninfected meals, o and o·5 per cent of flies were infected. When the infective meal was the first, the corresponding figures were 3·5 and 4·1. This illustrates the first point about the age of the fly taking the infective meal. But with monkeys, infective meals preceded by several meals from clean monkeys gave rates of o·9 and 2·3 per cent, but when the infective meal was the first, the corresponding figures were 23·5 and 59·2 per cent.

Van den Berghe, Chardome, and Peel (1963) infected a guinea pig from wild *G. morsitans* captured in Rwanda. A single *G. morsitans* reared from a puparium in the laboratory was then given its first meal on the infected guinea pig, which had shown a parasitaemia 7 days after it had been fed on by the wild flies. After the single tsetse, No. 17, had had its first infected meal it was fed on an uninfected guinea pig until that one too showed an infection. The period between the fly's first infected meal and the appearance of trypanosomes in the second guinea pig was 50 days. Temperature of maintenance of the fly was 20–22°C, a low temperature in comparison with the work of Burtt (1946a) mentioned above. Once the second guinea pig had become infected, the infected fly was fed successively on 13 different animals belonging to 11 different families. The fly died on the 96th day of its life, and on dissection was found to have its hypopharynx full of metacyclics and the salivary glands also very full of trypanosomes.

The next stage was to feed batches of clean, laboratory-bred *G. morsitans* on the animals that had received an infective bite from the single fly No. 17. These batches of laboratory flies then developed infections as follow: 20 per cent with Suidae (pig), 16·6 per cent with Felidae (cat), 14 per cent with Canidae (dog), 12·5 per cent with Hystricidae (porcupine), 10 per cent with Spalacidae, 7 per cent with Cercopithecidae (monkey), 6·2 per cent with Myoxidae, 6·0 per cent with Caviidae (guinea pig), 3·6 per cent with Procaviidae (hyrax), 3·2 per cent with Leporidae (rabbit), and 2·4 per cent with Muridae (rat). These figures support the evidence of Van Hoof, Henrard, and Peel (1937) that the animal host may influence the infection rate in the flies. But a comparison of the two papers also shows the difficulty of defining the behaviour of trypanosomes. From the earlier work it might be deduced that monkeys were far superior to guinea pigs as infecting hosts, but the more recent study shows hardly any difference between the two. (In both studies the monkeys were of the genus *Cercocebus* and although Van den Berghe and his colleagues do not mention the species, it is likely that it was the same as that used by their predecessors, *C. galeritus*.)

Transmission from tsetse to vertebrate

The chances of a tsetse becoming infected when it feeds upon a host with trypanosomes in its blood may depend upon the environment in which its developmental stages were passed. We have also seen, at least with trypanosomes of the *Trypanozoon* subgenus, that the age of the fly may be a major factor controlling its acquisition of a mature trypanosome infection. Besides this, some animals transmit infection to the tsetse more readily than others, although it is certainly not yet possible to relate this factor to the apparent differences in proportions of parasitaemias seen in wild animals and summarized in Table 4.2. Nevertheless it will be found, in Chapter 5, that high infection rates in nature may be positively correlated with the proportion of blood meals taken from antelopes, as opposed to other animals, and that this effect overrides the predisposition to infection provided by hotter climates. It seems likely that tsetse which happen to feed on an animal with abundant trypanosomes in its peripheral circulation are more likely to become themselves infected than others that feed on hosts in which the flagellates are rarely seen. But it is not yet proven.

When David Livingstone left Great Britain to explore the Zambezi river in 1858, he was urged by the great anatomist, Richard Owen, to observe, as carefully as possible, the numbers of tsetse-bites required to kill an ox (Livingstone 1956). At that time it was thought that *Glossina* injected a poison with their saliva and that sufficient of this had to accumulate in order to cause death. Translated into modern terms the question resolves itself into the measurement of the size of the infective dose of trypanosomes, that is, the number of parasites that must be inoculated to establish an infection.

When blood from an infected host is inoculated by syringe into an un-infected animal, the parasites may establish themselves in the circulation of the latter if there are enough of them. Many workers have measured this infective dose, the most recent being Willett (1956) and Baker (1960). The larger the number of trypanosomes inoculated, the shorter the prepatent period, that is, the period between inoculation and appearance of trypanosomes in the circulation of the recipient host. Baker's conclusion, from observations on two strains of *T. brucei* (one infective to man) in rats, mice, and guinea pigs, was that the prepatent period bore an inverse relationship to the logarithm of the number of trypanosomes inoculated. Willett's work had shown that there was a minimal infective dose of *T. brucei rhodesiense* below which it was not possible to infect a human volunteer. Fairbairn and Burtt (1946) had already shown that a dose of 300–450 metacyclic trypanosomes was required to infect the average man, but some men required more than this. These observations were in keeping with the experiences of the early explorers, condensed in Professor Owen's question. One might ride one's horse into a fly-belt for a short time and get away with it. If one kept him there, he would die.

The investigation in nature of the problem of metacyclic dosage is still in its infancy. In a series of studies of *G. pallidipes*, *G. brevipalpis*, and *G. fuscipes* in the Lugala sleeping sickness focus on the north-east corner of Lake Victoria (see Chapter 15), Harley first explored the relationship between the age of tsetse and the incidences of their infections with trypanosomes, especially the *Duttonella* (*vivax*) and *Nannomonas* (*congolense*) *groups*. These trypanosomes do not have to overcome the difficulties presented by the peritrophic membrane and therefore it would be supposed that the greater the mean age of a tsetse population, the higher its infection rate.

In his first study Harley (1966*a* and 1966*b*) showed that *G. pallidipes* were more heavily infected (with *T. vivax* and *T. congolense*) than *G. fuscipes*, and that the latter were more heavily infected than *G. brevipalpis*. In all three the older flies were more often infected than the younger, although in *G. brevipalpis* the regression of infection rate on age was not significant. The incidence of infection in *G. pallidipes* and *G. fuscipes* was highest in or immediately after the month of greatest rainfall, though with *G. brevipalpis* there was a lag of one more month before peak infection was reached. Over 80 per cent of infections in all three species were in flies of more than average age.

The high infection rate in or just after the rains was a consequence of the longer life of tsetse at that season. The largest contribution to the seasonal fluctuation was made by the commonest trypanosomes, those of the *vivax* group. *Congolense* group trypanosomes varied less in frequency through the year; but in a later paper (Harley 1967*a*) it is shown that they too become more frequent with increasing age in the tsetse population. The age factor is influenced by the sex of the fly. Females live longer than males, and Table 4.3, extracted from Harley's work, shows that females of all three species of *Glossina* at Lugala show higher infection rates with all three trypanosome groups than do the males.

Table 4.3 also draws attention to an aspect of cattle trypanosomiases that will appear on several occasions during discussion of the histories of these diseases in different parts of Africa. This is the paucity of *congolense* group infections in cattle subject to attack only by *palpalis* group tsetses. The very low rate of infection in cattle in Teso, a district of Central Uganda, mentioned in Chapter 5, is a reflection of their very narrow contact with

TABLE 4.3

Infection rates of tsetse flies at Lugala in Uganda, 1964–5†

		Infection rates		
	No. dissected	vivax *group* (%)	congolense *group* (%)	brucei *group* (%)
G. *pallidipes* males	1809	16·4	2·6	0·22
females	3451	22·1	4·2	0·29
G. *fuscipes* males	2199	9·3	0·8	0·05
females	1974	19·2	1·2	0·15
G. *brevipalpis* males	1378	5·1	2·2	0·07
females	538	6·1	2·6	0·19

† From Harley (1967*a*).

G. *fuscipes* on the Lake Kyoga shores. Only *Trypanosoma vivax* is found. Elsewhere, when other species of tsetse are present, *T. congolense* as well as *T. vivax* is found in the local cattle. This could, in turn reflect different opportunities for feeding. In Teso, with large populations of people and of cattle there are few wild hosts other than reptiles, and it is virtually certain that they, plus man and his livestock, supply most of the blood taken by *Glossina* on the Kyoga shores.

From Table 4.3 we can discover that for every infection by *T. congolense* in G. *brevipalpis* there are 2·39 infections by other trypanosomes. In G. *pallidipes* the ratio is 1 : 5·59 and in G. *fuscipes* 1 : 13·98. These ratios might again indicate different feeding habits (see Table 5.7 in Chapter 5). Kleine, whose views on the identity of the various human trypanosomiases we have already noticed, showed that '*T. gambiense*' could be transmitted by G. *morsitans*, and it was in line with his general thought that 'under suitable conditions every known species of trypanosome can develop in every species of *Glossina*' (Kleine and Fischer 1912). It is only recently that the proof that G. *fuscipes* at Lugala is a vector of *T. brucei rhodesiense* has brought about a change in thinking on the epidemiology of trypanosomiasis in that very long-lived focus of infection (see Chapter 14).

Harley's data in Table 4.3 (and there is ample other evidence) make it clear that G. *fuscipes* can develop an infection of *T. congolense*. It would seem, then, that different food habits are likely to be the controlling factor in determining the nature and extent of infection in populations of different species of tsetses found in the same area.

The most recent study to emerge from Lugala shows that this is not so. But the experiment was one that could hardly have been performed before the introduction by Lumsden of the virological methods already mentioned. These must therefore be examined briefly now.

Quantitative techniques in the study of trypanosome infection

Morphology, as revealed by the compound microscope, fails to distinguish strains of *T. brucei* infective or not infective to man. Among cattle trypanosomes, different strains of the same species may kill an ox in a few weeks or produce an infection of which the symptoms can barely be distinguished from the effects of overwork. Lumsden introduced two new ideas. The first was a method of measuring the infective dose of trypanosomes; the second was the concept of the *stabilate*. It is logical to begin with the second.

Isolates, strains, and stabilates

Lumsden's definitions are quite clear:

'*Isolate*: a section of a wild population separated off by transference into artificial conditions of maintenance, usually by inoculation into cultures or into laboratory animals.

'*Strain*: a population, derived from an isolate, maintained in captivity by inducing it to reproduce continuously by serial passages in cultures or in laboratory animals.

'*Stabilate*: a population whose reproduction has been arrested by viable preservation on a unique occasion. In stabilate material, selection of a continuously reproducing population, such as occurs in a strain, is avoided and selection is restricted to that exerted by the processes of preservation and retrieval from preservation' (Lumsden 1965; Lumsden and Hardy 1965).

Preservation, for all practical purposes, means deep freezing; retrieval is the process of thawing and inoculating into a host. The notion of freezing blood, other tissues, or suspensions of trypanosomes in artificial media was first thought of as a much more economical way of preserving strains than that of continuous passage from one animal to another by fly-bite. But, as Lumsden (1963) pointed out, a more important feature is that it provides a store of 'unaltering standard material to which recourse may be had for study or comparison over extended periods'. An extreme case of the sort of error that Lumsden's use of stabilates is designed to avoid was that reported by Fairbairn (1956). *The Wellcome (C) strain* was originally a *T. brucei rhodesiense* from an infected man in Tanzania. It was preserved by syringe passage from rat to rat for $18\frac{1}{2}$ years in England where it served as material for numerous experiments. Fairbairn inoculated 25 000 000 trypanosomes of this strain into himself, and although there was a marked reaction at the site of the inoculation, no infection developed. Furthermore, not only had the trypanosomes lost their virulence for man, but their morphology had altered and stumpy forms were no longer to be seen.

The isolate, then, is preserved by freezing as a stabilate and the vicissitudes through which a strain population must pass are avoided; but it has yet to be shown that freezing over long periods does not also produce other, if different, changes.

Measurement of the infective dose

Different species of animals are refractory or susceptible to infection. If susceptible, then the degree of susceptibility can be assessed by clinical observation, by assessment of physiological change, and by the degree of parasitaemia. The analogous property of the trypanosome is its power to infect. It may fail entirely to do so or, as we have seen, there may be a minimum infective dose. Willett (1956) showed that 80 000 blood forms of the Tinde strain of *T. brucei rhodesiense* would infect man, but that 20 000 failed to do so. At that dosage the trypanosomes were eliminated by the defence mechanism of the body. The infective dose is estimated by counting the trypanosomes in a known volume of suspension in a suitable fluid and then by inoculating equal volumes of serially proportional diluent into the chosen host, to discover at what point inoculation ceases to infect.

This process is relatively simple when dealing with blood forms, because comparatively large quantities of blood can be obtained from the infected host. When it is required to measure numbers of trypanosomes extruded by tsetse in its saliva when feeding, the technical difficulties are greater. An early attempt was made by Belgian parasitologists in the Congo. They placed a known quantity of blood in an appropriate container, and covered its open surface with a membrane through which a tsetse was induced to probe. They found that a single *Glossina palpalis* might inject as many or more than 1562 metacyclics at a single feed (Rodhain, Pons, Vandenbranden, and Bequaert 1912). Half a century later, Cunningham and Harley (1962) adapted their procedure to obtain and then make stabilates of metacyclics.

It is not necessarily the quantity of metacyclics that is important. Either every one is capable of multiplying in the host's blood, although many more than one may be required to overcome the host's defence mechanisms, or else the metacyclics vary in their ability to establish themselves. In the latter case the actual number would not provide a measure of the infective dose. The object in measuring infectivity of isolates is to discover whether it is a property constant within a species or within a strain, or whether it may vary in the course of evolution of trypanosome populations.

To measure infectivity, the frozen stabilate is thawed and diluted serially with ten-fold dilutions of a suitable fluid (phosphate-buffered saline pH 8·0). Equal quantities of each dilution are then inoculated intraperitoneally into groups of six standard white mice. The greater the dilution the smaller the chance that all mice in the group will become infected. It

has been demonstrated on more than one occasion that a single trypanosome will infect a mouse. If this is so then it is to be expected that when
there is an average of one infective trypanosome inoculated per mouse, 63
per cent of the mice will receive an inoculum of infective trypanosomes.
(The assumption is made that the distribution of trypanosomes among the
individual inocula follows a Poisson distribution.) The estimated numbers
of infective doses in 1 ml of trypanosome suspension for 63 per cent of the
mice, each given a standard quantity of the inoculum, provides a measure
of infectivity (ID_{63}) which can be used to compare stabilates either from
different strains or from the same stabilates under different treatments.

Using this method, Southon, Cunningham, and Grainge (1965) measured
the number of ID_{63}s of *T. brucei rhodesiense* for mice from nine feeds by a
single *G. morsitans* and obtained figures ranging from 5000 to 63 000, with
a mean of 23 000. Later Harley, Cunningham, and Van Hoeve (1966)
obtained a mean of 3200 ID_{63}s per feed, but numbers per feed varied from
0 to 40 000. These figures compare reasonably well with figures of up to
11 600 trypanosomes extruded in saliva probed on a slide (Fairbairn and
Burtt 1946), but are much larger than the early estimate of Rodhain, Pons,
Vandenbranden, and Bequaert (1912).

Work of this sort has only just begun to be applicable to the sort of
phenomenon described in the following chapters, but a return can now be
made to the problem of the apparent paucity of *congolense* group trypanosomes transmitted by *G. fuscipes*. It will be recalled that evidence suggested
that this might be due to lack of opportunity given by the food host of these
tsetse.

The infectivity of *Glossina morsitans*, *G. pallidipes*, and *G. fuscipes* with identical stabilates of *Trypanosoma congolense*

Harley and Wilson (1968) summarized a number of surveys beginning
with that of Jackson (1943) in Busoga (see Chapter 15) in which *G. fuscipes*
and *G. pallidipes* were fed on rats in order to isolate trypanosomes. In all,
32 707 of the former species produced only three *T. congolense* infections,
a proportion of 0·009 per cent; 14 085 *G. pallidipes* produced 92 infections
or 0·65 per cent. All these surveys were done around the north-east corner
of Lake Victoria, in Busoga in Uganda, or Central Nyanza in Kenya. They
suggest that the average wild *G. pallidipes* is 72 times more likely to infect
a rat with strains of *congolense* group trypanosomes than the average
G. fuscipes.

The next step was to inoculate *T. congolense* group stabilates into various
laboratory animals on which batches of three species of tsetse, *G. morsitans*,
G. pallidipes, and *G. fuscipes* were fed. Subsequently the flies were fed on
defibrinated blood through a rat-skin membrane. After two weeks (sufficient
time for trypanosomes ingested by the flies almost to have completed their
development cycle) blood left unconsumed after each meal was inoculated

into mice. This blood might thenceforward contain any metacyclics ejected with the saliva of those flies that had acquired mature infections. At 23–24°C, the trypanosomes took 15–20 days or more to produce mature metacyclics. The flies were now separated and kept in single tubes and encouraged to probe on warmed glass slides. This method of demonstrating the presence of trypanosomes in the saliva of tsetses is due to Burtt (1946b). Five infected *G. morsitans*, seven *G. pallidipes*, and two *G. fuscipes* were then fed through membranes on separate blood pools. The remains of 91 pools from each of which a single feed had been taken were available to make estimates of ID_{63} in mice. It had been shown separately that 16 mouse ID_{63}s were needed to infect a cow. On 58 occasions no mice were infected. In 16 feeds, 10 or less ID_{63}s were extruded, and therefore produced inocula with too few trypanosomes to infect a cow. Only 17 of the 91 feeds would have established a bovine trypanosomiasis (Harley and Wilson 1968).

The main interest of the experiment from the present viewpoint lies in the contribution to this result made by the different species of tsetse. *G. morsitans* and *G. pallidipes* continued to extrude infective trypanosomes throughout life, although not, of course, at every meal. But each of the two *G. fuscipes* produced infective trypanosomes at one meal only and thereafter not at all. In spite of this, however, when dissected at the end of the experiment they were found to have abundant trypanosomes both in the hypopharynx and in the gut. But this was not the only distinction. Other flies fed on animals infected with the same stabilates were dissected in adequate numbers. *G. pallidipes* showed an incidence of 13·2 per cent mature infections and *G. morsitans* 11·6 per cent, but only 2·9 per cent of *G. fuscipes* had trypanosomes in gut and proboscis. The immature infections showed a similar discrepancy: only 1·2 per cent of *G. fuscipes* displayed trypanosomes in the gut only. The corresponding figures for the other species were 6·6 and 13·0 per cent respectively. This must mean that *G. fuscipes* is less susceptible to infection by *congolense* group trypanosomes than the other flies and that its low incidence of mature infection is not caused by any stoppage of the development cycle. As the opportunities for infection were equal, the idea must be abandoned that *G. fuscipes* does not transmit *T. congolense* because of lack of opportunity imposed by its feeding habits. In the next chapter we shall find that from Uganda westwards to Senegal, in the zones where *palpalis* group tsetse alone are found, the incidence of *T. congolense* infection in cattle is negligible. It is also important to note that tsetse frequently inoculate sub-minimal doses of trypanosomes.

In an earlier experiment, using similar methods to measure the infectivity of a stabilate of human-infective *T. brucei rhodesiense* transmitted by *G. morsitans*, it was also shown that in 25 per cent of feeds no trypanosomes were extruded and that in a further 15 per cent too few were extruded to produce infection. Only 60 per cent of feeds would have resulted in establishment of human trypanosomiasis (Harley, Cunningham, and Van Hoeve 1966).

It will be observed that in these experiments we have come around to the essentials of the hypothesis propounded by Richard Owen to David Livingstone in 1858.

Immunity to trypanosome infection

The problem of infectivity has only recently begun to be investigated along lines that allow us to apply the results of research to situations long familiar in the field. Much the same may be said of the study of the physiological defences to infection developed by the vertebrate hosts. Once again promising early beginnings, long ago abandoned, have been revived by the invention, in other fields of research, of new techniques. New methods for the diagnosis of the human infections are beginning to produce evidence for the existence of epidemiological situations long suspected but unproven. On the other hand, much intrinsically interesting research now in progress has not yet reached the point where it can offer detailed explanations for what may be seen in the field.

The search for immunological and serological techniques for diagnosis of the human infection has for long been the preoccupation of French and Belgian workers. Where policy has been directed towards elimination of the disease by therapeutic sterilization of the infection in whole populations, it has obviously been essential to diagnose every case. When, as we have seen, a proportion of infected persons may be in apparently good health and show no clinical signs of disease and no parasites in the peripheral circulation, this may be a matter of some difficulty. The improvement of diagnostic methods is still the first object of immunological research. The second is an extension of this objective: to provide more precise methods of classifying trypanosomes than have yet been given by morphological study. It would be of immense value to find a simple means of distinguishing between strains of *T. brucei* infective or non-infective to man. Thirdly, though without great hopes of success, research may be directed towards the artificial immunization of people and of livestock (Gray 1967). Lumsden (1967) has also pointed to the possibility that antigen–antibody complexes formed in response to infection may themselves trigger off cell reactions that have pathogenic effects in certain organs.

In the course of an infection the trypanosomes multiply, and as the parasitaemia increases the patient suffers from a fever which denotes a crisis after which the population density of trypanosomes declines. This decline is associated with production of antibody in the blood serum. The parasites soon begin to multiply again and this relapse population produces antigenic material against which the antibodies that overcame the first crisis are ineffective.

New antibody is produced in response to this second growth of antigen, and again the parasitaemia is reduced, and yet again recovers in a third antigenic form, and so on until, in the case of the human infection, the patient dies, or recovers, or remains in a state of adjustment with the parasite. This continuous production of antigenic variants was demonstrated long ago by Ritz (1916) who showed that a single parasite could, in the course of its multiplication, give rise to at least twenty-two different antigenic types of trypanosome. However, whatever antigenic variants may appear in a strain of *T. brucei* during the course of infection in the mammal host, its original antigenic properties are restored when, at any stage, the trypanosomes undergo cyclical development in *Glossina*. Moreover, when a strain is divided into a number of substrains, at least one antigen is retained that is common to them all. This is the basic antigen. There is evidence that different basic antigens characterize strains from different areas. The hope that this would lead to a means of strain classification has so far been nullified by the discovery of variable antigens additional to the basic antigen in cyclically transmitted strains (Gray 1962, 1965, Brown 1963). The likelihood of producing a vaccine to overcome all possible antigenic variants also seems remote.

Some people, apparently, overcome infection in nature, as do cattle, and we have seen that there exists a minimum infective dose of trypanosomes. One trypanosome may set up an infection in a mouse, but 16 *T. congolense* may be the least that can overcome the initial resistance of a cow. In man the '*rhodesiense*' infection needs an inoculation of 300–450 trypanosomes to become established.† These are, perhaps, merely the numbers needed to avoid consumption by phagocytes long enough for multiplication to begin. (See Gordon, Crewe, and Willett 1956, and Gordon and Willett 1958 for an account of the development of a parasitaemia from the moment of the infected bite.) In animals like the baboon and man himself, refractory to all or nearly all trypanosome infection, the attack on the invading flagellates is obviously immediately successful.

Desowitz (1960), in his study of infections in antelopes, measured antibody production in each as well as changes in serum proteins. All five animals, including those that were refractory to infection, produced antibody suggesting that the refractoriness was, indeed, due to a defence response to the trypanosome. In all animals also, the levels of β-2-globulin and γ-globulin rose in proportion to other serum proteins. The globulins are serum proteins particularly associated with antibody formation. Desowitz's study provides evidence that the immunity of wild animals is associated with acquired characters as well, possibly, as with innate factors. In Chapter 3 we followed Baker (1963) in suggesting that parasitization of

---

† But since this was written Bailey and Boreham (1969) have presented evidence which suggests that trypanosomiasis in man may follow inoculation with as few as 10 mouse-infective trypanosomes.

mammals through tsetse-bite was a secondary phenomenon, and tentatively extended his thesis to suggest that the savanna-dwelling antelopes were still in the process of achieving adjustment to the flagellates. This adjustment must be achieved by selection which leads to the survival of individuals in which the faculty of appropriate antibody formation is best developed.

Lourie and O'Connor (1937) worked with a strain of *T. 'rhodesiense'* which had a prepatent period in their laboratory mice of five days or less, even in infections started by inoculation of single trypanosomes. But over a period of eight years, in which some five thousand mice had been experimentally infected, five had resisted the initial infection and it took seven or more days for trypanosomes to appear in their blood. On two such occasions these late-appearing parasites were studied. Lourie and O'Connor had first shown that a normally infected mouse, when cured by drugs, was immune for a time, from re-infection by the same strain. It was, however, fully susceptible to trypanosomes from a relapse in another mouse which had been infected with that same strain. Conversely if a mouse was inoculated with a relapse parasite and cured it developed a temporary immunity to the relapse strain but not the parent trypanosomes. Those parasites that appeared after seven days in one mouse in a thousand were found to have the immunological characteristics of relapse strains and not of the initial parasite populations in normal mice. These rare mice were therefore spontaneously resistant to the original strain, although the latter eventually overcame this resistance by altering their own immunological properties. One may wonder if the descent of primate ancestors from the forest canopy to the ground which led to the evolution of both man and baboon was accompanied by the selection for survival of refractory individuals. The other larger and partly terrestrial primates (gorilla and chimpanzee) which are susceptible to fatal infections tend to be limited, at least in the present day, either to areas in which tsetse that readily feed on man are rare (low level moist forest) or else to areas above the altitude limits of *Glossina*.

Wild animals produce antibodies in response to tsetse infection; so do men and so do cattle but to varying degrees in different ecological zones. Some antibodies are not protective and, generally, those that do protect, either against overwhelming multiplication of the antigenic strain or against infection by other strains, are limited in their effectiveness. Immunity against trypanosome infection is a complex process and is far from fully understood. The reader who wishes to pursue the subject further will find starting points in Weitz (1958), Soltys (1963), Weinman (1963), Lumsden (1967), and, especially, Gray (1967).

It is frequently asserted that because of tsetses and trypanosomes vast areas of Africa are closed to cattle. Other lesser but still large areas are dangerous to man himself. Nevertheless, more than one example will be given later of the contact of human societies with these infections that can only be explained by the assumption that physiological defences in man and domestic animals are by no means entirely useless. Hornby (1952), out of an immense experience of veterinary trypanosomiasis, mostly acquired in the days before drugs capable of widespread application were available, remarked: 'What is of importance in relation to trypanosomiasis control is the knowledge that every beast puts up a fight for life that is frequently successful, but that in every case the success is qualified.'

Some of the qualifications were clear in Hornby's descriptions of cattle infected with *T. congolense* or *T. vivax*. The course of the infection, whether towards eventual death or towards a self-cure, was conditioned not only by the properties of the infecting strain, but also by the nutrition level of the animal infected and the stresses to which it was subjected. One may suppose that qualifications of this kind affect the course of any potentially fatal infection.

With them in mind we may summarize factors contributing to survival of animals with trypanosome infection as follows:

Variation in host response. Different animals react differently to infection. They may be completely refractory; for example, man to *T. congolense*, or baboons to all trypanosomes. If susceptible, the infection may be mild; for example, *T. vivax* in horses, or *T. brucei* in cattle. But often, when the animal is susceptible, there is much variation in the virulence of the disease; for example, *T. vivax* in African zebu cattle.

Individual susceptibility. Some individuals of the same host species will throw off an infection by a strain of trypanosome that produces a disease in other individuals. This, perhaps, has led through natural selection to:

Racial immunity. Certain races of African cattle are much less liable to develop a pathological condition from trypanosomiasis than are others, although they can easily be infected. The best known are the N'Dama and Muturu cattle of West Africa (see Chapters 21 to 24), but Hornby (1947) described locally immune cattle in the Maputo district of Mozambique, and there is historical evidence for the phenomenon in other areas (see Chapter 17). There is also some evidence for local or 'racial' immunity in man (Chapter 24). Racial immunity is generally only developed against infection by local trypanosomes. It breaks down when the animal is subjected to infection by heterologous strains.

Local immunity. A population of cattle may be able to withstand a light, but intermittently continuous, infection by local strains of different species of trypanosomes, but collapses when exposed to heavy, sustained inoculation. 'There is a great deal of difference between the demands on the body imposed by a single infection due to a single inoculation, and the ability to withstand the multiple inoculations inescapable in a heavy fly-belt. It is a common experience to find recovered animals *near* a fly-belt; rare to find immune animals within a belt' (Hornby 1952).

Acquired immunity. Sera from animals infected with trypanosomes may contain protective antibodies. According to Soltys (1963) this was first reported by Rouget (1896) who showed that serum from rabbits and dogs infected with *T. equiperdum* inoculated into mice protected the mice from infection with the same strain. The technique has little value in practice because of the multiplicity of species and of strains of species in nature.

An important aspect of this phenomenon is the natural transfer of protective antibody from immune mothers to their offspring probably via the colostrum. By this means calves of N'Dama and Muturu cows are protected from the harmful effects of infection while they build up their own store of antibody.

Premunity. The gross effect of these various processes may enable a cattle population to live indefinitely in apparent good health, while subjected to continual infection. So long as the infection persists the animals can resist further infection by antigenically related organisms. This is the condition of premunity or premunition. It may end under the stress of other infections or when the challenge of new strains becomes too severe. It is terminated when the infection is cured by drugs. Individual predisposition to develop the premune state with relative ease may lead to the evolution, by natural selection, of immune or partially immune 'types' of cattle as well as of people. This is perhaps also the basis of survival of susceptible species of wild animals.

5

GEOGRAPHICAL PATTERNS OF TRYPANOSOME DISTRIBUTION

ONE maps the distribution of tsetse flies by catching them, determining their species, and plotting where each specimen is caught. Later one draws a line around the areas in which the capture records are marked. It is less easy to do this with trypanosomes, except those found in people. It is not too difficult, given an adequate organization of technicians, to do the same for the trypanosomes in cattle. But by far the greater part of the population of African tsetse-transmitted trypanosomes lives in the wild animal population and survey of their infections is very difficult indeed, although now that techniques of wildlife management are being developed, including the use of tranquillizer projectiles, one looks forward to greater progress in a not too distant future.

With the human trypanosomiases it is relatively easy to find out where people become infected and to plot this information on a map. When this has been done in the past, what is known as 'rhodesian' trypanosomiasis appears in various localities in eastern Africa from the Zambezi valley to Uganda, and what is known as 'gambian' sleeping sickness occupies much of the Congo basin and the countries of West Africa. But it becomes increasingly difficult to sustain these distinctions.

As in the previous chapter it would be logical to begin with trypanosome distributions in the natural hosts, but so far it is only possible to make tentative guesses about which are the important natural reservoirs of some species of trypanosome. It seems best to discuss the distributions of the cattle trypanosomes first, to go from them to the evidence about distribution in the tsetse flies, and from them to pass to the wild natural hosts, and so to man.

The geography of trypanosomiasis in cattle

In 1952, the International Scientific Committee for Trypanosomiasis Research decided that it would not sponsor a geographical study of the trypanosomiases of domestic animals. It was an unfortunate decision. A map that displayed the proportions in which the principal cattle trypanosomiases had been diagnosed in different provinces, or even in different countries, would have shown what foundation existed for the widely held belief that in eastern Africa *Trypanosoma congolense* caused most cases of cattle trypanosomiasis, while in West Africa this role was held by *T. vivax*. It might have made clearer what a student of trypanosomiasis meant by

East and West Africa. The paradox that trypanosome infections in domestic animals were only to be found where there were no tsetse flies and that in the fly-belts there was no trypanosomiasis problem because there were no domestic animals to suffer from it is especially an East African phenomenon. In West Africa the annual migration of Fulani cattle southward into the *Glossina* zone produces a situation not found east of longitude 20°E. A map might have provoked a debate on the differences in the epizootiology of East and West African trypanosomiases in the attempt to explain the differences in revealed patterns.

That the geographical approach could be valuable was evident from the Belgian contribution to the debate. Colback (1952) pointed out that trypanosomiasis was enzootic even among cattle living far from *Glossina* in the mountains of the eastern Congo, and supposed that transmission of the disease must therefore be effected by bites of Tabanidae and probably also of Stomoxydinae. In the heavily stocked regions of the eastern Congo and in Ruanda-Urundi the percentage of *Trypanosoma congolense* infections rose with increasing proximity to the fly-belts, while *T. vivax* infections became proportionately less. Colback was puzzled, however, that while *T. brucei* infections in donkeys and dogs were only found near the national parks thus showing the importance of the wild mammal reservoir, cattle in the same neighbourhoods had never shown *T. brucei* infections.

Classical East and West African diagnostic pictures

Mornet, of the Laboratoire Fédérale d'Élévage at Dakar, published maps of the distribution of trypanosomiases of domestic animals in what was then French West Africa (Mornet 1954, Mornet and Morel 1956). These maps showed whether or not a specific trypanosomiasis had ever been recorded at official veterinary centres since 1904. For all French West Africa, infections appeared in the following proportions:

Trypanosoma vivax	40 per cent
T. congolense	34 per cent
T. brucei	14 per cent
T. evansi	3 per cent
Mixed infections	1 per cent

This was the classical West African picture. Unsworth (1953) collected 965 records of infections in Zebu cattle in Nigeria during the years 1941–53 and obtained a similar result:

Trypanosoma vivax	68·7 per cent
T. congolense	26·0 per cent
T. brucei	0·4 per cent
Mixed infections	4·8 per cent

Mornet's records included livestock other than cattle. Camels account for records of *T. evansi* infection, while his 14 per cent of *T. brucei* infections as opposed to Unsworth's 0·4 per cent may have been due to inclusion of diagnoses of trypanosomiases in horses, donkeys, and dogs.

The Uganda tsetse-fly belts, for the most part, belong to the East African complex. In the years before drugs for cattle trypanosomiasis became easily available, it was the practice to record outbreaks rather than cases of the disease. Blood slides were taken from a proportion of the animals in a herd in which one or more individuals showed clinical signs of infection. A single positive blood slide indicated an outbreak in the herd. In the years 1931–4, 48 outbreaks were attributed to *T. congolense*, 11 to *T. vivax*, and 13 to *T. brucei*. There were also 353 outbreaks with infections of all three or combinations of two of these trypanosomes. In these *T. congolense* occurred in 345, *T. vivax* in 306, and *T. brucei* in 209. In 1932 and 1933, the Research Laboratory at Entebbe diagnosed in cattle 36 *T. congolense*, 21 *T. vivax*, and 8 *T. brucei* cases. The preponderance of *T. congolense* in Uganda seems clear. This was the East African picture.

Limitations of the data

The Colonial Civil Service data have their limitations. Most of the figures come from *Annual reports*. These documents served as records of achievement, as repositories of scientific data, and as vehicles of propaganda with the small interested public and with the Treasury. Figures may be misleading. For some years the records from one government laboratory showed disproportionately numerous diagnoses of *T. congolense* as compared with other trypanosomes. Eventually one perceived that the figures included not only records from the field, but also from slides obtained from laboratory cattle experimentally inoculated with this trypanosome. Publication of the data perhaps served to suggest the need for another microscopist on the laboratory staff, but otherwise only led to confusion.

More important are the difficulties of complete diagnosis. The trypanosomes demonstrable in an infected animal differ according to the techniques used. *T. brucei* may be difficult to find unless blood is inoculated into a suitable laboratory animal. Cunningham and van Hoeve (1965) have shown by serological methods that a high proportion of cattle in Western Uganda with negative blood slides either had been, or were perhaps still, infected with this trypanosome. Deom (1949) used protein shock to bring into the peripheral circulations of Eastern Congo cattle trypanosomes that were living cryptically in other organs, a condition that was then being studied in Kenya by Fiennes (1950).

Godfrey and Killick-Kendrick (1961) examined 298 zebu cattle in the Benue province of Northern Nigeria. They took thick and thin stained blood films and also inoculated the blood of their cattle into rats. By combining the results from all three methods they showed that 9·7 per cent of the animals were infected with *T. vivax*, 79·5 per cent with *T. congolense*, and 20·4 per cent with *T. brucei*. This was a surprising result in view of the almost universally accepted opinion that *T. vivax* was the dominant pathogen in West Africa.

They next examined 193 zebus among the migrating herds which annually traverse the *morsitans* fly-belts of the Zaria province (Killick-Kendrick and Godfrey 1963). These animals had been brought by their owners to inoculation centres, and on this occasion a fourth diagnostic method was employed, the examination of wet fresh blood films. This method and the thick stained film were equally good for the detection of *T. vivax*, but for *T. congolense* the latter was far superior, yielding 28·6 per cent infections against only 15·6 by the wet films. This second survey, again combining all methods, gave 10·4 per cent *T. vivax*, 34·2 per cent *T. congolense*, and 2·1 per cent *T. brucei*. They did not believe that their results revealed any change in the proportions of *T. vivax* and *T. congolense* in recent years, but, in part at least, attributed them to alterations in the practice of blood examination. They pointed out that earlier workers only took thick films for staining from those animals which had already shown themselves to be blood positive by the wet film method. This, as they had demonstrated, is a poor technique for revealing the presence of *T. congolense* and therefore the proportions of thick smears positive for *T. vivax* was artificially raised.

This explanation implies that veterinarians in eastern Africa did not carry out a preliminary wet film examination to select those animals from whom stained slides should be made. It seems unlikely that there was a consistent difference in the techniques practised on either side of the continent. What is more probable is that on both sides a variety of methods were used according to the facilities available, and that the geographical variability has a true epizootiological basis.

Killick-Kendrick and Godfrey (1963) offered another explanation. Homidium, then a very widely used drug in Northern Nigeria, is more effective against *T. vivax* than against *T. congolense* and so filters out the former trypanosome from the cattle population at a rate faster than the latter. In East Africa a reverse action favouring the survival of *T. vivax* has been attributed to the widespread use of another drug, antrycide. Finally, the distribution of *T. brucei* in Northern Nigerian cattle may be uneven, for earlier workers in other parts of that country had obtained relatively high infection rates with this trypanosome by use of the thick film alone. Unsworth and Birkett (1952) obtained 5·63 per cent of *T. brucei* infections, and Macfie (1913*a*) 5·4 per cent, suggesting that had they used the method of sub-inoculation into rats *T. brucei* infections would have been even more numerous.

Infections and vegetation in West Africa

Mornet's maps showed that *Trypanosoma vivax* infections in West African cattle had been recorded not only throughout those countries widely infested with *Glossina*, but extended north into the sub-Saharan herds for distances of 500–600 km beyond the fly-belts. *T. vivax* infections seemed to be limited in their distribution only by the boundary of northern pasture at the Sahara edge at about 18°N. This trypanosome had been discovered by Cazalbou in the Sudan in 1905, outside the *Glossina* boundary. Ziemann, who had found it a little earlier in the same year in the Cameroons, also thought it was transmitted independently of tsetse flies. The northern limit of *T. congolense* lay much closer to the known northern limit of *Glossina*. *T. brucei* also appeared, with one exception, only at stations within

TABLE 5.1

Trypanosome records at stations in the former French West Africa (Mornet 1954) related to West African vegetation zones

Vegetation	Stations at which T. vivax recorded	Stations at which T. congolense recorded	% of stations with T. vivax records
Wooded steppe . . .	6	3	67
Undifferentiated dry types .	13	11	56
Abundant *Isoberlinia* . .	10	10	50
Undifferentiated moist types .	3	6	33
Forest–savanna mosaic . .	1	2	33
Moist forest . . .	2	2	50

the *Glossina* zone. Trypanosome infections of domestic pigs (probably *T. simiae*), also within the *Glossina* zone, are absent from Muslim areas.

Table 5.1 has been compiled by superimposing Mornet's data on the vegetation map of Africa (Keay, Aubréville, Duvigneaud, Hoyle, Mendonca, and Pichi-Sermolli 1958). The numbers of stations in the two southern vegetation zones are too few for comparison, but from the wooded steppe (Sahel) southward into the undifferentiated moist vegetation (Southern Guinea zone) there is a distinct decrease in the proportion of *T. vivax* as compared with *T. congolense*.

Glover (1965) tabulated by provinces the distribution of 2704 positive slides from Fulani nomadic cattle collected during the rainy season of 1955–6 in Northern Nigeria. One may assign the various provinces to three main vegetation zones, although in some there is overlapping. In the Sudan zone are Sokoto, Katsina, Kano, Bornu, Bauchi, and Adamawa. Zaria and Plateau provinces are in the Northern Guinea zone, and Ilorin,

TABLE 5.2

Nigerian provincial infection data arranged according to the predominant vegetation type†

Province	Slides examined	T. vivax	T. congo-lense	T. v.–T. c. mixed	T. brucei
Sudan vegetation zone					
Sokoto . . .	377	66	18	9	—
Katsina . . .	690	93	67	6	—
Kano	977	181	133	18	—
Bauchi . . .	845	152	71	6	—
Adamawa . . .	736	210	55	3	—
Bornu	310	32	121	—	—
	3935	734	465	42	—
Northern Guinea vegetation zone					
Zaria	1836	159	154	6	3
Plateau . . .	1012	279	323	42	4
	2848	438	477	48	7
Southern Guinea vegetation zone					
Niger	287	24	85	—	—
Benue	809	98	201	14	2
Ilorin	160	21	48	—	—
	1256	143	334	14	2

† After Glover (1965).

TABLE 5.3

Summary of infections by T. congolense *and* T. vivax *in Northern Nigerian cattle according to vegetation zones*

Infection	Sudan zone	N. Guinea zone	S. Guinea zone	Totals
T. congolense . .	507	525	348	1380
T. vivax . . .	776	486	157	1419
Totals . . .	1283	1011	505	2799
% of T. vivax infections	60·5	48·1	31·1	50·7

Niger, and Benue in the Southern Guinea zone. The last three provinces extend also into the more southerly forest–savanna mosaic or derived savanna vegetation, while Bornu reaches north into the dry Sahel. Glover's figures are rearranged in Table 5.2. There is a slight predominance of *T. vivax* infections in the country as a whole, but the geographical relationships are made more clear in Table 5.3 in which the totals for mixed *T. congolense/T. vivax* infections is added to each of the total of the single infections of these trypanosomes. It is now seen very clearly that, as in Mornet's data, the proportion of *T. vivax* infections decreases as we pass from the dry north to the more humid south. We have, however, no reason as yet to postulate any causal connection with the climatic gradient.

The vivax *ratio*

In Table 5.3 a statistic has been used which is a useful one when discussing the geography of the cattle trypanosomiases. This is the *vivax* ratio which gives the proportion of infections ascribed to that trypanosome expressed as a percentage of the total of *T. vivax* and *T. congolense* diagnoses. When double infections are recorded they are counted as one of each for the purposes of calculating the ratio. The agreement between Mornet's and Glover's data is good. The latter, however, gives no information about the infections in cattle in the forest zones, and Mornet's information is clearly inadequate. The principal reason, of course, is that in forest country one does not find cattle in large numbers and the only animals to be seen are the various types of dwarf cattle. These are of little commercial importance and in any case are tolerant of infection by local strains of trypanosomes. One recent examination of cattle living in the forests or in the savanna derived from forest by cultivation was made by Foster (1963) in Liberia. He took slides from 1765 animals and obtained only 66 infections of which *T. vivax* comprised only 11·8 per cent.

Infections in East African countries

The diagnostic records for outbreaks in Uganda cattle in the 1930s showed a preponderance of infection caused by *T. congolense*. The low *vivax* ratio, characteristic of East Africa, persisted after introduction of widespread drug therapy. Between 1949 and 1956 inclusive (but excluding 1953) the totals of positives from 47 240 slide examinations of cattle were as follows:

T. congolense	*T. vivax*	*T. brucei*	*T. theileri*
1470	817	753	600

The *vivax* ratio here is 35·7 per cent. In Kenya, records published in *Veterinary department annual reports* in 1949 and 1950 and from 1957 to 1961 inclusive gave a *vivax* ratio of 46·6 per cent. In Tanganyika territory (Tanzania) the *vivax* ratio from records of 1412 infections published in

Annual reports between 1948 and 1956 was only 27·2 per cent. Shaw (1958) published incidence figures for various animal trypanosomiases in Zambia (Northern Rhodesia) from which it can be estimated that the *vivax* ratio from 1946 to 1956 was only 7·2 per cent, although in the year 1956–7 this figure had more than doubled to 16·8 per cent. The corresponding figure for that year in Southern Rhodesia was 23·5 per cent (Lawrence and Bryson 1958). These authors obtained the same ratio among 11 300 head of specially sampled cattle in the areas of Chikwizo and Urungwe. Some years later the Southern Rhodesian *vivax* ratio rose, and combined data for the years 1961 and 1962 amounted to 33·0 per cent (Federal Ministry of Agriculture 1962, 1963).

While the limitations of data of this kind must be borne in mind, as well as the difficulties of obtaining complete and accurate diagnoses, the marked downward trend of the *vivax* ratio, as distance southward from the equator increases, is impressive.

Uganda, with a fairly high *vivax* ratio, lies on the glossinological boundary between East and West Africa. In the latter a high *vivax* ratio is associated both with proximity to the more arid north or, perhaps, with the zone in which *G. tachinoides* alone is able to penetrate into a climate intolerable to other tsetses. A large part of the cattle population of Kenya is also pastured in the semi-desert country of its Northern Frontier province, while both it and Uganda have fairly extensive contacts, not with *G. tachinoides*, but with *G. fuscipes*, another widespread tsetse of the *palpalis* group. In short, these two countries that show an intermediate value in their *vivax* ratio share some of the environmental characteristics of Africa west of Cameroon.

The pattern of cattle trypanosomiasis in Uganda

The first of the drugs that subsequently were to alter the whole approach to domestic animal trypanosomiasis first became available in 1949. In Uganda, large-scale block inoculation campaigns were inaugurated during the next half decade. The numbers of slides taken and of those showing the three pathogenic trypanosomes as well as the non-pathogenic *Trypanosoma theileri* are given in Table 5.4. It is divided into two sections. The first summarizes figures published from 1949 to 1955 (but excluding 1953) for seven districts. Five more district figures were published in 1954 and 1955 and these are given separately. In two districts, Mbale and Teso, *T. vivax* infections preponderate and, indeed, in Teso, there were no records of *T. congolense*. The proportion of pathogenic positives to slides examined in these two districts is low; there was little trypanosomiasis of any kind except that due to the harmless *T. theileri*, which, especially in Teso, is more frequent than elsewhere. Differences in the total numbers of blood slides examined in different districts reflect not only the general incidence of local infection, but also local policy regarding the disease. Where

TABLE 5.4

District infections in Uganda, 1949–55†

District	T. congo-lense	T. vivax	T. brucei	T. theileri	Total slides	vivax ratio	Positives (ex. theileri) (%)
(1) Complete period, excluding 1953							
Buganda .	819	388	363	173	14213	32·1	11·0
Busoga .	362	170	159	48	11034	31·9	6·3
Mbale .	38	79	50	122	6609	67·5	2·5
Teso .	—	15	7	214	5967	100	0·4
Lango .	38	22	7	4	889	36·7	7·5
Ankole .	48	10	20	1	763	17·2	10·2
Karamoja	7	1	6	4	246	14·3	5·7
	1312	685	612	566	39721	34·3	6·6
(2) Districts only published for 1954–5							
Kigezi .	48	42	44	12	1246	46·7	10·7
Toro .	74	52	57	6	1770	41·2	10·3
Bunyoro .	1	—	5	2	617	0	1
Acholi .	9	3	—	—	94	25	12·8
West Nile	7	—	—	—	37	0	18·9
	139	97	106	20	3764	41·1	9·1

† *Uganda Veterinary reports.*

infection is widespread and has a high incidence, slides are taken frequently. Where special campaigns were being run, as they were in the early 1950s in Buganda and Busoga, blood examinations were frequent and regular. In other districts the number of slides indicates, in some degree, the interest of the stock owners in the health of their cattle. The figures for Ankole are not complete because at the time trypanosomiasis in that district was only partly under the direct control of the Uganda Veterinary Service (Chapter 9, also Ford and Clifford 1968).

The Uganda infection records show that a high *vivax* ratio is associated with a low overall incidence of pathogenic trypanosomiasis. Under natural conditions this occurs either where there are no *Glossina* at all or only *G. fuscipes*, as in Teso and Mbale districts. The proportion of *T. vivax* infection is also raised when the natural incidence of trypanosomiasis is reduced either by massive campaigns of antrycide injection or by successful attack on the vectors other than *G. fuscipes*.

The cattle population of Busoga district fell from 126 000 head in 1943 to 88 000 in 1949. An antrycide treatment campaign in 1950 was followed by growth of the population to 156 000 head in 1958 (Randall 1958). The

TABLE 5.5

T. congolense *and* T. vivax *infections and totals of negative slides taken in Busoga, 1949–55†*

	T. congolense	T. vivax	vivax ratio	Negative slides	Positive/ negative ratio
1949	172	49	22·2	1278	17·3
1950	6	4	40·0	791	0·01
1951	8	23	74·1	1015	3·0
1952	12	21	63·6	2173	1·5
1953			Figures not available		
1954	92	2	2·1	2403	3·9
1955	52	24	31·6	2952	2·6

† *Uganda Veterinary reports.*

Busoga data are given in Table 5.5. High incidence of infection with a low *vivax* ratio in 1949 changes with drug treatment to a low incidence of infection and high *vivax* ratio in 1950. This persists for two years. The gap in 1953 is unfortunate, because in 1954 and 1955 the total infection incidence (ratio of positive to negative slides) remains low, although by now, especially in 1954, the majority of infections are of *T. congolense* and there is a low *vivax* ratio. After the treatment campaigns it was the practice to treat relapses, which were nearly always due to *T. vivax*, with a second dose of antrycide. This was effective in removing infections from the cattle population as a whole. The relatively few animals that continued to show trypanosomes, among which *T. congolense* predominated, may have been recently infected from the *G. brevipalpis* and *G. pallidipes* fly-belt in the south of Busoga. It will be necessary to continue this discussion of trypanosomiasis in the Busoga cattle in Chapter 16.

West African trade cattle and the *vivax* ratio

More light is thrown upon the proportions of *T. vivax* and *T. congolense* infections by studies of trypanosomiasis in West African trade cattle. These are animals trekked southwards from the tsetse-free pastures of the Sudan and Sahel zones of West Africa, through the *Glossina morsitans* infested Guinea zone, for sale and slaughter in the densely populated areas near to the West African coast where cattle raising is difficult. This cattle trade was reported upon in some detail by Mittendorf and Wilson (1961) and their maps are also reproduced by Wilson, Morris, Lewis, and Krog (1963). From the countries to the west of and including the Republic of Chad that lie along the southern borders of the Sahara, over 500 000 cattle are sent every year, for the most part on the hoof (though some go by rail), to the southern markets. Many still die of trypanosomiasis *en route* or would do if not slaughtered for sale of meat at bargain prices. Those that reach their destination are nearly all infected. The stresses of travel and emaciation from diseases are responsible for the loss of thousands of tons of meat.

Unsworth and Birkett (1952) took a herd of 30 cattle from Kano in Northern Nigeria to Ilorin, south of the Niger river, a distance of 450 miles. Twenty of these animals were given a protective drug injection of antrycide pro-salt at Kano and 10 were used as controls. Of these 10 all became infected and 2 died before the end of the journey, which lasted for 45 days. This was 15 days longer than would normally be taken by trade cattle, but on days on which blood smears were taken the cattle were rested. All the cattle were free of parasites at Kano and remained so until the first infection was observed on day 24, after negative examination on days 4, 8, 14, and 19. Table 5.6 is modified from Unsworth and Birkett's tabulated

TABLE 5.6

Infections observed in ten cattle trekked from Kano to Ilorin in Northern Nigeria†

	Days after leaving Kano					
Observations	24	29	34	39	43	45
T. vivax	1	2	5	7	6	6
T. congolense	—	—	—	1	6	7
T. brucei	—	—	—	6	1	—
Total infections	1	2	5	14	13	13
Negatives	9	8	5	1	0	0
Deaths	—	—	—	—	2	—
Cattle surviving	10	10	10	10	8	8
Double infections	—	—	—	5	5	5

† From Unsworth and Birkett (1952).

results. First observed contact with tsetse (*G. morsitans*) was made on days 12 and 13, and from day 26 onward the herd was subject to a severe challenge from the same tsetse plus *G. palpalis* and *G. tachinoides* at river crossings and an occasional *G. longipalpis*. The first animal to show an infection evidently received it on days 12 or 13, and parasitaemia may have been patent at any time after the negative examination on day 19. From the infective bite to the appearance of trypanosomes in this first case could have been at most 12 days and at least 7. The second infection, observed on day 29, if received during the first contact with *G. morsitans* could have taken between 11 and 17 days to appear, or, though this is unlikely, if received on the second entry into tsetse bush on day 26, only 3 days. On day 34, with 5 animals positive, 3 of these might have been infected 8 days earlier on day 26. So far all infections had been of *T. vivax* (save for a single, transitory *T. theileri* infection in one animal on day 24). The *vivax* ratio on this more northerly portion of the route was 100 per cent.

On day 39 there was a sudden appearance of six infections of *T. brucei*, plus two more of *T. vivax*, and the first *T. congolense*. The *vivax* ratio was reduced to 87·5. On day 43 *T. brucei* had nearly disappeared from the peripheral circulations and the *vivax* ratio was reduced by the appearance of *T. congolense* in 6 out of 8 surviving cattle to 50 per cent. On reaching Ilorin all surviving cattle were infected; none showed *T. brucei*, but *T. congolense* now predominated to give a *vivax* ratio of 46·2 per cent. If the numbers of positive diagnoses made are added up, a typical West African picture again emerges: *T. vivax* 56, *T. congolense* 29, and *T. brucei* 15 per cent.

Godfrey, Killick-Kendrick, and Ferguson (1965) repeated Unsworth and Birkett's work on a larger scale. Their diagnostic methods were more precise for they inoculated blood from their cattle into rats as well as examining stained smears. Simultaneously a survey was made of the tsetse flies encountered on the route from Jibiya, near Katsina close to the Nigerian boundary with the Republic of Niger, south to Ilorin, a distance of 415 miles. In this survey samples of tsetse caught were dissected to obtain estimates of their infections with *T. vivax* and *T. congolense* (Jordan 1965c). The experimental herd of 30 animals was trekked along the trade route at the speed normally followed by trade cattle, except that two days of rest were interposed to enable more detailed examinations of the animals to be undertaken. They were thus 28 days *en route*. Unsworth and Birkett had rested their cattle on 15 days and took 45 days along a route somewhat different, except on the last section after crossing the Niger river.

T. vivax was first seen on the 24th day of the trek and *T. brucei* on day 28. *T. congolense*, however, was not seen until day 37. Infection might have been acquired in a sparse infestation of *G. morsitans* traversed on days 13 and 14 although dense populations of this tsetse were not met with until day 20. Essentially the two experiments give the same result. They show that where in West Africa infection comparisons are based on examinations of southward trekking slaughter stock, the geographical zonation in trypanosome records may be an effect of differences in the prepatent periods for the three species and to the comparatively brief life of *T. brucei* in the peripheral circulation.

Effects of drug treatment on the *T. vivax* ratio

Boyt, Lovemore, Pilson, and Smith (1962) introduced 10 cattle into a mixed *G. morsitans* and *G. pallidipes* fly-belt in Rhodesia. The animals were examined daily and treated with the drug berenil as soon as trypanosomes appeared in the blood. Under this regime the *vivax* ratio was 97·6 per cent. In untreated cattle the mean prepatent period of *T. vivax* was 20·7 days. When the infection was allowed to persist without treatment, *T. congolense* appeared with a mean prepatent period of 32·2 days.

The *vivax* ratio can therefore be influenced by the frequency of treatment, for if blood examinations are made sufficiently often and the appearance of trypanosomes is followed by cure, *T. congolense* and *T. brucei* will not have the opportunity to show themselves.

Infections in tsetse: the climatic correlations

The incidence of tsetse-borne trypanosomiasis of any kind must be related to its incidence in the vector. The results of many surveys, made over a period of 45 years, in which some 66 000 *Glossina morsitans*, 14 000 *G. pallidipes*, and 8000 *G. austeni* were dissected, were reviewed by Ford and Leggate (1961).

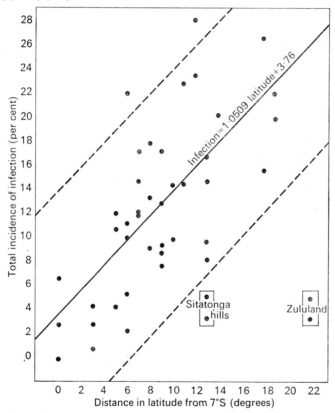

FIG. 5.1. Correlation between percentage of the tsetse populations infected with trypanosomes and distance from the *Glossina* equator. The points for the Sitatonga hills and for Zululand are omitted from the regression.

$$r = 0·6990. \qquad P < 0·001.$$

They showed that a positive correlation exists between gross infection rates (all species of trypanosome combined) and distance from the median (7°S.) of the *Glossina* belt in Africa as a whole. This correlation, they suggested, was in fact a correlation with increasing mean annual temperature, which rises with greater distance from the equator, as far as the tropics, although greatly modified locally by orographic features and other elements affecting climate. Thus the positive correlation with distance from the *Glossina* equator breaks down in Zululand and in the Sitatonga hills in Mozambique but not when infection rates are plotted against temperature (Figs. 5.1 and 5.2).

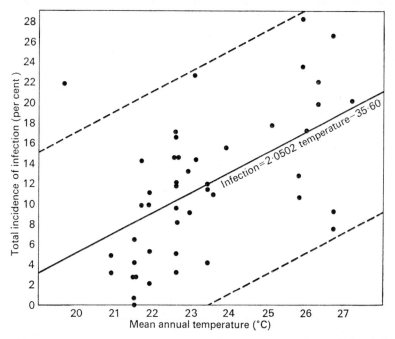

FIG. 5.2. Correlation between percentage of *morsitans* group tsetse-fly populations infected with trypanosomes and mean annual temperature.

$r = 0.5416.$ $P < 0.001.$

These correlations were to be expected. Burtt (1946*a*), Fairbairn and Culwick (1950), and Fairbairn and Watson (1955) had all demonstrated that tsetse bred in the laboratory were more easily infected when they had emerged from puparia that had been incubated at high temperatures (at 30°C rather than at the customary 27°).

Even so it was difficult to believe that temperature could alone be responsible for maintaining the levels of the infection rates. The tsetse receives its infection from a mammal host and various authors had drawn a conclusion similar to that of Ashcroft (1959*b*) that 'Both the number of infected tsetse and the species of trypanosome with which they are infected will be found to be related to their hosts.' It was therefore supposed that if temperature controls the predisposition of the *Glossina* population to infection local variations may well result from the differences in the wild animal populations in different areas.

Influence of the natural hosts of trypanosomes upon infection rates in *Glossina*

Leggate (1962) failed to demonstrate any direct relationship between changes in mean monthly temperatures and the infection rates in *Glossina morsitans* and *G. pallidipes* at Rekomitje in the Zambezi valley in Southern Rhodesia. Instead she found that during the rainy months of December to March (total rainfall 25·2 in) the infection rates were significantly lower than in the remainder of the year (total rainfall 1·0 in). High temperatures at the end of the dry season had no influence upon the infections in *Glossina* in the subsequent rains. Evidently other factors obscured the direct effects of climate. Leggate showed, as had earlier workers, that two species of tsetse fly living in the same area could have significantly different infection rates. In particular she demonstrated a marked contrast between the infections of *G. morsitans* collected in evergreen woodland growing along the banks of the Rekomitje river and the infections of the same tsetse collected in a nearby area of mopane (*Colophospermum mopane*) woodland. In the former the infection rate rose from 21 to 31·5 per cent between June and September and then dropped rapidly to 10 per cent in November. Flies in the mopane woodland, however, showed a falling infection rate, from 11 to 5 per cent between June and September, and thereafter rose to 19 per cent in December. For the rest of the year (January to May) infection rates in both communities fluctuated irregularly between 7·5 and 18 per cent, without any significant trends or differences between the fly populations of the two vegetation communities. It was only in the dry months that the opposing trends were evident.

There was no direct information available about what the Rekomitje flies were feeding on. However, by re-analysing blood meal data obtained in the Lubu valley (which, although some two hundred miles away from Rekomitje has a similar fauna and flora) Leggate demonstrated that the ratios of feeds from Bovidae and from Suidae and other mammals produced a seasonal curve which was a very close parallel to her Rekomitje tsetse infection rate curve. This suggested that her high infection rate in riverine tsetse in the hot weather was a direct consequence of a diet in which Bovidae predominated, and the lower infection rate of the wet season to a diet in which Suidae were the most frequent food source.

Jordan (1964) studied trypanosome incidence in *G. m. submorsitans* in Nigeria, adding the results of his own surveys to those of earlier workers, especially Lloyd and Johnson (1924). Like Leggate he was unable to demonstrate any positive correlation with local temperature. In particular he examined infections in three places, Mando and Gamagira in the Northern Guinea zone, and Yankari in the sub-Sudan zone. Flies from Yankari, a game reserve, showed a significantly higher infection rate than flies from Mando and Gamagira which did not differ significantly from each other. On the other hand, *T. congolense* infections were proportionally more frequent at Gamagira in relation to *T. vivax* than at either of the other places.

Jordan now related his infection data to the blood meal analyses of gorged flies collected at each place (Table 5.7). With regard to *T. congolense* infections at Gamagira, he drew attention to the high proportion there of

TABLE 5.7

Infections in and natural hosts of G. m. submorsitans in three areas of Northern Nigeria†

	Gamagira	Mando	Yankari
% flies infected with trypanosomes . .	3·0	5·0	12·0
% feeds on			
Bovidae . . .	8·6	15·5	52·8
Primates . . .	14·4	17·7	0·9
Suidae . . .	66·6	51·2	33·3
% *congolense* group trypanosomes amongst infected flies . .	81·2	44·8	36·8

† After Jordan (1964).

blood meals from Suidae (in this case warthogs) and suggested that the *Nannomonas* type infections contained not only *T. congolense* but many *T. simiae*, a trypanosome particularly associated with pigs and known to occur at Gamagira. Ashcroft, Burtt, and Fairbairn (1959) had shown that infections of *T. brucei* remained positive in the blood of various antelopes for long periods, but that although Suidae could be infected, trypanosomes were only rarely found in their blood. Jordan's own earlier work (Jordan 1961) had shown that trypanosomes were most abundant in those species of *Glossina* that obtained most of their food from Bovidae.

His general conclusion was that the low rates of infection at Mando and Gamagira did not fit the pattern demanded by the temperature correlation because Bovidae (other than the duiker, *Sylvicapra grimmia*, which is seldom fed upon by any tsetse) were extremely rare. At Yankari, where the overall infection rate fits the diagrams of Ford and Leggate, wild Bovidae were readily available. Thus locally the incidence of trypanosome infection in the principal food host will override the influence of temperature on the receptivity of the insect to infection. Jordan's study therefore supported Leggate's deductions as to the importance of the Bovidae in controlling the general level of infection in *G. morsitans* and the relative lack of importance of the Suidae.

When assessing the influence of climate and diet in determining incidence of infection in tsetse, it is necessary to recall Harley's (1966a and 1966b) demonstration that incidence is higher in populations of long mean life than in those that are short-lived. This correlation with age was reflected in seasonal change, for more flies were infected in or just after the rains, when life expectation is long, than at other seasons when it is shorter. Mean age reflects the rate at which the insects are living and this, in turn, is also a response to climate.

Distribution of trypanosomiasis in wild animals

A crude picture of the variations in patterns of *T. vivax* and *T. congolense* type infections in the continental population of cattle can be visualized. It is doubtful if this could be done for sheep and goats, and with swine the only sure fact is that trypanosomiasis of domestic pigs is unlikely to be seen in Muslim regions. Is there any evidence of geographical variation in the infection incidence in populations of wild animals?

When the causal organism of human trypanosomiasis in the Zambezi basin and its environs was declared to be a separate species and it was obvious that it must be transmitted by tsetse of the *morsitans* group because *Glossina 'palpalis'* was absent from the region, considerable alarm was felt. This alarm was not lessened when one expert suggested that human trypanosomiasis might even be spread through South Africa by mechanical transmission through *Stomoxys*. General Botha, then Prime Minister of the Transvaal, put pressure upon the British South Africa Company to take appropriate steps to deal with the menace in the territories for which it had assumed responsibility (Gelfand 1961). A team was sent to Northern Rhodesia (Zambia) by the Liverpool School of Tropical Medicine. Its members set themselves the task of comparing infection incidences at two climatically contrasted stations. They showed that the incidence of infection in *G. morsitans* was lower at Ngoa, the cooler of the two stations, and they estimated that some 35 per cent of the local animals carried trypanosomes in their blood. At Newalia, in the Lwangwa valley, already a well recognized focus of rhodesian infection, 50 per cent of the animals were infected and the infection incidence in *G. morsitans* was also high. By inoculating blood from 56 different animals shot near Newalia into monkeys or rats, they obtained 9 infections, but blood from 60 animals shot around Ngoa only yielded 2 infections (Kinghorn, Yorke, and Lloyd 1913).

Enough has been said in Chapter 4 to show that results of this nature should be interpreted with caution. One other variable not appreciated in 1913 that may or may not have affected the outcome of these early experiments is that Ngoa and Newalia are infested by different subspecies of *G. morsitans*.

The effects of technique upon the diagnostic outcome of examination of cattle blood has been stressed. No doubt variations due to similar causes affect the data given in Table 4.2. However, this table summarizes nearly all the information available. Most of the surveys on which it was based took place between 3°N. and 7°S. but it also includes data collected by Sir David Bruce and his colleagues in Malawi at about the same time that the

TABLE 5.8

Infections of all trypanosome species in wild animals obtained (A) by Bruce et al. (1913) in Malawi and (B) by other workers elsewhere†

	(A)			(B)		
Genus	*No. examined*	*No. infected*	*% infected*	*No. examined*	*No. infected*	*% infected*
Tragelaphus .	10	7	70	45	10	22
Kobus . .	13	9	69	97	48	49
Strepsiceros .	3	2	67	37	16	43
Redunca . .	19	12	63	20	5	25
Taurotragus .	10	6	60	53	12	23
Sylvicapra .	7	2	29	34	4	12
Syncerus .	9	2	22	78	4	5
Phacochoerus .	33	7	21	121	8	7
Alcephalus .	35	6	17	41	4	10
Ourebia . .	26	4	15	4	0	0

† Lumsden (1962), omitting Bruce's data.

Liverpool team was working in Zambia. A comparison can therefore be made between the incidence of infection (by any species of trypanosome) in the Malawi collection and the data remaining in Table 4.2 after Bruce's data have been extracted. Only genera common to both collections can be compared and this is done in Table 5.8. Again the data must be interpreted with many reservations, but the consistency with which the infection rates obtained in the more southerly habitat exceed those obtained elsewhere is impressive as is the similarity in the order of magnitude of infection rates in each list (Bruce, Harvey, Hamerton, Davey, and Bruce 1913, Lumsden 1962).

Collections of stabilates of trypanosomes from various sources are now being made at several centres. In due course, parasitologists may evolve a system of classification based upon the immunological and serological properties of the flagellates, upon their infectivity to different hosts, and upon their pathogenic properties as well as their morphology. When this has been done it will be possible to look again at the problem of the geographical distribution of tsetse-borne trypanosomes and the diseases they cause, whether in wildlife, in domestic stock, or in man.

The distribution of the human infections

Many maps have been made to show the distribution of human trypanosomiasis in Africa. A recent example is that of Potts (in Ady 1965). It shows the rhodesian disease variously distributed in large or small areas from the Okovango delta in Botswana north-east to the Zambezi valley and thence into Mozambique, or northward through Zambia into Western Tanzania and so to the northern corner of Lake Victoria. Quite recently the first cases have been diagnosed in western Ethiopia (Balis and Bergeon 1968). The gambian infection is also shown just north of Lake Victoria in small, isolated pockets. Moving westwards into the Congo the infected areas become larger, until passing into West Africa almost the whole of the area of countries west of Nigeria is shown to be infected. Perhaps if this map were to be redrawn now it would show the eastern or rhodesian area divided into two, with the southern portion, comprising at least the central Zambezi valley and Botswana, infected with a separate strain (Ormerod 1967).

6

ENVIRONMENTAL CONTEXTS OF
THE SAMPLE AREAS:
INTRODUCTION TO FIVE NARRATIVES

IT is useful, as an introduction, to bring together some of the natural links between the five sample areas in which the history and ecology of trypanosomiasis is to be described. Selection is necessary and super-ficiality of treatment is unavoidable. Although the three areas in the Victoria basin are very different in character, they are biologically and environmentally linked and this linkage can be extended to cover the other more remote sample areas of Rhodesia and Nigeria. Other connections will emerge in the course of the various narratives.

A brief account of the major events contributing to the evolution of the Victoria basin is followed by an even more brief glance at its climate. These sections provide an introduction to a consideration of the distributions of some of the tsetse species of the region, and their connections in time and space with the fly-belts of Rhodesia and Nigeria. In the chapters that follow it will emerge that these five sample areas share much that is common in their recent biological history. The concluding chapters will take up again this problem of the common ground of tsetse-borne disease in lands thousands of miles apart. At present it seems not impossible that epidemics and epizootics as violent as any that accompanied the beginnings of the colonial era may yet also follow rapidly upon its closure. On the other hand in many respects independence appears to offer conditions far more favourable for progress in the struggle with zoonotic infection than any that obtained under the most benevolent of colonial regimes.

Geology and topography of the Lake Victoria basin

Lake Victoria lies at 3717 ft above sea level. In the extreme north-west of the interlake area (Chapters 7–10), the peaks of Ruwenzori rise to 16 794 ft, more than 2000 ft above its own snow line. To its south-east, Sukuma-land (Chapters 11–13) drops down to Lake Eyassi below 3500 ft (Map 6.1). Although the main features of the Victoria basin have received their present-day form chiefly as a result of changes that have taken place since the Miocene, its rocks belong to periods of immense antiquity. The Pre-Cambrian series are divided into several age categories, three of which underlie the greater part of the basin.

Both north-eastern Ankole, invaded as recently as 1958 by *Glossina*

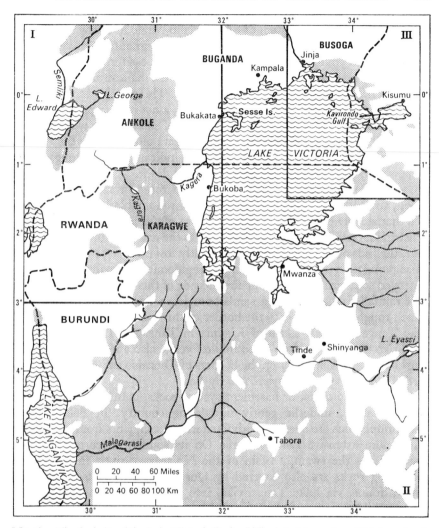

MAP 6.1. The fly-belts of the Lake Victoria Basin. I The interlake region; II Sukumaland III Busoga and Nyanza.

morsitans, and Sukumaland in the south where the *G. morsitans* and *G. swynnertoni* fly-belts are receding, are underlain by a basement system or complex of Pre-Cambrian rocks. Laid down originally as sediments beneath vast seas thousands of millions of years ago, they were folded, eroded, and intruded by later igneous rocks to form, over a period of some 3 000 million years, a rock layer of immense depth which forms the basic framework of the continent.

The great hills of north-west Ankole, overlooking the Western Rift, are formed from Pre-Cambrian rocks of the Nyanzian system of somewhat lesser age, 1800–2800 million years. Nyanzian rocks also to some extent interrupt the basement system of Sukumaland, while in Busoga (Chapters 14–16) they are widely overlain by later intrusive granites.

A third, still younger, series of Pre-Cambrian rocks forms the steep hills of Karagwe and southern Ankole and provides the main structural basis for the *G. morsitans* fly-belt in the interlake zone. These rocks were called by Speke (1863) 'beef-sandwich clay sandstones', a not inappropriate description for the alternating pink and white bands of shales and phyllites which they display. They are about 1000 million years old and form the Muva–Ankolean system. Stromatolites (fossil algae) indicate the beginnings of life in the seas beneath which they were first laid down.

Lastly, the youngest of the Pre-Cambrian rocks in the Lake Victoria region, the Bukoban system, is named from the double line of sandstone hills that steeply overlook the western shore of the lake. By confining the lacustrine forests of this high rainfall zone to the narrow shores beneath the cliffs, the hills of Bukoba contributed greatly towards the protection of the dense population of that region from the epidemic of trypanosomiasis that destroyed southern Busoga in the first decade of this century. South of this high rainfall area the Bukoba sandstones leave the Victoria margin and stretch roughly south-west to the border of Burundi to reach the shores of Lake Tanganyika just south of Kigoma in Tanzania. These upper pre-Cambrian rocks, of age 500–1000 million years, also appear in the neighbourhood of the Mara river on the borders of Tanzania and Kenya near the northern limit of the *G. swynnertoni* fly-belt.

In general the oldest or basement system rocks, both south of the lake and in Ankole, underlie gently undulating country. In Sukumaland, these undulations are overlain with Quaternary sediments from a formerly much more extensive Lake Victoria. On its south-west corner the lake basin adjoins the swampy basin of the Malagarasi river, in which the underlying rocks are also covered by Quaternary sediments. This river system drains, via Lake Tanganyika, into the basin of the Congo. The watershed between it and the Victoria basin plays an important role in the history of trypanosomiasis in Sukumaland.

Also of comparatively recent date are the volcanoes along the eastern wall of the Western Rift. The smaller of two volcanic areas, now inactive, lies on either side of the Kazinga channel between Lake Edward and Lake George in the north-west corner of the interlake zone. Here the country is pitted with craters, many of them with a small lake at the bottom. The larger area contains the Virunga volcanoes, on the border of Rwanda, Congo, and Uganda. They rise to great heights (Karisimbe 13 728 ft) and some are still active. They make an immense barrier of lava across the Rift Valley behind which Lake Kivu is dammed. On the east of Lake Victoria extinct volcanoes and volcanic soils help to determine the form of the *G. pallidipes* belts around the Kavirondo gulf and so contribute to the geography of the series of epidemics and outbreaks of sleeping sickness that have beset that region since 1901.

The topographical forms into which these various rocks have been shaped and which determine the appearance of the modern landscape derive mostly from three processes, warping of the earth's surface, rifting, and erosion, which have continued sometimes with greater and sometimes with lesser intensity from the Jurassic onwards into the Pleistocene.

Faulting had already occurred along the line of the Western Rift in the immensely long period of the Pre-Cambrian. The faulting that took place twice in post-Jurassic times followed the earlier lines. Another period of rift faulting was quite recent. The vast block of Mount Ruwenzori arose by an upthrust of rocks of the basement and Nyanzian systems in Quaternary times. Although Mount Ruwenzori hardly lies within the interlake zone, since it overhangs Lakes Edward and George from the north, the main floor of the Western Rift passes to the west of it and forms the valley of the Semliki river running north from Lake Edward into Lake Albert. It is the geographical starting point to one of the epidemic spreads of trypanosomiasis with which this account is concerned.

Lake Victoria had its origin in extensive warping of the earth's surface during the Miocene period. Before this event the great basin that later became the Congo extended further to the east and its rivers had their origins in a watershed in Kenya and Tanzania. A downward warping trapped the upper sources of these rivers and reversed the direction of flow of their middle courses. In Uganda, the Kafu and Katonga rivers that had once run westwards into the Congo basin now ran east, the one to fill up the newly drowned valleys of the Kyoga lakes, the other into the new-formed Victoria basin. The Kagera river, which was to become the largest influent of the lake, was also reversed and its new headwaters, now cut off by upthrust in the centre of the interlake zone which was a compensating movement for the down-warping of the Victoria basin, built up into a series of lakes and swamps before cutting back through the narrow gorge along which, between 1907 and 1913, *G. morsitans* moved west into Mutara in north-west Rwanda. The Miocene warping that reversed these rivers occurred after the first of the post-Jurassic tectonic movements that led to the formation of the Rift Valley, but before that which gave the valley its final form.

While these two processes of rifting and warping were taking place over some 600 million years, though mostly in the last 100 million, four great cycles of erosion occurred. These successively flattened the surface of the country which, in the intervals, was again broken up under the various tectonic forces already noted. The surfaces of ancient peneplains are most easily observed in the flat-topped hills of Central Uganda and in the level crests of the hill ranges of the interlake zone. Associated with the processes of alternate peneplain formation and erosion is that of laterization.

Laterites are formed in hot wet climates with hot dry intervals in which evaporation is intense. Under these conditions weak solutions produced by leaching from underlying rocks are concentrated and redissolved. This process extracts the more soluble salts but leaves the less soluble, especially hydroxides of iron and aluminium, near the surface. Here they accumulate as a reddish deposit of laterite which, in contact with the air, becomes very hard and may eventually form a shield several feet thick.

Laterites are important in determining the pattern of the tsetse-fly habitat in many areas, principally because the soil overlying them is shallow, or sometimes has been completely washed away. They therefore break up the otherwise even distribution of trees and shrubs and are covered by open grassland. Laterites and other formations associated with impeded drainages, where trees cannot grow, are often important in creating the patterns of host animal and tsetse behaviour described in Chapter 2 as having led to the concept of 'feeding grounds'.

The pattern of *Glossina morsitans* distribution in the Muva–Ankolean hills of Karagwe and Ankole is also influenced by the distribution of ancient laterite shields. Probably during a sub-Miocene peneplanation, under a hot wet climate, lateritic shields were formed in the valley floors. In a later cycle of erosion the intervening hills were flattened once more so that when peneplanation was complete, strips of laterite alternating with strips of rock not covered by laterite, marked the positions of earlier valleys and hills respectively. With the recommencement of intense erosion in the late-Tertiary the laterite shield of the former valley floors gave protection to the rocks beneath them. The erosive forces now acted upon the alternating exposed rocks which were worn away to produce valleys lying between flat-topped, laterite-capped hills (Fig. 6.1). It lightened the burden of exploring the patterns of tsetse-fly distribution in these great hills to appreciate a little how the framework on which those patterns were arranged had developed over such an immensity of time.

In this very cursory account of the geological background of the Victoria basin one has thought of the processes described as providing the environmental framework upon which the pattern of disease has evolved. But before passing on to look at other factors that have contributed to the geography of that pattern, there remains to note the significance of certain aspects of recent geology and palaeontology.

In the north-east corner of Lake Victoria, at the entrance to the Kavirondo gulf, lies Rusinga island. Here, in deposits of the lower Miocene, were discovered the remains of the ape *Proconsul*. If the account of the zoogeography of *Glossina* and of its development as a vector of salivarian trypanosomes given in Chapter 3 approximates to what in fact happened, then it may be supposed that the evolution of man from terrestrial apes took place over the same period and, perhaps, in the same environment. Man is refractory to all trypanosomes save some rarer strains of *T. brucei*; the

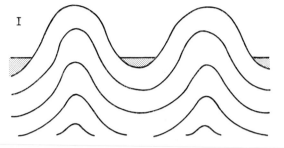

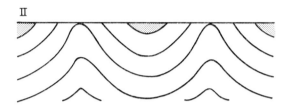

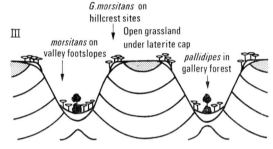

FIG. 6.1. Highly schematic diagram to illustrate formation of the geological substrate of *G. morsitans* and *G. pallidipes* distribution in Karagwe. I Folding of Pre-Cambrian sediments and formation of laterites in valleys; II Peneplanation; III Erosion with laterite caps acting as protection.

baboon is refractory to all. The similarity of response to infection in these two distantly related primates may have its origin in the adjustments to infection that the ancestors of both had to make in descending from an arboreal to a terrestrial habitat. The discoveries at Rusinga, at Olduvai (just outside the limits of Sukumaland), and elsewhere in East Africa at least show that prehistory does not nullify the hypothesis. Of equal significance are the remains in these and other sites, particularly the Kaiso deposits around Lakes Albert and Edward, of many species of larger mammals, extinct as well as modern. They include no single specimen of any animal that could be regarded as ancestral to the domestic ox, and so confirm the evidence from other sources that cattle entered tropical Africa in recent times and probably not more than 2000–3000 years ago. Domestic

animals have by no means reached the same degree of adjustment to trypanosome infection as has been achieved by man.

Climate and land use

The general pattern of tropical climate is controlled by the movement of
the inter-tropical convergence zone of low pressure that moves north and
south and back again in response to the seasonal change in relative position
of the earth and sun. The trade winds are drawn into this moving equatorial trough, bringing rain with them. In the Lake Victoria basin, as in
many other parts of East Africa, pronounced topographical features, the
mountains, the great Rift Valley faults, and the large water surfaces of the
lakes all break up and warp this basic weather pattern.

Total rainfall varies considerably. On the west of the lake the town of
Bukoba, with 80 in of rain, just falls within a band of high rainfall
centred over the Sesse islands. This zone of higher rainfall extends north-
east to cover most of the second sample area of Busoga and the adjoining
Nyanza province of Kenya, but here has already fallen to a mean of
50–60 in. The northern limit of this area, at the level of Tororo, where
the present East African Trypanosomiasis Research Laboratory is built,
is also influenced by the neighbourhood of Mount Elgon, fifty miles to the
north-east.

Westward from Bukoba the mean annual rainfall is halved in a distance
of 20 miles and the spread of *G. morsitans*, described in Chapter 9, has
taken place in country enjoying 25–35 in of rain running from north to
south through the middle of the interlake region. Further west the wet
climate associated with the eastern wall of the Western Rift, which limits the
potential area of spread of *G. morsitans*, is sharply broken in the valley south
of Mount Ruwenzori to provide a narrow channel of arid climate overlying
what were once the pastures of Busongora, and now form the centre of
the tsetse-infested Queen Elizabeth national park. On the west of the Rift
Valley, the edge of the high rainfall area of the Congo basin is encountered.

South of the lake, Sukumaland provides the driest of the three sample
areas. On its northern limits the lake shore lies between the 40- and 50-inch
isohyets, but the greater part of this densely populated region enjoys about
30 in of rain a year. In its extreme south-east a zone of arid country, with
less than 20 in annually, overlooks Lake Eyassi from the north.

It is frequently pointed out that what is important in comparing precipitation in two areas is not its total amount, but its distribution throughout the year and its reliability. Thus, although the mean annual rainfalls
of Sukumaland and of the central zone of the interlake region are much the
same, the latter may expect precipitation to exceed 30 in in four years out
of five, but in Sukumaland this expectation applies only to excesses over
20 in. In the Busoga–Nyanza fly-belts, for the most part, the inhabitants may expect to receive 40–50 in in 80 per cent of years.

Rainfall probabilities in relation to tsetse distribution in East Africa have been examined briefly. Of the total land surface of Uganda, Kenya, and Tanzania (640 080 mile^2) about 280 000 or 43 per cent were infested by *Glossina* in 1958. Land with a good prospect of obtaining 30 in of rain, which will permit of arable farming, formed only 10 per cent of the fly-belts. Land with a poor prospect of obtaining 30 in, on which arable farming was unlikely to succeed commercially, formed 34 per cent of the fly-belts (Ford 1958b). The intermediate 56 per cent of tsetse-infested bush occupied areas 'where the indifferent reliability of a 30 inch rainfall produces marginal conditions of a kind which do not necessarily preclude arable farming, but which place distinct limitations on the likelihood of its success' (East African Royal Commission 1955).

One of the principal points that will emerge from this study is that much of the deterioration in the situation of the tsetse-borne diseases that has taken place during the last century has been a consequence of large-scale depopulation brought about by other diseases or by social disorganization followed by famines. Where officials concerned with projects to eliminate tsetse have been most successful and their efforts have been followed by favourable responses in rural development, they have generally been operating in land which was occupied in recent historical times. Often, however, there has been no response because the practical glossinologist must, of necessity, operate in land that is either marginal, poor, or bad. This trend will, inevitably, become more pronounced, for many of the residual foci of infection are located on land that for one reason or another is unusable.

Climate influences, but does not always fully control, the usages to which its occupants put their land. The main forms of agriculture practised in the sample areas will emerge in the following narratives, but in underdeveloped countries the economic and ecological pressures have not, except in a few instances, reached a level which forces the inhabitants to a full exploitation, by whatever techniques they may command, of the terrain. The usages to which land is put may derive from historical as well as environmental factors. The point was well made in a study by Beguin (1960) on the land use practices of five ethnic groups in a comparatively small area in the southern Congo, where neither climate nor soils could afford any explanation for marked variations in human population density. The overriding factor was the social and historical role of the dominant tribe. Such factors greatly influenced the course of events to be described in the interlake region.

The tsetse belts

In Chapter 3 a broad outline of the distribution of the main groups of tsetses was provided, and in the narratives to follow further details will be given. Also in Chapter 3 the attempt was made to view the evolution of the genus *Glossina* and the pattern of its present distribution as a single process that was related, also, to the evolution and distribution of the trypanosomes. It seems desirable to attempt a similar outline for the small portion of this process which is in progress around Lake Victoria and, at the same time, to draw attention to its relationship with the situations described in Rhodesia and in Nigeria.

Glossina fuscipleuris provides a convenient and illuminating starting point. It is found in the interlake region in the forests that clothe the wall of the Rift Valley overlooking Lake George. Until recently it appeared from maps of tsetse distribution in Uganda that *G. fuscipleuris* and *G. fusca* were both somewhat indiscriminately to be found in forests overlooking Lakes Edward, George, and Albert, and that they linked across the valley to the tsetse of the Ituri forests to the north of Ruwenzori. They were, in short, part of the peripheral Congo tsetse population. Quite recently Wooff (1968) has prepared a map which shows clearly that in this Rift wall fly-belt, through most of which *G. pallidipes* and *G. fuscipes* are to be found, the distribution of *G. fuscipleuris* is quite separate from that of *G. fusca*. The former reaches from the south up to the line of the road between Fort Portal and Mubende; the latter comes down from the north as far as this road. There is no obvious climatic, vegetation, or faunal barrier and the only natural feature that coincides, more or less, with the divide between the two species is the watershed between the Muzizi river basin, draining into the southern end of Lake Albert, and the basins of the Mpanga and Katonga rivers draining respectively into Lake George and Lake Victoria. There is nothing topographically spectacular about this watershed.

The Uganda and Tanzania tsetse maps also show that although *G. brevipalpis* reaches up through the interlake zone as far as the Kagera river at 1°S., it does not cross the barrier of the hills in south-west Ankole and the neighbouring district of Kigezi to overlap with *G. fuscipleuris* on the Rift wall. *G. brevipalpis* in the Kagera valley feeds on hippopotamus and is found on both banks of this not very wide river. An animal that has not been able to cross it is the rhinoceros, very common until recently in Karagwe south of the river but absent from Ankole, and indeed only appearing in Uganda in northern districts adjoining the Sudan.

Elsewhere, *G. fuscipleuris* may overlap with *G. brevipalpis*, for example in the valley of the Lukuga river and the forests on the slopes of the Mitumba mountains west of Lake Tanganyika and even just south of Lake Edward around Rutshuru (Evens 1953). This latter record suggests that it is still possible that *G. brevipalpis* may be found in the Rift Valley forests of Uganda in the same locality, but that the valley of the Kagera does mark its northern limit in most of the interlake region seems to be well established.

In the same way, although the boundary between *G. fuscipleuris* and *G.*

fusca on the Muzizi–Mpanga watershed seems to be quite clearly defined, yet on the western side of the Rift Valley the two species overlap along the northern edge of the Congo forest as far west as the Cameroon Republic.

There is little doubt that the district of Ankole lies in a region of well-marked biogeographical discontinuity. Moving northwards from the *Brachystegia* woodlands of western Tanzania one sees that commoner species disappear one by one. *Brachystegia* and *Julbernardia* indeed cease on the line of the Bukoba sandstone hills that have been noted as running south-west between Lake Victoria and Lake Tanganyika. Other common or spectacular trees of the *miombo* reach northward through Karagwe as far as the Kagera valley. One of these is *Afrormosia angolensis* which may be encountered not infrequently a few miles south of the Kagera but was not recorded among the trees of the Uganda Protectorate by Eggeling and Dale (1951). An early paper by the German forester Holtz (1911) mentions it by its local name in the Minziro forest just north of this river, in the portion of Tanzania bounded by latitude 1°S. The small but spectacular *Dalbergia nitidula*, a not uncommon flowering tree of the *miombo*, has just succeeded in reaching across the river into Ankole. White (1962) has discussed this 'Lake Victoria interval' as it affects the distribution of the widely spread forest and forest-edge evergreen tree, *Diospyros mespiliformis*, commonly found in Northern, Central, and Eastern Uganda, but missing from the interlake area, although common in the central and southern portions of the western *miombo*.

It appears probable that this gap had its origin in diastrophisms and climatic changes during the orogenic phase of the Quaternary (Boughey 1957). In the neighbourhood of Uganda and Lake Victoria it divided the great *miombo* woodland into two. The greater portion belongs to the south and east, with its abundant species of *Brachystegia* and *Julbernardia*. The West African Northern Guinea zone, that stretches from the West Nile district of Uganda westwards to Senegal is dominated by the very closely related *Isoberlinia doka* and *I. dalzielli*. With this separation came the splitting of *Glossina morsitans* to form the northern and western *G. morsitans submorsitans* and the southern and eastern *G. morsitans morsitans* and *G. morsitans centralis*.

It is of some significance to note that by 1960 the latter subspecies, in its rapid spread to the north described in Chapter 9, had reached to about 60 miles south of the eastern extremity of the West African *G. morsitans submorsitans*. In about 1890 the gap must have been in the neighbourhood of 260 or even as much as 400 miles. Whether or not these East and West African fly-belts might have united but for the efforts of the Uganda Tsetse Control Division is a matter for speculation only. But the rapid move towards union showed that whatever natural features in the past brought about the division of the subspecies, their continued separation during the long period before the biological catastrophe of the colonial impact was sustained by human activity, aided perhaps by elephants, in controlling vegetation and faunal successions.

Glossina fuscipleuris east of Lake Victoria

In 1913, Woosnam (1914) collected a number of large tsetses in the south-west corner of the Masai reserve in Kenya near where the Mara river crosses the Tanzania border. These proved to be *Glossina fuscipleuris*. Later Lewis (1934, 1937, and 1939) added much to our knowledge of the species in the area and showed that not only did they infest the gallery forests near the headwaters of the Mara river, but also of the Oyani river, an upper tributary of the Kuja and Migori rivers. Some attention will be given to this area in Chapter 16, for in it there are five species of tsetse, *G. fuscipleuris*, *G. brevipalpis*, *G. pallidipes*, *G. swynnertoni*, and *G. fuscipes*, and both the rhodesian and the gambian forms of human trypanosomiasis have been and continue to be diagnosed.

G. fuscipleuris on the Mara–Oyani headwaters is chiefly of interest because it is almost certain that there is no intermediate infestation between it and that found on the hills of north-west Ankole. It must be regarded as a relic of a much wider distribution that no longer survives.

Buxton (1955) mapped, unfortunately without comment or reference, a single record of *G. fuscipleuris* near the border of Tanzania and Mozambique and not far east of Lake Nyasa. Because of the limited possible habitats for the species and the intensity of entomological survey over many years, one can be reasonably confident that the gap between the *G. fuscipleuris* belt of Kenya and its main distribution area further west is real. The same cannot be claimed for Buxton's record in the south. In the vast expanse of Tanzania links might yet be found.

Buxton's record became more interesting when Santos Dias (1962) carried out a search for tsetse puparia in the riverine forest of the Uanetse river in southern Mozambique, an area known to have been infested before 1896 but since then free of tsetse. He found puparia of *G. morsitans*, *G. pallidipes*, *G. brevipalpis*, and *G. austeni*. These finds were of considerable interest, but were not extraordinary because the three latter species either still survive or did so until comparatively recently at no very great distance from the Uanetse river, while the former presence of *G. morsitans* in the basin of the nearby Limpopo is well established (see Chapter 17). A single puparium of *G. fuscipleuris* was a more notable discovery. An isolated record of this nature, of the puparial shell of a fly that probably died seventy years earlier and of which the nearest known modern records are some 1500 miles distant, must be accepted with some caution but it is not impossible.

The distribution of East African vegetation has been much studied by Moreau whose most recent conclusion is that during the glacial periods of the Pleistocene a continuous block of country, from Abyssinia to South

Africa, lay under a montane climate. 'Of the actual extent to which ever-green forest occupied the montane block during any stage of the glaciation it is impossible to be sure' (Moreau 1967). It is, however, certain that at times during the Pleistocene much greater areas than exist today were covered with closed forest. A vegetational and faunal continuity existed that would have allowed *fusca* group tsetses and their hosts to have spread along the forest edges associated with the highlands of both the Western and Eastern Rifts to the Lake Nyasa region. The distribution of *G. brevi-palpis* along these routes is still quite clear (cf. Evens 1953 and *Tanganyika Atlas*), but this species has, as it were, lost its geographical connection with the Congo forests. It has also used, between north and south, the route provided by the scrub and thicket of the East African coast that is also occupied by *G. austeni*.

These connections have an intrinsic interest, but they are important also for the light they throw upon the means by which cattle, on at least two occasions (a third is still in progress), penetrated the tsetse-infested African tropics to reach the fly-free pastures of South Africa. It is a process which, in the first sample area to be described, the interlake region, appears to have been halted by events that began some eighty years ago.

7

KARAGWE AND ANKOLE BEFORE
THE RINDERPEST

ONE cannot describe the effects of the spread of tsetse flies on a land and its inhabitants unless one knows what they were like before these insects arrived. If most of the 'advances' of *Glossina morsitans* observed by men like R. W. Jack in Rhodesia and C. F. M. Swynnerton in Tanzania were merely its reoccupation of areas it had infested before the rinderpest, descriptions of land before and after will not tell much. We are interested in the replacement of long-established human communities by a fly-belt. There are not many areas of which much is known before the appearance of the rinderpest in the 1890s. One is that which the Germans, who began to occupy its southern half in 1891, called the *Zwischenseengebiet*, from its position between Lake Victoria and the lakes of the Western Rift Valley, Lakes Tanganyika, Kivu, Edward, and George. Today it comprises the Bukoba and Karagwe areas of Tanzania, the countries of Rwanda and Burundi, the district of Ankole and Kigezi in south-west Uganda, and part of the eastern boundary of the Congo Republic. It has a wide range of climates and a varied and spectacular topography. There are three, or perhaps more, main ethnic groups representing three separate cultures; and a very wide spectrum of plant life, from the semi-arid thorn bush around a minor lake, Burigi, to rain forest on the one hand and montane forests and alpine vegetation on another. No area has a better claim to lie at the heart of the continent, and of all Africa south of the Sahara no part has so long focused the imagination of the outer world, for here are the Mountains of the Moon and the ultimate source of the Nile.

The interlake area, especially that part of it which became involved in the spread of *G. morsitans*, has the great advantage that it was visited and described at length by two of the earliest of the explorers, Captain Speke and Captain Grant, as long ago as 1861, and after them in 1876 by H. M. Stanley. In 1889 the latter was back again with Emin Pasha, an able and observant naturalist, among his companions. In 1891 Emin returned with the German biologist, Franz Stuhlmann, in time to see the beginning of the series of events with which this account is chiefly concerned. Another acute observer following a different route, Captain H. M. Lugard, was also present in 1891 to record the dramatic event of the rinderpest panzootic. These men were followed by a long series of scientists, travellers, and administrators, many of whom wrote accounts of the interlake area, so that there are few parts of tropical Africa so well documented from the viewpoint of the student of trypanosomiasis.

Speke and Grant, 1861

After the long traverse of the caravan road to Tabora and then northwest from there, passing from one rapacious chief to the next, Speke and Grant entered with relief the last stage before arriving in Karagwe. 'We now had nothing but wild animals to contend with before entering Karagwe. This land is "neutral", by which is meant it is untenanted by human beings.' Speke was a felicitous observer, who thus in his first sentence about Karagwe mentions a feature of African geography that has been of great importance in preserving both the wild fauna and its attendant parasites. Countries, tribal areas, and kingdoms did not confront each other across boundaries, but kept themselves separate by more or less wide zones of uninhabited 'no-man's-land', the *Grenzwildnisse* of German writers. These boundary wildernesses were, and still are, reservoirs of infection. Speke also drew attention to the geology of Karagwe. He and Grant crossed the southern neutral zone which separated it from the most northerly of the *miombo* chiefdoms, Usui or Busubi, and reached the shallow lake of Burigi (Urigi) 'around which herds of hartebeest and fine cattle roamed'. Then:

Rising out of the bed of the Urigi, we passed over a low spur of beef-sandwich clay sandstones, and descended into the close, rich valley of Uthenga, bounded by steep hills hanging over us more than a thousand feet, as prettily clothed as the mountains of Scotland; whilst in the valley there were not only magnificent trees of extraordinary height, but also a surprising amount of the richest cultivation, amonst which the banana may be said to prevail. . . . Leaving the valley of Uthenga we rose over the spur of Nyamwara where we found we had attained the delightful altitude of 5,000 odd feet. . . . Tripping over the greensward we now worked our way to the Rozoka valley (Speke 1863).

After the long monotony of *Brachystegia* woodland and dry thornbush, the green hills of Karagwe must have seemed very welcoming. Others, indeed, crossing these hills of 'beef-sandwich clay sandstones' at other seasons have found them wearisome. From the accounts of Speke and Grant and their successors it is possible to put together a picture of a society and the land it occupied before the biological consequences of the infiltration of European culture brought about its collapse.

Grant (1864) described Karagwe:

With respect to the habitations of the people, suppose that on the face of a bare hill overlooking a lake we place forty or fifty dome-looking huts of cane covered with grass; divide them into sets of two or threes by screens and gates of cane; throw an embankment round the whole, and have a dense hedge of euphorbia trees on the top of the embankment, screening the view of the lake and the country round, and you have the Palace of Rumanika, containing his five wives, sons, four hundred cows and their calves, etc. Except a hut or two outside this 'bomah' nothing but a curl of smoke in the valleys showed there was any population in the country. Descend to the valleys and you find neatly formed huts of grass inside the plaintain groves.

Care is needed in accepting such statements without other confirmation. A view from a hill crest looking down upon acres of bananas may have made a vivid impression and, coming to mind later, formed the basis for a generalization that may not be valid. In eastern and central Karagwe, by 1940, the bulk of cultivation was on the ridges and the valleys were bush filled; but in north-western Karagwe the people lived at the foot of the hills and there was evidence of high-level cultivation that had disappeared. Evidences of settlement confirming a general reversal of the pattern described by Grant were easily to be seen in Karagwe twenty years ago.

The Ihangiro depression

Between the Kagera river, where it runs northward between Rwanda and Tanzania, and the Lake Victoria coast, the geological and climatic processes noted in Chapter 6 produced a series of great hill ridges and deep valleys running roughly south to north along the length of the modern districts of Bukoba and Karagwe. In the east three such ridges, rising in places to over 5000 ft, of which the most easterly appears only as a chain of islands parallel to the Bukoba coast, are formed of Bukoba sandstones, the extremely poor soils of which manage under a high rainfall to support the dense populations of what were once a chain of six little kingdoms. The high coastal rain belt is about 20 miles wide and is bounded along its western length by the Ihangiro depression, also about 20 miles wide, containing in the south the lake and swamps of Burigi from which the Mwisha river runs north below the scarp that bounds the depression in the west. At the corner opposite to Lake Burigi, under the shadow of the coastal hills, is another lake, Ikimba. Both it and Burigi are the last relics of a much larger lake that filled the Ihangiro depression during part of the Pleistocene.

Speke, followed some months later by Grant who had been sick, walked across the northern end of the Ihangiro depression to Kitangule where he saw the 'thousands and thousands of cows' belonging to the Mukama of Karagwe, Rumanyika. Grant estimated the number at about 10 000.

He left a description of his walk from the capital of Karagwe to Kitangule. By 1947 only some enormous plants of *Euphorbia tirucalli*, descendants doubtless of those that had formed hedges around the kraals, remained as a sign of former glory. Cattle are again to be seen in Kitangule now, but of another breed. But in general, and especially in the central part of the Ihangiro depression, there has been little change. Grant's paragraph would almost suffice today.

On emerging from these to the river plain, the flat country became studded with mounds from six to eight feet high, raised by the ever-working white ants. Thorny scrubs, cactus, climbing aloes with pink flowers covered them, or the jungle or grass was varied by circles of brushwood, giving shade to the rhinoceros; the older trees were veiled over with silvery grey moss, which drooped gracefully, like the pendent branches of the weeping willow. The plain extended for ten miles, with several 'back-waters' upon it, covered with thorny mimosa and papyrus, through which we had to cut our way. Emerging from it and going towards the river, we came upon higher land—a dry grassy plain three miles across, kept short by cattle, and just the ground on which to find a florikan. There were several huts which gladdened the eye after a dreary march.

In 1911 the German geographer, Hans Meyer, crossed the Ihangiro depression and by then most of the cattle had gone. He gives an account of the bush through which he passed between Lakes Ikimba and Burigi.

At Ndama we left the road and began our march through the uninhabited wilderness of lower Ihangiro to Burigi. Sometimes we followed the tracks of the native Wakyanga along which they went through the savanna hill country to hunt or to seek honey or to get smoked fish from Burigi which they bartered for millet and banana meal. The people of Ndama take three days to reach the northernmost point of Lake Burigi. At first, in the low lying parts south-south-west of Ikimba the breast-high reeds were so thick that the leaders had to break a road through forcibly and the long caravan moved endlessly winding and twisting through the thick grass that was scattered over with little hillocks or old termite hills covered with a growth of thicket species from 5 to 20 metres high, of Leguminosae, Commiphoras, Phoenix palms, tree Euphorbias and the felt like interlacings of the branches of *Euphorbia tirucalli* etc. Soon after, with our entry into hilly country the vegetation changed to the less dense 'orchard steppe' of the same type that covers the southern foot of Kilimanjaro. . . . The soil is predominantly covered with grasses of the genus *Andropogon* among which the 2 m. high *A. rufus* with its violet, light brown, sheen, *A. cymbareus* with its thick, oat-like bushy inflorescences and *Tricholaena dregei* with its fine, silky, delicate rose-red flowers most strike the eye. Among these grow low bushes, up to a metre high, of the genera *Aerua, Hibiscus, Ipomoea*; Labiates of the genera *Pychnostachys, Ocimum, Geniospermum*; Composites of the genera *Gutten-bergia, Vernonia, Elephantopus, Pluchea, Melanthera, Berkheya* and others are widely scattered. Almost all, in the middle of the dry season, had flowered and dried up—grey-brown like the whole grass cover, except where they are in the neighbourhood of water holes and strips of gallery forest. Only occasional Liliaceae of the genera *Sanseviera, Chlorophytum, Kniphofia* and *Aloe*, with a presentiment of the approaching short rainy season, had put out their succulent leaves and highly coloured slender shoots from the grey-brown monotony of the soil. Commonest among these are the *Aloe* species, *A. saponaria* and the larger *A. laterita*, of which the spotted leaves and orange to deep red panicles, shine like flames among the tall withered grasses (Meyer 1913).

It will be necessary to look again at the Ihangiro depression which is comparatively waterless in the dry weather and inhospitable except around

Ikimba and Burigi and along the Mwisha river, for it lies in the rain shadow of the Bukoba coastal hills. In part it belonged to the two largest of the coastal kingdoms, Kyanja and Ihangiro, and in part to Karagwe, but in fact was a *Grenzwildnis* between the three. Karagwe proper is bounded in the east by the great scarp called the Migongo (the backbone) that over-looks the Ihangiro depression from a height of about a thousand feet.

Kollman stood on the crest of the Migongo and later wrote:

The edge of the plateau of Karagwe rises abruptly in a steep ascent up to 1000 feet. On attaining this height one is rewarded by a glorious view. At one's feet lies the wide, apparently endless, well wooded, Kagera Plain, closed on the distant horizon by masses of mountain gleaming indistinctly, and to the west the eye sweeps over mountains and valleys in rich succession. In the valleys and gullies lie the banana groves and huts of the Karagwe people. The hills and mountains generally are covered with low grass, forming good pastures for cattle. Further on in the country we find wide plains, generally with high jungle or stretches of primeval forest,—a haunt of numerous rhinoceros (Kollmann 1899).

Karagwe: the Butenga valley

Karagwe is made up of three ridges on a somewhat larger scale than those of the coastal belt, and formed of the Muva–Ankolean pre-Cambrian sediments that Speke described as 'beef-sandwich clay sandstones'. The valley bounding the western ridge contains the chain of swamps and lakes through which flows the Kagera river. It is broadened, especially in the north-west of Karagwe where the Kagera turns east towards Lake Victoria, by 'arenas' formed by intrusive granites that carry wide areas of often treeless grassland.

The Butenga valley that gave Speke and Grant their first glimpse of Karagwe behind the eastern scarp serves well to illustrate the sort of information available from the early travellers. Speke wrote that 'notwith-standing the apparent richness of the land, the Wanyambo living in their squalid huts seemed poor'. The Nyambo of Karagwe, like the Hutu of Rwanda and the Iru of Ankole, were Bantu descendants of the inhabitants of these lands before the arrival of the half-hamite Tusi (in Rwanda) and Hima in Ankole and Karagwe who reduced their agricultural predecessors to a servile status, while they themselves continued to live upon the milk and blood of the long-horned Sanga cattle they had brought with them some five or six hundred years earlier, from the north.

The first European visitor to Karagwe after Speke and Grant was H. M. Stanley in 1876. On that occasion he did not pass through Butenga, but he did so in 1889 accompanied by Surgeon Parke (1891) and Emin Pasha (Stuhlmann 1916–27). Again the difficulty of interpreting the accounts of travellers is apparent. They followed Speke's route in the opposite direction, from Rozoka to Butenga. The hills over which their predecessors had 'tripped' were now 'dreary wastes of sere grass in valley and mountain' (Stanley). Parke wrote, 'We marched today over very rough, gravelly ground, and then up precipitous hills, which we found extremely laborious work. . . . This is very barren, dried up, uninteresting country.' We are told nothing about Butenga itself, except that the party left there on 10 August 1889. To Stanley and his companions, looking forward to the end of their immense journey, and all three suffering from malaria, the steep hills of Karagwe doubtless seemed even grimmer than they are in mid-dry season today. When the grass has not yet begun to recover from the season's fires, the lumps of schist and phyllite and quartz that interrupt the skeletal soils of the steep slopes make climbing in and out of the valleys a burden that, at the end of the hot day, is difficult to bear. In the early rains, when Speke and Grant triumphantly near their goal, the Nile source, had climbed into the cool green grassy hills, the impression was a very different one. Both are true.

The English botanist Scott Elliot (1896) saw Butenga in 1894. 'The really fertile parts are the narrow ravines at the heads of the minor valleys, for instance at Mgara and Butenga, where a little stream of water drops down three or four miles through a narrow valley covered and shaded by banana plantations and then forest.' By this time Karagwe had fallen into the depths of the miseries from which it is still recovering.

The pastures

The inhabitants of Butenga were agricultural Nyambo. It was not a cattle area. Two main pastures of eastern Karagwe were the low-lying lands around Burigi and at Kitangule, at either end of the Ihangiro depression. Another cattle area was in the north-west corner of the country, known as Bugoye (Wugoye or Wagoya). Here the Muva–Ankolean hills rise to well over 5400 ft and look over the Kagera winding through papyrus-filled swamps and lakes a thousand feet below. The steep slopes of these westward-facing hills do not confront an equally high valley wall on the other side of the river. They are separated from hills of the same geological formation in the Kigezi district of Uganda and, somewhat to the south, those of Rwanda, by wide arenas. These are, in parts, still treeless and, where there are no trees, there are still cattle. The earliest record we have of this area comes from Emin Pasha who, in company with Dr. Franz Stuhlmann, was on his way to his death at the hands of Arab slavers in the Congo.

While still at Bukoba Emin received a message, on 20 January 1891, from Ankole. Its king, the Mugabe Ntare, sent an embassy of 40 men to invite Emin 'to go and assist him against his enemies. A cattle plague has been decimating his livestock, and he now insists that his neighbours have bewitched his cattle, and he desires to avenge himself.' The plea was ignored.

Emin and Stuhlmann left Bukoba on 12 February and had reached Bugene on the Karagwe Migongo by the 21st, having discovered Lake Ikimba *en route*. On the 24th they arrived at the Arab trading centre at Kafuro and remained there for a month. Stuhlmann described the country around Kafuro which lay about a mile from the present county head-quarters at Nyabionza.

The vegetation of the country is, comparatively speaking, poor. Mountains and valleys are covered throughout with grass 50–80 cm. high, among which, during the wet season, appears a splendid flowering of bulbous plants, bind-weed (*Ipomoea*), yellow composites, *Senecio*, *Crozophora*, with blue veronica-like flowers, *Coleus*, *Chenopodium*, and other plants. During the dry season the grass dries to yellow straw, which is often ignited by the natives and transformed into black charcoal. On the appearance of the rains, however, of which the main period here seems to be from the beginning of January to the beginning of May, the country clothes itself, as if by a stroke of magic, with the most splendid green. These extensive grass plains form a magnificent pasture land and the hand-some long-horned cattle of the natives bear witness to the nutritive quality of the soil. Here and there a great fig tree stands out in these grassy plains, from its branches hanging long aerial roots, an acacia, or, perhaps, a *Dracaena*. On the whole, however, the tree growth, which is mostly confined to the valley floors, is so sparse that building wood can only be obtained, by great pains, from afar off. The low bush, in which *Erythrina* predominates, scarcely suffices the sparse population for firewood. Only where, in the depths, the water stands longer, or where little streams flow, which incidentally all go to the north, is luxurious vegetation found. In thickets of Juncaceae and *Amomum* grow the handsome wild banana (*Musa ensete*) which, with their gigantic bright green leaves, are visible afar off. Violet blossoming *Epilobium hirsutum* and Heliotrope, as well as *Moschoma*, blackberries and 'cow-cabbage' form a bright picture, intertwined with tendrils of *Clematis grata* and *Ipomoea*.

During our stay in Kafuro, we had the opportunity to observe some of the customs of the country. As already mentioned, the whole of Karagwe is a grass covered plateau, cut through by numerous, chiefly meridional, valleys, on which here and there great fig trees and *Erythrina* bushes stand; only in the valleys is there any thick tree growth. The villages, like those near the lake, stand in large banana plantations in which the conical huts are scattered, or else as kraals in the open. In the first type the aboriginal people mostly live; in the latter the ruling class who are almost entirely engaged in cattle rearing. The kraals comprise a number of huts which are surrounded by a hedge of thorn. There, in the yard which is stiff with dirt and vermin, the cattle are bivouaced at night, and by day the dried dung is gathered together to make a fire at night, the smoke of which keeps away the insects. The cattle, without exception, belonged to the longhorned humpless, Hima race, and are looked after with great care. They are driven to pasture in herds of 100 to 1000 by men armed with spears, the milch cows usually separately, and these are milked after an hour's grazing. Milk only is taken from them and with few exceptions, only sick beasts are slaughtered. The milk itself is consumed almost all in the liquid state or is made use of for the production of butter (Stuhlmann 1894).

Emin on the first stage of the journey north from Kafuro wrote:

22.3.91. From Kafuro we proceeded in the first place over the hills, which were now clad in pretty green, back towards Njakigandu, where we camped when we first came here, and crossed the little watercourse, but went on from there on the road to Kjivona, which I had traversed with Stanley. The continual rain has favoured vegetation, and pretty gaily coloured blossoms are now seen everywhere, some exhaling beautiful perfumes, as, for instance, the carissa and the acacias. Nevertheless on the whole it is monotonous,—up hill, down hill, and along mountain slopes, over slippery red laterite soil which clings to the boots like lead. Although now and then a banana plantation, clad in fresh green, a small village, a herd of cattle, and wide fields with standing crops introduce some variety into the landscape, the almost complete absence of all trees rather spoils the effect. But in place of trees there are ample thistles of various kinds, which make themselves very unpleasantly perceptible. . . . There is not much to be got here; the village is wretched and nothing can be had for love or money. . . . Kakikondyo, the King's brother, is to meet me here and accompany me as far as the boundary.

We started at 6.7 a.m. . . . We crossed the bare crests of the hills and then descended a gentle slope. Here we again saw some trees, viz. Acacias with completely flat tops, such as are frequently met with in South Africa; this is a sign that the hills of Karagwe would be capable of producing trees but for the fact that their growth is stopped by fortuitous agencies—such as being nibbled off by goats, or destroyed by fire, or on account of agriculture; this ought to be noted for the future. At the present moment Karagwe is only suited for cattle breeding. . . . Doubtless there is a deep swamp in the valley when the rainy season is at its height, but today there was only thick grass and cutting reeds. After passing these we commenced a rather arduous ascent over small blocks of rock, finally arriving on a plateau. We then crossed a slight depression covered with fragments of rock, and ascended to a second plateau called Busese. . . .

We had the pleasure of seeing a rhinoceros in the valley, but we only just caught sight of it and it disappeared immediately. A number of small green parrots with yellow breasts were flitting past overhead. Francolins were calling each other and pairing in all directions, but there was no sign of guinea fowl. Various kind of 'honey suckers' . . . are very frequent, glittering . . . in beautiful metallic colours.

A man coming from Butumbi brings fresh reports of ravages caused by the Nkole in Mpororo and Butumbi. They are said to have carried off women and children, burnt down the huts, cut down the bananas—in short, done all the harm they could and then returned home, though not without the loss of a good many of their number . . . (Stuhlmann 1916–27).

This was the first indication of the effects of the rinderpest. The Ankole cattle by now were mostly dead and the Nyankore were raiding south into the little buffer state of Mpororo and from there into Rwanda in an attempt to replace the lost herds. They carried the infection with them.

Continuing northward, the travellers now entered the third main cattle-raising area of Karagwe. Leaving Kyivona they eventually reached the plain of Btohssi:

The wide plain of Btohssi, covered with short grass, with here and there a few bushes, forms a very broad defile between the hill chains on either side. It is only frequented by Wahuma cowherds with their splendid herds of cattle, but it is not inhabited or cultivated, because the people prefer to build their dwellings in the hollows between the hills and on alongside of brooks, as tilling the soil is there less laborious than on the parched plain, where even yesterday no rain appears to have fallen . . . Three rhinoceros (Stuhlmann 1916–27).

Stanley had explored some of this route in 1876:

In our march of ten miles from Isossi to Kasya I counted thirty-two separate herds of cattle, which in aggregate probably amounted to 900 head. We also saw seven rhinoceroses (Stanley 1878).

The frequency with which rhinoceros were seen before the use of fire-arms began to drive them into the denser thickets and forests in which they are now found is one of many indications of changes that were to come. But the most striking passages are those that refer to the sparseness of tree growth. Emin had first discussed this in a note about his entry into Karagwe with the Stanley expedition in July 1889. They had crossed the Kagera from Nsongezi by canoe. On both sides of the river valley the deserted *Grenzwildnis* was inhospitable.

Five and a half hours through completely withered, dried up country without a drop of water. Steppe bush, thorn thicket, dust and the charcoal of burnt grass, and withal, many people sick.

Emin, describing the march into Karagwe wrote:

An apparently straight valley, with steppe vegetation leads into the mountains, in and around which we have followed a very stony path; on the whole the country gives a yet more inhospitable impression than Ankole. Here is both long and short dry grass, with scarcely a tree on the mountain ridges, over which a cold wind blows. That tree growth can thrive is proved by the appearance of solitary, though admittedly, 'stunted' trees and the rich wooding in the ravines; it is owing to the fires, which, every year, driven by tumultuous winds, sweep over these high plateaus, that no higher vegetation can grow; it is the deficiency of water, the thinness of the earth cover (the ashes are dispersed by the wind), the goats, which prevent the up-growth of bush. The vegetation in a ravine reminds one, by the height and slenderness of occasional trees, of western areas; the components belong, however, to our northern and north-eastern primitive forests. I noted *Afzelia, Khaya, Vitex, Calophyllum, Ficus, Myrsine*, etc. (Stuhlmann 1916–27).

Just as today a quite false impression of the general aspect of some parts of Africa, especially the less richly endowed, may be given to the traveller who sees from the tarmac road on which he is motoring the frequent villages that lie along it but cannot see the vast emptiness behind, so it is necessary to recall that the early accounts were made up from what was seen from the main footpaths. To this information may be added archaeological evidence and the evidence provided by plant indicators which may sometimes substantiate the spoken recollections of older inhabitants.

Emin and Stuhlmann on their way north to the Kagera were conducted by a relation of the Mukama whose name was Mukakikonjo (Kakikondyo, the king's brother in Emin's account). They noticed the herds and the somewhat poor huts in which their owners lived. There was little cultivation around the arenas that provided the principal pastures. Stuhlmann wrote, 'The population of this district, which is known as Wugoye, belongs to the pure Bahima tribe.' In 1947 the present writer was fortunate in encountering Mukakikonjo's son, Rutalindwa, who had been a young man when his father had seen the two travellers out of Karagwe. Rutalindwa confirmed that in those days only the Hima and their cattle occupied the plains and the surrounding hill slopes. Observing the belt of banana gardens that now lined much of the road along the foot of the hills and knowing that the Hima depended for many services upon the Nyambo serfs, one asked where these people had lived at that time. Rutalindwa pointed to the steep slopes of the arena wall and said, 'The beer came from over the top.' Later, ascending these hills by the road leading to the tin mines at Kyerwa, one crossed into the wide Kishanda valley. No early written account of this valley has been found. It is separated from the Sina and Ibanda arenas by a ridge of hills that rise sharply on their western slopes to over 6000 ft at the highest point, Kichware, but slope down more gradually to form its western wall. The upper slopes of this western wall of Kishanda are now covered by dense forest from which the tin miners cut pit props of *Markhamia platycalyx*. Woodmen engaged in this work were asked if they had seen signs of former habitation. Without speaking one of them pointed to near the questioner's feet and there, half buried in leaves, lay a large grindstone. Later one learned that the dominance of the *Markhamia* in these forests derived from trees of this species that are planted along paths through the banana gardens in this part of the interlake zone. Occasional castor-oil plants among the secondary thickets had a similar origin.

Ankole

The Hima invasion of the interlake area took place 500–600 years ago. Descendants of Ruhinda, founder of the ruling clan the Hinda, gained control not only of Ankole and Karagwe, but of areas as far round Lake Victoria as the island of Ukerewe on its east coast. In Ankole they settled around the lakes in the south-east quarter of the present district, using them as a dry-season water reserve, but moving each year, during the wet season, further into the surrounding grasslands.

They had come from the north-east, and they brought their cattle with them. On arrival they must have found adequate pastures and comparative freedom from disease. It seems likely that their entry in a country hitherto inhabited by cultivators was a peaceful one. They were, perhaps, welcomed by the inhabitants as are the Fulani of West Africa, who also migrate in search of pasture. It was not until the eighteenth century that they became politically organized and began to govern their predecessors in the land, turning them into serfs.

When Stanley arrived in Ankole in 1889, its area was much smaller than it became under British rule. It is convenient to speak of it then as Nkore, a spelling used by early writers, reserving Ankole to indicate the modern district.

Nkore, based upon the lakes, the papyrus swamps that surround them, and the lower reaches of the river Ruizi that flows into them, was a country of grasslands, for the most part dominated by red oat grass, *Themeda triandra*. Some parts carried a woodland of *Acacia gerrardii* and *A. hockii*; other places were dotted with abundant large termite hills usually carrying a single candelabra *Euphorbia*, a bush of evergreen *Rhus glaucescens*, and often a *Grewia bicolor*. These comparatively open savannas occupied the eastern half of the modern district. They enjoy an annual rainfall of 25–40 in. Dry seasons are seldom severe and in most years rain falls in every month, although not sufficiently to prevent extensive grass fires in July, and also, to a lesser extent, in January.

Stanley descended into the Ruizi basin, having crossed the great hills of Buhwezu.

In the valley between the Denny and Iwanda Ranges (*Mawangara and Ibanda*) we passed over 4000 cattle of the long-horned species. The basin of the Rwizi, which we were now in, possessed scores of herds (Stanley 1890).

This part of Ankole (Kashari and Shema counties) is not greatly different today, at least superficially.

There are thousands of cattle roaming over this region: they present a great variety of colours, and the full grown ones are usually about the size of an English three-year old. . . . We met large herds of them, at intervals of a couple of miles or so, grazing near our path. . . . There is little or no firewood to be found anywhere in these parts. . . . The natives, although friendly, are very stingy with us. There are so many thousands of cattle about in all directions, yet they will not bring us a scrap of either milk or butter: not even to *sell* (Parke, 1891).

Stanley was well received and the expedition rested from 15–20 July not far from the site of Mbarara. On the 24th they entered the settlement of Mavona.

The principal pastures of Nkore lay in the central area called Nshara. This was also called Karo Karungi, the good or beautiful land. South of the lakes in central Nshara were the high hills of Bukanga and Ngarama which, on their southern slopes, overlooked the Kagera valley and Karagwe on its southern bank. North of the lakes the home pastures of Nshara occupied the drainage basin of the lower Ruizi and other smaller rivers emptying into them. Across the watershed in the north, the areas of Nyabushozi and Mawogola provided additional grazing for the wet season or for longer periods of shortage of pasture, as for example when Nshara became un-usable by accidental over-burning of grasslands or by locally severe out-breaks of disease. The eastern half of these northern pastures drains into the Katonga river. This formed the boundary with Toro, a buffer state between Nkore and its powerful northern neighbour, Bunyoro. The north-western corner of Nkore abutted on two other small tributary chiefdoms, Buzimba and Kitagwenda. They were drained by tributaries of the Mpanga river, flowing over the wall of the Rift Valley into Lake George, then called Ruisamba. Buzimba is now united with the north-western corner of the old Nkore to form the county of Mitoma. Kitagwenda, once so populous that Stanley could not persuade his army to approach it, has disappeared (Stanley 1878).

Buzimba was not a country of the dry acacia savannas and grasslands. Its people lived on the east wall of the Western Rift, under a relatively high rainfall, in deeply dissected valleys in Muva–Ankolean mountains more massive than those of Karagwe and southern Nkore. The rain forests rise, at the highest levels, to altitudes at which they give way to a sub-alpine vegetation. People also live on the tops of the flatter hills at lesser heights.

Kitagwenda lay on the lower slopes of the Rift wall and its cultivation extended to the shores of Lake George. Its chief sat on a political fence between the Mugabe of Ankole in the south and the Mukama of Bunyoro in the north, and his little country survived because of its commercial importance.

Also in the great mass of Muva–Ankolean mountains that now form most of the north-western quarter of modern Ankole were the lesser kingdoms, tributary to Nkore, of Buhwezu and Igara.

The south-west quarter of modern Ankole consists of two counties, Rwampara and Kazhara. The first, Rwampara, was already a part of Nkore in 1890. It is a mountainous area, its northern face overlooking the Nkore pastures, and its southern face forming part of the more or less empty frontier zone of the Kagera valley. In the far south-west, the county of Kazhara came into being when the country of Mpororo was divided between the British Uganda Protectorate and German East Africa. Its southern half today belongs to the Republic of Rwanda. On its eastern borders Nkore adjoined the powerful country of Buganda, from which it was separated around the eastern end of the Nshara lakes by the little country of Koki, a dependency of Buganda.

Evidences of trypanosomiasis in Karagwe and Nkore before 1890

So far we have been concerned solely with the general appearance of the interlake countries of Karagwe and Nkore before they were taken over by the colonial powers. In the next chapter the immediate sequels of the European impact are described; then follows a description of the invasion of the interlake region by *Glossina morsitans*. Chapter 10 will relate the changes that took place in the same period in some of the little countries on the northern borders of Nkore which were followed by a spread of *G. pallidipes*. It will become evident that in those countries the three species of tsetse that transmitted the trypanosomes that caused the depopulation of the Rift Valley, both of its people and its cattle, must have been established there for centuries.

This deduction cannot be made about *G. morsitans* in Karagwe and Nkore. Its invasion of the interlake region after 1891 was a new event. But trypanosomiasis of cattle was not unknown. The first modern record comes from the first Anglo-German boundary commission of 1903 when a horse belonging to the leader of the British team died of a trypanosome infection near the Kagera river (Delmé-Radcliffe 1947). The disease, *omurasho*, was familiar to Hima cattle owners in both countries. It was not associated with tsetse. People thought that in certain places the grass was poisonous and that cattle entering them would die. These foci of infection were well known and avoided. One was at Buhamira on the eastern borders of Karagwe, in the middle of the Ihangiro depression and about 15 miles south of the Kagera river. This was recalled by people in Karagwe in 1947. Ten years later informants in Ankole stated that cattle were never taken to Nsongezi on the Kagera because of *omurasho*, and another added that there was also a focus of the disease on the Kakitumba river. These three sites are shown on Map 7.1. It was characteristic of the infection at these places that it did not spread and it was not greatly feared because it could be avoided. The three sites have a feature in common. All lie in the frontier zones described by Speke as 'neutral', meaning they were untenanted by man, and by German administrators as *Grenzwildnisse*.

In 1926 a single specimen of *G. pallidipes* was captured in riverine bush on the Kagera river near the confluence of the Kakitumba (Simmons 1929). Although the valley was intermittently under observation by veterinarians and entomologists it was not until 1953 that the next specimen was recorded (van den Berghe and Lambrecht 1956). *G. brevipalpis* also occurs in the Kagera valley as well as in the Ihangiro depression. Both of these flies can live in quite small populations in restricted habitats, provided the latter are also frequented by suitable hosts. Bushbuck, buffalo, and bushpig are now common in parts of these valleys and perhaps range more widely than they did in the last century. In the Kagera hippopotamus provides blood for *G. brevipalpis*.

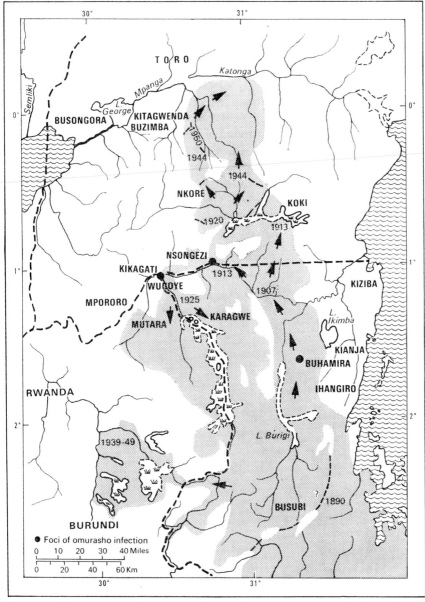

MAP 7.1. The spread of *G. morsitans* through Karagwe into Burundi, Rwanda, and Ankole.

When *G. morsitans* appeared in these areas the accompanying spread of infection seemed to the local people to cause a disease they had never seen before. It moved gradually, but not too gradually for its movement to be imperceptible. Like the rinderpest it was new and it seemed to bear no resemblance to the stationary *omurasho*. They used a new name for it, *rwakipumpuru*, not belonging to the Nyankore language, and now thought to have been introduced by veterinary officials who had met it in Buganda.

Somewhat in the same way one found that the Nyankore used the Ganda word *ebivu*, meaning any large biting fly, for *G. morsitans* (at least in talking to officials), although there was a local word, *enkurikizi*, that was said to refer specifically to tsetse. The existence of this word was explained by its reputed attribution to *G. fuscipes* which must have been long familiar to people living in the neighbourhood of the Rift lakes and streams.

The interlake countries, with their immense populations of semi-nomadic cattle, were not then entirely free of trypanosomiasis. The disease was known, at least locally, and foci of infection were avoidable. They tended to lie in the *Grenzwildnisse* and did not spread through the land as did the *G. morsitans* fly-belt when it appeared so suddenly at the end of the nineteenth century.

8

THE COLLAPSE OF KARAGWE AND NKORE: WARS; RINDERPEST; SMALLPOX; JIGGER FLEAS; GERMANS AND BRITISH

Succession and other wars

ALTHOUGH Speke and Grant thought that the Nyambo in their huts in the midst of banana gardens seemed poor, they nevertheless left an impression of a flourishing community governed by a wise and benevolent monarch. The Mukama Rumanyika was still ruling from Bweranyange when Stanley made his first visit to Karagwe in 1876. The 'gentle' Rumanyika was then about sixty years old, but soon afterwards he committed suicide, the usual end for divine kings when their powers began to fail. The ensuing struggle for the throne between the dead man's sons sounds, in Stanley's prose, barbarous enough. But Stanley was a journalist. The story of the seventeen sons who were slaughtered by their brother, who also blinded the eighteenth, is almost entirely untrue. Fighting between the sons of a Hinda king was a normal way of settling the succession. It was hardly war; rather a series of murders carried out by small rival gangs. Rumanyika himself had failed to slaughter his brother Rwegira, who set himself up as ruler of the north-western corner of the country, Bugoye, relying upon the uninhabited bush of the *Grenzwildnis* to fall back upon if danger threatened. An early German administrator thought poorly of warfare between the kingdoms of the Victoria coast. 'The battle opens with an exchange of prodigious insults, for there is no proper war cry. Angry tongues maintain and the pombe flask stimulates battle among the Wahaya' (Richter 1899). Elsewhere in the same article he refers to the son of Rumanyika's rival brother who kept up the struggle and continued to be at war with Rumanyika's successors, 'if one wishes to designate as war the harmless nightly cattle thieving of a quarrelsome people'. Ceremonial boasting songs were, and still are, one of the Hima arts but the singers magnified trivial events into powerful dramas. Grass fires that led to quarrels about grazing became the theme for passionate recitals about imaginary battles (Ford 1953), and almost any public occasion provoked exaggerated declamations that were artistically splendid but could be misleading when taken as history (see, for example, Morris 1964 for specimens of Hima dramatic poetry). One account (*Bukoba district book*) states that in one of the battles waged against Rumanyika's brother by the Mukama's son, Kakoko, four piles of testicles, each 4 ft high, were brought back as trophies of victory. A rough calculation suggests that this might have been achieved by the slaughter of some 75 000 men. (In the 1948 census there were under 13 000 males over 16 years old in the whole chiefdom.) Sometimes, no doubt, there was fierce fighting and there were also occasional massacres.

In 1887, according to Stanley, the Ganda, who claimed suzerainty over the countries west of the lake, including Karagwe, made a comparatively large-scale invasion. Two years later, he arrived at the shore in the southwest corner of Lake Victoria and was astonished at the number of human skulls lying about. They remained from a battle in which the local Zinza tried to oppose the Ganda. In Karagwe the Ganda were said to have murdered a number of the Arab traders at Kafuro, although in another passage one finds that one of the Arabs was murdered by his own son. Certainly, there need be no doubt that the small Arab trading community at Kafuro broke up before 1889. It is also certain that the succession struggles after the death of Rumanyika were prolonged and, perhaps, unusually vicious. One reason for this was that the son best qualified to succeed was unable to do so because he was left-handed (see Grant's account of Kakoko in 1861), a blemish that unfitted him to rule as a 'divine king'. He therefore, until his own murder in about 1885, was forced to rule through one or other of his brothers. In 1890 or in early 1891 when the rinderpest epizootic killed the cattle and smallpox developed into a severe epidemic, the country was under another regent who was remembered over fifty years later for his barbarous cruelties. In 1947 the present writer was shown a place where this Kaketo had ordered the slaughter of the inhabitants of one village to be continued until the blood flowed from the place of execution, on top of one of the larger hills, to the valley beneath. Barbarities occurred, wars were fought, but except on rare occasions it seems unlikely that they were a principal cause of depopulation. Rather, perhaps, they tended to accompany and, possibly, even relieved some of the effects of more powerful agents of population control.

The Great Rinderpest

Lugard's belief that Great Rinderpest began with an infection brought into Africa in cattle imported by the Italians during the occupation of Eritrea still seems acceptable.† What is certain is that the disease that entered tropical Africa in 1889–90 and by 1896 had spread to the Cape was extremely virulent. Not only cattle were killed but several species of wild animals suffered severely, especially buffalo, eland, bushbuck, and giraffe as well as the pigs, warthog, bushpig, and forest hog. Lugard (1891), reporting on its effects in Uganda, said that, 'In some districts almost all the game including the small antelopes, seem to have perished, with the exception of the hartebeest class, the waterbuck, and the zebra—and of

† Another version is mentioned in Chapter 22.

course, the elephant and hippopotamus.' In Karagwe, as elsewhere, the rhinoceros also escaped.

A very virulent epizootic of rinderpest had attacked the British cattle population in 1865. The disease was enzootic in the cattle of the steppes of eastern Asia and from time to time, for instance during the reign of Charlemagne, caused very heavy losses in eastern Europe. In the thirteenth century there were serious epizootics in France, while during the Napoleonic wars it spread throughout Europe. The Crimean War was blamed for the spread of the virus that reached England in 1865. According to Salem (1930) rinderpest may have reached Egypt for the first time in 1841 from southern Russia or from Rumania and Asia Minor. On that occasion 665 000 head of cattle were lost. In 1863, 784 642 head were supposed to have succumbed to an infection brought from the Danube basin. It seems likely that this was the parent strain of that which reached England two years later and, according to one authority, caused the deaths of 420 000 head of cattle (Hall 1962) before it was controlled by a policy of slaughter. In Africa there was no policy, except to fly from infected areas and to attempt to replenish losses by raiding neighbours not yet afflicted. To these causes of wider spread of infection was added the infection of many species of wild game. In most of the larger pastoral areas it was usually estimated that 90–95 per cent of the cattle died. (A good general account of the panzootic is to be found in Simon 1962.)

Emin received information of the rinderpest in Ankole in January 1891. Early in April he and Stuhlmann found that the infection had reached the Kagera river via Mpororo, possibly having been carried there by a war party from Ankole sent to replenish the Ankole herds. In June it reached Bukoba where Langheld had been left in charge by Emin. He later wrote:

Our cattle, which were at first in excellent condition, showed signs of sickness. Already before my arrival a disease had destroyed a large number, but the remainder had recovered. Now the animals showed a diminished appetite, they became very weak, excreted abundant urine and their excrement was liquid and mixed with blood. I gave the beasts some salt water, which produced only a temporary apparent improvement. Moreover the natives were unable to give me any remedies. Their magic charms, which they besought me to use, I rejected. In my diary I find the following entry:—

                June 29th— 2 head died
                      30th— 9   ,,   ,,
                July 1st—18   ,,   ,,
                      2nd—12   ,,   ,,
                      3rd—34   ,,   ,,

among them my best bull. It was a pitiable sight, as the handsome, powerful, completely snow-white animal, one morning was unable to get up and, two hours later, died. I had hopes that his great strength would have enabled him to withstand the disease. [In the station herd] . . . of over 600 there remained to us only thirty-five (Langheld 1909).

These figures approximate closely to the mortality levels noted elsewhere, about 95 per cent. When infection reached a herd, deaths followed in very rapid succession. An inquiry carried out in 1924, and recorded in the *Bukoba district book*, concluded that in the two districts of Bukoba and Biharamulo there had formerly been a cattle population of about 400 000 and that this was reduced by 95 per cent, i.e. to 20 000 in the two years 1891 and 1892. There is no reason to suppose these figures are exaggerated.

Famine and smallpox

The first effect of the rinderpest was famine among the pastoral people, among whom were the ruling clans. Hitherto the Hima in Karagwe and Ankole, and the Tusi in Rwanda and Burundi, as well as in the minor kingdoms like Mpororo, Igara, Buhwezu, and the Bukoba coastal kingdoms, had lived almost entirely on a diet of milk and blood. Secondly, the famine disorganized government, for the ruling Hinda clan as well as the ordinary pastoral Hima were forced to turn to the agricultural Bantu tribes to obtain food which was sufficient only for the needs of the growers. The oligarchs became dependent upon their serfs who, compelled to dispense their own food reserves, brought famine upon themselves as well. The shame involved in these happenings induced many Hima to commit suicide. Under famine conditions endemic diseases became epidemic. Smallpox, in the opinion of early medical men in Africa always the most dangerous of African infections, grew very prevalent, not only in the interlake area but in other parts of Africa as well, especially where pastoral milk drinkers were suddenly deprived of their basic diet. In Karagwe so virulent was the smallpox that it seemed to the people that its effects were as dreadful among themselves as was the rinderpest among their cattle, so that they called both by the same name, *mubiamo*.

Lugard saw but did not recognize the smallpox. The rinderpest had reached the countries east of Lake Victoria six months before it reached Karagwe. In Kamasia, Lugard noted that 'The vultures and hyenas were too surfeited to devour the putrid carcases, which lay under almost every tree near water.' He reflected that the rinderpest 'in some respects . . . has favoured our enterprise. Powerful and warlike as the pastoral tribes are, their pride has been humbled and our progress facilitated by this awful visitation. The advent of the white man had not else been so peaceful.' When in June 1891 Lugard visited the interlake area, he sent messengers to the Mugabe of Nkore, but they returned saying that as all his cattle were dead, Ntare was ashamed that Lugard should visit him in his poverty and starvation. Of the Hima in general he wrote that they

were driven to eat of what the agriculturists could provide, and to endeavour themselves to follow their arts, for the terrible plague had swept off their cattle

. . . Large numbers of the people, too, had died, unable to procure food or to accommodate themselves to an unwonted diet. The remnants are thin and half starved and much liable to a loathsome skin disease or 'itch' which breaks out in large scabby sores and is most contagious (Lugard 1893).

The panzootic continued to flow southwards through the savanna and savanna woodlands, generally first through the domestic cattle population, because its arrival provoked flight from areas in which deaths first occurred. Later the Hima realized that running away from rinderpest was useless and they spoke of this as a distinguishing characteristic of the disease when comparing its effects with those of trypanosomiasis from which it was wise to flee.

One effect of the extreme virulence of the rinderpest was that it tended to eliminate not only itself but other diseases as well. With mortality approaching 100 per cent, the very few survivors that escaped infection were free to multiply unencumbered by any disease burden and without any competition for pasture. This is not the place to review the steps taken in later years to control and eventually eliminate rinderpest from most of Africa south of the equator. Ankole had its last outbreak in 1944 (*Uganda veterinary report*), but between the passage of the panzootic and the final disappearance of the disease there were frequent epizootics, some localized, some widespread; some in which the virus was relatively mild in its effects, others in which mortality was very high. The rinderpest of 1889–96 was a natural catastrophe that not many Europeans witnessed and few at the time understood.

Carmichael (1938) reviewed its effects in game. Buffalo, giraffe, eland, bushpig, and warthog were highly susceptible, but the Uganda kob varied in its response to infection. Wildebeest, kudu, and giant forest hog were also susceptible, but the response of impala, oribi, and duiker varied. Elephant, rhinoceros, hippopotamus, roan antelope (perhaps very slightly), waterbuck, hartebeest, and topi were not affected.

Jigger fleas

The rinderpest and smallpox did not complete the tale of biological catastrophe that overwhelmed the interlake area as well as the rest of Africa in the decade before sleeping sickness emerged as the disease that most struck the imagination of the invading European. Another earlier invasion had been approaching for many years. The South American jigger flea, *Tunga penetrans*, seems to have become established in West Africa at least by the beginning of the eighteenth century. But a new and evidently very vigorous invasion began with the arrival at Ambriz in Angola of a ballast-laden British ship from Rio de Janeiro, the *Thomas Mitchell*. This newly introduced population of jiggers spread very rapidly (Hoeppli 1969). Baumann encountered it in Uzinza on the south-west corner of Lake

Victoria in 1892. The chief had made a request, common enough then, for help against enemy tribes.

Besides these human enemies, Mtikiza and his people had an animal foe not so easily attacked. It was known to me of old in West Africa and I found it here for the first time and cannot say I was overjoyed at the renewal of acquaintance. I mean the sand-flea, *Pulex penetrans*, that disgusting insect which buries itself in the toes and other parts of the human body. When, in 1885, I travelled through the Congo, the sand-flea which, as is well known, originates in Brazil and was brought by ships in sand ballast to West Africa, was only at Stanley Pool. It reached Stanley Falls in the Congo steamers and spread itself over Manyema, whence it gradually came to Ujiji and Tabora. It was carried directly to the west coast of the Nyanza by Stanley's expedition. It will certainly not be much longer before it reaches the east coast of Africa, indeed, perhaps we shall see it make its way from there to India in its triumphant progress throughout the world.

He who keeps his feet clean and daily searched in order to extract the recently entered animals, has little to fear from the plague. Should, however, a sand-flea—which once fully established ceases to smart—be left, it swells to the size of a pea and produces finally an abscess, which, if they occur in large numbers, may cause blood-poisoning and death. Especially in regions where this animal is recently arrived and thus, where its treatment is not understood, it produces real disaster. We saw people in Uzinza with whole limbs rotted off, indeed whole villages, following the plague, have died out (Baumann 1894).

Langheld (1909) saw its effects in Karagwe, when he went there in 1893.

In earlier years it was well populated. Now, perpetual quarrels over the throne and the resulting wars, smallpox, the rinderpest and, in some parts also, a plague of sand fleas, had cleared out the population, so that I found great banana plantations, that must have fed many people, completely abandoned.

His successor at Bukoba, Hauptmann Herrmann, described the people of that country as having been 'warlike, numerous people, at present decimated by smallpox; the sand fleas in 1892 were so vicious that a harvest had to remain standing because of lack of labour' (Herrmann 1894).

One consequence of these catastrophes was that they helped to amplify the effects of language difficulties and exacerbated the non-comprehension that developed between the Africans and the Europeans. The jigger fleas did not take long to circumvent Lake Victoria and were so bad among the Kikuyu in Kenya in 1898 that the name given to the circumcision age-group of that year, *nothi*, was the name also given to the jiggers. Father Cagnolo (1933), in his curious English, comments as follows:

The natives pretend that before the coming of the European their country was free of this insect. It is said to have been imported by black troops, but the low [*i.e. uneducated*] people at present have already built on it a legend that explains how, in their opinion, the Akikuyu fell under the British dominion. The European could not have occupied their country with arms only, so he had recourse to wile. He sent along by night a few trusties with kris [*karais* = *basins*] full of seed of pulex penetrans for distribution in various places in Kikuyu. The insect spread. The Akikuyu, unaware of the fact, soon got infected, their feet got diseased, and the warriors were outvied and subdued.

If the Europeans did not send in men to sow the seed, they nevertheless imported these fleas very effectively. In this account we are concerned to relate the material effects of the European invasion. Ignorance on both sides led to mistrust and failure of understanding. This, of course, later helped towards misunderstanding (among other problems) of the ecology of trypanosomiasis.

'Law and order'

A young Mukama, Ndagara II, had emerged from the succession struggles in Karagwe and, for a short time, reigned at Bweranyange. He died of smallpox in 1893 and the power contests began again. To the German administration in Bukoba the first step to recovery was the restoration of 'law and order'. This they achieved by exiling one successor and hanging another and installing a foreigner as their puppet ruler (Ford and Hall 1947).

Like their British neighbours across the Kagera in Ankole the Germans looked upon themselves as saviours of people sunk in centuries of barbaric misery. Few realized that they were the prime cause of the suffering they tried to alleviate. This is clear, for example, in the record of the British botanist, Scott Elliot, who, three years after the rinderpest, travelled down the Kagera valley along the western border of Karagwe.

The country of Karagwe was in a marked decline as I passed through it. When the master hand of Rumanyika was removed, and a youth Kajeti, brought up in a dissolute and licentious court, came to the throne . . . things at once fell to pieces. [There was no such person as Kajeti. He meant Kaketo who, after the death of Ndagara II, was regent for his nephew Ntare, grandson of Rumanyika.]

Along the whole western border, that is along the Kagera River, the country is completely uninhabited. I passed numerous banana plantations, which are neglected and becoming overgrown with weeds, and destroyed. The two fringing semi-independent states on the west bank of the Kagera . . . have by their continual raids produced this effect. The people received no protection and were obliged to go.

Oppressions and robbery of the poorer people, as well as licentious and drinking habits in the King's entourage, are an inevitable consequence of a warlike and raiding state. They have, in Karagwe, as usual, produced utter destruction of the community after a very few years (Scott Elliot 1896).

It did not occur to this botanical moralist that Great Britain was, and would continue for several years to be, a warlike state in Africa.

It is not inappropriate to end this narrative with an African account of these events, not in Karagwe, but in Kiziba, one of the smaller kingdoms of the Bukoba coast. It was taken down during the first decade of this century by Rehse (1910).

The Europeans came to the country. They settled in the country of Kyamtwara at Bukoba. The first to come there was Herr Basha (Emin Pasha). Mukotani (chief of Kyamtwara) went to him and libelled Mutatembwa (of Kiziba). Herr Basha came to make war against Kiziba. He put the King's stronghold to flames and stole cattle. Then he went away. Scarcely two days after he had left the country the cattle began to die and the sand fleas (*jiggers*) came to the country. The cattle nearly all died till only a few remained and the sand fleas killed the people. Also a sickness broke out which killed the people. Many, many died. We sat with our few cattle, which we had bought in Isheshe, when another European, Herr Korongo (Richter) made war on us. He stole the cattle and went home. After he had returned to Bukoba Herr Kama (von Kalben) made war on Kiziba. He came before dawn. Karutasigwa was alone in the fortress. We sang and played and did not worry about the Europeans until they were near us and fired a salvo. Many people died.

Mutual misunderstanding was almost total.

Nkore after the rinderpest

The first news of the rinderpest had reached Emin at Bukoba in January 1891 and therefore it had presumably begun to affect the Nkore herds in 1890. The country was ruled by a firmly established Mugabe, Ntare V. When Emin ignored his plea for help he raided the heavily stocked pastures of Mpororo and Rwanda. This achieved nothing except to hasten the spread of infection which reached cattle watering on the Kagera in northwest Karagwe in April 1891. (The Rwanda people made a return raid in 1895 after the Nkore herds had begun to recover.)

The British in Nkore had an easier task than the Germans in Karagwe. Stanley had made blood-brotherhood with a cousin of Ntare in 1889, and Lugard had arrived over six months after the onset of rinderpest and smallpox and so did not get blamed for them. Ntare, who had lost a son in the smallpox epidemic, died himself in 1895. A nephew, Igumira, successfully supported the claim to the throne of a youth, Kahaya, who may have been Ntare's son, but some said his own. The Enganzi (chief minister) was in favour of collaboration with the British and it was he who successfully negotiated an agreement with them and obtained their support for Kahaya (Morris 1962). The assumption of power by the Uganda Protectorate government was not entirely peaceful. One administrator was murdered (Morris 1960) and there was a considerable amount of movement by leading Hima with their cattle, either to get away from the British and their protégé Mugabe or as part of an attempt to readjust pasture as the cattle population began to recover from the panzootic. These movements often involved transference of herds from one country to another. Somewhat naively, German and British officials regarded these activities as smuggling.

Oberleutnant von Stuemer reported on the cattle south of the Kagera in 1902:

As to the cattle population it is better than before but nevertheless is not large enough to provide adequate numbers for unlimited export. To that extent the raising of the export duty on cattle last year was fully justified. A lively cattle smuggling trade is in progress west of the Kagera from Rwanda through Mpororo to Uganda. It has been partially controlled but will only be fully suppressed by the erection of the projected Mpororo frontier post (von Stuemer 1904).

The Anglo-German boundary commission completed its work in the Kagera valley in 1902–4 (Delmé-Radcliffe 1947). For some two thousand years African agricultural and pastoral people had gradually eliminated their hunting and gathering predecessors and had achieved a mobile ecological equilibrium with the wildlife ecosystems and their associated diseases. It is a fruitless exercise to guess how, if left to themselves, they would have dealt with the epidemics and epizootics that beset them at the end of the last century. But if it is possible to point to any single factor that ensured the destruction of that ancient ecological equilibrium it was the imposition of international boundaries to replace frontier zones. The mechanisms of adjustment provided by the *Grenzwildnis* were eliminated by the surveyor's theodolite and the lawyer's pen.

9

THE SPREAD OF *GLOSSINA MORSITANS* INTO ANKOLE

IN 1909, Uganda veterinary officials found that cattle were dying in the Ngarama and Bukanga areas of south Ankole and demonstrated infection by *Trypanosoma congolense*. Simmons (1929) adds that there was evidence that cattle had begun to move away from the new infection in 1907; local Ankole historians suggest 1908. The Mugabe had sent a herd of his cattle to Bukanga (Map 9.1) and took some of them with him when he went on a safari to Mombasa in 1907. Shortly after his return, a year later, cattle began to die in Bukanga.

The first observation of *Glossina morsitans* in the interlake region was made by Hans Meyer who crossed the Ihangiro depression from Lake Ikimba to Lake Burigi (Map 7.1) in 1911:

Not one of the earlier travellers through this bush had mentioned a little animal that gave us a great deal of trouble: the tsetse (*Glossina morsitans*). On our first day's march (*after leaving Lake Ikimba*) through low lying country where the rainy season had brought on a thick growth of bush and high reeds, these well-known large biting flies were seen swarming around the men and animals of the caravan. Normally they suck the blood of wild animals. Evidently they were not infected, for our mules were still well and active for months after they were bitten and only succumbed much later from infection acquired in Usumbura or Unyamwezi. At Burigi Lake itself, where the natives had cleared the bush, I saw no tsetse. In the low lying depression they reach north to the lower Kagera, but have not yet reached the plateau overlooking Lake Victoria (Meyer 1913).

The first sentence in Meyer's account is the important one. It is very unlikely that Speke, Grant, Emin, Stuhlmann, Langheld, Hermann, and Richter, all of whom crossed the depression before 1900, would have failed to report the presence of the flies.

The spread of *Glossina morsitans* through Karagwe after 1891

An informed veterinary estimate, made in 1924, put the pre-rinderpest cattle population of Bukoba, Karagwe, and Biharamulo districts at 400 000 head (*Bukoba district book*). It is not unreasonable to assess the cattle population of Nkore and the neighbouring small countries since absorbed in Ankole district at 250 000. This may well be an understatement. In Rwanda and Burundi the cattle may have reached a total of more than a million.† The majority of this vast population was exterminated by

† In 1919, before the rinderpest epizootic of that year there were thought to be 1 000 000 head of cattle in Rwanda alone. In 1954 the census total was 580 631 (Adamantidis 1956).

the rinderpest. In Nkore, Mpororo, Rwanda, and Burundi recovery was rapid, but in Biharamulo and Karagwe a rapid spread of *G. morsitans* had occupied all but a few thousand acres of pasture by the mid-1920s.

Evidence for the presence of a large cattle population in Karagwe before the rinderpest lies not only in the records of travellers and in the oral tradition of local people (Ford and Hall 1947) but also in the relics of old kraals. These were easily to be found in the tsetse-infested bush in 1947 and must have been much more obvious in 1924. The Ankole and Tusi cattle are varieties of the so-called Sanga breed. They are quite distinct from other Sanga types and are even more clearly distinguishable from other main breeds (Faulkner and Epstein 1957, Joshi, McLaughlin, and Phillips 1957), and there is no question of the relative antiquity of the Hima and Tusi in the interlake region. At the latest their presence there dates from the end of the sixteenth century, and a period of 600 years is likely. It must also follow that when they arrived they found disease-free pastures. They brought their long-horned cattle with them and there is some evidence that they displaced other cattle-owning people.

What factors prevented *G. morsitans* from spreading through the *Grenzwildnisse* at some earlier date, before the arrival of the rinderpest and other coincident disasters? Did it actually invade the Ihangiro depression between 1891 and 1907 or was it, along with *G. pallidipes* and *G. brevipalpis*, confined to very small fly-belts in the *omurasho* foci at places such as Buhamira? Speke's 'neutral' zone, south of Lake Burigi, could also have contained a small fly-belt. The difficulty about this hypothesis is to imagine any method by which a species such as *G. morsitans* could have been prevented from spreading when not surrounded by an abundant agricultural population. We know from accounts of the vegetation of the Ihangiro depression and from Speke's note that the neutral land south of Burigi was inhabited by wild animals, and extensive high-density agricultural populations were not present. One must postulate a barrier further south (Map 7.1).

An ecological limit to the interlake region is provided by the Bukoba sandstone hills, already described as running in a south-westerly direction from the Lake Victoria coast to Lake Tanganyika. Occupying this line of hills was the country of Usui or Busubi. Two Germans passed through it just after the passage of the rinderpest.

On the 23rd August [1892] we climbed over two high rocky crests between which lay gently rolling inhabited and cultivated land. From the last height we descended into a wide valley, which was covered on its slopes by banana plantations and fields. On the other side lay the great 'hut-complex' of Kasasura, chief of East Usui, one of the mightiest potentates of German Africa. . . . On August 25th we went through the village of Nyaruvongo, Kasasura's residence, which though rich in banana gardens did not appear to be very thickly populated; we climbed over a mountain ridge and entered into grassland with open

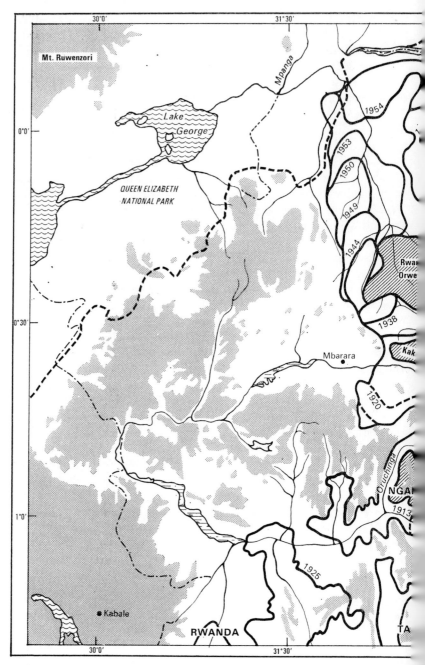

MAP 9.1. Successive stages in the spread of *G. morsitans* in Ankole u
and *G.*

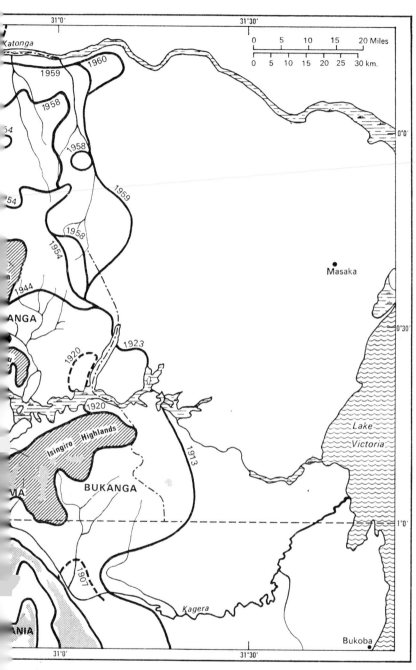

000-ft contour. Broken line indicates eastern limit of *G. pallidipes*
...s of the Rift Wall.

bush, broken up by sorghum fields, banana plantations and friendly huts. Here and there grew a large broad leafed tree indicating an earlier forest cover. Climbing higher one reached the plateau country at Msenyi, which is cut through by deep valleys in which the water runs towards Lake Urigi (Baumann 1894).

Two years later Graf von Götzen followed a similar route.

On the borders of Usambiro and Usui a complete change in the formation of the whole country was noted. Along slippery loam paths one enters a heavily populated land. A broad well cultivated valley floor leads to a small saddle-plateau. The habitations of the people here are extraordinarily scattered; one no longer sees the regular lines of *Euphorbia* hedge with which the Wanyamwezi and Wasumbwa shut in and protect their village enclosures. . . . In the meadows, in which the ground colour almost disappears under a thick carpet of yellow flowers, we saw the first herd of Hima cattle, distinguished by their gigantically big horns.

Kasasura's residence at Nyaruvongo was near the modern town of Biharamulo.

A new luxuriance, much greater than that shown by the vegetation hitherto, now surrounded us. Dracaenas sprang up abundantly and a tree with leathery, shining leaves and large red flowers added much to the colourful liveliness of the scene; in the valleys sparkled rapid torrential streams. . . . The number of settlements, banana shambas and fields of beans, potatoes and sorghum was astonishingly great (von Götzen 1895).

There is little to be gained by speculation about the origin of the spread of *G. morsitans*. Until the rinderpest there were abundant cattle around Lake Burigi, and the same breed of long-horned Sangas was associated with the settlements along the Bukoba sandstone hills that formed the northern boundary of the *Brachystegia* woodlands of Western Tanzania. Some cattle survived around Lake Burigi until 1935 when 1700 animals were moved away with their owners as part of a resettlement scheme to prevent spread of human trypanosomiasis from the south (Maclean 1935).

Busubi and neighbouring countries suffered the same series of epidemics following close upon the rinderpest as were seen elsewhere. There was a lively fear of smallpox, for Kasasura, like other rulers of the interlake region a divine king, would not allow himself to be photographed: 'If he did smallpox would break out in the land' (von Götzen 1895). Reference has already been made to Baumann's account of the jigger plague in Uzinza, a country adjacent to Usui. It is also possible that a contributory factor encouraging the spread of tsetse had been the Ngoni invasion of the northern countries of the *Brachystegia* woodlands (Chapter 11).

The most northerly point reached by the *Brachystegia* woodlands of Tanzania is just inland from Ruiga bay on the Victoria coast at approximately 2°S. It is about 65 miles south of the point on the Kagera where the cattle of Bukanga were infected in 1907 or 1908. The first map of the

Bukoba district (including Karagwe and Biharamulo) was made in 1893–4 and published five years later by Herrmann (1899). It plots in some detail the locations of banana gardens which are easily visible over considerable distances. The southern limit of the comparatively dense population of the coastal portion of Ihangiro is clearly marked by the change in size of these gardens. This change corresponds closely to the limits finally reached by *G. morsitans* in this area. The change in mean area of the banana gardens is not necessarily indicative of change in population density. It indicates primarily a change in the crops cultivated. A basic diet of plantains is replaced by one of cereals and root crops, annuals requiring cultivation, planting, and harvesting every year, instead of the perennial banana which although also requiring proper management does not immediately fail if unattended. In short, the failures of harvests recorded by Langheld and Herrmann in 1892 and 1893 would have had a more rapid effect south of Ruiga bay than north of it. It is unlikely that *G. morsitans* would have spread across this line of settlement immediately after the disasters of 1891. Even if there had been a major collapse of population, the effect of rinderpest on the natural hosts of this tsetse would have brought about a recession rather than a spread. In the comparatively narrow corridor provided by the Ihangiro depression, with a suitable vegetation already present, a rate of spread of six or seven miles a year is not impossible. This would imply a break-through from the *Brachystegia* woodlands into the *Acacia gerrardii* and termitaria thicket of the depression in about 1897.

Tsetse were first seen in the Kagera valley in the Ngarama area (see Map 9.1) in 1913. Veterinarians, however, had reported the presence of bovine trypanosomiasis near the Kakitumba river in 1912, but this, as we have seen, was a known focus of *omurasho* in which, subsequently, *G. pallidipes* was discovered. In 1947 it was stated by local informants in the Bugoye area of north-west Karagwe that, like the rinderpest before it, the tsetse had come down the Kagera valley from the north, from Ankole. This happened in about 1925. From this point the tsetse moved southwards up the Kagera valley and spread throughout the *Acacia* savanna of the Mutara area of north-east Rwanda (Lambrecht 1955, van den Berghe, Lambrecht, and Christiaensen 1956, van den Berghe and Lambrecht 1962).

A second expansion of the fly-belt into Rwanda was first recorded by Belgian authorities in 1939. In the following decade this invasion increased to occupy an area of approximately 1000 mile^2 known as Bugesera adjoining the country of Burundi (Buyckx 1964). If the assumption is correct that *G. morsitans* did not occur north of the Bukoba sandstones of Biharamulo and outside the *Brachystegia* woodlands of Western Tanzania before 1897 one may calculate its total area of spread to 1960 at 9500 mile^2. Of this area some 2500 mile^2, comprising the greater part of the old country of Nkore, was infested between 1907 and 1960. This indicates a much slower rate of spread at a rate of 49 mile^2 a year as against 150 mile^2 a year for the whole fly-belt assuming that the spread began in 1897. The greater part of the spread in Karagwe took place in fully grown tree savanna, but as the fly-belt grew so its expansion had to await the growth of trees in what was formerly open grassland, and then the populating of the new woodlands by a suitable host fauna.

In Ankole as well as Karagwe the spread of *G. morsitans* was assisted by the movement of cultivation away from the foot-slopes of hills and valley floors. In part this was an effect of population decline, but during the troubled years after 1890 people tended to congregate on the hill crests for mutual protection.

In 1934, two immigrant labourers to Uganda were picked up not long after they had passed through Ankole. Both were suffering from an infection of rhodesian trypanosomiasis and both had come from country just south of the interlake region where the infection had been first encountered in about 1930. This greatly alarmed the Uganda authorities who urged the government of Tanganyika to take steps to prevent the further spread of the disease towards Uganda. In 1935, therefore, the surviving population of Karagwe was concentrated in five separate sub-chiefdoms. This removed yet more people from the foot-slope and valley sites to the summits, making available more land suitable for occupation by *G. morsitans* and its hosts (Maclean 1935).

The spread in Ankole between 1907 and 1920

Veterinary observation of cattle trypanosomiasis has been continuous in Ankole since 1909. The infected cattle in Ngarama had been watered on the Kagera river near the confluence of a tributary called the Ikariro. Ngarama was in the Uganda Protectorate. The Ikariro confluence (though not its source) now lay in German East Africa, for civil servants in London and Berlin had decided that the boundary between these two newly defined countries should follow latitude 1°S. westwards from the Lake Victoria coast until it intersected with the Kagera. It is possible, but not certain, that had this arbitrary excision of Ankole pastures not been made, veterinary attention might have been drawn earlier to the epizootic. With the memory of the rinderpest of the nineties fresh in their minds, local cattle owners regarded the new disease as yet another example of European malevolence.[†]

Deaths from trypanosomiasis in Ngarama and Bukanga in southern Ankole had accounted for about 75–80 per cent of the herds by 1910. By 1911 only 1000 head remained from a former population of about 10 000. No wild animal deaths were seen and it was therefore judged that rinderpest was not involved.

---

† There was much misunderstanding. The Ikariro river appears in all earlier accounts and maps as the Kafunzo. This merely means a place with papyrus. Mbarara, principal town of Ankole, was named in the same way. The inquiry through interpreters, 'What is this place called?' became, 'What is this called?' The answer, Mbarara, was the local name for *Themeda triandra*, the pasture grass that covered most of the landscape.

Bukanga and Ngarama are hill pastures. The wide, flat, hilltops more than 5000 ft above sea level, relics of a Miocene peneplain, fall away abruptly in the south to the Kagera, about 1000 ft lower. On their northern slopes the drop to the Ankole lakes is not so far. Springs and ponds sufficed for a permanent population of only about 1000 head on the hilltops in the dry season. The greater bulk of the cattle, as elsewhere in Nkore, engaged in a seasonal transhumance and in the dry weather moved off the hills into the valleys to water in the Kagera to the south or in the lakes to the north. The thousand survivors of the tsetse invasion were those that found enough water at the higher altitudes. A population of about this number maintained itself until 1950, after which it began to multiply rapidly under the protection of new prophylactic drugs that allowed animals to use pastures that were still infested with tsetse.

Glossina morsitans spread westwards along the Kagera valley, the empty *Grenzwildnis* between Nkore and Karagwe, and as each tributary valley was reached it, in turn, became infested as far as it provided a suitable habitat and food supply for the tsetse. In fact there was only one route through the high south Ankole hills. The variously named Oruchinga, Ebitatenge, or Nshen valley enters the Kagera floor at Nsongezi, where in Stanley's time a ferry carried travellers between the two countries. The valley runs north, climbing for about 10 miles and then slopes down to the most westerly of the Ankole lakes, Nakivali.

In 1889 a large population had lived in the valley at Mavona. Emin had written:

July 24th. We often pass stretches of light *Acacia* bush and then again luxurious thorn thicket and bush-forest. Only the occasional steep hills are covered with nothing but grass; the mountains are usually up to two-thirds bushy and then nearly bare. Finally the route leads down a long valley, for a change, through banana plantations, harvested fields (durrah, beans, a little maize, eleusine) and villages where, an unusual thing, much manioc was planted (Emin in Stuhlmann 1916–27).

The settlement at Mavona produced abundantly quite a variety of garden produce, such as peas, beans, tomatoes, potatoes, manioc, cucumbers, banigalls, bananas and plantains (Stanley 1890).

Mavona was much diminished by the plagues that shortly afterwards beset all Africa, and in 1914 *G. morsitans* penetrated the Oruchinga valley, to reach the southern shore of Lake Nakivali. By this time the danger to the pastures of central Ankole had been realized. When the First World War broke out it was anticipated that traffic along the military lines of communication between Entebbe and the British forces facing the Germans across the Kagera would carry the tsetse all over the country.

The military road led south-west from Masaka through Koki up into the heights of Bukanga and Ngarama and then descended to the Oruchinga valley where it branched, north to Mbarara and south to Nsongezi and the military front. In 1915 the army headquarters moved to Mbarara. Traffic between there and the Kagera consisted mainly of pedestrians and motor and ordinary cycles. Simmons (1929) relates that 'An immediate result of this traffic was a rapid and marked increase in the range and density of the fly, which became apparent first in the south and spread northwards, the greatest degree of concentration appearing to be on the road.' The sentence describes a situation common enough but still not fully understood.

Two attempts were made to block movement of tsetse through the valley. Refugees were encouraged to settle at its head, to re-create the old Mavona, and form a barrier of cultivation. A primitive de-flying chamber was made—a grass hut through which all pedestrians and vehicles had to pass and submit, inside it, to fumigation by smoke from burning grass blown by a mechanical bellows.† These measures did not stop the spread of the tsetse. In 1916 the Germans evacuated Bukoba. Military activities ceased and traffic between the Kagera and Mbarara was much reduced. Nevertheless by 1920 *G. morsitans* was taken within 12 miles of that town.

Local opinion inclined to the view that road traffic was responsible for the spread. Casual observers failed to note tsetse flies away from the roads while hunting, although eland, oribi, impala, warthog, and zebra were common. The apparent freedom of these and other animals from the attentions of the tsetse was puzzling, especially in areas where the flies existed in such numbers that progression, whether on foot or by motor cycle, was a painful experience (Simmons 1929).

Recession: 1919–20

In 1919 another disastrous epizootic of rinderpest entered Ankole. There were very heavy losses among the cattle. Eland, buffalo, and warthog were markedly depleted in numbers. The cattle population was reduced from an estimated 300 000 to 80 000 and it was later recalled that 'Miles of road or wide plains were littered with carcases or dying cattle and the overpowering stench caused physical nausea' (*Uganda veterinary report*, 1930). In 1920, the year that tsetse reached within 12 miles of Mbarara, a reduction in the density was noticed and by next year it was clear that a recession was in progress although there had been no change in the bush cover and some animals, such as hartebeest and waterbuck, were not scarce. A further shrinkage was seen in 1922 when these other species became scarce because local hunters now concentrated upon animals not susceptible to rinderpest. This received official encouragement because it was thought that it would hasten the end of the rinderpest epizootic. The consequence of the simultaneous reduction of the wild ungulate populations and the cattle was a

† The technique may have been suggested by the Hima practice of fumigating their cattle to free them of *Stomoxys* by driving them through grass smoke before they enter the kraals in the evening.

particularly unpleasant outbreak of man-eating by the now half-starved population of lions.

The Great Rinderpest had provoked at least two outbreaks of man-eating. The best known was that at Tsavo in 1898 (Patterson 1907). In Chapter 11 reference will be made to an outbreak of man-eating as one of the causes of depopulation in the Shinyanga district. The man-eating in Ankole in 1922–4 has been well described by Pitman who was intimately concerned in dealing with it.

It began in the Sanga chiefdom (see Map 9.1). The lions were not aged toothless creatures.

These Sanga man-eaters were virile, breeding animals which eventually were killing human beings from inclination . . . as opposed to the more ordinary type of man-eater which is driven to prey on man through inability to kill game. Their activities can be attributed to the state of semi-starvation to which they were reduced consequent on the practical extermination of their normal food supply, the game; and the rapidity with which they embarked upon a career of general man-killing was presumably a result of their joining in troops to hunt for food (Pitman 1931).

They killed 33 people in the first quarter of 1924 in Sanga. One lion was known to have killed 84 people and another 44.

It is impossible to realise the horror of such a situation until one has come into direct contact with the murderers and their victims. Death may lurk in every patch of grass, in each thicket, behind any bush whether in the gloom of night or in the reassuring light of day. A friend may be struck down at one's side, a herdsman tending the cattle, a woman filling water-pots or—worst of all— stealthily during the hours of darkness, lions may break into a hut and deliberately butcher the inmates (Pitman 1931).

Pitman mentions, without specifying where they lay, 'considerable tracts of country where every village had been abandoned owing to the depredations of lions' and where 'impenetrable undergrowth is now all that remains to mark the scene of the tragedy'. Presumably this was in south-west Uganda for it is stated that in a neighbouring mandated territory slaughter of antelopes was taking place on a vast scale. An alternative possibility suggested was that the attack might have been made by a troop of lions from the Sanga area.

The Sanga lion episode has been mentioned at some length because it was a fragment of the ecological system in which the spread of tsetses also took place. Similar happenings seen elsewhere on more than one occasion may be an expected part of the pattern of events that follow the reduction, either from disease or deliberate slaughter, of natural prey populations.

By 1925 tsetse had disappeared from areas that had been heavily infested in 1915, and the northern part of the Oruchinga valley became fly-free. It was therefore planned to inaugurate control measures which would restrict *Glossina* to the more or less uninhabited Kagera valley and prevent it from invading the northern pastures again. Surveys were being undertaken with this in view when tin was discovered in south-west Ankole at Kikagati in the Kagera valley. Traffic again became frequent and the antitsetse operations were now replanned because it was thought that the mining community working and living in the valley would risk infection from sleeping sickness. This work had some success (Simmons 1929) but by the time it was finished the Oruchinga was again fully infested and Mavona once more lay in the fly-belt.

Emin's and Stanley's accounts of Mavona have been quoted, and the unavailing attempts of veterinary officials to reconstitute it to block this entry for tsetse into Ankole in 1914 and 1915 have been mentioned. It is not outside the scope of this book to note its subsequent history. I was sent to Ankole in 1944 to inaugurate the fifth campaign against *Glossina morsitans* and looked forward to eventual success. My recommendations included a programme for resettling Mavona and the northern end of the Oruchinga valley so that when the last tsetse had gone there would be no danger of reinfestation from the Kagera valley. Although *G. morsitans* continued to spread so that in the next 15 years almost the whole of the old country of Nkore had disappeared, the project remained in the district development plan. A dam was constructed to improve the water supply and a system of branch roads was made to facilitate access. Various inducements to settlers were offered. A mission built a splendid agricultural training college.

Probably these efforts would, in time, have been crowned with success and the fruitful gardens of 1889 restored; as, in a sense, they were although not in a way that might have been predicted in 1944 or even as late as 1960 after much development work had been done. In 1962 the Hutu in the neighbouring country of Rwanda overcame their rulers and expelled the pastoral Tusi. Several hundreds of these people, with their followers and nearly 14 000 head of cattle, fled to Ankole. Immense clearings were bulldozed for the cattle along the southern shores of the Ankole lakes and the people were accommodated in the Oruchinga valley which, in a very short time, was converted from tsetse-infested woodland to treeless, fly-free cultivation.

The further spread of *G. morsitans* and its effects

The lower Ruizi basin and the country around the western end of the Nshara lakes was the heartland of Nkore. In this area the Mugabe usually lived and pastured his personal herd. Here also, in a pasture called Masha, were kept the cattle assigned to the royal drums, Bagyendanwa. The Bagabe were buried at| Ishanzu on the southern shores of Lake Nakivali. These places were infested by *G. morsitans* between 1914 and 1920. The cattle were moved away and the western lakes ceased to be available for watering. In 1920 a focus of *G. morsitans* infestation was found in the south-east of Nshara. This was thought to have been introduced by the military traffic in 1915, but an inquiry made in 1944 suggested that it was the front of another area of natural spread that had circumvented the eastern end of the Bukanga hills and entered the country of Koki in 1913. This focus did not disappear between 1920 and 1925 when the depopulation of tsetse hosts by the 1919 rinderpest brought about the recession of the fly front at the western end of the lakes.

The recession was temporary. As the warthog and other favoured host populations recovered, so did the tsetse. The recovery was all the quicker because the human populations were still greatly depleted from the effects (as elsewhere) of the epidemics and famines of the previous three decades. The Veterinary Service had completed its protective clearings around the tin mines of south-west Ankole by 1930. By this time the shores of the lake were once more infested and the cattle had again been driven from the Masha pasture. It was here that the main effort at control, financed by special funds from the British government, was centred (Poulton 1938). The infested area was surveyed to discover where the main concentrations of *G. morsitans* were located. When these 'concentration areas' had been defined the trees in them were felled by local axemen. In Masha, the main area treated in this way was along the course of the Lugeye river. This river (dry during much of the year) receives water draining from a number of valleys on the slopes of hills that bound the western margin of Masha. One of them into which the axemen were sent to fell the bush was named Viaruha or Byaruha. In 1889 Stanley had come here to make blood-brotherhood with the Mugabe (who, however, had preferred to send a nephew as his deputy).

The next day (22 July 1889) we started at dawn to continue our journey . . . In an hour we turned sharply from E. by N. to S.E. by S. down another valley. Herd after herd of the finest and fattest cattle met us as they were driven from their zeribas to graze on the rich hay-like grass, which was green in moist places. After a short time the course deflected more eastwards until we gained the entrance of a defile, which we entered to ascend in half an hour the bare breast of a rock hill. Surmounting the naked hill, we crossed its narrow summit, and descended at once its southerly side, into a basin prosperous with banana plantations, pasture and herds, and took refuge from the glaring sun in Viaruha village (Stanley 1890).

Emin wrote, 'We then descend steeply and go through a large banana plantation with many huts. This place is called Viarua' (Stuhlmann 1916–1927). Surgeon Parke (1891) commented, 'We have a splendid supply of bananas here.' By 1930 Byaruha was populated only by wild game, living in a woodland dominated by *Acacia gerrardii*. In 1944 a dense stand of *Acacia hockii* had replaced the *A. gerrardii* which had been felled a dozen years before.

In Karagwe there was no doubt at all that many parts had been depopulated before the arrival of the tsetse flies. The insects and their host animals had been able to occupy country formerly kept as cultivation or as relatively open grassland by human activity. *G. morsitans* did not drive out the population of Karagwe; its disappearance allowed the tsetse to enter. The abandoned villages that Scott Elliot had seen in 1894 in west Karagwe did not become engulfed by the spread of *G. morsitans* until sometime between 1912 and 1920 or even later. In 1915, 7000 head of cattle were taken by their wealthy owner from Ankole into central Karagwe and in the same year a somewhat smaller herd of Karagwe cattle crossed the Kagera into Ankole (Kamugungunu 1946). These movements were not initiated by flight from trypanosome infection but they show that the western portion of the Kagera valley had not become dangerous. They also show that the central and western pastures of Karagwe were still free of *G. morsitans*.

In Nkore the case was otherwise. The people were becoming accustomed to the new rule; they had survived the smallpox and had learned how to deal with jiggers. The cattle, in spite of recurrent rinderpest and infection with East Coast fever were multiplying rapidly. But the appearance of *G. morsitans* put an end to the recovery and, in the course of half a century, extinguished the country of Nkore.

The attempt to stop the spread of tsetse into the Ankole pastures between 1930 and 1936 failed, as did several later schemes. Between 1907 and 1960 the infestation by *G. morsitans* grew until it occupied an area of 2587 mile^2 north of the Kagera river. Expansion therefore averaged 49 mile^2 a year, but there was much variation in the growth rate of the fly-belt. Apart from the period of recession in 1920–5, rates varied between 20 mile^2 a year in 1930–44 to 312 mile^2 a year in 1953–4 (Ford and Clifford 1968). Between 1959 and 1964 a large part of the most recently invaded portion of eastern Ankole was freed of tsetse, partly by fauna destruction and partly by use of insecticides (*Uganda Tsetse control reports* 1960, 1961, Wooff 1964).

Although in the old days the Hima cattle aristocracy did not cultivate and the agricultural Iru serfs were not permitted to own cattle, the two societies were interdependent and long after the Protectorate government had introduced new laws, the old relationships persisted. As the tsetse moved north into the Nkore pastures, the cattle moved away to escape infection. The less mobile Iru, living in their plantations of bananas, were left behind; but in time they moved as well. During the 1940s it was possible to see this process in operation.

Cattle and their Hima owners left an area when the animals began to show symptoms of trypanosomiasis. This happened 2–5 years before it was possible to capture a tsetse fly by the routine methods then in use for survey. Movement of cattle did not merely mean their removal from the infected area. It was necessary also to find new pastures not already filled to capacity by other herds. This often meant removal into another river basin with access to dry-season water supplies as well as room for seasonal changes in grazing areas and adequate reserves of grass during the grass-fire seasons. Migration away from infection therefore meant that much larger areas had to be abandoned than was necessary merely to escape trypanosome infections.

Evacuation of the land by cultivators was a more gradual process. Cultivators still living in an area from which their neighbours were gradually departing, or people who had recently left to settle elsewhere, were usually quite unaware that their difficulties had anything to do with the departure, perhaps five or more years before, of the Hima and their cattle. Two reasons were commonly given for movement. Either the water-holes were drying up or the raiding of their crops by wild animals had increased beyond their capacity to keep the marauders away. Often both reasons were given. A variant on this theme was that a herd of buffalo had begun to use the communal water-hole and the women of the household were frightened to go to draw the day's supply of water. One had the evidence of one's eyes to show that these were valid reasons.

Disappearance of cattle meant that young trees (*Acacia hockii* or *A. gerrardii*) were no longer felled for kraal building. The periodical burning of grass was discontinued or its regime was changed. Some Iru were servants of the Hima and followed the migrating herds. Others were craftsmen who supplied the cattle owners with milk pots, carved from the trunks of *Albizia coriaria*, or furniture of other kinds; smiths who made spears or brewers who sold banana beer, and others dependent upon the herdsmen, followed their customers.

Water-holes were always carefully looked after by the herdsmen. Some were derived from small hillside springs which ran intermittently to fill small tanks dug below them. Others were scooped out in the valley floors where subsoil water accumulated and revealed itself by patches of hygrophilous plant life. Cattle were not allowed to drink from these water-holes; instead the herdsmen made (and still make) oval tanks with mud walls about a foot high. They filled the tanks themselves by throwing in bucketfuls of water from the water-holes. The cattle would then be called up by name, in groups of about six at a time, to drink. The remains of these artificial watering tanks, slightly raised ovals about 12 ft long by 6 broad, could be seen in the tsetse-infested bush ten to twenty years after the cattle had gone. The water-holes from which they had been filled were by then usually marked only by a thicket. In 1944 it was decided to clear the bush from a valley some 18 miles east of Mbarara which was known to have been invaded by *G. morsitans* in 1935. Plant indicators of previous cultivation were still visible, but it was not possible to begin work until a water supply had been created for the labour gang of about one hundred men. The site of the former water-hole was found, some of the bush around it removed and the hole re-dug. After the next rains had filled it it was possible to bring in the men and begin work. In part the disappearance of the water-holes was caused by the use made of them by wild animals that moved in as the cattle moved out. Buffalo, pigs, and other animals found their range enlarged by the departure of cattle and the water-holes, no longer carefully tended, were churned to mud by trampling and gave a foothold to thicket-forming shrubs.

Changes in flora and fauna

A South African veterinarian with much experience of rinderpest who visited Uganda as an adviser after the First World War predicted that one consequence of the panzootic would be the growth of bush in areas that had formerly been open grassland (Montgomery 1923). In 1944 there were many witnesses to affirm that the county of Nyabushozi which contained much of the old pastures of Nkore had once been treeless. At that time, indeed, most of the low hills that form the watershed in eastern Ankole between the drainage basin of the Katonga river in the north and that of the Ankole lakes in the south were still without trees. Only a narrow salient of *Acacia gerrardii*, about 5 miles wide, ran northward along the western edge of these grasslands to join another bank of *Acacia* and other light woodlands nearer to the Katonga. In the main Nyabushozi pastures there were few large trees, nearly all of them *Albizia coriaria* with an occasional *Acacia sieberiana*. Termitaria (*Macrotermes* sp.) are numerous in Ankole pastures and here carried one or two shrubs of *Rhus* and *Grewia*, with sometimes a candelabrum *Euphorbia*. *Acacia hockii* formed dense stands on many hillsides, but were all 5-6 ft tall. Among them, in places, one found young *A. gerrardii* of about the same height. Only in the western salient was this species to be found fully grown. It seemed evident, and local people maintained, that these patches of young acacias were new and expanding.

In 1944 it was confidently expected that *G. morsitans* would be controlled long before these trees were big enough to provide them with a habitat. Six years later the spread of tsetse had not been halted and the infested salient was 7-10 miles wide. Then, suddenly, in 1953 and 1954, *G. morsitans* overran some 600 miles of the country that ten years earlier had seemed quite unsuited to it. By this time the *Acacia hockii* was 12-18 ft high and there were extensive areas covered by *A. gerrardii* woodlands well over 20 ft in height. The open grasslands of Rwanda Orwerwa (*the treeless country*) were now reduced to a small area of about 120 mile^2 not far north-east of Mbarara. At the same time that the trees had been growing many of the pasture grasses on which the cattle had grazed had disappeared, to be replaced by the unpalatable *Cymbopogon afronardus*.

Three factors seem to have contributed to the changes in the vegetation. The first was the retreat of cattle from sources of infection and their replacement by wild animals such as buffaloes and various antelopes. Water-buck were a particular nuisance as crop raiders to surviving cultivators and to newcomers who were induced to settle in the hope of forming a barrier to the spreading tsetse. The disappearance of people meant that the continual felling of trees, for various household purposes as well as the clearing of land for cultivation, ceased. The shrubs on the termitaria, no longer browsed upon by goats, grew and multiplied. Banana gardens, which unlike the ground cleared for cereals are perennial foci of meso-phytic vegetation, collect year by year their mulch of fallen leaves and stalks and develop a rich soil on which dense thickets soon develop when they are abandoned. These changes, initiated by the removal of cattle, must have been very widespread after the Great Rinderpest and concurrent depopu-lation by smallpox and famine. The invasion by tsetse prevented full recovery and once more removed the vegetation controls that had been partly resumed.

A second cause of the proliferation of *Acacia hockii* may have been the changes in grass-burning practice inaugurated by the veterinary services in 1930-6 when much thought was given to the problem of controlling bush. *G. morsitans* was especially associated with well-grown *A. gerrardii* wood-land in which there were abundant termitaria thickets. One of these foci of dense tsetse population was in the Byaruha valley where 41 years earlier Stanley had found banana gardens and many cattle. Once the trees had been felled in these 'concentration sites' it seemed necessary to prevent their regrowth and also gradually to destroy the still unfelled woodlands. To do this a strict control was imposed over grass burning and fires were forbidden in the tsetse-infested area until the last possible moment before the rains broke, when the whole countryside was ignited.

In spite of early signs of apparent success with this measure against *A. gerrardii* (Poulton 1938) it now seems probable that the proliferation of *A. hockii* was encouraged by the fires. This happened in two ways. When growth above ground is suppressed by intensive burning of partially pyrophytic trees like *A. hockii*, it is encouraged below. There is extensive suckering from which, in due course, new shoots appear at a distance from the parent plant. In addition, as Harker (1959) showed, brief exposure of the seeds of this tree to high temperature improves the chances of success-ful seed germination.

Man, as an agent of vegetation change, is rivalled only by elephants. In 1944, and doubtless for years afterwards, elephant bones were easily found in the Nyabushozi grasslands. They were relics of a government-sponsored campaign of elephant control throughout the Protectorate. The widespread human mortality from various causes in Uganda in the first two decades of the century had much diminished an important agent of control on populations of elephants. This was especially the case in Western Uganda, where, between 1910 and 1920, people were removed as a prophylactic measure against sleeping sickness from most of the Western Rift Valley. The territory available to elephants was greatly enlarged and they became pests over a very large area. To deal with this situation the government created a number of large reserves, mostly in Western Uganda, in which elephants were protected, and at the same time encouraged their slaughter elsewhere. Brooks and Buss (1962) have compared the distribution and migration routes of elephants in 1929 and 1959, at the beginning and at the end of the elephant control work. They describe an annual movement of elephants through eastern Ankole between the Katonga and Kagera valleys. This finally ceased as a result of intensive hunting in 1937.

Because of the disordered condition of the country after 1890 it is not possible to know what had been the natural condition of the elephant population earlier in the nineteenth century. But it seems not unlikely that the annual migration between the Katonga and Kagera valleys, the northern and southern *Grenzwildnisse*, had been a long-standing event and one to which the local cattle owners were well accustomed. Swynnerton (1923c) who was engaged by the Uganda government to report on its elephant problem was told that in June 1923 a herd of approximately 100 elephants was seen sharing a water-hole with 400 head of cattle in eastern Nyabushozi. The control exercised by elephants on tree growth in fire-maintained savanna is well known (see, for example, Buechner and Dawkins 1961, Buss 1961). The situations most favourable for growth of trees are the valley floors in which drainage is good or on the lower foot-slopes of hills. Travellers through east central Ankole in the beginning of this century commented upon the open savanna, the bare slopes of the bigger hills, and the dense woodland in the valleys leading off them.

One traveller, Sir William Garstin, a hydraulic engineer surveying the Nile headwaters for the Egyptian government, described elephant damage to woodlands near the eastern border of Ankole:

Throughout the country signs of elephant are very numerous and the damage these animals do to the forests is amazing. Large trees are snapped off near the roots, and others are uprooted and tossed about, apparently wantonly as frequently the branches are not even stripped of their leaves. [This passage was inspired by what had been seen at Nsonge, 5 km inside the Ankole border with Buganda.] For the next 40 kilometres or so of the journey to the west the character of the country is extremely uninteresting and most monotonous. Low ridges and broad swamps alternate with maddening regularity. These ridges are sparsely wooded and the reedy swamps generally border a sluggish stream flowing in a channel blocked by tall grass. . . . At kilometre 150 from Lake Victoria a welcome change appears in the landscape. The hills are high and more resembling mountains than any met with since leaving the lake. They are bare and grass covered. The absence of trees is very striking. The valleys are full of dense jungle and in the dry season water, in this part of the route, is a serious difficulty. A few kilometres further on banana plantations recommence on the lower slopes of the hills (Garstin 1904).

Bush-clearing activities of elephants sufficiently intensive to eliminate *Glossina* has been observed in recent years in at least two national parks (Ford 1966). It seems probable that the halting of the annual migrations of elephants through the Nyabushozi grasslands was an important factor in releasing the woodland succession.

It is relevant to recall Grant's walk in 1861 across the Ihangiro depression to Kitangule and its dry grassy plain 'kept short by cattle' where, he estimated, Rumanyika kept about 10 000 head of cattle (p. 124). Speke, a few months earlier, had also seen the cattle and added, 'In former days the dense green forests peculiar to the tropics, which grow in swampy places about this plain, were said to have been stocked by vast herds of elephants; but since the ivory trade had increased, these animals had all been driven off to the hills of Kisiwa and Uhaiya, or into Uddu beyond the river, and all the way down to the Nyanza.' At this time only a few Arabs had reached Karagwe or Uganda and one doubts that the ivory trade had had so devastating an effect. It seems more probable that at the time of Speke's visit the elephants were, indeed, north of the Kagera on one of their periodical migrations. Whatever the explanation, the association of elephants with the neighbourhood of cattle in open grasslands is interesting.

Langdale-Brown, Osmaston, and Wilson (1964) consider that the dry *Acacia* savanna, dominated by *Acacia gerrardii*, has been derived from a thicket climax by burning and grazing. They draw attention to instances of thicket regeneration and to the role of termitaria in providing foci for growth of thicket species. The invasion of relatively treeless grasslands by *Acacia* may, indeed, find its explanation in the reasons already advanced and one can agree with these authors in supposing that suppression of grass fires would lead to proliferation of a thicket climax or sub-climax vegetation. But the account of vegetational changes given in this chapter suggests that the *Acacia* savanna is an intermediate seral stage between open grassland and thicket. If this is so, and since they are obviously not climax grasslands, the problem is raised of their origin. To this problem, which is fundamental to the ecology of the cattle populations of Africa, it will be necessary to return later.

Effects of the spread of *Glossina morsitans* on the Ankole cattle

The series of epizootics that beset the Ankole cattle as *G. morsitans* spread throughout the pastures of the south and east of the country have been analysed (Ford and Clifford 1968). Once the main features of the disease when carried by this tsetse had been recognized, cattle owners reacted to it by moving away from the pastures in which their beasts showed symptoms of infection. Fig. 9.1 plots cattle population estimates recorded in *Uganda blue books* (1909–20), in *Annual reports of the department of veterinary services* (*Uganda veterinary reports* 1920–64), and for the years between 1933 and 1953, which are omitted from the latter source, in

TAE—M

Watson (1954). The earliest figure is given by Meldon (1907). Not much reliance can be placed on the figures before 1920. It is likely that the very rapid increase between 1910 and 1912 was in part due to the incorporation of the northern half of the old kingdom of Mpororo, now divided between the British and the Germans, into Ankole, where it became Kazhara county. This would not account for all of the 1910–12 increase and it seems likely that the fall from 330 000 in 1915 to 230 000 in 1916 may represent a more sober guess at numbers. (However, from August 1914 to the end of 1915 a small army was stationed in the area waiting to invade German East Africa.) In 1919 occurred the severe rinderpest epizootic already mentioned, when the countryside was littered with carcases (*Uganda veterinary report* 1930). In 1920 the last of the *Blue book* reports gave a figure of

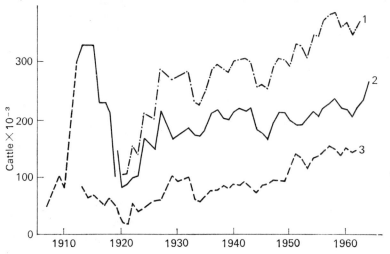

FIG. 9.1. Estimates and counts of Ankole (2) and Masaka cattle (3) and of the combined cattle population (1) of both districts.

144 000 head of cattle for the year ending 31 March 1920. The first *Veterinary report* (1920) for the same year, ending 31 December, gave a figure of 81 924 head. A protective inoculation campaign was carried out during the year and it is known that the second total was obtained from a census completed in December. It is therefore likely that the difference of 62 000 between the two assessments of 1920 is a fairly accurate measure of mortality in that year.

This 1919 epizootic was, as we have seen, followed by a recession of the fly-belt. The surviving cattle, freed of rinderpest, and relieved of the pressures of the fly-belt, and with virtually unlimited grazing, increased from just over 80 000 in 1920 to 217 000 in 1927. But in the next two years numbers dropped to 167 000. By this time *G. morsitans* was spreading again, but it would be wrong to attribute this decline to mortality from trypanosome infection. This was the period in which the Masha pastures watered by the Ruizi river, and the dry-season grazing around the south Nshara lakes, became cut off by the encroaching tsetse. The only other source of water within the bounds of the old Nkore (for the Kagera had long been cut off) was the drainage basin of the Katonga. Two eastern chiefdoms of Nkore, Mawogola and Kabula, had been excised from the domains of the Mugabe and presented by the British administration to the more powerful neighbour, Buganda, as a punishment to Ankole for the murder of an official. This did not stop the Hima herdsmen from using it, and the decline of 50 000 head observed in Ankole between 1927 and 1929 was paralleled by a rise of 42 000 head in the cattle population of Masaka district which now included Mawogola and Kabula. Similar compensating movements can be detected in 1944–6 and in 1949–51. The first was reputed to be a response to an unpopular attempt by officials in Ankole to promote a ghee industry. The second followed the demarcation of a danger zone in central Ankole into which *G. morsitans* was then spreading. The general trend of this cattle population is therefore best shown by the curve for the two districts of Ankole and Masaka combined. From this it is clear that the population density scarcely changed between 1927 and 1950, but varied about a mean of 280 000 head. The two fluctuations observed during this period can probably be associated with rinderpest. The virus re-entered Ankole and Masaka from the north in 1930, when it was estimated that it killed about 15 000 beasts in the two districts. In 1931 and 1932 mortality was negligible, but in 1933 a very virulent epizootic entered south-west Ankole. Fifty thousand animals were inoculated, of which some 15 000 died from the effects of the inoculation. In addition many animals died in naturally infected herds. Although the reported deaths do not account for the drop of 49 341 head between the totals for 1932 and 1933, it would seem likely that the rinderpest, or its side-effects, accounted for most of it. Most of this fluctuation was recorded in Masaka, whereas the centre of the 1933 epizootic was in Kazhara on the western side of the district. Those cattle that had crossed from north-east Ankole into Masaka in 1927–9 returned in 1933 and thus masked, in the population estimate for Ankole alone, the fluctuation due to the rinderpest. There were occasional small outbreaks during the next decade. The most severe was in 1937, when deaths after inoculation amounted to 3700. Finally, the last Ankole epizootic took place in 1943, when 132 000 head were inoculated in the two districts. The disease was last observed in Ankole in 1944, although a small outbreak in Masaka in 1950 was controlled without any loss.

After the 1919–20 rinderpest outbreak and the declines in 1933 and 1943, recovery was very rapid, but ceased abruptly at about the same level on each occasion. Between 1920 and 1927 the cattle population grew at a rate of approximately 15 per cent per annum, but from 1927 to 1932 it did not grow at all. From 1934 to 1937 the growth rate was almost 10 per cent per annum, but from 1937 to 1942 the total increase was only 4·4 per cent. Again, from 1946 to 1948 the increase was also at 10 per cent per annum, but by 1950 the combined cattle population of the two districts was less than 5000 above its 1927 total (Ford and Clifford 1968).

This pattern of growth will be observed again in Sukumaland (Chapter 11) and in Rhodesia (Chapter 20). But in those areas, fluctuations after attainment of stability were due to starvation, assisted in Sukumaland by theileriosis. The latter disease does not now occur in Rhodesia, and in Sukumaland it exerts its effect on the population by periodical epizootics. In Ankole it is enzootic throughout.

The control of cattle population density in Ankole

The old country of Nkore covered a region of grass savanna dominated by the red oat grass, *Themeda triandra.* The assumption, made on page 146, that its cattle population totalled about 250 000 was based upon a supposed stocking rate of about a beast to 10 acres. As the fly-belt grew in area cattle were forced eastwards into the northern half of the county of Nyabushozi or else into the south-western quarter of the district. Movement towards the north or west was impossible, for since 1934 the pastures of the northern portion of the old Nkore, in the modern county of Mitoma, had been invaded from the west by *Glossina pallidipes*. This was a separate event and is described in Chapter 10.

In 1942 the 60 000 head of Nyabushozi cattle occupied about 820 mile^2 of pasture (8·7 acres per beast). Twenty years later, when nearly all had emigrated (partly voluntarily and partly compulsorily under the necessities of tsetse control) only some 120 mile^2 of country (Rwanda Orwerwa in Map 9.1) was not engulfed in the fly-belt. With only 8814 head remaining (Table 9.1) the stocking rate was then 8·8 acres per beast. At the mid-point between these years the figure of 24 211 head in about 730 mile^2 of tsetse-free country gives a much lower rate. This was shortly after one of the largest emigrant movements when, between 1949 and 1952, the Nyabushozi cattle were reduced by 20 000 head and the Masaka district total rose by 44 000. Another county, Mitoma, was also involved in the movement. After the completion of tsetse reclamation work in northern Nyabushozi (Bernacca 1963, Wooff 1964) its stock population rose to 66 000, yielding a stocking rate of 9·2 beasts per tsetse-free acre. It is clear that in spite of the vicissitudes of the period and, after 1950, a widespread use of prophylactic drugs, there was a continual trend towards density adjustment at just under 10 acres per beast. But it is also clear that this could not have been maintained had there been no pasture reserve available in Mawogola and Kabula.

Other evidence of balance between population and pasture availability is given by the data for the county of Shema which, in sixteen counts between 1942 and 1965 yielded a mean population of 23 461, with maximum

TABLE 9.1

Changes in distribution of Ankole cattle, 1942, 1952 and 1962†

Counties	1942		1952		1962	
	Population	%	Population	%	Population	%
Nyabushozi . .	60 200	27·70	24 211	12·64	8 814	3·97
Kazhara . . .	42 300	19·47	55 401	28·92	76 385	34·42
Rwampara . .	32 700	15·05	41 747	21·80	46 107	20·78
Shema . . .	23 600	10·86	21 775	11·37	20 445	9·21
Kashari . . .	19 700	9·06	22 526	11·76	27 967	12·60
Igara . . .	17 700	8·14	14 160	7·39	14 947	6·74
Mitoma . . .	12 900	5·94	2 708	1·41	12 431	5·60
Buhwezu. . .	7 100	3·27	7 427	3·88	6 474	2·92
Isingiro . . .	1 100	0·50	1 575	0·82	8 326	3·75
Totals . . .	217 300	99·99	191 530	99·99	221 896	99·99

† From Ford and Clifford (1968).

fluctuations to 28 662 in 1955 and 19 865 in 1961. The central position of this county should be noted. It will be seen in Chapter 13 that in Sukuma-land the central district sustains a stable density of human population while the populations of peripheral districts fluctuate.

Figure 9.1 shows that after 1950 the steady state of the combined Ankole–Masaka population was not maintained. Numbers rose and continued to rise to 1960. This was attributable to several factors. The most important of these was probably the use of prophylactic drugs against trypanosomiasis which not only enabled cattle to remain in closer juxtaposition with the fly-belts, but also increased the birth rate by reducing calf loss due to abortions caused by trypanosome infection. A second factor was the effect of the Protectorate government's action in preventing the Hima aristocracy from continuing its monopoly of cattle raising and encouraging the cultivators to keep herds (Randall 1944). An increasing portion of the cattle population thus became stabilized in small herds attached to individual farms, instead of enjoying a semi-nomadic life in relatively large herds. The effect of this was to increase available pasture.

The pattern of Hima nomadism was determined not only by the need to find fresh pastures, but also by the geographical disposition of water. The stress of seasonal migration in search of water was believed to be responsible for many calf deaths. A large number of dams, with a total capacity of 1500 million gallons, were constructed between 1944 and 1951 in the portion of north-east Ankole at that time still free of *G. morsitans*. At the same time a tick control campaign was begun in the south and west of Ankole, where theileriosis was most prevalent. In 1949 over 19 000 cattle deaths from notifiable diseases were reported, amounting to 9·04 per cent of the estimated cattle population for that year. Of these deaths 65 per cent were caused by *Theileria* infection and 33 per cent by trypanosomes. Other diseases, which included anthrax, foot and mouth disease, and blackquarter were of trivial importance. Three years later, when trypanosomiasis was much reduced by drugs, tick incidence had also fallen and the stresses on calves (among which the mortality due to *Theileria* chiefly occurs) had been relieved by well-distributed artificial water supplies, the death rate from notifiable disease had fallen to 3·78 per cent, with 56 per cent of these deaths due to *Theileria* and 41 per cent to trypanosomiasis.

It is a Hima custom to slaughter male calves not selected for breeding. This is a means of population control against which official propaganda has long been directed. In 1942 Hima herds showed only 7·4 per cent of males, as against 19·4 per cent in herds belonging to Nyankore cultivators. As the latter then owned 41·6 per cent of Ankole cattle, whereas in 1935 they had owned only 26 per cent, it would appear that slaughter of male calves as a means of population control was diminishing (Randall 1944).

Export of cattle for trade was small. In the five-year period 1939–43, cattle exports from Ankole only amounted to a mean of 2·8 per cent of the cattle population, and this had risen to 3·1 per cent for the five years 1949–53. In Ankole itself in 1953, an average meat consumption was 8·4 lb per head per annum as against a mean of 18·07 lb for Uganda as a whole (Watson 1954). In pre-colonial times population control by export and sale of butcher's meat did not exist; but its place may have been taken by losses through raids from the neighbouring countries of Buganda and Bunyoro.

Although trypanosomiasis exercised a direct effect on Ankole cattle, its main influence lay in reduction of area of pasture. Before the invasion by *G. morsitans*, population control was exercised by slaughter of male calves and death of calves by *Theileria* infection. The influence of *Theileria* varied according to stresses imposed by pasture shortage and transhumance migrations, which acted both directly and indirectly through milk supply. The milk had to feed the Hima cattle owners and their families as well as the calves. This need supplied the *raison d'être* for killing male calves. There were periodical epizootics of other infections. One veterinary investigator recorded that there were outbreaks of a disease called *suna*, which may have been malignant catarrhal fever, in Karagwe in 1855, 1867, and 1876 (*Bukoba district book*), but we are not told how this precision in dating was achieved. Contagious bovine pleuropneumonia was said to have appeared in 1880 and 1884. Lugard (1891) mentioned what may have been the same epizootic of pleuropneumonia as having passed through Nkore in 1887.

An essential requirement for survival was abundance of pasture. Poor management of seasonal grass fires could lead to acute shortages only to be offset by removal to another district or even another country. Although warfare and cattle raiding between the countries of the interlake region were by no means unknown, in times of adversity the less afflicted might offer hospitality to the cattle of its neighbour. A study of the ecology of the interlake pastures would have to regard the cattle of Ankole, Rwanda, Burundi, Karagwe, and their satellite countries as a single population. If this were done it would be found that another factor of population control had to be taken into account. This is the creation of new pasture by the destruction of wildlife ecosystems through human activity.

10

THE ANTECEDENTS OF TRYPANOSOMIASIS IN NORTH ANKOLE AND THE RIFT VALLEY

B Y 1944, cattle in the county of Mitoma on the north-western border of the old country of Nkore had been dying of trypanosomiasis for about ten years. Several surveys had failed to discover any tsetse and it was thought that the infection was brought in sporadically by *Glossina morsitans* carried up from the fly-belt in the south by motor traffic. In January 1945 we found a single female *G. pallidipes* in gallery forest at the head of a minor tributary of the Mpanga river (Map 10.1). This was 25 miles east of and 1500 ft above any earlier record of this species. Soon afterwards *G. fuscipes fuscipes* was taken on another river, and *G. fuscipleuris* was caught in a nearby outlier of the dense forests that cover parts of the Rift wall in this region. The historical antecedents of this second invasion of tsetse must now be examined.

The Rift Valley at the end of the nineteenth century

Stanley had looked down on Lake George (Ruisamba) in 1875. This lake lies in a branch of the Rift Valley that forks north-east from Lake Edward under the south-eastern slopes of Mount Ruwenzori. The explorer had added 2000 fighting men from Buganda to his expedition and had marched westwards from the Nile source on a route just north of the Katonga river. He crossed the Mpanga and entered Buzimba, a little satellite chiefdom of Nkore. From a height of 5000 ft one looks across, in good weather, to the snows of Ruwenzori, 16 763 ft above sea level and 45 miles away to the north-west. In the Rift floor is Lake George at a fraction under 3000 ft, joined by the 20-mile-long Kazinga channel to Lake Edward (Lutanzige in some older writings). Stanley hoped to press on westwards to the Congo, but the people of the little country of Kitagwenda at the foot of the Rift scarp were unwelcoming. Two emissaries sent down to the lake below returned to report that the descent was so steep and the people so numerous that it would not be advisable to attempt the passage. The expedition turned back. They had learned of the Katwe salt trade and reported that the salt was hoisted up the precipices wrapped in bull-hides. 'Great stores of salt had been seen, which came from Usongora [*the plains north of Lake Edward and the Kazinga Channel*] and abundance of Indian corn, millet, sweet potatoes, bananas and sugar cane had also been seen at the lake shore.'

In 1889 Stanley was back again, this time from the north in company

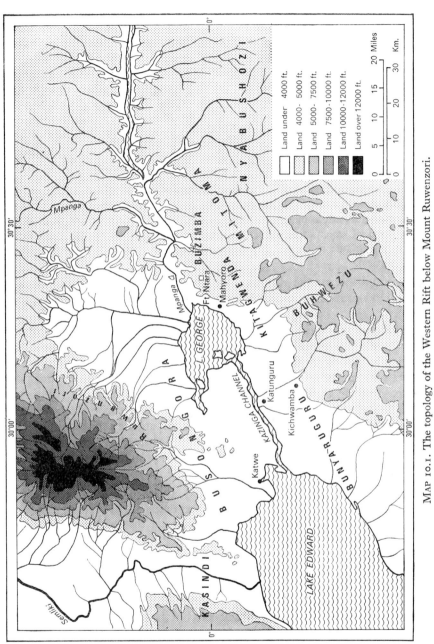

MAP 10.1. The topology of the Western Rift below Mount Ruwenzori.

with Emin. They came down the Semliki valley from Lake Albert, under the western face of Ruwenzori to the centre of the salt trade, the lake at Katwe. From here the salt was taken to Kitagwenda in canoes. This time Stanley was not deterred and marched through Kitagwenda. To this entrepôt of the salt trade and its market came 'people from Uganda, Karagwe, Mpororo, Kitara [*Bunyoro*] and Ankole' (Emin in Stuhlmann 1916–27). In a discussion about the disappearance of Kitagwenda in the events to which we are now leading, Père Gorju (1920) put its population at about 30 000.

In 1891, two years after Stanley and Emin, Lugard crossed northern Nkore to Buzimba on top of the Rift, thence down into Kitagwenda and on to Kichwamba.

I marched round the south of Mount Kibinga to Ibanda which is the frontier village of Ankole towards Kitagwenda and Unyoro. Here there was an enormous amount of cultivation, mostly mtama. [At Kichwamba] we halted some days to collect food, of which there was a very great quantity (and largely exchanged for salt, which in turn is carried to Ankole and Uganda and exchanged for other commodities).

He noted that on the Rift wall 'were very extensive forests full of elephants and probably yielding rubber, etc., extending for miles' (Lugard 1891).

Lugard traversed the Rift floor and the Kazinga channel and went on to the Semliki. He crossed to its western bank and marched 20–30 miles to the north, crossed again to the east bank, under the western slopes of Ruwenzori, and then south again. It is clear that dense populations of banana-growing people lived on both sides of the valley in its southern portion (its northern half is covered by part of the Ituri forest). Lugard made no mention of people living near the river, and he saw elephants near it both when crossing to the west and at the more northerly crossing to the east. But marching northward up the western side on the foot-slopes of the Mitumba mountains he wrote:

All the country was densely inhabited and cultivated, bananas, grain of all kinds and beans seem the staple food. [And on the southward return, along the foot of Ruwenzori] I have never seen anything like the cultivation. As far as the eye can see, endless acres of plantations extend, all looking most luxuriant —bananas, grain and beans. . . . The fields are wonderfully well kept, not a weed to be seen. I am told that a vast quantity of food is grown, in order to be exchanged for salt. It is a wonderful granary, and if we hold the salt lake we tap all this endless supply.

In the event the British got the salt lake, but the Belgians took the Semliki.

The dense cultivation lay on the foot-slopes of the Rift wall or of Ruwenzori and pushed up the hillsides where the valleys were wide enough and not too steep; or, in suitable topographical situations (as around Ibanda or Kichwamba) occupied parts of the top of the Rift wall.

Elsewhere, where the mountains did not rise above its altitudinal limit, there was, and still is, forest.

Below, in the floor of the Rift, on either side of the Kazinga channel, the moist climate of the mountains gives way abruptly to a semi-arid climate with less than 30 in of rain. Here, in the flat grasslands dominated by *Themeda triandra* with a sparse woodland of acacias, early travellers found cattle. Stanley (1890) and his companions indeed saw few, because the plains of Usongora had recently been raided by Kabarega, Mukama of Bunyoro, and the herds had been driven into hiding. He described the deserted kraals as *zeribas*, every one of which, 'besides being protected by an impenetrable hedge of thornbush, had within a circular dyke of cattle dung, rising five feet high. These great circular heaps of refuse and dung were frequently met in Usongora and will remain for a century to indicate the sites of the settlements when village and generation after generation have disappeared.'

The expedition marched around the northern end of Lake George, and the surgeon, Dr. Parke (1891), recorded in his diary that, among other animals, they saw 'a few giraffes'. These later disappeared, presumably victims of the rinderpest. Near one camp on the east of Lake George, Emin saw many buffaloes and wrote, 'They belong, like those found west of the lake, to the small, red, western species. Antelopes also are abundant; elephants, very big, carrying large trunks. In this country there appear to be large numbers of goats and sheep but few cattle.' They went on up through the gap through which the road from Mbarara now runs north to Fort Portal and, on 5 July 1889, in the valley between Ibanda on their left and the mountains of Buhwezu on their right 'the first herds of the Wanyankori were discovered' (Stanley 1890). Emin noted, 'We march steadily round the mountains of a steep slope. In the depths bananas and huts.' Surgeon Parke added, 'The country here is abominably hilly and wearisome to march over.' A commentator on these records remarked that the march from the shore of Lake George into the hills of Buhwezu would today take more than the few hours that Stanley took because of the entanglements of forest that have replaced the settlements and open grasslands of 1889 (Lukyn Williams 1935).

Either the rinderpest was late in arriving in the Rift Valley or else the cattle made a very rapid recovery. Scott Elliot recorded that shortly before his arrival there in 1894 Kasagama, Mukama of Toro, who had been offered the overlordship of Usongora and Kitagwenda by Lugard (Macdonald 1897), had sent an expedition to assert his authority over various chiefs living to the south-west of Ruwenzori. This expedition 'performed its duty by seizing the cattle of everybody' who possessed any. He observed that cattle 'appear to be very easily kept over the whole country around the Albert and Albert Edward Nyanzas; those I saw being in the very best condition' (Scott Elliot 1896).

Cattle were still doing well on the plains of Bunyaruguru south of the Kazinga channel in 1905. 'Between the hills and the north-east end of the Nyanza is a plain of great fertility, if one may judge from the fatness of the great herds of cattle which feed there' (Wollaston 1908). There were also swarms of small antelopes, the commonest being Uganda cob and reedbuck.

In 1945 it was not difficult to convince oneself that circular rings of dry thicket, each some 20–40 yd across and composed of *Grewia, Capparis, Euphorbia, Sanseviera, Erythrococca*, and similar shrubs, often overgrown with creepers such as *Cissus quadrangularis*, were indeed relics of the kraals that Stanley had seen.

Three botanists made notes on the vegetation of the Rift in the early years of the century. Dawe (1906) crossed the high hills of western Ankole from the south. Coming down from the heights he noticed successively: the sub-alpine 'tree lobelias', *Lobelia gibberoa* and the arborescent heather, *Phillipia*; the forests of the intermediate levels dominated by *Parinari mobola*; the densely populated banana belt in the deep valleys and on the steep slopes around the crater lakes; and then the hot dry plains studded with candelabrum euphorbias and acacias. Near the Kazinga channel, around the small fishing village of Katunguru, was a denser bush mainly of the shrub *Capparis tomentosa*. Dawe was chiefly interested in finding plants of economic potential, but his successors, the German botanist Milbraed and the Swede Robert Fries, had wider interests. From their observations it is clear that the various shrubs and thicket-forming species which have since proliferated in the national parks were already present. But they were confined to naturally sheltered areas and escaped the fires that annually kept open the main plains. Milbraed, a member of an expedition led by the Duke of Mecklenberg in 1907 (Mecklenberg 1910), wrote that these plains were of little interest to the botanist but 'on the other hand, the eyes of the sportsman are delighted with the great herds of *Adenota* and *Damaliscus*' (Milbraed 1914). The latter's description of Lake Edward is valuable, because it shows that on its western shore, under the wall of the Mitumba range, the same zone of cultivation that British travellers had observed south of Lake George was also present:

On the west side, especially towards the north, one finds on the sandy beaches great walls of *Phragmites vulgaris* which are decorated with the violet flowers of *Ipomoea cairica* (L.) Sweet and a yellow *Phaseolus*. Between the beach vegetation and the steep, high, bare mountains of the west coast (on the slopes of which the grass *Trichopteryx arundinacea* (Hochst) Benth. is abundant) the land, in so far as it is not under cultivation is, for the most part, composed of secondary vegetation, of elephant grass, large shrubs and several trees.

The list of trees and shrubs that follows, as well as the presence of elephant grass, suggests that the cultivated area was already diminishing.

In 1954, below the Rift scarp south of Lake George and east of the protected area that later became the Queen Elizabeth park, was another wide zone of elephant grass that marked the site of the former cultivation of Kitagwenda. Today, in 1969, the elephant grass (*Pennisetum purpureum*) is disappearing and banana gardens are again to be seen. But in the Rift floor, where early visitors had seen not only herds of antelope but fat cattle as well, the over-protected wildlife of the Park has converted much of the once open plains to a mass of untidy thicket.

Fries described the open plain in the southern part of the Semliki valley in 1912.

The grass steppe covers the whole plain between the hills. It was composed of a very uniform vegetation of few species [and was] completely treeless and shrubs also were lacking. The principal grass was the metre-high *Themeda triandra* which so completely dominates that one can call this community a *Themeda triandra*-Association. *Andropogon contortus* was also characteristic. . . . Here and there on the steppe green spots were to be seen which showed up even from a distance, by their bright, fresh colour. They formed, however, no remarkable interruption in the uniformity of the steppe. The reason for their appearance was the moisture which gathers during the rains in shallow depressions here and there and which, during my visit, were quite dried out.

One cannot, of course, be sure, but the botanical description that follows is so characteristic of comparatively recently deserted Hima kraals that one may still see in many parts of Ankole that it seems very likely that these were, indeed, what Fries was describing.

The bright green colour is due principally to *Panicum maximum*, the dominant plant. A few other grasses also belong to the *Panicum maximum*-Association, *Andropogon halapensis*, *pertusus* var. *insculptus*, *Nardus* var. *validus* and *Panicum brizanthum*. Intermingled with these there grew in addition *Achyranthus aspera* var. *argentea* (common), *Oxalis stricta* (sparse), the Euphorbiaceous *Acalypha bipartita*, *Tephrosia barbigera*, *Hibiscus cannabinus*, *Barleria ventricosa* (Acanthaceae) and *Cassia mimosoides* (Fries 1921).

Sleeping sickness in the Rift Valley

By 1905, when Wollaston noticed the fatness of the herds in the Rift floor, sleeping sickness on the shores of Lake Victoria had already killed many thousands of people. There was much anxiety lest it should appear in the rest of the country. In 1906 Dr. Bagshawe caught *Glossina fuscipes fuscipes* ('*G. palpalis*') on the shores of Lake George. There was some concern because he also found its puparia under leaf litter in banana gardens near the lake. But there was no evidence of an epidemic.

In 1910, however, Dr. van Someren 'reported that many villages around Katunguru on the Kazinga channel had now become infected and thought that the infection had come from Kyango on the Congo side of Lake Edward'. The greatest mortality 'was amongst natives of the islands and van Someren decided that the salt trade was responsible for the spread of the epidemic' (*Sleeping sickness bulletin* 1911).

During his survey, van Someren collected some tsetse near Lake George that he identified as *G. morsitans*. He also found that cattle near Mahyoro, on the eastern shore of the lake, were infected with *Trypanosoma congolense* ('*T. nanum*') and noted that the natives were aware of the dangers of this place to their cattle. It seems almost certain that the tsetse seen by van Someren were *G. pallidipes*. The species was collected in 1911 in the Semliki valley by Neave (1912). In the next year Duke collected trypanosomes from game animals in the Rift. He mentioned van Someren's report and took the trouble to write, 'concerning *G. morsitans* I can say that I did not meet with this fly during my investigations' (Duke 1913). *G. pallidipes* is now widely spread throughout this area.

As a result of van Someren's report the policy of evacuation of infected areas was applied in the Rift as it had been in Buganda and Busoga. In February 1912, Western province officials reported that all natives in sleeping sickness areas had been removed to fly-free areas; but in the next month Dr. McConnell found much human trypanosomiasis in the Ankole crater lake area. In 1913, more people were moved and the canoes of fishermen and salt traders were burned. New routes were opened so that people could travel without coming into contact with tsetse.

The evacuation of infected villages and the defining and redefining of prohibited areas continued throughout the war years. Among the evacuees from the plains south of the lakes were 900 Hima who took with them about 10 000 head of cattle (*Ankole district book*). In 1920, Dr. Hale Carpenter took charge of sleeping sickness control in Uganda and, finding that the epidemic had subsided, began to relax restrictions. Encouraged by this, certain Ankole chiefs obtained permission to reintroduce cattle to the Rift pastures. A trial herd of 150 animals was brought in. By 1923 all were dead and where, for as far back as there are written records (i.e. since 1889) and, in local tradition very much longer, cattle had flourished, the country became infested throughout by *G. pallidipes*.

Origins of the Rift Valley epidemics

From cattle dying in 1934 in pastures above the Rift wall we have arrived at the death of other cattle in 1923 in the valley floor. This was traced to the spread of *G. pallidipes* that had followed the evacuation of populations among which an epidemic of human trypanosomiasis had developed between 1905 and 1910. The story can be carried further back in a study of sleeping sickness in the Semliki river valley made by Dr. van Hoof in 1926–7. In this he recorded the history of the valley as given him by the local district commissioner, M. Hackaers. There was a tradition that in the distant past a succession of tribes had settled in this very fertile valley. Lugard's account of it in 1891 has been mentioned on page 172.

These immigrant tribes had each remained but a short while and then moved on again after having been decimated by the disease.

The Mabudu, for example, who now live in the Nepoka, were settled over 200 years ago in the Semliki, to the north of Ruwenzori; they abandoned that part of the country, so they say, to escape the ravages of sleeping sickness.

Similarly the Bakuma or Babira, whose vanguard, coming from the east, passed round to the south of Ruwenzori and then spread northwards and westwards, to the districts of Uvumu and Mombasa, only remained for a short time in the Semliki valley where the dreadful disease killed more of their people than the wars they had had to wage in order to force their way across the high plateau dominating the fatal valley.

The European occupation of this territory assumed an administrative character in 1896.

The Belgians, as ignorant as their predecessors, built their administrative headquarters at Beni on the Semliki banks. They completed their task of 'pacification' of the tribes and thereafter an active traffic set in between the various occupied posts. This contributed greatly to the spread of the disease. Then, as the population of the plains seemed too scattered, some of the tribes which had settled on the spurs of Mounts Ruwenzori and Mitumba, and were as yet untouched by the ravages of the disease, were urged to move nearer to the administrative centres.

[The administrative centres] became the most dreadful foci of infection, since it was impossible to approach them from any side without crossing countless streams and marshes infested with tsetse. It is not surprising, then, that practically nothing remains of the population which had settled round these stations, and that in some cases, especially in the Kasindi plain, whole villages should have disappeared.

At the first news of the epidemic, the Belgian medical services organised a systematic campaign and an enormous lazaret, built of durable materials, was established close to Beni. The atoxylisation of patients and isolation of advanced cases, however, did little to improve the situation. The contact between the natives and the glossinae and the opportunities of infection remained unchanged and defeated all prophylactic measures.

In the course of a few years, from 1915 to 1923, M. Hackaers was able to estimate the extent of the catastrophe. In the Kasindi plain, whole villages had disappeared and a chief who, in 1923 had buried twenty-seven out of his one hundred and seventy-five subjects, including women and children, asked permission to settle elsewhere. Of the regular boatmen in the Lake Edward service, every single one almost was suffering from trypanosomiasis and, in spite of atoxyl treatment, five or six out of every twenty died each year.

To quote M. Hackaers, 'settlements were strung out all along the valley on the banks of the Semliki, where the people lived by fishing, and along the tracks close to rivers infested with glossinae'. There was an active canoe traffic on the Semliki and on Lake Edward.

The lazaret itself was situated in the midst of villages where at least 40 per cent of the population was suffering from the disease. The census of population was very incomplete, many tribes indeed refusing submission. In this dense scrub, it was impossible to hope for any supervision over traffic without the assistance of a large staff or recourse to coercive measures. All this time there was a shortage of labour, the upkeep of ways of communication became exceedingly precarious, and both for the members of the Medical Service and for the administrators of the territory the supervision of the native districts involved not only hard work but also considerable danger (van Hoof 1928a).

This account by one of the most distinguished of Belgian medical workers on sleeping sickness has been quoted at length because it brings out three points that are relevant to the present study:

(1) The history of successive epidemics among invading people who, like the Belgians themselves, settled in the floor of the valley.

(2) The attribution of the epidemic to movement of the indigenous people nearer to the administrative centres—i.e., nearer to the valley floor.

(3) The opposition of these people to the Belgians and the contrast with the flourishing communities seen by Lugard in 1891.

The first two items point to a problem still not settled. They suggest that the disease had been endemic in the area for centuries. An alternative theory had first been set out by Drs. Dutton and Todd who were sent to the Congo Free State by the Liverpool School of Tropical Medicine in 1903. Dutton died of relapsing fever during the course of the journey around the Congo basin, but his name precedes that of Todd in the *Fourth progress report* of the expedition prepared by the latter (Dutton and Todd 1906). In it the view is taken that gambian sleeping sickness had been endemic for an indefinitely long period in the lower Congo basin and that it spread eastwards when the eastern part of the Free State was pacified between 1885 and 1895 and people began to move up and down the river and its tributaries. Beni, the administrative centre on the Semliki that the Belgians had built in 1896, is described as 'harbouring imported cases of trypanosomiasis' in 1905. It will be necessary to examine the hypothesis of the eastward spread of the epidemic in Chapter 14.† Here it needs only to be observed that evidence that infection reached the British side of the border from the Belgian is not strong. The first cases on both sides were seen in 1905. Epidemic conditions were reported at Lake George in 1910, but by then Dutton and Todd's theory was well known and, indeed, a very similar hypothesis had already been put forward to account for the Busoga epidemic (page 242). All that is really certain is that on both sides of the

---

† Morris (1963), who summarizes evidence supporting this hypothesis, gives van Hoof (1928a) as an authority for the appearance of the disease 'on Lake Edward and the Semliki River in 1896, possibly earlier'. This is not so. Van Hoof's mention of that year refers to the commencement of European administration in the area. Elsewhere Morris (1960a) appears to accept the idea that the epidemic was provoked in the way described by M. Hackaers.

Rift Valley and within it there had been the most widespread and profound political disorder that brought acute misery to the ordinary peasantry.

Lugard had set up a series of forts in Western Uganda, but the religious wars in Buganda itself absorbed all the military and administrative man power available so that they had to be manned by Sudanese soldiers who at once began to plunder the people in their vicinities. One of these forts was at Ntara overlooking Kitagwenda. There was another at Katwe. According to one contemporary observer these soldiers not only 'laid waste Kabarega's provinces for two days' march to the north but they had been equally successful in converting the province of Kyaka and the greater portion of Kitagwenda, south of the line of forts, into a desolation' (Macdonald 1897). A colleague, Major Owen, with whom Macdonald worked, reported to him that

> Fifteen hundred square miles in Southern Unyoro were desolate, . . . Kitag-
> wenda had been rendered actively hostile and . . . in Usongora the people
> would gladly be without us. In fact, he estimated that all the friends we could
> reckon in those regions, . . . amounted to two thousand Wanyoro settled at the
> forts, and Kasagama of Toro with, he estimated, five thousand people. The
> remaining population of the great extent of the country we were occupying, at
> considerable cost in blood and money, would, he considered, be far from averse
> to our departure (Macdonald 1897).

The forts were evacuated in September 1893, and Kasagama of Toro was given 200 muskets to help him to look after himself. Shortly after this he carried out the cattle raid that Scott Elliot reported in 1894 (page 173). The wars against Kabarega of Bunyoro (who certainly must now be looked on as a patriot king) were begun by Colonel Colville in November 1893, partly because of fears in London that the Belgians, now beginning to establish themselves in the Eastern Congo, would push on into Western Uganda. Macdonald, whose account has been used here, was a professional soldier who for a short time was in charge in Uganda and would not deliberately have emphasized that the British were unwelcome if it were untrue. A more recent account of the devastation made in Bunyoro by the conquest of that country is to be found in Dunbar (1965). Large areas were depopulated, and where people remained famines and social disorder were widespread for some years before sleeping sickness was recognized. The botanist, Dawe, who was in the neighbourhood of Kitagwenda in 1905, remarked that the natives 'away from the road are extremely timid, and it is with the utmost difficulty that food is obtained here, . . . on emerging from the forest and reaching the inhabited parts, everyone ran away and hid in the tall grass with their spears.' In Kitagwenda itself 'the natives were rather troublesome, and caused considerable confusion by blocking up the foot-tracks that led to their somewhat secluded gardens' (Dawe 1906).

The British portion of the Western Rift was devastated by the colonial wars but its people's miseries were trivial compared with the horrors that were endured by the inhabitants of the Eastern Congo. The confrontation of the Europeans and the Arab slave traders set in motion the most appalling outbreaks of inter-tribal strife on top of genuine attempts by the inhabitants to preserve themselves from one or other of the invaders. In the eastern parts of the Congo cannibalism had been known at least since the end of the sixteenth century (Pigafetta, trans. Cahun 1883). However, one has only to read, for example, Grogan and Sharp's (1900) story of the invasion of Mushari, between Lakes Kivu and Edward, by the Baleka, which they interrupted in 1898, or Slade's (1962) account of the pacification of the country just west of the Rift, to appreciate that these were not normal times. Large-scale destruction of human communities can only take place after relatively long intervals in which they have had time to grow and establish themselves. It is evident that the stresses to which the indigenous peoples were subjected between 1885 and 1895 had a profound effect upon the epidemiology and epizootiology and trypanosomiasis in the Rift. The first cases of sleeping sickness were identified in 1905. Before that date a handful of soldiers, administrators, missionaries, and adventurers found themselves involved in confused and barbarous conflicts that had been provoked by their arrival but which they could neither understand nor control. The virtual disappearance of cattle from the county of Mitoma in north Ankole between 1934 and 1952 was one of their lesser consequences.

Recent sleeping sickness

Sleeping sickness was still present in the Semliki valley in 1952 (Neujean and Evens 1958) but had been reduced to a very low level, if perhaps only doubtfully eliminated, by 1960 (Neujean 1963). On the Uganda side of the border small communities living in valleys on the southern slopes of Mount Ruwenzori just outside the boundary of the Queen Elizabeth national park were free of infection, or seemed to be so, in 1956 and 1957, and Morris (1960a) tentatively suggested that the disease may have been eliminated. He summarized the incidence of sleeping sickness in the Lakes Edward and George area from 1925 onward and showed peaks of infection in 1927, 1932, 1942, and 1947. The peak years of 1932 and 1942 were preceded by years, 1930 and 1938, in which incidence was so low that no cases were recorded. Morris asked himself the question of how the epidemic could be maintained at such a low level. In part it was likely that the efficiency of surveys varied. When an epidemic had been reduced by treatment, inspection in these remote areas became slack. On the other hand the disease was extremely mild. 'The patient may not feel sick until a year or two after his initial infection, and even when he begins to have symptoms they may not trouble him greatly, he will not distinguish them from the many fevers and feelings of malaise and inertia to which he is so accustomed' (Morris 1960a).

The people suffering from this very mild disease were living on the mountain slopes between the plain and the upper forests in the situation in which Lugard found his densely populated and very prosperous communities in 1891. Morris makes the point that the riverine *G. fuscipes* must feed almost entirely on man himself and his small stock, since there are no crocodiles in Lake Edward or its environs and he saw no *Varanus*. Further, 'Although game is very plentiful in the National Park and penetrates some way up the valleys . . . it is completely absent from the occupied and cultivated zone.'

If the normal condition of the disease in this area is so mild that sufferers do not distinguish it from their other fevers then it is not impossible or, indeed, it is very likely that the earliest travellers in the area would not have noticed it and the people themselves would not have identified with it the cause of the heavy mortality in the epidemics that followed the population displacements by the Belgian administration after 1896.

The present position

The story may, very briefly, be brought up to date, but obviously not to its final conclusion. In the Uganda Protectorate the people who had survived the consequences of British hostility to Bunyoro were, within a decade of 'pacification', afflicted by widespread epidemics of human trypanosomiasis. They affected the whole Rift Valley from Lake Edward to the Sudan border. The evacuation policy was carried out, leaving large areas of empty land around the forests of the Rift wall. The forests were designated as forest reserves and the empty peripheral savannas became game reserves of various kinds (*Uganda atlas* 1962). One of the largest of these is the Queen Elizabeth national park.

South of Lake George, but outside the Park boundary lies the land once occupied by the people of Kitagwenda. Their banana gardens at the foot of the Rift wall were replaced by the high grasses of a moist *Acacia* savanna, which adjoin *Albizia–Markhamia* forests, also successional to banana-dominated cultivation. Up to ten years ago these areas were a favourite elephant-hunting area, for animals found there were not within the protected zone. During a visit in 1965 one saw that the high grass savanna at the foot of the Rift wall had disappeared and it was again covered by banana gardens. But the erstwhile pastures of the valley floor, where cattle shared the *Themeda* with Uganda cob and topi, are still, as they have been since 1920, infested by *G. pallidipes*. The denser bush that Dawe noted in 1905 near the village of Katunguru is now greatly extended, perhaps as a consequence of overprotection of hippopotamus and elephants.

In the Semliki valley, where the Belgians reversed their first policy of inducing people to congregate near the river, the central Kasindi plain was again evacuated and people once more congregated on the lower slopes of Ruwenzori and of the Mitumba mountains. In these conditions the epidemic was brought under control. By 1959 cases were too rare for Neu-jean (1963) to regard the area even as a *foyer silencieu*. No report is available since that year.

Final note on the Semliki focus

One note remains to be made. In 1926, Drs. Van Hoof and Duke found a woman named Risiki dying of trypanosomiasis in spite of a variety of treatments, at Bambu near Kilo, a mining settlement to the west of Lake Albert. By every diagnostic criterion she was infected with *Trypanosoma* '*rhodesiense*'.

This woman moved in native mining circles and never left the neighbourhood of Kilo and its mining camps and the country of Babira and the region round Mombasa and Irumu, where *G. morsitans* has never yet been reported. In this region, rare sporadic cases of *T. gambiense* infection have been found near the Chari and its tributaries, where *G. palpalis* and a big tsetse of the *fusca–brevipalpis* type are found. The place where she was most probably infected is Nyankunde, her birthplace, which is included in the sleeping sickness area of Geti-Boga, to the north of the Semliki Valley (Duke 1928).

The tsetse of this region are, in modern terminology, *G. fuscipes*, *G. nigrofusca hopkinsi*, *G. fuscipleuris*, and as Lavier (1928) who also examined the trypanosome pointed out, *G. pallidipes*. The Risiki strain was forgotten for many years, for it did not fit into the pattern of accepted theories. It was not until 1942 in Busoga that the role of *G. pallidipes* as a vector of trypano-somes between the wild animal reservoir and man had to be accepted (Chapter 15).

The history of the Rift epidemics suggests that an endemic mild, chronic disease was present among the dense populations of the Rift wall, where *G. fuscipes* alone maintained transmission between people. The con-dition will be encountered again in the story of trypanosomiasis around the north-east corner of Lake Victoria and yet again in Southern Nigeria where the vector is *G. palpalis*. Where, for any reason, this physiologically and ecologically balanced system, comprising human infective trypano-somes, riverine tsetse, and man, is broken down and involved with the spread of other tsetses dependent primarily upon wild animals, then the disease takes on an acute form giving rise to disruptive epidemics. In normal circumstances the sporadic, solitary appearance of a *rhodesiense*-type strain passes unnoticed. It is a rare event when a village woman like Risiki is seen by men like Drs. Duke and van Hoof.

II

SUKUMALAND: ANTECEDENTS OF
EPIDEMICS AND EPIZOOTICS

The Sukuma and associated tribes

BY 1960 the pastoral Hima societies of Nkore and Karagwe had almost disappeared and their grazing lands were infested by *Glossina morsitans*. In Rwanda and Burundi the same tsetses had begun to invade the pastures of the Tusi, carrying with them not only the cattle trypanosomes, but also the human parasite, *T. brucei rhodesiense*.

In Sukumaland, a near neighbour of the interlake countries, the same series of biological and social catastrophes that preceded the break-up of the Hima and Tusi societies also initiated widespread invasion of tsetse and epidemics of sleeping sickness but had a sequel, at the end of the colonial era, very different indeed. Here the confrontation between the bush–wild mammal–tsetse and the man–cultivation–cattle ecosystems has resulted in expanding human and cattle populations and retreating fly-belts.

The Sukuma who lived immediately to the south of Lake Victoria are the largest tribe in Tanzania. They numbered 1 093 767 people in the 1957 census. They are a northern branch of the Nyamwezi groups of tribes whose territory stretches from Lake Victoria in the north to Lake Rukwa in south-west Tanzania. Immediately south of the Sukuma are the Nyamwezi proper, who numbered 363 258 people in 1957. They are mainly concentrated around Tabora, where, in the early nineteenth century, Arab traders founded their settlement of Kazeh in the chiefdom of Unyanyembe. South of the Nyamwezi two more small sub-tribes together amounted to 51 628 people. They live outside the area now to be discussed. Finally, on the west of Sukumaland, around the small town of Kahama, were 76 435 Sumbwa (Abrahams 1967).

These Nyamwezi tribes compete for their existence with the flora and fauna of the *Brachystegia* woodland, the *miombo*, which supports the *Glossina morsitans* fly-belt of western Tanzania over an area of about 90 000 mile². The Sukuma, in the north, also push eastwards into the drier *Acacia–Commiphora* thornbush of north central Tanzania. This is infested with *G. swynnertoni*. Both fly-belts also contain local aggregations of *G. pallidipes* and, in patches of more mesophytic vegetation near the lake, *G. brevipalpis* as well. Parts of the lake shore carry a population of *G. fuscipes fuscipes*.

There are other tribal groups living in this region who do not belong to the Nyamwezi. The small tribe of Bahi, also called Hadza or Kindiga, live in the far south-eastern corner of Sukumaland, overlooking Lake Eyassi. They are survivors of an earlier culture who do not cultivate or raise cattle and whose existence by hunting and gathering gives them a relationship with the tsetse-borne diseases quite different from that suffered by the technically more advanced Nyamwezi. More important in the recent history of the southern part of the Victoria basin are the Zinza. They occupy, but are being displaced from, the country west of Sukumaland between the Sumbwa country and Lake Victoria. They are a southern branch of the interlake tribes and they are diminishing in number. Between the censuses of 1948 and 1957 their numbers dropped from 62 794 to 55 187, a decline of 12·1 per cent. Their neighbours on the west, whose country lies between that of the Zinza and Karagwe, the Subi, did even less well in the same period. They decreased from 74 052 in 1948 to 61 384 in 1957, a loss of 17·1 per cent. Such figures do not necessarily mean that people of certain genetic characteristics are dying out. They may be, but much of the decline is due to people abandoning old loyalties and for reasons of convenience calling themselves by the tribal name of another group. The Sukuma increased by 23·1 per cent between 1948 and 1957 and some small part of this increment (of 204 967 people) may have been contributed by Zinza who decided to become Sukuma (*Tanganyika census* 1963).

The first written information about the Sukuma comes from Speke and Grant who here, as in Karagwe, were followed by Stanley and Emin. Their writings again provide an introduction to the study of trypanosomiasis in an area which, for several years, was a centre of research on *Glossina* and on sleeping sickness.

Speke's traverse of Sukumaland in 1858

Speke left his companion Richard Burton lying sick at Kazeh (Tabora), on 9 July 1858, and went north to discover Lake Victoria. He published a map of his route and a diary of what he saw (Speke 1864). In it are notes on the human population, on cattle and crops or, on occasion, bush and wildlife. According to Speke's own figures the distance between Kazeh and Mwanza (Map 11.1) was 213 miles. From Kazeh to the second stop at Ulekampari (18 miles) Speke's safari marched over woodland-covered hills and he saw a herd of zebra. There were cattle at Kazeh and at Ulekampari. For the next 90 miles, to Kahama (probably nearly 20 miles north of the modern town), the way led through well-populated and cultivated country. In particular the people of Msalala were very numerous; Speke wrote, on 19 July:

Ugogo, on the highway between the coast and Ujiji, is a place so full of inhabitants compared with other places on that line, that the coast people quote it as a wonderful instance of high population; but this district astonished all my retinue. The road was literally thronged with a legion of black humanity so exasperatingly bold that nothing short of the stick would keep them from jost-

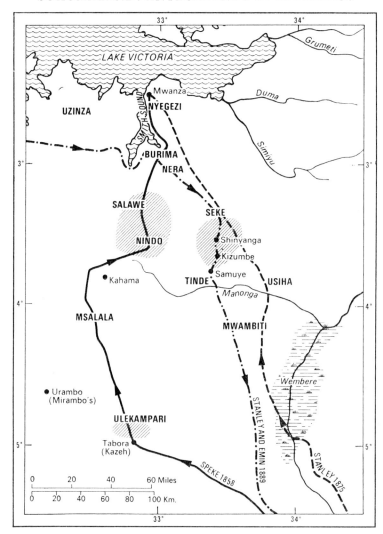

MAP 11.1. The routes of Speke 1858, of Stanley 1875, and of Stanley and Emin 1889, through Sukumaland. Hatched areas show where bush was encountered.

ling me. Poor creatures! they said they had come a long way to see me and now must have a good long stare; for when was there ever a Mzungu here before.

The village of Kahama itself was deserted although the country round about was much cultivated. But 19 miles after leaving it the explorer entered 'the jungle of Nindo, with its abundant game' and, until Salawe was reached, passed for three days through a waterless wilderness of thorn and tree forest. There were some villages, but no milk, for the people 'fearing the Wamanda, had driven off their cattle to the northward', but in Salawe,

Speke saw a herd of cattle being driven south to Tabora. On the return journey, in the Nindo wilderness, there were 'troops of zebra and giraffe, some varieties of antelopes roaming about in large herds, a buffalo and one ostrich' as well as 'the fresh prints of a very large elephant'. Before the safari came in sight of Smith Sound they were once more in cultivation, among many people. Apart from the short stretch through wooded hills just north of Tabora, and about 45 miles through Nindo, the country was well populated and carried an appreciable cattle population. There was little bush. Fifteen miles south-west of Kahama, Speke remarked that 'the quantity of cattle surpasses anything I have seen in Africa'.

A map drawn 65 years later (Swynnerton 1925*a*) showed that all the route traversed by Speke, except for about 60 miles, of which 40 are taken up by the northern section around Mwanza, was infested either by *G. morsitans* or *G. swynnertoni*. Swynnerton's map also shows the outlines of the fly-belts as they were known to the Germans in 1913. South of Kahama the chiefdoms through which Speke had passed were all engulfed in the east-ward-spreading belt of *G. morsitans*. The Nindo jungle, recognized in 1913 as a fly-belt, was, however, still isolated. Potts (1926) showed it to be infested with *G. swynnertoni*, thus demonstrating that its origins lay in the east of Sukumaland.

Stanley's first journey

The next visitor to Sukumaland was Stanley (1878) whose route, 50 miles east of Speke's, is also given on Map 11.1. On 9 February 1875, he reached the village of Mombiti (Mwambiti) 'in the rich country of Usu-kuma, where the traveller, if he has resources at his disposal, need never fear starvation'. Fifty years later Swynnerton's map showed that *G. morsi-tans* from the west and *G. swynnertoni* from the north and east had met not far from here and that the Mwambiti area was in course of invasion. Travelling northward Stanley crossed the Manonga river, near which he saw many giraffe 'feeding on the dwarf acacia, but the country was too open' to allow an approach to them. On 17 February he arrived in Usiha:

> The commencement of a most beautiful pastoral country, which terminates only in the Victoria Nyanza. From the summit of one of the weird grey rock piles which characterise it, one may enjoy that unspeakable fascination of an apparently boundless horizon. On all sides there stretches toward it the face of a vast circle replete with peculiar features, of detached hills, great crag masses of riven and sharply angled rock and outcropping mounds, between which heaves and rolls in low broad waves green grassy plains whereon feed thousands of cattle scattered about in small herds.

From Usiha north-north-west to Mwanza the landscape has scarcely changed in ninety years.

Stanley and Emin in 1889

When Stanley made his next traverse, in 1889, he was travelling south with Emin Pasha. They entered Sukumaland from Uzinza. Their route crossed the chiefdoms of Burima, Nera, and Seke and so avoided the Nindo bush. The Sukuma were now hostile and there were several skirmishes. In Seke everybody had disappeared. Emin found two huts filled with hides and sheep and goat skins and supposed that many cattle had died recently; nevertheless, he wrote, 'the cattle population is considerable'.

Leaving Seke they entered an area of thornbush where the Pasha saw 'Acacias of three or four species, *Albizia, Dalbergia melanoxylon, Boswellia papyrifera* (frequent), *Adansonia* (frequent and fine specimens), some occasional miombo. . . . The majority of the trees and shrubs are Papilionaceae.' (*Boswellia* does not occur in this area. Perhaps a *Commiphora* was meant.)

Later we crossed open country with groups of large rocks strewn about very picturesquely; here and there a great shade giving tree—Tamarind or *Ficus*—and obviously new huts and groups of huts scattered about relieve the view and, into the bargain, groups of natives, women and men, were evident, who did not run away from us but shouted and gesticulated. . . . We were . . . in new country and soon pitched our camp near a fairly high group of rocks at the foot of which were water holes, whilst round about lay many groups of huts. The place (or district) is called Sinyanga or Unyanga, belonging to Chief Udirerua, and is independent of the places and people behind us (Stuhlmann 1916–27).

From Shinyanga they made two short marches to Kizumbe, near the place that became New Shinyanga. The second of these marches took them for two hours through bush 'made up of *Acacia* and *Dalbergia*. . . . Spoor of zebra and buffalo were common.' The route from Seke had led through country that subsequently became the experimental blocks of the Tanganyika government's Tsetse Research Department.

Half a century after Emin wrote his description, glossinologists of the Shinyanga team held the view that a major cause of the spread of tsetse fly was a cyclical process of depopulation followed by bush regeneration followed by tsetse-fly advance that in turn caused more depopulation. This was the view of Swynnerton, first director of tsetse research, formed after studying the country crossed by these earlier travellers. It is therefore important to note that most of the country covered by Swynnerton's reclamation schemes was bushland, well populated by game animals in 1889. Among these animals were buffaloes. They disappeared when the rinderpest arrived two years later and have not yet returned.

The caravan travelled on through Samuye. On 28 September 1889:

After about half an hour's march we entered the bush and, although all was dry as broomsticks, had the satisfaction now and then, of meeting a green *Acacia* —harbinger of Spring. Here also we found in great numbers the 'Arak' of the

Arabs [*Salvadora*] out of which they make teeth scrubbers [*miswak*] a substitute for our toothbrush. The peppery fruits were still green. The bush was extensive and in front of us large hills raised themselves and our way led towards them. Isolated open spaces penetrated into the bush; somewhat later came stubble fields and fields prepared for cultivation and here we found quantities of young plants of a *Hyphaene*, such as we had seen in Usambiro; three fairly well grown examples of the same tree were found in the neighbourhood of the village of Samuye, behind which we camped. . . . Round about all is cut down and only the hills are covered with scrub and bush (Stuhlmann 1916–27).

Samuye also was later engulfed in a fly-belt and then became the site of a succession of experiments in tsetse control.

The Ngoni, Mirambo, and Langheld

Emin Pasha refused to be taken to Europe as a trophy by Stanley and instead joined the service of the new government of German East Africa. He was sent back to establish German rule over the territories west and south of Lake Victoria, with the biologist Franz Stuhlmann as his companion. They were given a detachment of native troops under the command of Lieutenant Wilhelm Langheld. Eventually Langheld arrived in Bukoba, the station founded by Emin on the west coast of Lake Victoria, and there recorded his account of the arrival of the rinderpest panzootic (Chapter 8).

Langheld (1909) had followed Emin and Stuhlmann along the old route from Tabora in 1890. Cattle were abundant in the inhabited areas and in good health. Langheld's importance to this narrative lies in the battle he fought at Tinde, 30 miles south-west of Shinyanga. This battle was one of several fought during the last decade of the nineteenth and the first of the twentieth century that put an end to that remarkable phenomenon, the *mfecane*, the great outpouring of the Ngoni peoples that was initiated by the political and military genius of the Zulu tyrant, Shaka.

The *mfecane* (Omer-Cooper 1966) impinges at several points upon the modern history of African trypanosomiasis. It began about 1820 in Zululand. In forty years the Ngoni had spread throughout most of southern Africa and had reached the outskirts of Sukumaland. It is one of the most frequently encountered explanations for the spread of human trypanosomiasis after the arrival of the Europeans, that because they pacified the country, people were able to move about in a way never done before. The Ngoni invasion is evidence to the contrary. The Ngoni certainly moved widely about the country and they provoked other movements. There is no evidence that epidemics of trypanosomiasis followed in their wake.

Zwangendaba, who had led one branch of the Ngoni on a great migration from Zululand, died in 1845 near Ufipa in central Tanzania, and his heirs and their followers left the tribal centre to carve out new realms for themselves. A group that called themselves Tuta were raiding as far north as the Zinza country in 1860 (Speke 1863). Not far from Tabora they captured a young chief, Mirambo. This remarkable man learned the military techniques of the Ngoni and later, from his place at Urambo, came to dominate a great area north of Tabora. His troops, numbering several thousands, were called *ruga-ruga*.

Mirambo's power grew through his opposition to the Ngoni and the Tabora Arabs. He set himself up as a commercial rival to the latter and fought a war with them in 1871. He died in 1884, but his army of *ruga-ruga* remained at Urambo. Langheld estimated their strength at 3000 warriors. A missionary account puts the population of Mirambo's capital at 10 000 inhabitants, with another 5 000 living around the walls (Oliver and Matthew 1963). Langheld wrote of hut upon hut stretched across the plain as far as the eye could see. Emin Pasha had arranged an alliance with these people and with their help Langheld broke up the Ngoni power. The main action took place at Tinde. Langheld commanded a force of 35 *askari* and 700–800 *ruga-ruga*, mostly armed with muzzle-loaders. Their firing set fire to the thatched roof of the enemy headquarters. Many women and children, as well as cattle, were collected in these buildings. As the unfortunate people and animals struggled out they were shot down. However, at this moment the arrival of more Ngoni forces compelled Langheld to retire to his base at Samuye to await the arrival of reinforcements. Eventually another detachment of regular soldiers, plus a quick-firing gun and a cannon, were brought up and the Ngoni forces were overcome and dispersed.

The battle at Tinde extinguished the most northerly focus of the *mfecane*, some 2500 miles from its point of origin in Zululand. Forty years later Corson began one of the great classical experiments on human trypanosomiasis at the Tinde Sleeping Sickness Laboratory.

The Germans soon afterwards had to turn against the Nyamwezi. Mirambo's successor, Siki, who had taken over his armies and who, since 1885, had been building up opposition to the Europeans in the same way that Mirambo had tried to control the Arabs, was finally destroyed after two days of fighting at Tabora. This account is concerned with Sukumaland, the country north of Tinde. But it is not out of place to notice the destruction of Siki by the Germans, for it is evident from Nyamwezi history (see, for example, Oliver and Matthew 1963) that the prosperous communities that Speke had observed in 1858 were, indeed, a cross-section of what had once been a large and flourishing military and commercial country.

The Nindo bush

Swynnerton (1925a) investigated the past history of Shinyanga, the southernmost chiefdom of the Sukuma people. According to Wamba, chief at Shinyanga in 1925, the chiefdom had been founded by Mwola, a hunter from Mwanza on the southern shore of Lake Victoria, and his wife Giti, who being of royal blood, was the first chief of the line. Wamba was the nineteenth of her successors. The essential part of the story is that since the time of Mwola and Giti (perhaps to be dated at around 1700) the population had expanded and had subdivided itself into other chiefdoms as well as Shinyanga. The bush had gradually disappeared and cultivation and cattle husbandry developed more or less steadily. This continued until about 40 years before Swynnerton's conversation with Wamba; i.e. until about 1885. At that time 'only a portion of Nindo, the mbugas of Seke and an area in Seke, Mwadui, Uchunga, and Usiha, contained appreciable bush'.

Swynnerton attributed the survival of bush in Nindo to two local wars, the second of which was actually a raid by an alliance of local chiefdoms to clear out a gang of cattle thieves. Later, 'the demands made by the earlier German safaris to and from Mwanza were so excessive in relation to its small population that many of the people remaining migrated to more heavily populated parts, and man-eating lions more than once hastened the process and so assisted the tsetse to dominate' (Swynnerton 1925a). It may be, however, that there were other factors accounting for the emptiness of Nindo. The first is time. If, indeed, the Sukuma had been expanding southward away from the lake for two hundred or more years, the population pressures that had converted central Sukumaland to treeless 'cultivation steppe' may not yet have developed sufficiently to engulf this area as well. The second factor is topographical. Nindo is situated upon the watershed between the Lake Victoria drainage and the drainage eastwards to Lake Eyassi. Its natural water supplies are poor and its soils unattractive to farmers. Finally, although to a great extent the Sukuma and the Nyamwezi may be looked upon as the northern and southern branches of a single great tribe, nevertheless they are separated and Nindo lies close to or upon the boundary between them—in short, it is part of a *Grenzwildnis*. It seems likely that it remained a 'jungle' because it was environmentally and politically unfavourable for settlement and because of this was suitable as a refuge for criminals as well as for game and tsetse fly. We have the evidence of Speke that Nindo and adjoining Salawe were, respectively, a 'jungle' and 'a waterless desert of thorn and small trees', bounded on the north and the south by densely populated country. This was nearly 20 years before the various disturbances to which Swynnerton attributed the depopulation of Nindo.

Rinderpest, jiggers, famine, man-eating lions, and the First World War

The biological disasters that swiftly followed upon Langheld's 'pacification' of Sukumaland must often have seemed worse than the violence that had preceded it. Langheld left Sukumaland for Bukoba in January 1891. In that year the rinderpest panzootic arrived, probably through Masailand on the east. Lieutenant Werther, of the German anti-slavery commission, walked north through Shinyanga and Sukumaland in 1893. Most of the cattle were dead and only chiefs and wealthy persons owned any. He also met with jigger fleas and found that the inhabitants of Nyegezi, on the east side of Smith Sound, were emigrating in hopes of finding new homes free of this pest. He saw people not only without toes but with more than half the foot eaten off (Werther 1894).

It may be supposed that the loss of their cattle did not bring complete disaster to the Sukuma as it had to the Hima. They were primarily cultivators, using their cattle 'as an investment at a very high rate of interest' (Malcolm 1953), but not relying on them to provide their basic diet. Nevertheless, the rinderpest cannot have been lightly regarded for, again in Malcolm's words, 'the Sukuma are kind to their animals and go to immense trouble to ensure that their cattle obtain adequate pasture and water. One might almost say that the Sukuma looks upon his cattle, of which all the adults are named, with the same affection shown by an Englishman for his dogs.' If the bond between the Sukuma and his cattle is less than that between the Hima and his, it is still almost a symbiosis, and the rinderpest must have had profound effects in Sukumaland.

An indirect effect of the rinderpest came from the east. The *Glossina swynnertoni* belt in Maswa is a buffer between central Sukumaland and the vast grazing lands of the Masai. Even worse hit than the Hima, for they had no subject Iru to turn to for help, the Masai were soon in a dreadful state.

In February 1892, Baumann (1894) was camped by a stream leading off the great extinct volcano of Ngorongoro.

Earlier this had been a favourite watering place of the Masai, now, nobody was to be seen, only an emaciated half-imbecile Masai woman who tottered with staring eyes through the camp. This was the first sign of that frightful famine which we were to see daily in Masailand.

We met a wandering troup of Masai, warriors, elmoruo, and women, all starving and wretched, with donkeys on which their pots and all sorts of articles were piled, with a few goats and sheep. . . . We found two Masai children, who, left by their tribe, were near to death by starvation.

A year later, March 1893, Langheld (1909) met some Masai who begged him, so acute was their misery, to accept their children as a gift.

While the settled populations, to whom the products of agriculture remained for nourishment, were able to recover [their stock] by breeding from the few surviving animals, the Masai had consumed these also, so that today scarcely any cattle remain. At the first onset colossal numbers of the Masai, at least two-thirds of the whole tribe, were destroyed. The warriors were at first able to carry themselves through by hunting and petty thieving, but the women, children and old men were completely abandoned to misery.

Reduced to skeletons they tottered through the steppe, feeding on honey of the wild bees and on nauseating carrion. All warlike undertakings went awry and the elmoran were simply thrown back and often did not return home, but starved on the way. Only in a few areas kraals remained with sheep, goats and asses, and as a result of hunting, wide stretches of country became empty and the Masai lived as beggars among the surrounding settlements.

Many agriculturists, like the Wambugwe and their neighbours, will not assist their old enemies and slaughter all Masai. In Usukuma, Ushashi, in Irangi, Unguu and Usagara, as well as in the Kilimanjaro district, however, they find shelter and alms of food (Baumann 1894).

The Masai, of course, like the Hima, first attempted to replace their stock by raiding their neighbours. Cattle rustling was, in any case, a way of life for them. But now their attempts to recoup their losses only spread the disease further afield and brought them no relief. According to Percival (1918) the rinderpest had been brought into Masailand in looted stock:

The first outbreaks in Masailand were among the Loi-tok-i-tok on the slopes of Mount Kilimanjaro. Here it had been brought by Masai raiders, who had visited the coast about 1890 and brought back a quantity of looted cattle . . . in a short time the Loi-tok-i-tok had no cattle left. [They therefore] made a joint stock raid upon the Wakamba, to find that the Wakamba cattle were dying. However, they brought some looted stock back with them, only to start disease amongst their own cattle, which so far had been clean.

There seems no record that the Masai raided into Sukumaland as they had tried to do in Ukamba and, indeed, Baumann's account even suggests that they received hospitality from the Sukuma. But for many years the Sukuma are said to have avoided the eastern parts of their territory. Mac-Coll, the first veterinary officer in the newly mandated Tanganyika Territory, described (*Tanganyika veterinary* 1921) the remains of so many kraals in the south-east of Sukumaland, in the area called Meatu, that he thought there must have been very large-scale depopulation. This may have been a consequence of Masai raids, for Malcolm (1953), thirty years after MacColl's account was written, speaks of some Sukuma who had migrated to Kanadi, an area just north of Meatu 'in spite of a very real fear of the Masai'.

The rinderpest had scarcely spent its first violence when there was a very severe famine in 1900. It is remembered by its Nyamwezi name of *nzala ya mitundu*, the hunger of the *miombo*, for people were reduced to chewing the inner bark of *Brachystegia spiciformis*. Malcolm (1953) does not mention its cause, but Kollmann (1899) wrote that the Sukuma said, 'Before the white man arrived there were no locusts; with them the locusts came to devour our fields.' There is nowhere any evidence that locusts were, like the jiggers, a European importation; indeed, it is certain that they were not. But the concurrence of these afflictions seemed to the sufferers to find their cause in the arrival of the white man.

The spread of tsetse fly was noticed early in the new century. Swynnerton

(1925*a*) spoke to old men in Nindo who told him that the chiefdom was infested with tsetse before the great rinderpest, but that after it the fly disappeared (as it did in Ankole in 1919 and as it had done, in 1896, in Rhodesia). But on recovering tsetse began to invade areas that, before the rinderpest, had been free of them. A scheme was proposed by a German administrator at Shinyanga for a barrier clearing, but nothing was done and the fly eventually infested all the available bush until it came up against the barrier of denser human settlement. Then this barrier began to collapse.

This was near Shinyanga itself, where, in 1909, four man-eating lions became so troublesome, killing in all about thirty persons, that a great number of people deserted. Bushes grew up on their gardens and grazing land, and the tsetses, arriving later and pushing into these, made the ground to right and left of the gaps untenable by the cattle owners living there, and these also fell back. The first very general retreat in the face of the tsetse occurred ten years ago, [i.e. 1915] and since then the progress has been continuous. The tsetses unaided have proved amply sufficient to keep the people in steady retreat, but in point of fact they have been assisted, and retreats locally precipitated, by all of the many reasons which cause a native to evacuate his garden or his grazing. In one place it is the drying up of water-holes; in another the mere need for shifting that is necessitated by the native's impermanent methods of cultivation; in yet another the repeated early burning-out of grazing by irresponsible honey-hunters in the neighbouring bush; and in another [Usule and Usanda] proximity to a depot, and therefore forced labour, during the war; and the methods of Wamba's predecessor helped to expel population. In every case the small local evacuation had been seized on promptly by the tsetse and wider retreat brought about (Swynnerton 1925*a*).

This is an interesting passage for it reveals several features in common with the retreat of cultivators in Ankole. In both countries man-eating lions were an aftermath of successive rinderpest epizootics and the drying up of water-holes was associated with the growth of bush.

The disadvantage of proximity to a labour recruitment depot, especially after 1914, is clear from the records of another early student of trypanoso-miasis. In November 1917 Dr. G. D. Hale Carpenter was medical officer at Lulanguru, 17 miles west of Tabora. He was attached to the Belgian force and had the task not only of running a hospital but of examining 'recruits'.

Since the middle of October, when I got here, three batches of Congolese of about 450 each have arrived, and I have examined all of them and rejected some for apparent early Sleeping Sickness. . . . It is said that altogether 15 000 are coming through here, but though that sounds a large number it is only enough to make good the wastage of *all* porters for *one month*. I have about 60 in hospital; every batch that arrives leaves me with cases of Pneumonia and Amoebic Dysentery, but thank goodness they seem free of Cerebrospinal Meningitis, which has been a great scourge in some parts (Carpenter 1916).

It is not to be supposed that Carpenter's figure of 15 000 wastage indicated that all these men were killed or wounded.† The majority no doubt deserted. However, losses among the carrier corps certainly were heavier than losses among the troops. Carpenter's patients were Congolese. The German forces had already taken their quota of Sukuma.

The main effect of removal of numbers of able-bodied men from their villages was to prevent the proper cultivation and harvesting of crops. This may have been a contributory factor to another very severe famine which began in 1918 and continued into 1920. Swynnerton (1923a) and Duke (1923) were both in the north-east corner of Sukumaland two years after the famine. Duke thought that thousands had died from want of food and that hookworm infections must have spread enormously during that time. In 1919 the world pandemic of influenza had unusually severe effects because of the undermining of the general vitality of the inhabitants by the famine.

The demographical condition of the Sukuma in 1920

The outbreak of sleeping sickness in the Maswa district in 1922, described in Chapter 13, was one of the events to which the story given in this chapter has been leading. Writers like Kuczynski (1937) and his successors, who were responsible for drawing attention to the need for properly conducted enumerations of colonial populations, were doubtless correct when they maintained that there was no valid evidence for population change during the early years of colonization. But it would be wrong to suppose from this that changes had not taken place. It was even more wrong to suppose, as did many colonial officials, that their coming must have evoked an immediate beneficial response. In Sukumaland, it is true, the processes by which the Germans established 'law and order' were comparatively benign; they had not, as they had done in southern Tanzania in 1905–7, made a solitude and called it peace (Moffett 1958). At the same time, as in the interlake area, the succession of epidemics, epizootics, and famines that the coming of the European provoked brought down upon populations as uncomprehending as themselves a biological warfare that had devastating consequences.

One would have liked, instead of this historical outline, to have produced a graph to show the changes in growth rate of the Sukuma and Nyamwezi populations over the years 1880–1920. That such a curve would have

† Rodhain (1919), who was in charge of the medical service with the Belgian troops, records that their force consisted of some 10 000 men, of whom 1000 were whites. In addition there was a corps of native carriers whose numbers were constantly varying between 10 000 and 15 000. The death rate among the carriers was four or five times greater than among the combatants. They were mostly killed by dysentery, especially in the 1917 campaign, and mortality in some hospitals was as high as 61·6 per cent. Carpenter's figure was exaggerated, but the losses of able-bodied men from some areas must have been sufficient to affect the prospects of the following year's harvests.

shown a continuous decline seems quite certain. It is also equally certain that this decline was the direct consequence, not as Swynnerton and nearly all Europeans thought, of the disorders inherent in barbarism, but of the ecological catastrophe of their own arrival. It is not possible to understand the sequence of epidemiological and epizootiological events except in the light of the events that preceded them.

12

THE RECOVERY OF SUKUMALAND

The ideas of C. F. M. Swynnerton

IN a classical study of the methods of another branch of the Ngoni peoples who invaded and settled in the neighbourhood of the Sitatonga hills in Mozambique, Swynnerton (1921) showed that the human activities of bush felling, burning, cultivation, and hunting could eliminate tsetse flies. In 1921 he was appointed game warden in Tanganyika Territory with the double task of protecting the wild game animals and solving the tsetse problem. He was convinced that this was possible without wholesale slaughter of the wild animal hosts of *Glossina*, a method then beginning to be used as a protective measure in Rhodesia. He needed an area in which he could put into practice the Ngoni technique and in 1923 selected the Shinyanga district in southern Sukumaland for his first large experiment. He summarized the situation there as follows:

> Except in one respect the position in the open country is ideal. There is complete segregation of tsetse and people, and a situation exists, in consequence amounting, for practical purposes, to control of the tsetse. All the people are able to keep cattle and all the children to get milk, tsetse are excluded, and, owing to the compactness of settlement, mammalian pests are excluded except from the margin, and the people generally are accessible for purposes of administration, medical treatment, education and agricultural development.
>
> The exception is this. The tree roots survive in the open country and wherever population thins for a time, shoot up into trees and bushes. Where they are adjacent to tsetse bush, the fly is carried into them, while they are still small, on persons passing to and fro, and cattle begin to die. The people then fall back, allowing new bush to spring up and the process to be repeated. In Shinyanga this retreat and the reconquest by fly has been for some time at the rate of a mile a year and new 'fronts' have been formed, so that cattle areas are now nearly surrounded (Swynnerton 1925a).

Swynnerton had already visited Sukumaland to study the entomology of an epidemic of rhodesian trypanosomiases around the *G. swynnertoni* infested country east of Mwanza. His first map of Sukumaland accompanied his report (Swynnerton 1923a) and a second map was published two years later (Swynnerton 1925a). The maps indicate that in southern Sukumaland particularly, people were retreating from its periphery, and that from the east *G. swynnertoni* and *G. pallidipes* and from the west and south *G. morsitans* were invading the evacuated lands and provoking further retreats in the way he had described. The spread of tsetse was most rapid in the Shinyanga chiefdom and it was estimated that 20 000 people had left between 1912 and 1921.

The organization of voluntary turn-outs of the people of the district to fell the trees and clear the bush, their resettlement in the reclaimed areas, and the construction of defence lines along which periodical slashing of regenerating shrubs and trees prevented a repetition of the process have been fully described (Swynnerton 1936, Napier Bax 1944). Between 1923 and 1930 bush was felled over 118 mile^2 and the spread of tsetse was halted.

In 1929 Swynnerton resigned his post as game warden in order to form a new Department of Tsetse Research. In 1930 this department set up its headquarters at Old Shinyanga, in a fort built by the Germans as an administrative centre. The work of clearing went on into the 1930s and a great area of tsetse-infested bush lying west of Shinyanga was divided up into blocks to serve as experimental areas. The research that was conducted here is well documented and has been summarized by Glasgow (1960, 1963a).

Swynnerton (1925a) described his discussions with the people of Shinyanga. He saw no end to the processes that the earlier depopulations had initiated. Bush regeneration in lands emptied by war, disease, famine, and flight from German labour conscription depots had allowed the tsetse to spread. Cattle died and their owners moved to save the survivors. In moving they provoked further invasion of tsetse.

The natives, till we turned them, were definitely 'on the run'. Everywhere on the edges of the cattle-areas there was the same advance of the young bush, and the tsetse, and everywhere inside them are still the live roots of the suppressed bush. The natives themselves were highly alarmed, and some said to me, 'Where will the end be?' I replied, 'Unless you stand firm and yourselves attack, the end will be in little more than twenty years with the death of your last beast somewhere in Uchunga.'

The cattle threatened then numbered about 345 000.

At that time and for many years after it was thought that what was then going on in Shinyanga and elsewhere in Tanzania was a normal condition of African life. The majority of officials concerned, in one way or another, with problems of land use believed that agricultural malpractice led, through soil impoverishment, to abandonment of exhausted lands. This was another way to start the processes that Swynnerton had described. Indeed, after the passage quoted above he went on to relate how the retreat in front of the fly had brought about a congestion of cattle in the country still not infested. This in turn was leading to over-grazing and over-grazing caused erosion. The idea was put forward (though not by Swynnerton) that tsetse infestation was, in the long run, beneficial and that trypanosomiasis, by preventing invasion of the bush, preserved it unharmed for future, wiser generations. By driving people out of country they were in process of ruining, tsetse infestation enforced a period of fallow and allowed impoverished soils to recover. One veterinarian remarked that the fly-free areas of most African countries would meet their existing needs for stock if they were used economically. They were not, but were abused abominably. 'We must not', he said, 'be content to get rid of tsetse at any price' (Hornby 1930). Later he changed his opinions (Hornby 1948), and adopted the view that *Glossina*, by crowding people into the fly-free areas, was a principal agent in causing erosion.

Recession of *Glossina swynnertoni* in Maswa district

Up to the outbreak of war in 1939 tsetse reclamation and defence works were carried out at several points around the periphery of Sukumaland. In June 1939, a visit was made to one of these peripheral areas in the district of Maswa, at the southern end of what is conveniently referred to as the Simiyu salient, from the name of the river that traverses it in a roughly northward direction to Lake Victoria (Map 12.1). *G. swynnertoni* were easily caught on the fly-rounds. In 1947 the visit to the Simiyu salient was repeated. It was difficult to recognize much of it as the same country. Not only were there no tsetse flies, but the bush also had gone. Where fly-round paths had been followed through *Acacia–Commiphora* thorn savanna and game animals had been seen, there was cultivation and pasture, and the treeless landscape was varied only by scattered villages and herds of cattle. In some parts the process of take-over of the land was still in progress; huts were being built and patches of bush were still standing.

In that particular area control work had been abandoned in 1935 because of lack of popular support and it was certainly not possible to claim that the elimination of the tsetse had allowed the people to occupy land formerly closed to them. Administrative and agricultural officers also were of the opinion that no anti-tsetse measures were needed before people could occupy the bush. In the first year settlers would mark out their plots, fell enough bush to cultivate a crop and build a house. In the second year they extended their cultivation and brought in their sheep and goats. In the third year they brought their calves and finally, in the fourth year, the whole family with all their adult cattle moved in.

The expansion of Sukumaland

The experience at Maswa led to an examination of the changes that had taken place during the interval between Swynnerton's survey in 1923–4 and the preparation of a map of tsetse distribution in 1947. Swynnerton's map distinguished between cleared settlement or 'cultivation steppe' and various categories of natural vegetation. Not all bush was infested with tsetse and where there were indications of this an approximate limit of

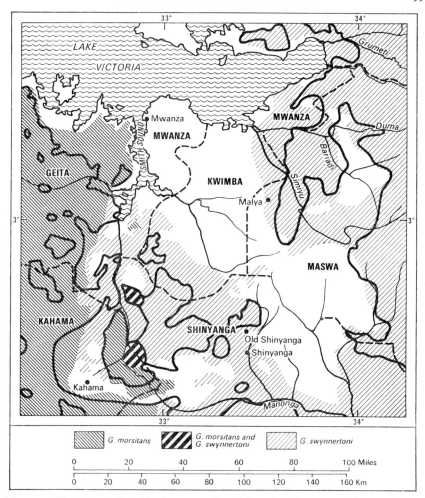

MAP 12.1. The tsetse-infested bush surrounding Sukumaland in 1925 and in 1947 (heavy outline), with district boundaries.

infestation was drawn. The 1947 map, on the other hand, distinguished between fly-belts and fly-free land. It is probably that Swynnerton's map slightly exaggerated the extent of tsetse infestation; the 1947 map may have exaggerated the areas free of tsetse. The area scrutinized was bounded by parallels 32° 15′ and 34° 5′E. and 2° 00′ and 4° 00′S. Small sections of the neighbouring districts of Nzega and Ukerewe included in these parallels were left out of the calculations.

The result of the comparison was surprising. It was known from official records, many of them published by Swynnerton (1936) and Napier Bax (1940), that about 800 mile^2 within the rectangle had been reclaimed from tsetse infestation by bush clearing and other techniques in programmes organized by the Tsetse Research Department. It was therefore startling to find that the area of tsetse-free settlement had increased, during the period of 23 years, by over 3000 mile². Tsetse had disappeared from some 2400 mile² without any organized attack on it.

Table 12.1 gives the 1924 and revised 1947 figures together with others. Great accuracy cannot be claimed. The 1924 map not only plotted bush rather than tsetse, but it was also drawn on a base map often locally inaccurate. If the first map overestimated tsetse infestation, the second for 1934, like that of 1947, may have underestimated it. Gillman (1936), who

TABLE 12.1

Approximate areas and rates of change of area of tsetse infestation in Sukumaland from 1924 to 1966; area bounded by longitudes 32° 15′ and 34° 15′E. and latitudes 2° 00′ and 4° 00′S.

	Tsetse infestation: mile²				
District	*1924*	*1934*	*1947*	*1955*	*1966*
Geita	2091	2132	1512	1475	1145
Mwanza Cent. . .	76	109	217	101	109
Mwanza NE. . . .	431	189	185	202	90
Kwimba	378	428	122	213	119
Maswa	2756	2011	2084	1906	1295
Shinyanga . . .	2017	1377	714	403	199
Kahama	2051	1261	1742	1377	1504
Total tsetse areas . .	9800	7507	6576	5677	4461
Tsetse reclamation . .		350	450	623	82
Tsetse infestation + reclamation . . .		7857	7026	6300	4543
Gross rate of change % p.a. . . .		2·7	1·0	1·8	2·2
Net rate of change % p.a..		2·2	0·8	1·4	3·0

drew it, obtained his information from the Tsetse Research Department but it is clear that he did not include as infested some of the areas under experimental treatment by that department. The 1955 and 1966 areas suffer because they are estimated from the small-scale map published in the *Tanganyika atlas* (1956) and its revision in 1966 (Turner 1967). Other factors also detract from accuracy. Different glossinologists have different standards by which to judge if tsetse have been eradicated from an area; in any case it is difficult to determine when this has happened. Boundaries between chiefdoms and hence of districts may change slightly from time to time.

There is no question that the area of Sukumaland has at least doubled itself since 1924. If we are to regard the growth of the human population together with their livestock as the principal factor in bringing about this change, then it is necessary to make adjustments for the land reclaimed from tsetse fly by work specifically directed to that end. The remainder can then be attributed to the agricultural effort of the Sukuma peasantry, assisted by the various government departments.

Tsetse reclamation in Sukumaland

Swynnerton's initial experiment in 1923–4 at Shinyanga led to the recovery of 24 mile² of land, and yearly turn-outs of able-bodied men from the Shinyanga chiefdoms continued to enlarge this area. In 1927 this work ceased to be the responsibility of the Tsetse Division of the Game Department (forerunner of the Tsetse Research Department) and was taken over

TABLE 12.2

Reclamation from tsetse infestation, 1923–38 (in mile²)

District	1923–30	1931	1932	1933	1934	1935	1936	1937	1938	Total
Shinyanga	24	6	44	57	57	4	8	3	6	209
Maswa .	—	—	3	3	23	?	—	—	—	29
Kwimba .	—	—	—	35	3	7	—	—	—	45
Mwanza .	—	—	—	—	2	?	—	—	—	2
Kahama .	—	—	—	—	—	3	—	—	5	8
Totals .	24	6	47	95	85	14	8	3	11	293
Shinyanga†	94									94
Huruhuru‡					– – – 250 – – –					250
Running totals .	118	124	171	266	351	365	623	626	637	637

† Clearings between 1926 and 1930 under control of district administration.
‡ See Napier Bax (1944).

by the administration. A record in the *Shinyanga district book* states that 86 mile² had been cleared by felling or ring-barking by the end of 1927, and that as a result of this about 200 mile² of country had been thrown open for grazing. From 1927 to 1930 new clearing amounted to 'nearly 32 square miles'. However, in one area (Ilola in Lohumbo) it was necessary to clear up regeneration of bush cut in 1927 and 1928, and people were still leaving this area up to 1933 (Napier Bax 1944).

In 1931 the newly organized Tsetse Research Department took over control of clearing work from the administration. Records of areas cleared between then and 1938 are tabulated in Swynnerton (1936) and Napier

Bax (1940). Activity in clearing was concentrated in two periods, 1924–5 and 1932–4 (Table 12.2).

An appreciable proportion of this clearing was done to create corridors for cattle where the spread of tsetse had cut off access to large seasonal grazing grounds. Comparatively little reclamation work was done during the war years in Sukumaland (Table 12.3). An epidemic of *T. 'rhodesiense'* sleeping sickness began in Ukerewe, just outside the north-east corner of the area of the present study, and this absorbed most of the available resources of the department. Thus although it was reported in 1946 and

TABLE 12.3

Recorded estimates of tsetse clearing, Sukumaland, 1939–66 (in mile²)

District	1939–49	1950	1951	1952	1953	1954	1955	1956	1957	1958	1959–66	Total
Shinyanga	— — — — — — — —			600	—	—	—	—	—	—	50	650
Geita .	—	?	2	3	5	4	5	6	1	—	—	26
Maswa .	?	—	—	—	—	—	—	2	15	8	—	25
Kwimba .	—	—	—	—	—	4	—	—	—	—	—	4
Running totals .	?	?	2	605	610	618	623	631	647	655	705	705

1947 that 105 mile² of country had been reclaimed in the Lake province, almost all of this was outside Sukumaland (*Tanganyika Tsetse* 1949).

A revision of the data collected in 1947 confirms the estimate (admittedly rough) that was then made. Some 837 mile² of country had been reclaimed in Sukumaland by activities specifically directed towards removal of tsetse fly.[†] Of this area about 387 mile² could be taken as the result of destruction of the *Glossina* habitat, mostly by sheer felling of bush, and about 450 as land not providing a suitable environment for tsetse, but denied to cattle either by its proximity to tsetse or by lack of access routes free of infection.

Of this 837 mile² about 350 was cleared by 1934 and the remainder, most of which was grazing land, between 1934 and 1938. Table 12.1 also shows the effect of adjusting for active tsetse reclamation, including that achieved in more recent years.

Interpretation of tsetse reclamation data

Before making a final interpretation of the information given in Table 12.1 it is necessary to explain the difficulties of assessing the results of tsetse reclamation. The classical case was the successful elimination of *Glossina*

[†] Napier Bax (1944) reported that 1000 mile² of tsetse-infested land had been reclaimed in the whole of Tanganyika.

pallidipes from Zululand. After many years of failure, by a variety of methods, this species was finally killed out by aerial fogging with insecticide in 1952. By this time the tsetse habitat had been reduced to the three fauna reserves of Umfulosi, Umkuzi, and Hluhluwe. Their combined area was about 200 mile². The cost of applying the insecticide and ancillary work was £2·5 millions. Using the conventions customary among the Shinyanga glossinologists this worked out at a cost of almost £20 per acre. The South Africans claimed, however, that the three reserves together formed a focus of infection for cattle in 7000 mile² of surrounding farmland. That this infection was spread by dispersing *G. pallidipes* had been established many years earlier by Bedford (1927). On this basis the cost per acre is reduced to 12s., but it was claimed, with some justice, that the work had been experimental and that in the light of what had been learned, costs could be reduced to under 2s. per acre (du Toit 1959).

Difficulties of this sort also affect the estimation of results achieved with the less sophisticated hand axe. Tables 12.2 and 12.3 show the recorded achievements of tsetse reclamation within the area under examination. Table 12.2 summarizes the detailed tables given by Swynnerton (1936) and Napier Bax (1940). Table 12.3 shows the estimated areas of clearing given in the *Tanganyika Tsetse Reports* (1949–58) in the districts of Geita, Maswa, and Kwimba, plus 600 mile² in Shinyanga and Kahama districts cleared of tsetse between 1948 and 1952 by game destruction (Potts and Jackson 1952). This area includes Speke's 'Nindo jungle'. In 1958 the last of the experimental blocks, No. 9, was abandoned. Encroachment of settlement appeared to have eliminated the tsetse in it by 1965. This accounts for the 50 mile² shown in the last column of Table 12.3.

Apart from 650 mile² shown for Shinyanga, most of which are attributable to the experimental work of the Tsetse Research Laboratory in that area, the amounts of clearing reported are very small. Most of the areas shown are estimates from the number of 'men/days' of work recorded in the *Tanganyika Tsetse Reports*. A rough average of 4500 men/days per mile² was used to determine them. Some clearing was done in Geita in 1950 and some in Maswa in 1942, but it is very doubtful if the decade 1940–50 would have shown more than 20 mile² of clearing specifically against tsetse.

The differences between Table 12.2 and Table 12.3 represent a change in policy. Up to the beginning of the Second World War it was held, at least by tsetse 'experts', that in order for the African peasant to take over new land it was necessary for tsetse flies to be eliminated. The estimates made in 1947 had shown that, at least as a general proposition, this was not true. The Sukuma were taking over land rapidly, unaided by entomological expertise. Then in 1949 rhodesian sleeping sickness broke out among settlers in the van of the immigration movement into Geita. This will be examined in the next chapter, but the relatively small clearings shown for

Geita in Table 12.3 represent the effect of applying a policy of bush clearing in foci of high density of *G. morsitans*. This reduced the risk of infection and the settlement movement continued. The final elimination of *Glossina* was now always an effect of settlement and cultivation.

It is appropriate at this point to note that when, in 1947, attention was drawn to these effects of population expansion, colleagues asserted that they would have been on a far smaller scale and, indeed, might not have happened at all, if it had not been for the demonstration by Swynnerton and his team at Shinyanga that the spread of tsetse flies could be halted and that they could be exterminated by the efforts of the people themselves. This view is unacceptable. If it were true there could never have been cattle owners and cultivators in tropical Africa.

Growth of the cattle population

Before attempting a reassessment of the trypanosomiasis problem on the peripheries of Sukumaland it is necessary to examine the populations affected by these diseases. Cattle figures are more complete and, over a longer period, more reliable than the human data.

A series of counts and estimates of the cattle population of Tanzania is contained in the *Annual Reports of the Department of Veterinary Services*. There are gaps, but from 1921 to 1957 we have figures not only for the country as a whole, but also for the provinces. The number of cattle in Sukumaland is included in the figures for the Lake province.† Livestock totals of cattle in the districts comprising Sukumaland for the years 1945 to 1957 (of which 1948 and 1949 are missing) were obtained from unpublished reports. For the last five of these years the cattle in the districts of Mwanza, Geita, Kwimba, Maswa, Shinyanga, and Ukerewe averaged 73·6 per cent of the Lake province population (limits 72·2 in 1957 and 74·3 in 1956). The residuum in 1957 was made up of 77 675 head of cattle in the districts of Bukoba and Karagwe west of Lake Victoria, and 644 957 head in the districts of Musoma and Mara east of the lake. The Bukoba and Karagwe group has fluctuated around 70 000 since 1913 when 66 590 were counted. Malcolm (1953) published for the years 1934, 1944, and 1947 the number of cattle units for the Sukumaland districts, Mwanza, which then included Geita, Kwimba, Maswa, and Shinyanga. He also published a map showing changes of distribution of cattle units between 1934 and 1947 (cattle units: 5 sheep or goats equal one ox).

The Lake province cattle population growth curve is given in Fig. 12.1. The 1913 figure (Hill and Moffett 1955) is the total of the two German districts of Mwanza and Tabora and covers a slightly larger area than the Lake province under the British. The province was also changed in 1931 when Shinyanga district was transferred from what became the Western province (formerly Tabora province) to the Lake province. This accounts

†Now the Lake and West Lake regions.

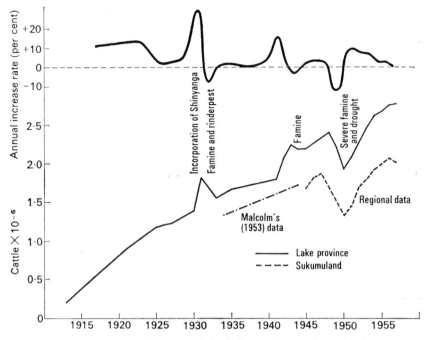

FIG. 12.1. Growth and rate of increase of the Lake province cattle population, 1913–57, with data for Sukumaland alone from 1934–57.

for the peak shown in that year. In 1931 and 1932, however, this apparent gain was lost as a result of drought and a severe rinderpest epizootic in which the district of Kwimba alone was said to have lost 100 000 head, and Bukoba half of its cattle amounting presumably to about 30 000 head. Before this, however, there had been losses from famine.

In November 1929 the district of Shinyanga appeared little better than an arid waste, overstocked by scabby, starved and debilitated cattle. On visiting Karita and Mihama the Veterinary Officer found a doleful and desolate state of affairs. At early dawn the emaciated and tucked-up herds trudged drearily for miles to the nearest bite of grass; some, only able to stagger a short distance, hovered around the bare land near the bomas where they lingered on and died. Others, reaching the water holes, too weak to crawl through the sticky mud, fell and died from exhaustion. Young calves left in the huts and bomas hardly had strength to call for the cows that might never return, or, if they did return, could not supply them with much-needed milk. These calves lay growing weaker and more exhausted daily, until death came to close the unhappy scene (*Tanganyika veterinary report* 1930).

There was another severe famine due to drought in 1944, but the worst drought and famine occurred in 1949 and in that year and the next numbers dropped by 482 051. It is possible that this loss was underestimated, for the total of hides and skins exported from Mwanza in 1949 suggests that over 500 000 Sukuma zebu died in that year (Newlands 1956).

It is remarkable that the general trend of the cattle population was upward in spite of periodical heavy mortality from drought and starvation, and in spite of the spread of tsetse around the borders of Sukumaland until the mid 1930s. To a great extent this increase is a measure of the tremendous losses due to the original rinderpest pandemic of 1891. It is indeed possible that the Sukuma cattle population had not recovered fully by 1960. No figures were published between 1938 and 1942, but at about this time the population growth rate accelerated, although increase was halted by famine in 1944 and, very severely, in 1949–50.

In 1937 the Veterinary Department recorded that control of rinderpest had been lost throughout large areas of Tanzania; but by 1943 the eradication of the virus from a large part of the territory had been achieved. The principal control over increase was now, and continues to be, availability of grazing. The year 1937, in which it had been noted that control was lost over rinderpest, was also a bad year for pleuropneumonia, and tick and worm infestation was unusually heavy. 'Yet, on the whole, . . . it was a good year for stock—of such importance is food in a country where disease slays its thousands and starvation its tens of thousands' (Hornby 1938).

East coast fever

While Hornby's dictum is true over sufficiently long periods, infections have reduced stock populations on a scale comparable to that produced by the more severe famines. The rinderpest panzootic was one example. Locally, *Theileria parva* infection (East coast fever) may have almost equally devastating results. In Ankole it exerts a far greater direct control over stock numbers than does trypanosomiasis. Throughout that area it is enzootic and calves that are unable to build up their immunities sufficiently rapidly, die. The survivors are immune through life. In Sukumaland the situation is different and is the subject of a recent study by Yeoman (1966, 1967). The disease is enzootic in the north and west of the area, but is absent in the south and east. This distribution is correlated with the distribution of the vector tick, *Rhipicephalus appendiculatus*, and this, in turn, seems to be associated with the higher rainfall of this half of Sukumaland.

Yeoman's maps show that, very roughly, the enzootic area for East coast fever extends from the lake shore southward to about the level of the 30-in isohyet. Nevertheless, he found no significant correlation between rainfall and tick infestation rates in any single locality. However, north and west of a line running from Salawe in the western extremity of Shinyanga district, to the lake shore some 60 miles east of Mwanza, cattle populations are subject to infection as calves and the adults are immune;

south and east of this line is a zone in which from time to time more or less severe epizootics break out.

Little is known of infection rates of *T. parva* in *R. appendiculatus*, even in enzootic zones; it may be only a fraction of 1·0 per cent. None the less, epizootics of this disease, causing severe losses, can occur where the tick infestation rate on cattle is as low as 1–4 ticks per beast. Outside the epizootic zone severe sporadic outbreaks appear in populations of cattle with tick rates ranging from 0·3 to 0·8 per beast. Where the tick rate is less than 0·2, the area is free of the disease. It is clear that quite small changes in the environments of the vector may lead to large changes in the epizootiological status of the disease.

Kwimba district lies athwart the zone separating the enzootic from the free area of Sukumaland and is therefore more subject than other parts to epizootics. Epizootic East coast fever in Sukumaland had been reported in 1934 and 1936, and in 1956 it was evident that an important epizootic was again developing. The district reports give the following stock totals:

1952	400 736
1953	377 694
1954	338 467
1955	362 378
1956	347 456
1957	325 596
1958	317 655

indicating a decline at the rate of 3·8 per cent per annum. There was an apparent rise of 23 911 head between 1954 and 1955. The figure for 1955 was obtained by direct counting of the entire stock population during a rinderpest prophylaxis campaign, suggesting that estimates for earlier years were too low. Taken together, however, these data reveal a continuous decline that contrasts with the rapid increase rate of 5·3 per cent per annum shown by the Sukumaland cattle population as a whole after the losses from famine in 1949–50 (cf. Fig. 12.1).

Yeoman's work dealt with three years from 1957 to 1960. But the epizootic condition in Kwimba persisted, with striking effects. During a visit to Sukumaland in early December 1965 the writer drove through it from Mwanza to Shinyanga. The part of the journey through Kwimba was remarkable not only for the almost complete absence of cattle, but for the effect this was having upon the grass cover. At that time of year one might expect to see new grass beginning to shoot from the roots that are all that survives from the dry season just ended. Instead, patches of last season's grass 2–3 ft high could be seen where they had escaped burning and this in a country where seasonal grass fires were hitherto unknown because the cattle never left enough to burn. It was estimated by the veterinary staff at Mwanza that about 200 000 head of cattle had died of East coast fever in Kwimba in 1963 and 1964.†

It was supposed that the epizootic that had, for some years, been developing in southern Kwimba had been exacerbated as a result of the unusually heavy rains that fell all over the Victoria basin in 1961–2. Yeoman's failure to demonstrate a correlation between rainfall in any particular year and infestation rates of *R. appendiculatus* has been mentioned. In discussing the water relations of *Rhipicephalus* he notes that rainfall could have indirect effects on humidity, pasture growth, populations of small (potential host) mammals, and on soil condition and its suitability for oviposition. An abundant and high persistent grass growth replacing a sparse short transient growth might conceivably produce microclimates of higher relative humidity without any change in the general climate. An epizootic sufficiently severe to kill enough cattle to allow tall grasses to replace close-cropped turf could, in that case, improve the vector environment and lead to exacerbation of the epizootic until a balance was restored as an increasingly immunized population of cattle recovered sufficiently to reduce the pasture again to close-cropped turf so that tick numbers were once more brought down.

The brief history of the disease in Kwimba outlined here suggests that its epizootic spread may be a consequence of severe cattle loss due to other diseases or to famine. The epizootics noted by Yeoman to have broken out in 1934 and 1936 follow closely upon the drought and severe rinderpest of 1932 and 1933 (cf. Fig. 12.1) in which 100 000 head of cattle are said to have died in Kwimba. There is some evidence to suggest that the East coast fever epizootic, first recorded in 1956, may, in fact, have begun in 1953. In the previous three years, the whole cattle population of Sukumaland had suffered the appalling losses of the 1949 famine and were then recovering from it. Hornby, who frequently deplored the 'overstocking of Sukumaland', more than once pointed out that the yearly grazing of the grass down to its roots kept down the tick population. When he became director of tsetse research at Shinyanga in 1939 he introduced a herd of cattle. The animals grazed on the open cleared areas between the experimental blocks, which had to be conserved as pasture. Their grasses were therefore not burned off, while cattle owned by local villagers were kept out by fences. Within three years *Theileria* infections appeared and dipping for tick control had to be instituted. It seems not improbable that the spread of ticks in Kwimba is a consequence of severe reduction in grazing pressure, brought about by deaths from famines or from other diseases. The infection may therefore be seen as supplementing the effects of death by starvation by prolonging the interval for pasture recovery.

East Coast fever is an indigenous disease of the East African tropics.

† McCulloch, Suda, Tungaraza, and Kalaye (1968) say that in 1962–4 some 300 000 head died from the disease. There were no reported cases of trypanosomiasis.

It plays an important role in African ecology, but has been relatively little studied and its interrelationship with trypanosomiasis in cattle population control has never been examined. It is clearly a potent factor in the conflict between the human and bush ecosystems in the Victoria basin.

Growth of the human population in Sukumaland

The first population distribution map of Tanzania was produced by Gillman (1936) using estimations made in 1931 and 1934 by enumeration from tax collection figures. Martin (1961) states that the 1931 census was held at the request of the Secretary of State for the Colonies, but that no instructions were given as to how it should be carried out. Gillman, unsatisfied with its result, persuaded the Tanganyika government to repeat the operation in 1934. On this occasion administrative officers were asked to provide details from the most recent census or from the tax assessment rolls, whichever was considered to give the more accurate data. In the latter case, the number of taxpayers was to be multiplied by the coefficient customary in the district, which usually varied between 3 and 3·5. Gillman was more interested in the distribution of population than in the accurate estimation of its true density. His figures for both estimates are given for each district and the total population for the whole territory in 1931, 5 022 700, was higher than that for 1934 by 197 974, about 4 per cent.

Martin (1961) compared the estimates of population of the three territories of Kenya, Uganda, and Tanganyika made in 1947 by the poll tax coefficient method, with the totals derived by direct count, carried out by trained enumerators during a specified week in 1948. In Tanganyika this census gave a total 1 415 000 greater than that which had been obtained by the poll tax method in 1947. Martin (1961) believed that during the nine years ending 1957, when a second census was held, the population of the three territories had increased at a gross rate of 1·75 per cent per annum. Allowing for such an increase between 1947 and 1948, one concludes that the 1947 estimate for the whole territory was short by 21·7 per cent.

In Table 12.4 various enumeration results, including the census data of 1948 and 1957, are given for the five administrative districts of Sukumaland. Unfortunately no figure was obtained for Kwimba district in 1947 and the totals excluding Kwimba are therefore also given, in brackets. Using these bracketed totals we find that the 1947 total for the four districts excluding Kwimba was 18 per cent underestimated as compared with the 1948 census count. That this deficiency should be less than for the territory as a whole might be expected, since Sukumaland was relatively intensively administered and communications are good.

It will also be observed in Table 12.4 that there are considerable discrepancies between the figures given for 1934 by Gillman (1936) and Malcolm (1953). It has not been possible to resolve them. Gillman, in 1935, was nearest in time to the 1934 enumeration, which he had initiated;

TABLE 12.4

District totals of the human populations of the five districts of Sukumaland from various sources

	Gillman 1936		Malcolm 1953			African census report	
	1931	*1934*	*1934*	*1944*	*1947*	*1948*	*1957*
Geita ⎫	254 500	287 900	55 600	87 200	108 200	139 028	268 846
Mwanza ⎭			146 600	156 200	161 000	178 761	176 344
Kwimba .	200 000	191 700	191 600	199 600	—†	237 962	241 340
Shinyanga	144 500	146 500	152 600	195 400	171 400	212 503	252 677
Maswa .	230 000	194 400	206 200	177 800	205 200	244 968	291 460
Totals .	829 000	820 500	752 600	816 200	—	1 013 222	1 230 667
	(629 000)	(628 800)	(561 000)	(616 600)	(645 800)	(775 260)	(989 327)

† No estimate is available for Kwimba in 1947. For the purposes of comparing population growth rates in Table 12.6, the bracketed totals, which exclude Kwimba, are used.

on the other hand, Malcolm, with a long experience of Sukumaland, must have had access to the original tax returns upon which the figures sent by provincial officials to Gillman were based.

Table 12.5 reproduces the data given for the whole of the Lake province in the *Tanganyika Census* (1963). These data are far less subject to error

TABLE 12.5

African population growth 1948–57 in districts of the Lake province

District	Population 1948	Population 1957	Net increase	% increase
Biharamulo . .	49 849	40 765	−9 084	−18·2
Bukoba . . .	299 860	367 962	68 102	22·7
Geita . . .	139 028	268 846	129 818	93·4
Kwimba . .	237 962	241 340	3 378	1·4
Maswa . . .	244 968	291 460	46 492	19·0
Mwanza (rural) .	178 761	176 344	−2 417	−1·4
Mwanza (urban) .	8 885	15 241	6 356	71·5
Musoma . .	142 062	200 564	58 502	41·2
Ngara . . .	104 706	102 148	−2 558	−2·4
North Mara . .	115 037	145 029	29 992	26·1
Shinyanga . .	212 503	252 677	40 174	18·9
Ukerewe . .	119 329	126 109	14 780	13·3
Total. . .	1 844 950	2 228 485	383 535	20·8

than were earlier enumerations. It is clear that the incremental rates of population growth varied greatly in different districts during the 9-year period. The population of Geita nearly doubled itself, as did the urban population of Mwanza town. Some districts declined slightly in the number of their inhabitants, but the overall increase in the Provincial population was 20·8 per cent, indicating a multiplication rate of 2·1 per cent per annum. This is somewhat larger than the figure proposed by Martin for the whole territory; but again it is an expected result.

In Table 12.6 the data of Table 12.4 are compared in terms of the geometric increment rates between paired groups of data. For reasons given above it will be clear that we cannot compare differences between data from different sources. The census returns of 1948 and 1957 may be compared,

TABLE 12.6

Mean annual rates (%) of geometric increase for human population in Sukumaland

	1931–4	1934–44	1944–7	1948–57
Geita ⎫ ⎬ . .	+6·4	+4·6 (+1·9)	+11·2 (+4·0)	+7·6 (+3·9)
Mwanza ⎭		+0·7	+4·8	−0·2
Kwimba . .	−1·4	+2·8	—	+0·1
Shinyanga . .	+0·5	+2·4	−4·3	+2·0
Maswa . . .	−5·4	−1·5	+4·9	+3·2
Mean . . .	−0·35 (−0·02)	+0·8 (+0·9)	— (+1·5)	+2·2 (+2·4)

Bracketed figures are either combined Mwanza and Geita rates, for comparison with the 1931–4 figure, or mean rates for all Sukumaland excluding Kwimba.

as may the three estimates for 1934, 1944, and 1947 given by Malcolm, and those for 1931 and 1934 given by Gillman.

Geita was not given separate administrative status as a district until after 1944, but as Malcolm tabulates his data according to chiefdoms, separate totals for Geita and the new Mwanza district can be given for all except Gillman's data, when both districts appear under one heading. The absence of a figure for Kwimba in 1947 also means that if we wish to compare that year with others, then totals for the whole of Sukumaland less Kwimba must be used. These totals are given in brackets in Table 12.4, and the increment rates derived from them are also in brackets in Table 12.6. The total increment rates after the excision of Kwimba make little difference in those periods in which it can be included. This is not surprising since Kwimba is the one district which has shown the least tendency to change its human population density throughout the period we are considering.

TAE—P

In Sukumaland as a whole the four periods show a continuing and steady risc in its population increment rates. Gillman's view that the difference between his totals for Tanzania as a whole in 1931 and 1934 is within the expected limits of error may be accepted. There is no acceptable evidence that the Sukumaland population as a whole increased between 1931 and 1934. We may be diffident, too, about asserting that a mean annual increment of 0·8 per cent per annum for the decade 1934–44 was evidence of a real increase, but are reassured when we find that the three years 1944–7 show a rate nearly double that of the preceding decade. Finally, in the intercensus period of 1948–57, the increment rate of 2·2 per cent per annum for all Sukumaland (2·4 if Kwimba is left out) we know to be acceptable, and this increases confidence in the earlier figures, especially as they are supported by the historical evidence of glossinologists, agronomists, and administrators.

Inspection of the individual district figures shows, however, that this steady rise in the increment rate for the whole of Sukumaland is not found everywhere. In the period 1931–4 the population of Maswa appears to have been shrinking rapidly, Shinyanga was just holding its own, Kwimba was declining, though less rapidly than Maswa, but Mwanza in the north seemed to be multiplying rapidly. At this time the expansion across Smith sound had not begun. Swynnerton's efforts in Shinyanga had, at least temporarily, stopped the evacuation of that district, but in Maswa people were still leaving, as they were from the north-eastern border of Kwimba near the Simiyu river, including that portion of its course where the 1922 'rhodesiense' epidemic had begun and which formed its boundary with Maswa district. The displaced people were moving north and west into Mwanza East and Mwanza Central.

In the 1934–44 decade the decline of the Maswa population, although continuing, had slowed down; Shinyanga and Kwimba were increasing, and so was the old, large, Mwanza district, but by now the bulk of the population growth was being absorbed by Mwanza West, soon to become Geita district.

In the next period of three years the trend in Maswa was reversed and its population grew rapidly. So did that of old Mwanza, especially in Geita. The increase rate there of 11·2 per cent per annum was due to people moving, with official encouragement, across Smith Sound. The Kwimba data are missing, but the Shinyanga population was once more declining quite rapidly.

The Shinyanga decline was caused by the presence of the tsetse research department in the district, for nearly half its area had been turned into a game reserve to provide room for field experiments. The experimental blocks were surrounded by 'defence lines', about a mile wide, in which the department organized periodic clearing of woody regeneration. This was comparatively effective in preventing tsetse from leaving the experimental blocks, while traffic that used roads traversing these infested areas was clear of *Glossina* in de-flying chambers. However, the population which, one may suppose, was growing at the mean rate for Sukumaland of 1·5 per cent per annum, now had no room for expansion. In 1944 Malcolm (1953) states there were 195 400 people in Shinyanga district. This means that every year 3000 people, perhaps 750 families, needed to find room to live. Moreover, although according to accepted dogma, protection from tsetse should have allowed people to cultivate and own cattle up to the edge of the defence lines, this did not work out in practice. The experimental blocks were also game reserves and no hunting was allowed within them. On the eastern edge of an area of about 40 mile^2 known as Block 9, many Sukuma who had settled in the areas reclaimed by their own efforts under Swynnerton's direction in 1923–5 found that the depredations of bushpig and various antelopes, plus the limitations imposed on shifting cultivators by the neighbourhood of the block, were forcing them to leave. One may suppose they emigrated to Geita.

Considerable political pressure was exerted by the Shinyanga chiefs to compel the department to give up some of its land and this was done, but the most desired area and the source of most trouble to the neighbouring Sukuma, Blocks 9 (40 mile^2) and 4 (5 mile^2) were retained. Block 11 (50 mile^2) and Block 10 (30 mile^2) were handed over, but the former was unattractive for cultivation and little of it was taken up. Block 10 disappeared when a large dam was built, in 1956, to provide water in an otherwise badly supplied area. The large area further east (Blocks 13, 14, 15, and 16) were cleared both of tsetse fly and of the majority of their larger wild mammal fauna between 1948 and 1951 (Potts and Jackson 1952).

These measures,† although not providing all that the people of Shinyanga wished for, had a beneficial effect and in the next decade the population increment rate for the district again rose to near the rate for Sukumaland as a whole. In this inter-census period the movement into Geita continued (in spite of the appearance there of rhodesian sleeping sickness); in Mwanza, east of Smith Sound, the population did not change appreciably in numbers and nor did Kwimba. The population of Maswa continued to grow at a rate rather faster than that of Sukumaland as a whole and the recession of the peripheral tsetse belts continued.

Comparison between Sukumaland and Unyamwezi

The recession of the tsetse belts around Sukumaland was a response to growth of the human population. If this is so what has happened to areas inhabited by people who have not increased in number? South of the

† In 1955 I had a conversation with an old man who had been headman at Old Shinyanga when the Germans fled in 1915 and had been left to receive the pursuing British force. (He still wore his moustaches in the manner of Kaiser Wilhelm II.) He asked why it was that ever since Swynnerton had been killed the department had ceased to help the people of Shinyanga. I could find no answer to satisfy myself.

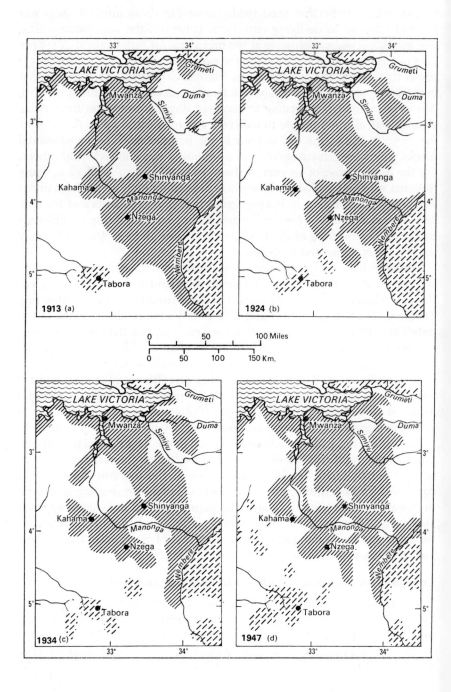

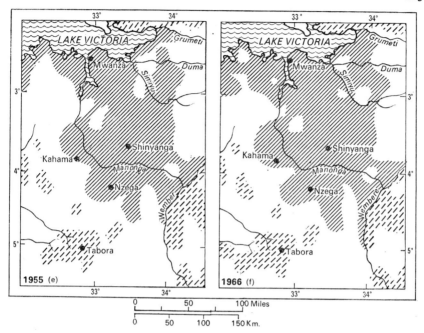

MAPS 12.2a-f. The distribution of *Glossina* around Sukumaland, Nzega, and Tabora in 1913, 1924, 1934, 1947, 1955, and 1966. Hatching indicates cultivation steppe. Broken hatched areas not included in area estimations.

Manonga river lies the district of Nzega, inhabited by Nyamwezi. This area, too, was subject to spreading tsetse belts in the first quarter of the century (Swynnerton 1925*b*). It is partly sealed off from Sukumaland by the Nindo *Grenzwildnis*, but the Manonga valley makes a less formidable frontier zone. It is not proposed to discuss the Nzega populations at length but to draw attention to the contrast that the Nyamwezi peoples as a whole present to the Sukuma. The people of Shinyanga district, immediately north of the Manonga river, increased by 18·9 per cent between the census years 1948 and 1957, and the Lake province as a whole increased by 20·8 per cent. The Nzega population, however, only increased by 9·2 per cent and the population of Western province, of which it is part, increased by 11·3 per cent. The Nyamwezi tribe, moreover, increased by only 0·1 per cent either because they did not in fact multiply or because they took other tribal names. The increase shown, for example, in Nzega is due almost entirely to multiplication of Sukuma immigrants and not to indigenous Nyamwezi (*Tanganyika Census* 1963).

Maps 12.2*a*–*f* show the change in tsetse distribution not only for Sukumaland but also for Nzega district and part of Tabora. The Wembere river which, with its wide swamps, separates the Nyamwezi from another tribal group, the Iramba, is taken as the south-eastern boundary. The amoeba-like outlines of the fly-belts around the Nzega population appear to have moved more often and more irregularly than in their continuations north into Sukumaland, but the total area of the fly-free inhabited portion of the district has hardly changed at all. Over the 42 years between 1924 and 1966 the Nzega settled area has diminished at a rate of 0·32 per cent per annum. The maps are taken from small-scale territorial tsetse distribution maps and there must be a large margin of error. We are perhaps only justified in saying that the populated area of Nzega has shown no measurable change in 42 years, although it has changed its shape considerably.

13

THE EFFECTS OF THE DECLINE AND REGROWTH OF SUKUMALAND ON THE TSETSE BELTS

Swynnerton's account of the Maswa *T. 'rhodesiense'* epidemic

AFTER about 1930 the growth of Sukumaland was controlled, on its southern borders, by the experimental activities of the Shinyanga Tsetse Research Department. Only on the eastern and western borders is it possible to study the behaviour of the tsetse-infested bush more or less, but still not entirely, free of entomological interference. In February 1922 the first case was reported of what became known as the Maswa *T. 'rhodesiense'* epidemic. Swynnerton's first map of Sukumaland, produced as part of his study of the epidemic, gave a 'rough indication of infected villages' (Swynnerton 1923*a*). The 1925 map was slightly more accurate, but did not show the situations of the infected villages. The outline of the epidemic area from the 1925 map together with the village sites from the 1923 map is given in Map 13.1.

Of the people of the area in 1922 Swynnerton wrote that:

[They] are to be distinguished into (a) cattle-keeping cultivators, who live relatively thickly in cleared areas, and who, where near enough, visit the woods for wood, bark rope, water, hunting, fishing, young birds and honey, medicines, ancestor worship, and material for the Ifubo or silver-leaf dance; and (b) hunting and fishing cultivators, who, owing to nagana, can keep no cattle, and who live in a more scattered fashion in the woodland area itself. It is a most interesting point that they have been enabled to do this, as they themselves state, by the freedom they have now obtained from the old tribal raids and clan warfare that forced on them the concentration that has usefully cleared so much country; and they have been induced to do so by the loss of their cattle in the epidemics that have accompanied the European regime during the past thirty years. Game skins and fish nets may be found in most huts of this section. The fruits of *Strophanthus eminii* Asch. & Pax., are used for the manufacture of arrow poison by every native in these parts and are found lying in the villages. Pits, game nets, and heavy rope snares are also employed. Along the whole lower course of the Simiyu and at the points at which we saw the Simiyu and Duma higher in their courses large stationary fish traps, often in the form of a ditch and protected against crocodiles by palisades, were abundant; fish baskets are in places supported against the current and floods by stone dams across the river; and during our canoe voyage we came on anglers with rods, one at least of whom had been extraordinarily successful. The Wantusu, in particular, whether in the clean

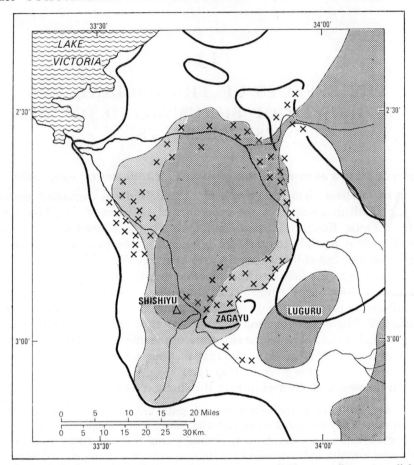

MAP 13.1. Outline of bush infested with *G. swynnertoni*. Heavy outline: 1925; light shading: bush in 1957, not tsetse-infested; heavy shading: bush in 1957 still infested; Crosses show sites of villages involved in the Maswa sleeping sickness outbreak.

areas or in the woodland, are clothed almost entirely in well-brayed skins of game; these also cover their beds. Long necklaces made from discs cut neatly from the shells of ostrich eggs are worn by everyone, and whole ostrich eggs are mounted as charms on the summits of the huts (Swynnerton 1923*a*).

Swynnerton described three villages. In one there were only four huts and the bush was growing all around them. It was easier to catch tsetse in the open spaces around the huts than in the bush itself. An old woman was seen with a dozen or more flies on her garments and skin. They followed her into one of the huts. One hut was deserted, the wife dead and the husband gone. In another he suspected, from the warmth of the bedding, a sick woman had been lying, but had hidden at his approach. A second village was larger, in better repair, and stood in natural grassland a quarter of a mile from the bush edge. A few tsetse were caught in it and it was thought they had been brought by persons who had visited villages further inside the bush, like the first one. Three or four people were dead and four were sick. Finally a third village, along with many others, lay in open country, about half a mile from the nearest bush which was, however, encroaching. There had been several deaths but no tsetse were seen. It was thought that the victims had become infected when on visits into the bush.

Swynnerton was always eager for evidence that tended to exculpate the wild game. He concluded that 'those people who live in the woodland, and those that live near it and enter it for the same purposes, are nearly as available to the tsetse as food-animals as the game itself; they are also far more available than the game when it is scarce, and must then carry great numbers of tsetse to their villages'. A medical officer, H. L. Duke, who later took charge of the Sleeping Sickness Laboratory at Entebbe in Uganda, and visited the Simiyu salient shortly after Swynnerton, did not accept these views.

The trypanosome population of the salient in 1922

Duke examined the blood of shot animals and found a '*T. vivax*-like' organism in a roan antelope and a *brucei*-type trypanosome either from a waterbuck or a warthog, for the blood of both was injected into the same

TABLE 13.1

Duke's (1923) dissections of G. swynnertoni in Maswa, 1922

	Localities			
Type of infection	*(A)*	*(B)*	*(C)*	*Totals*
Proboscis and gut . .	24	1	8	43
Proboscis only . . .	57	19	68	144
Gut only	8	1	6	15
Gut and salivary gland . .	2	1	0	3
Total infected . . .	91	32	82	205
Total dissected . .	819	722	665	2206

monkey. He also dissected 2206 *Glossina swynnertoni* obtained from three types of locality. His data, which he gave as percentages of flies infected, are reworked in Table 13.1 to give actual numbers.

In the (A) type localities the inhabitants were heavily infected and game and fly were both present, the latter in relatively large numbers. Class (B) were from less heavily infected villages near which game was scarce and tsetse 'not particularly numerous'. Class (C) includes places where there was game but no people. Flies were 'fairly numerous'. Proboscis and gut infections may have been (and probably chiefly were) *Trypanosoma congolense*, but with perhaps also some mixed *T. congolense–T. vivax* infections; proboscis-only infections were almost certainly very nearly all of *T. vivax*. Gut-only infections could have been immature *T. brucei* (and/or *T. 'rhodesiense'*).

Duke's purpose was to find what he called the 'game index' of the tsetse, that is the percentage of insects carrying trypanosomes which, in the absence of domestic stock, must have come from the blood of game; secondly he wished to know if the distribution of the pleomorphic trypanosomes bore any relation to the distribution of the infected villages. He added that domestic stock was so rare in the fly-belt that all trypanosomes must have been derived from game or man. With this Swynnerton would have agreed, for he regarded as potential hosts for the tsetse only man or the wild game.

It is unfortunate that no quantitative estimate of the infection rates in the various villages was published. If the totals of flies containing trypanosomes, regardless of the species of the flagellates, are compared, then Duke's figures establish his first point. The total of 91 infected tsetses in a sample of 819 dissected, from Class (A) heavily infected villages, is significantly greater ($\chi^2 = 22 \cdot 4072$; $P < 0 \cdot 001$) than the total of 32 infected flies in a sample of 722 from less heavily infected Class (B) villages, where there were fewer flies and game was scarce.

The percentage of tsetse with infected salivary glands was so small that it was impossible to suggest that in the more heavily infected villages the tsetse were themselves more heavily infected with *T. 'rhodesiense'* than were flies caught elsewhere. On the contrary Duke pointed out that his figure of 3 gut and gland infections in 2206 dissections (0·13 per cent) was very similar to the figures obtained by other workers. Bruce in 1912 in Nyasaland had obtained 0·1 gut and gland infections in 1975 dissections, and 0·09 per cent in 1060 dissections in 1913. Duke himself and Muriel Robertson, in Uganda, had had 0·19 per cent gland infections in 1562 dissections.

He concluded (1) that the main hosts of the tsetse and source of the trypanosomes were the game and not, even in the heavily infected villages, man and (2) that direct and not cyclical transmission was largely, if not solely, responsible for the spread of the trypanosome among the inhabitants of the area. This direct transmission was, to a large extent, performed by *Glossina* itself. Duke also came to a conclusion which, if it differed from that of Swynnerton, must nevertheless have been gratifying to him, namely that the wild game served as a valuable buffer between man and the tsetse and, in normal circumstances, preserved him from intense attack.

Duke's data have the interest of rarity. He continued for another decade to concern himself at Entebbe with the problem of trypanosome transmission, especially of the role of G. *fuscipes* in propagating *Trypanosoma* '*gambiense*'; but interest in tsetse infection rates in different epidemiological situations ceased almost entirely in East Africa when, by 1930, it had become generally accepted that elimination of the vector was the only satisfactory solution to the trypanosomiasis problem. It was over 30 years before Whiteside (1953) in the Lambwe valley in Kenya showed, as Duke had done, that local variations in the environment could affect the incidence rate of trypanosomes in the vector. The problem has since been further clarified by Jordan's studies already mentioned in Chapter 5.

The Maswa epidemic reached its peak in 1925 when 108 cases were diagnosed. It is possible that the first case was a man brought into Mwanza hospital in 1918. The last case in the area was a single one in 1938, though it may be that the majority of cases after 1931 came from the neighbouring area of Ikoma where another epidemic reached a peak in 1932. Altogether 564 cases were observed in and around the Simiyu salient between 1922 and 1938.

Evacuation of infected villages

Approximately 5000 people were moved out of the salient in 1922 and were resettled in the open country around its periphery. This resulted in considerable congestion, which was relieved by communal bush clearing in 1926–8 (Fairbairn 1948).

The removal of these people permitted a further expansion of the fly-belt. Montague (1926) surveyed the Simiyu salient and reported a widespread growth of thickets in the formerly occupied country. There had also been changes in the fauna. In 1923 hartebeests had been the second most abundant species in the area, but they had now left, 'most probably due to the "closing-up" of the country with thickets'. However, Montague observed that there had been a general increase in game which, he thought, had prevented even larger areas becoming almost pure thicket. In the extension of bush at the south-east corner of the Simiyu fly-belt a cattle ranch had been established in the 1920s. This Marialuguru (or Malya) ranch became infested with G. *swynnertoni* and G. *pallidipes*. Deaths from trypanosomiasis rose from 5 in 1187 head in August 1931 to 50 in 591 head in November. With the appearance of infection most of the stock were moved from the ranch. Between 1932 and 1934 various clearings (including the temporary reclamation of the Malya ranch) were made, amounting to some 32 mile^2.

In Maps 13.1 and 13.2 an outline of the Simiyu fly-belt prepared in 1957 (Barnes 1958) is superimposed on Swynnerton's map. In the 35 years that intervene the salient had become greatly reduced in area and almost completely isolated from the main G. *swynnertoni* fly-belt further east. The same species of game animals were present. Swynnerton (1923a) had recorded, 'in order of scarcity', situtunga, bushbuck, giraffe, reedbuck, waterbuck, duiker, impala, ostrich, roan antelope, eland, topi, hartebeest, and zebra. For a fauna that he maintained was exceedingly scarce, this was quite a comprehensive list. There was said to be one rhinoceros, but

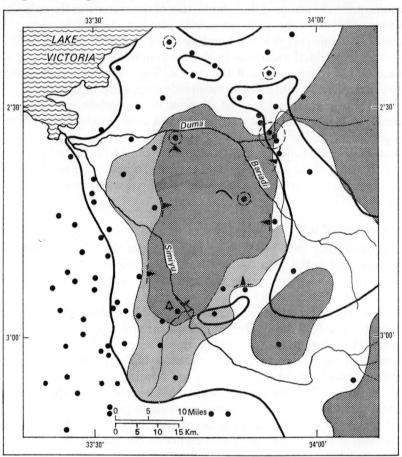

MAP 13.2. Outlines as in Map 13.1. Dots show locations of herds plotted by Yeoman 1958–9. Dots encircled by broken line indicate herds infected with trypanosomiasis. In the south and east many other herds were present as well as those shown on the map.

buffalo, formerly plentiful, had not recovered from the rinderpest. Warthogs were present, but bush-pigs were scarce.

Barnes in 1957 saw the same species of game, except for situtunga, bushbuck, and ostrich, and also recorded oribi, steinbuck, dik-dik, and elephants. Duke had dissected tsetse from localities where the inhabitants were heavily infected and game and fly were both present. Barnes, however, remarked that the larger animals tended to keep well clear of the settled area and around the edges of the salient the fly was either very light or non-existent.

The most marked instance of an area where an increase in settlement has had the result of driving out both the larger game and *G. swynnertoni* is in the bush to the south of the Shishio–Luguru road which has been settled intensively over the last few years. A great deal of this bush still bears the appearance of typical *swynnertoni* habitat but the fly is not there and the only game animals seen in this area are impala, reedbuck, duiker and dik-dik.

Barnes showed on his map not only the outline of the tsetse belt but, around it, a zone in which tsetse was absent or very scarce. It is in complete contrast to Swynnerton's and Duke's observations of villages that, in their day, occupied an outer zone of a much larger fly-belt and were heavily infested with tsetse.

One final piece of evidence for changed conditions is found in the distribution of the cattle population. At the time of the 1922 epidemic there were no domestic animals in the tsetse-infested villages. Cattle lived only in the open country away from the bush edge. In 1958–9, about a year after Barnes drew his map, Yeoman (during the study of East coast fever already mentioned) plotted the positions of herds of cattle in and around the Simiyu salient. It is true that since 1950 efficient drugs conferring some degree of temporary prophylaxis had become increasingly available, but a heavy risk of infection such as would be incurred by exposure of cattle to an obviously visible population of tsetse would have been an intolerable burden. Map 13.2 shows Barnes's tsetse outlines and the positions of herds plotted by Yeoman. Cattle owners were well aware of the effects of trypanosomiasis and the limits beyond which they would not graze their stock were recorded. There is a good correlation with Barnes's survey. Trypanosomiasis was noted as a particular problem for six herds pastured within the fly-belt, presumably owned by people carving out new homes for themselves. This is a very different situation from that noted at the government ranch at Marialuguru in 1931.

When the Sukuma population as a whole was in a state of decline, bush, game, and tsetse spread among the surviving villages, killing off and driving away both people and their cattle. In the subsequent reversal of the population trend, game animals and their attendant tsetse populations were kept at a distance from the bush edge. The encroaching settlement thus tended to be separated from the sources of infection by a zone of still unfelled bush in which the tsetse, the trypanosomes, and their hosts were rarely seen. In these conditions epidemics could not occur and locally enzootic cattle trypanosomiasis was not intolerable and, in any case, was a temporary phenomenon that disappeared as the pressure of human population increased.

The Uzinza (Geita) coast in 1922

On 18 July 1922, Lt. M. S. Moore, V.C., seconded from the King's African Rifles to Swynnerton's Game Department, left Mwanza by dhow, accompanied by a hospital dresser, to survey the country west of Smith Sound for tsetse flies and sleeping sickness cases and to collect any other information of epidemiological value. This was the country of Uzinza, home of the Zinza people. It was incorporated in Mwanza district, but later became a separate district after the discovery of gold at Geita. It was already known that the offshore islands were infested with *Glossina palpalis* (*G. fuscipes fuscipes*). Moore spent a week surveying the shore line and bush inland. *G. morsitans*, *G. pallidipes*, *G. brevipalpis*, and *G. fuscipes* were all collected. There was a mission in charge of an African priest at Buingo on the Rusenye peninsula, and a sparse population of 'very truculent' natives lived along the shore with their cattle. Of these there were a large number in the open country of the peninsula, but for the most part the bush edge came to within less than a mile of the shore and *G. morsitans* were abundant, as were game animals. Moore recorded that *G. morsitans* and *G. fuscipes* did not bite human beings. The only tsetse that bit him was, somewhat unexpectedly, a female *G. brevipalpis*. He saw one robber fly (Asilidae), of which there were many, with a tsetse in its jaws.

The local inhabitants, besides keeping cattle, fished, hunted with bows and arrows, and cultivated, chiefly bananas, cassava, and cotton. Wherever Moore found sleeping sickness suspects his assistant took blood slides, but these must all have been negative for there are no records of human trypanosomiasis at this time in Uzinza. The grass everywhere had been burnt or was burning. There were crocodiles and hippopotamuses along the lake shore, and inland were seen the spoor of topi, giraffe, roan antelope, duiker, bushbuck, impala, zebra, lion.

Apart from the missionaries near the lake shore, few Europeans can have seen much of northern Uzinza at the time of Moore's visit. The main road to Bukoba and the countries west of Lake Victoria followed the route that the Arabs, Speke and Grant, and their successors had used and although others (Stanley, for example, in 1889 and doubtless regular, if infrequent, German officials) had used more northerly routes, no path that Moore saw in 1922 was, as he said, fit even for a bicycle (Moore 1922).

West Mwanza (Geita) district in 1934 and 1937

In 1930 sleeping sickness (*T. brucei rhodesiense*) was diagnosed in West Mwanza (later Geita) district. In the years 1934–6 some 5400 people were concentrated in six settlements (Gillman 1936, Fairbairn 1948, Malcolm 1953). This prophylactic resettlement took place in the southern chiefdoms of the district. The northern chiefdoms, Karumo and Buchosa, must, at this time, have been free of apparent infection. Nearly all their people were living along the lake shore.

At about the same time that human trypanosomiasis appeared in the district, gold was discovered in comparatively large quantities at Geita. The need to establish a mining community with a main access road and the possibility, seemingly inherent in this new situation, of the development of epidemics led to a renewal of interest in tsetse. Surveys were carried out in 1935 and 1937 and from the last of these (Burtt 1937) the account begun by Lt. Moore can be continued. A description of some of the vegetation of the area at this time is also to be found in Burtt (1942).

There was still no road between Smith sound and Geita and an air reconnaissance confirmed that the country was largely uninhabited. The narrow coastal strip of settlement was seen, but inland there were only scattered villages of the Rongo tribe, many of whom were iron-smelters. They grew cassava and sweet potatoes as basic crops, with some maize, millet, eleusine, groundnuts, and beans. They were 'excellent porters and had a cheerful and intelligent disposition'. The country had formerly carried a larger population.

Between Kamchanga and Kawaba many old village sites were seen, one extensive abandoned village site being called Nyabazinza. I was informed that the path to Mazinda passes the abandoned village sites of Nakahama and Nyangendu. The extensive abandoned cultivation of Kawamba village also indicated a very much larger population in the past.

The word Nyabazinza suggests that it may not have been a village name, but that its inhabitants had been Zinza and not Rongo.

In another passage there is more evidence of former population.

Old village sites are frequent on the higher ground, the most recently inhabited being that of Isaka where huts, elaborate pig fences, and clumps of banana trees are still standing . . . At every village enquiries were made in order to ascertain if possible why so many villages had been abandoned and also where the former inhabitants had gone. In every case I was informed that the villages had been abandoned on account of the depredations of bushpigs and that the pig were able to break through the elaborate pig fences surrounding the gardens. The former population had in almost all cases moved to the lake coast (Burtt 1937).

In recent years a number of Sukuma had come to settle among the Zinza along the lake shore.

It is curious that although in the three years 1934–6 the sleeping sickness branch of the Medical Department had carried out the resettlement of people for sleeping sickness control, Burtt did not mention the possibility that human trypanosomiasis may have contributed to depopulation. The separation of entomology and epidemiology was complete. However, had the empty villages that Burtt described been evacuated at the orders of the Medical Department it is certain that the Rongo would have known about

it and would have told him. The key observation was that 'in every case
. . . villages had been abandoned on account of the depredations of bushpigs': the Zinza and Rongo had been losing in their confrontation with the
woodland ecosystem.

The Karumo chiefdom in 1947

In 1938 it was decided to encourage the Sukuma to colonize the empty
country west of Smith Sound. By 1947 about 300 mile², mostly in the chiefdom of Karumo, had been settled and *Glossina morsitans* had retreated.
The natural vegetation was woodland dominated by *Julbernardia globiflora*,
with *Brachystegia tamarindoides* occupying hilltops wherever rocky granite
outcrops occurred. The drainage lines were comparatively open wooded
grassland, with small trees among which *Combretum ternifolium* was the
most frequent species. There were scattered thickets on termite hills.
Where the drainage lines descended to lower levels and broadened out as
they flowed together, the valley floors opened out into more or less treeless
seasonal swamp grassland (*mbuga*), bordered by large *Acacia rovumae* and
the smaller *Lannea humilis*. At this level, the *Julbernardia* woodland was
replaced in places by a community in which the dominants were *Afrormosia anglolensis*, *Combretum grandifolium*, and *C. gueinzii* with many other
tree species. On the termite hills the thickets usually carried trees of
Albizia brachycalyx or *A. amara* with an undergrowth of *Rhus* and other
shrubs (Ford 1948).

A traverse of the edge of new settlement in this sort of country can be
described by use of a diagram prepared in 1947 (Fig. 13.1a). Roughly east
from a chief's house in the completely cleared and settled ridge shown on
the left of the diagram, the first *mbuga* was crossed to enter the bush on the
second ridge. On its crest a new house had been built and there was some
cultivation and cattle. In spite of this the chief expected to see tsetse here,
but it was a dull day and none was taken. A second *mbuga* led to the gentle
ascent of a third ridge not yet occupied by a settler. Here, at the junction
between the *Acacia rovumae–Lannea humilis* fringing woodland and the
higher level *Combretum–Afrormosia* woodland one male *G. morsitans* was
caught. At the edge of the third *mbuga* 7 males and 1 female were taken in
about 10 minutes. On the second *mbuga* an oribi (*Ourebia*) was seen and it
was said that topi (*Damaliscus*) were often seen in the third *mbuga*. Their
footprints, made in the rains six months earlier, showed that these antelopes
had, at that time, been frequent in the second *mbuga*. (In 1947 one had
not learned to inquire more intently into the abundance of animals like
the warthog and others now known to be favoured hosts of *G. morsitans*.)
This traverse had shown that *G. morsitans* could easily be caught less than
a mile from grazing cattle in country where most of the natural vegetation
was still standing and from which not all of the natural fauna had disappeared.

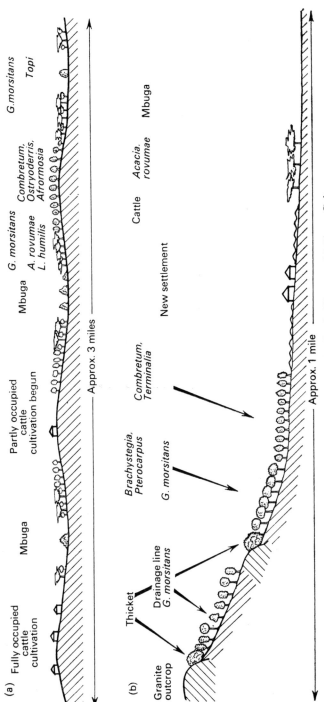

(a) Fully occupied cattle cultivation

Mbuga

Partly occupied cattle cultivation begun

Mbuga

G. morsitans
A. rovumae
L. humilis

Combretum,
Ostryoderris,
Afrormosia

G.morsitans
Topi

Approx. 3 miles

(b)

Granite outcrop

Thicket

Drainage line
G. morsitans

Brachystegia,
Pterocarpus

G. morsitans

Combretum,
Terminalia

New settlement

Cattle

Acacia.
rovumae

Mbuga

Approx. 1 mile

FIGS. 13.1a and b. Transects across the fly-line in Karumo chiefdom, Geita, 1947.

Fig. 13.1*b* illustrates the same thing happening in a different topographical situation around the rock inselberg of Kasamwa. In the crevices between the bare granite blocks of its summit were patches of thicket (*Cussonia arborea, Clerodendron myricoides, Canthium schimperianum, C. burtii, Markhamia obtusifolia, Annona chrysophylla, Lannea fulva, Ochna* sp., and *Strophanthus eminii*). Where there was deeper soil in the crevices stood isolated trees including *Pseudolachnostylis maprouneaefolia, Lannea schimperi, Afrormosia angolensis, Combretum grandifolium, Entada abyssinica, Psorospermum febrifugum, Pterocarpus bussei*, and *Ficus* spp.

Leading down from the Kasamwa hilltop a drainage line followed a shallow open glade some 70 yd wide by 200 yd long. A male *G. morsitans* was caught as soon as the glade was entered. At the edge of the glade were patches of thicket similar to that found on the hilltop above, while in it were scattered *Combretum ternifolium, C. grandifolium, Terminalia sericea, Dombeya* sp., and other small trees. At its lower end the glade ran into the *Brachystegia spiciformis* woodland that surrounded the hill. Here another tsetse was taken. The *Brachystegia* woodland at this point was only about 200 yd wide and gave way to secondary scrub dominated by *Combretum ternifolium* and *Terminalia sericea*. A short distance across this scrub led to cultivation, new houses, and cattle. The owners were Rongo who had lived here before and had been moved, in the early 1930s, into a sleeping sickness settlement. They had been back a year and had brought their livestock in only a few months before our visit. They knew that tsetses were to be found on the hill, but their cattle were still healthy.

The country seen in 1947 was being invaded by Sukuma, and wild animals were few. Ten years before, Burtt had also seen few animals and had attributed this paucity of fauna to the numbers of hunters armed with muzzle-loading guns. But he saw frequent signs of bushpigs. In 1937 *G. morsitans* had been exceedingly abundant throughout the *Julbernardia* woodland, although it was absent from the higher hills clothed with *Brachystegia tamarindoides*. The tsetses were most abundant along the margins of valleys flanking the woodland and they seemed to be concentrated in the short grass areas of the narrower valleys. It was here, especially, that Burtt remarked that bushpig tracks were always abundant. It is possible to confuse the tracks of bushpig and warthog, but whichever they were, Suidae were abundant and *G. morsitans morsitans* is more often a feeder on pigs than on other species (Weitz 1963).

A generalized vegetation catena showed, (1) *Brachystegia tamarindoides* on the more outstanding summits where the ground was broken by granite outcrops; (2) on lower, more gentle slopes still showing exposed rock in places, a woodland of *Julbernardia globiflora*, with some *Brachystegia spiciformis* and occasional *Pterocarpus bussei, Anisophyllea* sp., etc. This woodland continued lower down, (3) when exposed rock was no longer to be seen. Areas in the lower woodland carrying a mixture of *Combretum* spp., *Terminalia*, especially *T. sericea*, and *Afrormosia angolensis* indicated former settlements. On the margins of drainages (4) *Combretum ternifolium*, *C. grandifolium*, *T. sericea*, *A. angolensis* were interspersed with thickets on termitaria. In some situations the actual drainage line was occupied by more frequent termitaria thickets or continuous riverine thicket. In lower, wider drainages (5) *Acacia rovumae* and *Lannea humilis*, also with scattered termitaria, either clothed the whole valley floor or gave way (6) to more or less open *mbuga*.

The two upper sections of this catena could not be used for cultivation. The two lower were also not used except for occasional plots of rice where flood waters could be retained by low earth bunds. The main cultivation areas therefore were to be found either in section (3) the lower *Julbernardia* woodland or in (4) the *Combretum–Terminalia–Afrormosia* zone down to the edge of, or encroaching upon, (5) the *Acacia–Lannea* and termite thicket zone where this was not too subject to water-logging. In short, cultivation came down to and impinged upon the zone in which Burtt recorded abundant bushpigs and concentrations of *G. morsitans*. It has been observed in Chapter 2 that the interpretation of catches of *G. morsitans* by moving parties of men is not a simple matter; but occupation of zones (3) and (4) by cultivation must have interrupted the activities of the wild pigs. It seemed probable therefore that in this way both the habitat and the food supply of *G. morsitans* were eliminated by immigrant cultivators. One concluded, in 1947, that the ultimate safeguards against more epizootics were the continuing fertility both of the people and of the soil.

Sleeping sickness in Geita district

Trypanosoma brucei rhodesiense infections appeared among recent Sukuma immigrants in 1949. By August there were 11 cases. Records of

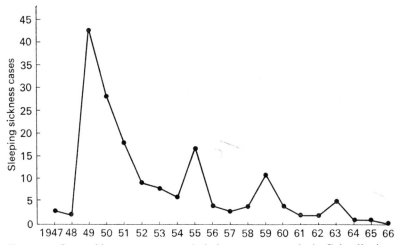

FIG. 13.2. Cases of human trypanosomiasis from 1947 onwards, in Geita district.

human trypanosomiasis for Geita district are shown in Fig. 13.2. The epidemic had broken out in the Isaka–Nyahunga area among people in the van of the immigrant movement who were still sparsely distributed. This area was one specifically mentioned by Burtt (1937) as having been abandoned because of the depredations of bushpigs.

The epidemic was welcomed by government agricultural officers. Immigration from Sukumaland had been proceeding very rapidly so that the controls on population density which seemed to them so essential, if soil exhaustion and erosion were not to overtake the area, had not been properly implemented. The appearance of the disease enabled the sleeping sickness ordinance to be invoked, under which legal restraint might be used to compel people to settle in places thought to be desirable. One difficulty was that the conservationists wanted to settle the new population at a density of 100 persons per mile^2.† The medical authorities, on the other hand, wished to see double this density, for 200 people to the mile^2 would ensure the rapid production of a more or less treeless cultivation steppe in which tsetse could not live. It was eventually decided to compel these sparsely scattered pioneers to retire behind a given line until the land was considered safe from reinfestation and then to open up another section of the front for occupation. In this process protection would be given to the earlier settlers by prophylactic partial bush clearing to reduce the density of the *Glossina morsitans* population. Under these conditions, with a watch kept upon the health of the people by the Medical Service, no serious epidemic ever developed. Exceptionally, since it is rare for them to contract trypanosomiasis, two members of the tsetse field staff were infected in 1950 during the first surveys made to plan clearing work.

Clearing began in 1952. The method adopted was selective felling of trees in the interzones between the alluvial and eluvial vegetation. Not surprisingly the anti-tsetse measures were popular among the immigrants,

---

† The administrative, agricultural, veterinary, hydrological, and engineering work associated with this expansion of the Sukuma people was, and is, considerable. Malcolm (1953) should be consulted. It is no part of the present study to describe it; but the 'Sukumaland agricultural equation' upon which the figure of 100 persons per mile^2 is based may be quoted from Rounce (1949); it is this:

'In ONE HOMESTEAD there are on the average TWO TAX-PAYERS or a total of SEVEN PEOPLE with an average of FOURTEEN CATTLE and TEN SMALL STOCK UNITS (at 5 small stock equalling one stock unit) equals SIXTEEN STOCK UNITS which produce altogether SIXTEEN TONS OF MANURE PER ANNUM. This manure is enough to manure EIGHT ACRES EVERY OTHER YEAR which is one acre more than the average acreage of arable for Sukumaland but the stock require TWO ACRES EACH OF PASTURE (the average for Sukumaland is 2½ acres) equals THIRTY TWO ACRES PLUS EIGHT ARABLE equals FORTY ACRES equals SIXTEEN HOMESTEADS PER SQUARE MILE equals 112 PEOPLE PER SQUARE MILE, say ONE HUNDRED. Three miles to walk to water is about THIRTY SQUARE MILES equals FIVE HUNDRED HOMESTEADS equals EIGHT THOUSAND STOCK × FIVE GALLONS OF WATER × 120 DAYS (August to November) equals FIVE MILLION GALLONS (to allow for evaporation) per 500 HOMES AND THIRTY SQUARE MILES.'

For more recent assessments of the Sukumaland problem reference may be made to Ruthenberg (1964, 1967).

for they lightened their own task of clearing land for cultivation (*Tanganyika Tsetse* 1954; also, for a summary of work done, *Tanganyika Tsetse* 1958). The process still continued in 1965. What would have happened had there been no preliminary reduction of the tsetse population by clearing and no medical surveillance cannot be known. It is not at all certain that human trypanosomiasis would have halted the expansion of Sukumaland.

Summing-up on trypanosomiasis in Sukumaland

The sequence of events described in this and the two preceding chapters runs as follows:

(1) Severe reduction of the human population began soon after 1890 and continued until about 1920. The evidence is abundant but not quantitative.

(2) In 1891 and the next few years the domestic cattle population was almost completely exterminated by rinderpest. Buffaloes in the bush around Sukumaland were wiped out and probably other species including the Suidae and some antelopes were nearly exterminated.

(3) As a consequence of (2) there was a recession of tsetse from the borders of the settled country, but recovery of the animal hosts was rapid and by 1913 the flies were spreading again and now invaded country, denuded of much of its human population, (1) above, which had previously been tsetse-free.

(4) An outbreak of rhodesian sleeping sickness in the Maswa district probably began in 1918 and reached a peak in 1925. It was controlled by evacuation of people and this, in turn, accelerated the spread of *G. swynnertoni*.

(5) The greatest spread of *Glossina* was in Shinyanga in the south of Sukumaland from an area of bush with abundant wild animals, the 'Nindo jungle', that had been extant at least since 1858. This area was part of a *Grenzwildnis* between the southern Sukuma and the northern Nyamwezi.

(6) Between 1923 and 1930 organized bush clearing halted the spread of tsetse in this area and the remaining bush was preserved for experimental purposes by the Tanganyika government Tsetse Research Department.

(7) The cattle population of Sukumaland probably continued to multiply very rapidly until about 1925 when the rate of increase diminished. In 1931 and 1932 famine plus a rinderpest epizootic brought about a decline, but thereafter the cattle population continued to rise, though increase again was halted by famine in 1942 and, very severely, in 1949.

(8) The human population ceased to decline in the 1920s and may have been showing a true increase by the mid 1930s (0·8 per cent per annum between 1934 and 1944).

(9) Until the mid 1930s, spread of tsetse fly around Sukumaland continued but was halted in some parts by bush clearing.

(10) After about 1935 the trends were reversed. The increase rate of the

human population may have reached 1·5 per cent per annum between 1944 and 1947.

(11) By 1947 the tsetse belts were receding all around Sukumaland, and the tsetse-free area of cultivation steppe had increased, as compared with 1924, by 3000 mile², of which only 800 could be attributed to direct entomological attack on the tsetse.

(12) The growing human population began, during the late 1930s, to reclaim bushland both on the east and west of Sukumaland. In the south, expansion was prevented by the preservation of about 1000 mile² of bush, much of which had earlier composed the ancient frontier zone of Sukumaland.

(13) The greater part of the excess population moved westwards into Geita district, where the population probably increased from about 60 000 in 1934 to 270 000 in 1957. The expansion eastwards began later and in the south only began when the preserves of the Tsetse Research Department were decontrolled.

(14) In 1949, epidemic human trypanosomiasis appeared among immigrant people in the van of the westward movement into Geita. This was easily reduced by preventing scattered settlement and by reduction of tsetse density by partial bush clearing. The medical coverage was also greatly superior to that which it had been possible to provide in the 1922 epidemic.

(15) Apart from sleeping sickness, there was considerable evidence that, in contrast with the situation in the 1920s, cattle trypanosomiasis was less of a problem. In Geita, even without drug therapy, immigrant settlers grazed their cattle quite close to bush in which *G. morsitans* could be taken. On both sides of Sukumaland cattle trypanosomiasis was not a serious obstacle to the occupation of bush and expulsion of the larger wild fauna by peasant farmers.

(16) The principal control over cattle population density is exerted by availability of pasture. Pasture is created by the destruction of bush by farming. This process, however, does not proceed rapidly enough to prevent overstocking. This leads in turn to heavy periodical mortality from famines and thirst in bad years.

(17) A further control over stock numbers is exerted by theileriosis, a tick-borne disease that spreads outside enzootic areas when heavy losses of cattle by starvation lead to temporary understocking. This causes more abundant grass growth than is usual and hence enlarges the environment available for the growth of tick populations. These, in turn, produce epizootic conditions. Development of immunity in the calves of surviving cattle assists in the build-up of the cattle population to a level at which pasture grasses are kept too short to support enough ticks to maintain an epizootic.

Gaps in knowledge

Lack of history

One cannot review the history of trypanosomiasis in Sukumaland without being conscious of how much information is lacking. History itself is lacking. What evidence there is suggests that Sukumaland may not yet have expanded sufficiently to occupy all the country that a hundred years ago was inhabited south of Lake Victoria.

There is no yardstick to measure achievement. The entomologists believed that without their efforts trypanosomiasis might have extinguished the Sukuma altogether (cf. Swynnerton's remarks on p. 197). This now seems a wrong view. We do not know, in fact, whether those devoted labours served any useful purpose at all. It seems likely that the retreat of the Shinyanga people, without the help of the tsetse control teams, would have continued until population pressures in central Sukumaland had become intolerable, after which they would, once more, have attacked the bush–wild animal–tsetse ecosystem as indeed their ancestors must have done in the beginning. The 'most beautiful pastoral country' over which Stanley had looked from the top of a granite inselberg in Usiha had been carved out of tsetse-infested woodlands hundreds of years before. The most that can be claimed is that recovery from the epidemics, epizootics, wars, and famines that the coming of the colonial powers had instigated was eased by the technical services that they later set up. Among these it is probable that medical services by their effect on the reproduction rate and the hydrological services by improving water supplies made a far greater contribution to the solution of the Sukuma trypanosomiasis problem than did the entomological attack on *Glossina*.

Trypanosome risk

The incidence of trypanosomiasis, whether human or in domestic animals, must depend upon the frequency with which their populations receive infective bites. Duke (1923) showed that the gross infection rate, inclusive of all trypanosomes, in *Glossina swynnertoni* in the Simiyu fly-belt, was 9·74 per cent. We do not know the infection rate of the flies that caused the evacuation of the government herds from the Marialuguru ranch in 1931. Still less can it be guessed what proportion of the Shinyanga tsetse were infected when Swynnerton began his clearing operations in 1923. Nor is it known what proportion of the tsetse are infected now, or at any time in the last twenty or more years in areas where they have been receding and people have taken their cattle, with little adverse effects, into bush still supporting tsetse. If, as Barnes's 1957 survey showed, the game animals were retreating from the advancing tide of settlement it might be supposed, in the light of Jordan's (1964 and 1965a) studies, that a diminishing game population would cause a reduction in the proportion of tsetse carrying trypanosomes.

Support for this notion is found in data published by Vanderplank (1947b) and by Robson and Hope Cawdery (1958). The infection rates in *Glossina swynnertoni* in the Shinyanga experimental blocks recorded by those authors are:

1941	6·3 per cent (Vanderplank)
1942	4·8 per cent (Vanderplank)
1943	4·1 per cent (Vanderplank)
1944	3·4 per cent (Vanderplank)
1957	2·4 per cent (Robson and Hope Cawdery).

Such evidence as there is, therefore, suggests that during the period of expansion of the Sukuma population, the infection rate of trypanosomes in *G. swynnertoni* was diminishing. It may be objected that the Shinyanga experimental blocks were game reserves and that the tsetse and trypanosome hosts were protected from the effects of human interference. However, during the years 1941–4 much experimental control work was in progress and it now appears probable that the adverse effects that this work had upon the tsetse populations was due to interference with their normal feeding routines. The figure obtained by Robson and Hope Cawdery (1958) was from tsetse captured on the western edge of a block of bush much subject to incursion by local Africans.

Effects of physiological adjustment to infection in cattle

One other point needs to be made. African zebu cattle are able to tolerate some degree of trypanosome infection. In the Shinyanga area, in drought and famine years, cattle owners drive their cattle to pasture in the fly-belts. They say that they know some will die of the infection whereas if they keep them in the tsetse-free lands all will die of starvation. Whiteside (1949) herded 340 head of local cattle in 5 mile^2 of *Acacia–Commiphora* bush at Shinyanga, infested with *G. pallidipes* and *G. swynnertoni*. He estimated that this herd outnumbered the larger wild animals (giraffe, greater kudu, and impala) about six times, but was less than the indigenous population of warthogs, bushpigs, and small buck. The experiment (to study the effect on the tsetse of insecticide sprayed weekly over the cattle) lasted for 5 months. Blood slides were taken from all animals showing signs of sickness. Of these 21·5 per cent showed trypanosome infections. These were treated with phenidium chloride. For comparison slides were also taken each week from 10 per cent of the animals that appeared to be perfectly healthy. It was found that 21·4 per cent of these also showed trypanosomes in their blood.† They were what, in some conditions of

† These blood slide data were not published but are preserved in a memorandum dated 29.4.46 in the E.A.T.R.O. archives.

human trypanosomiasis, are sometimes called 'healthy carriers'. No animals died of trypanosomiasis during the 5 months' exposure to tsetse and on the whole, because grazing inside the fly-belt was more abundant than in the tsetse-free pasture outside, they improved in condition. Only 2·15 per cent of them received treatment. One may ask whether this ability to survive in the fly-bush had any connection with a possible low frequency of infective bites received. It is a question yet to be answered.

Final conclusions on Sukumaland

The cause of the spread of tsetse around Sukumaland observed between 1913 and 1935 was the progressive reduction in human population density among the Sukuma people that had taken place from 1890 to 1920. In these conditions of spreading tsetse and increasing wild trypanosome host population, epidemics of sleeping sickness broke out and cattle could not survive in proximity to the tsetse belts. In the subsequent period of population increase among the Sukuma, the wild hosts of tsetse and their accompanying tsetse populations retreated from the spreading human population. The latter, when initially penetrating the fly-bush, encountered some risk of infection, but it cannot be stated what would have been the outcome of the Geita epidemic had no prophylactic measures been taken. The responses of the cattle, which could, in these circumstances, tolerate proximity to the tsetse, suggests that the human epidemic might have died down naturally to a level of easily tolerated endemism.

During these extensive changes in the interrelationships between the two ecosystems, bush, wild animals, tsetse, and trypanosomes continued to persist in three areas, the Nindo–Shinyanga frontier zone (*Grenzwildnis*) between the Sukuma and Nyamwezi peoples, the Simiyu salient on the east, and the hills of Buhungukira on the west of Sukumaland. These are natural foci of infection from which tsetse and trypanosomiasis will again spread if the present upward trend of human population is reversed without any fundamental change having taken place in the forms of land usage now practised.

In contrast to the *Grenzwildnis* is what may be called the 'heart' of Sukumaland, centred on Kwimba district. Here, throughout all their vicissitudes, the Sukuma people have maintained a more or less constant density of population. When people moved out of the peripheral districts of Shinyanga or Maswa they did not cram themselves into country already fully occupied as Swynnerton (1925a) and Hornby (1948) thought they must do; they went, no doubt under economic pressure, to under-developed areas and opened them up. When the adverse pressures were relaxed, in Maswa by reduction of incidence of human trypanosomiasis or in Shinyanga by removal of the Tsetse Research Laboratory and its game reserves, these areas also began to fill up once more. This process will be encountered again in the Tiv country of Nigeria where it has been defined as 'centrifugal expansion' (Chapter 22). It is of some interest to take a last look at Speke's 'Nindo jungle'. Tsetse reclamation workers are very often in doubt as to when they have finally got rid of the 'last fly'. No doubts were ever expressed about the success of the game destruction experiment of Potts and Jackson (1952). The 'Nindo jungle' was, perhaps for the first time ever, cleared of *Glossina morsitans*, *G. swynnertoni*, and *G. pallidipes*. According to the theories of those who established the Tanganyika Tsetse Research Department, this should have permitted the Sukuma and Nyamwezi to have occupied and developed it. In fact, although on several other portions of the periphery of Sukumaland the local peasantry had developed, unaided, large areas of tsetse-infested bush, they showed no interest in taking over the disease-free Nindo. In 1966 it was one of two areas only, in the whole of Tanzania, in which tsetse was known to be spreading (Turner 1967). The wildlife had recovered and the old focus of infection was re-establishing itself.

14

BUSOGA AND SAMIA AND
THE FIRST EPIDEMIC OF
GAMBIAN SLEEPING SICKNESS

Busoga and Samia before the epidemic

THE climate of the north-east corner of the Victoria basin, particularly the country north of the Kavirondo gulf, is strongly influenced by the high altitudes of the northern highlands of Kenya
and the great mass of Mount Elgon, 14 176 ft above sea level, as well as by
precipitation derived from the surface of the lake itself. From this wettest
of the three sample areas chosen around Lake Victoria, *Glossina morsitans*
and *G. swynnertoni* are absent and *G. fuscipes fuscipes*, *G. brevipalpis*, and
G. pallidipes only are found. The last of these, in Busoga as well as in parts
of the higher rainfall zones overlooking the Western Rift, has some habits
that are very different from those it displays at the southern end of the lake.
The Busoga–Nyanza epidemics involved both gambian and rhodesian
types of infection as well as two vectors, *G. fuscipes fuscipes* (*G. palpalis* in
earlier literature) and *G. pallidipes*.

As in the interlake area and in Sukumaland a background to subsequent
events is to be found in the records of early European visitors. A sharp contrast was plain to all travellers when they left the Luyia country and crossed
the Sio river, now the boundary between Kenya and Uganda, and entered
Busoga. A good account comes from a visitor in 1895, the title of whose
memoirs, *Some experiences of an Old Bromsgrovian*, gives little indication
of their value to the student of circumstantial epidemiology (Ternan 1930).

The boundary between Kavirondo and Usoga was very clearly marked, and
the difference between the two countries was extraordinary. Kavirondo, generally
speaking, a land of long grass and no trees and not very interesting. Usoga, a
mass of banana groves in every direction, interspersed with plenty of magnificent
forest trees, with lanes through the groves neatly fenced, and lots of shade.

The contrast between the two sides of the Sio river still persisted half a
century later, especially in those parts nearest to the lake, when much of
central Nyanza was no longer a country of long grass and no trees but a
mass of impenetrable thicket, and southern Busoga, now empty of bananas,
was covered either with thicket or secondary rain forest. The contrast is
very largely edaphic and only partly climatic. The soils of those parts of
central Nyanza adjacent to the lake have either impeded drainage or are

poorly drained and, for the most part, overlie a laterite horizon and comprise mainly sands or clays. In Busoga the soils are well-drained loams or friable clays (Scott 1962).

Another newcomer in the 1890s was Dr. Albert Cook, with whom the history of human trypanosomiasis in eastern Africa begins. He crossed the Sio river with a party from the Church Missionary Society on 10 February 1897. That afternoon a message arrived urging that a doctor should hurry on to Luba's, on the other side of Busoga, to attend a man hurt in a hunting accident. Cook, already having done the day's routine march of twenty miles, set off again at 5.30 p.m. and walked until 10 p.m. Towards sunset he crossed some hills from which he had his first view of Lake Victoria. Next morning he and his three carriers entered Busoga proper.

Almost immediately the aspect of the country changed; instead of the bare treeless hillocks of land, with here and there patches of sweet potatoes, we got beautiful trees and large gardens of bananas. . . . There were grand rocks and rocky defiles, and bogs of tall papyrus. . . . Just as the sun dipped [we] entered Wakoli's district. Half an hour later, as darkness was falling, we arrived at the great chief's village, an enormous place. . . . The next day we marched the twenty-nine miles to our Mission Station at Luba's. . . . All day long the walk had been lovely; at first we passed through miles and miles of banana plantations, and then through belts of forest land, with grand trees from one hundred to one hundred and fifty feet high, and wide spreading foliage in proportion with dense bush in between, and then a belt of pasture land with perhaps a swamp at the bottom through which a causeway ran (Cook 1945).

Evidently the Busoga forests, even if surrounded by miles and miles of banana plantations, were in existence in 1897. The use of the word 'pasture' suggests cattle. Roscoe (1923) notes that the cattle of Busoga 'were smaller than in other parts of Uganda; they were black or black with white markings, and had a small hump and short horns. . . . There were no large herds . . . but every peasant, however poor, kept at least one cow.' In southern Busoga the masses of bananas with islands of forest would scarcely have permitted any other form of husbandry. Most of the pasture must have been found in the valleys where, today, wooded grasslands with *Acacia campylacantha* lead down to a papyrus or *Miscanthidium* swamp in the valley bottom. It is to be supposed that these Soga cattle suffered the same fate as others when the rinderpest arrived in 1890. Dr. Cook did not specifically mention cattle, but only pasture. If he saw any they were the survivors of the great panzootic recovering their numbers, as elsewhere, very rapidly.

One other early account is concerned more with the differences in social organization in the two countries. Dr. Ansorge travelled up from Mombasa to Uganda in 1894.

On the overland journey to Uganda, the traveller on leaving Kavirondo enters Usoga, and he notices a complete and remarkable change in every respect. From the absolutely nude savages in Kavirondo he passes to a race where not even the youngest walk about uncovered; from a stingy and inhospitable tribe he joins one which greets him with a hearty welcome and extends to him a lavish hospitality; from treeless grasslands he finds himself in a well wooded country and under the shade of magnificent trees; from circular villages fortified with earth wall and trench he is among unprotected dwellings, of which a few of the better class have a fragile reed fence put up for privacy and ornament.—There is scarcely any other fruit to be had in the country except ripe bananas. But for this exception, Usoga is the nearest approach to what imagination pictures the Garden of Eden to have been (Ansorge 1899).

The Kavirondo (for the most part here are meant the people sometimes called Bantu Kavirondo but now called Luyia) were at that time undergoing the process of 'pacification', and the caravan with which Ansorge travelled had had to fight its way through their country. Hospitality seems a little much to have expected. The remains of walled and trenched villages may still be seen in the tsetse-infested thicket around the Field Station in the sleeping sickness focus at Lugala belonging to the East African Trypanosomiasis Research Organization.

By 1924 depopulation on both sides of the Sio river had occurred long enough ago for the regenerating vegetation to obliterate most of the cultivation seen by travellers at the end of the nineteenth century. 'At Mjanji one is between the two types of country, to the west the typical Uganda forests (here lying behind dense belts of papyrus), to the east the dreadful country of thorny bush and creeper, with the barren hills behind Sio' (Carpenter 1924). The lower Sio basin forms the country of Samia.

The great epidemic

On 13 February 1901, Dr. Albert Cook and his brother Dr. J. H. Cook, who were now established at the C.M.S. hospital in Kampala, saw two patients showing symptoms that recalled to the former what he had learned of the West African disease of sleeping sickness. The great tropical parasitologist, Manson, had recently suggested that it was a filiariasis. Cook examined the blood of his patients and found both to be swarming with filariae. Three months later, in May 1901, Forde, in the Gambia in West Africa, recovered from the blood of patients suffering from fever a trypanosome that was described by Dutton, in 1902, as *Trypanosoma gambiense*. The disease became known, for a time, as the 'Trypanosoma fever' but was not linked to the well-known West African disease of sleeping sickness or negro lethargy.

By the end of 1901 it was evident that a very serious epidemic of this supposed filiariasis was in progress. Cook reported to the Protectorate Government that over 200 natives had died on one of the larger islands of the Busoga coast and that thousands appeared to be infected.

In 1902 the Foreign Office arranged with the London School of Tropical

Medicine to send to Uganda a commission consisting of the English doctors Low and Christy, and the Italian parasitologist, Aldo Castellani. The latter made the first relevant observation when he demonstrated the presence of trypanosomes in the cerebro-spinal fluid of an advanced case. Lumbar puncture is still standard diagnostic procedure in treatment of sleeping sickness. In March 1903, a Royal Society sleeping sickness commission arrived, led by Col. David Bruce, and Castellani returned to Europe. In the remarkably short time of five months Bruce and his co-workers showed:

(1) That sleeping sickness is caused by the entrance into the blood and cerebro-spinal fluid of a species of trypanosoma.

(2) That this species is probably that discovered by Forde and described by Dutton from the West Coast of Africa and called by him *Trypanosoma gambiense*.

(3) That the so-called cases of trypanosoma fever, described from the West Coast, may be and probably are, cases of sleeping sickness in the early stage.

(4) That monkeys are susceptible to sleeping sickness, and show the same symptoms, and run the same course, whether the trypanosomes injected are derived from cases of so-called trypanosoma fever, or from the cerebro-spinal fluid of cases of sleeping sickness.

(5) That dogs and rats are partially susceptible, but that guinea pigs, donkeys, oxen, goats and sheep, up to the present, have shown themselves absolutely refractory.

(6) That the trypanosomes are transmitted from the sick to the healthy by a species of tsetse fly, *Glossina palpalis*, and by it alone.

(7) That the distribution of sleeping sickness and *Glossina palpalis* correspond.

(8) That sleeping sickness is, in short, a human tsetse fly disease. (Bruce, Nabarro, and Grieg 1903.)

Although, after Castellani's discovery of the trypanosomes in the cerebro-spinal fluid, Bruce, who a few years earlier had established the link between tsetse flies, trypanosomes, and nagana in cattle in Zululand, naturally at once began looking for similar links in Uganda, these eight conclusions, reached after five months' work, provide astonishing evidence of his genius. None is wrong and, sixty-four years later, only (5), (6), and (7) require any amplification.

Meanwhile the epidemic continued to develop. An official despatch to the Secretary of State notes that:

In 1900 there were 8430 deaths; in 1901, 10 384; in 1902, 24 035; in 1903, 30 411; in 1904, 11 251; and during 1905, 8003. This total of 92 544, however, only represents the loss of life during six years in the Kingdom of Buganda alone. The mortality in Busoga, where statistics have not been available, has probably been quite as great if not greater, and if we include the deaths that have occurred from sleeping sickness in Unyoro and the Nile District, it may be taken that the total mortality from this scourge in the Uganda Protectorate up to the end of 1906 considerably exceeded 200 000 (Bell 1909).

It will be observed that the figures given in this despatch include a total for the year 1900, although it was not until the next year that the Cook brothers examined the first two sufferers. Presumably the 1900 estimate was made by the method that Cook saw in operation.

In Busoga at that time the teaching of arithmetic had not gone very far, so the chiefs were bidden to bring in to the District Commissioner a twig for the death of every one known to have succumbed to this disease in his district. We met a train of men carrying in bundles in this manner. That first day the twigs totalled eleven thousand and the sad little processions continued for several days longer (Cook 1945).

In an earlier despatch the Commissioner had noted that the natives had been almost completely wiped out everywhere along the lake shore. Some of the Sesse islands had lost every soul, 'while in others a few moribund natives, crawling about in the last stages of the disease, are all that are left to represent a once teeming population' (Gray 1908). One Soga chief, Nanyumba of Bunyuli, had 17 000 fighting men at his command before the epidemic. In 1920 he had 105 taxpayers (Wallis 1920).

Christy told of an incident of a kind that must have been a commonplace experience for the men trying to control the epidemic.

At a shamba in Buvuma I saw three little children playing outside a hut in which the father was lying in an advanced stage of the disease; in an adjacent hut lay a woman in the last stage, with terrible ulcers on her thighs and ankles; while in a field close by was a youth, also in a late stage, unable to stand, crying and talking hysterically, as he endeavoured to scoop a hole in the sun-baked ground in the hope of finding one last remaining sweet potato in a patch long out of cultivation (Christy 1903).

In 1906, Sir H. Hesketh Bell decided that the way to end the epidemic was to break the contact between the population at risk and the vector. Survivors still living beside the lake were compulsorily moved two miles inland away from the tsetse. This measure was completed by December 1907. It was not possible to do this with the island populations, and at first clearings were made on the mainland shore so that they could still visit it without coming into contact with tsetse. An order was promulgated in 1908 for the registration of all canoes which thenceforth were supposed only to land at authorized places.

The totals of recorded deaths fell from 30 411 in Buganda in 1903 to 1546 in the whole Protectorate in 1910. The Director of the Sleeping Sickness Bureau, which had been set up in London to collect and circulate information about the disease, commented that it was unfortunate that there was no record of the population of the various districts nor of the case mortality, and added that it would have been difficult, as one may well believe, to obtain accurate returns of either (*Sleeping sickness bureau* 1909a).

Efficiency of collecting and recording data increased yearly and the decline in the number of deaths each year owed much to the activities of the medical services. The removal of sick persons to isolation camps must have done much to reduce the frequency of transmission of the trypanosomes, but not every one that was infected died and there is no means of telling whether the proportion of cures either with or without the aid of various drugs changed over the decade. There is some indication in the published figures that the evacuations had a beneficial effect. In 1904 the total of deaths fell by 63 per cent as compared with 1903. In the next three years the decline was comparatively steady at 29, 34, and 36 per cent of the deaths for the preceding year, but in 1908, after the completion of the mainland shore evacuations, the figure rose to 49 per cent and in 1909 was 46 per cent.

At about the time that the Lake Victoria epidemic seemed to be coming under control, widespread infections were found around the Rift Valley lakes and along the Nile, and the same policy was applied. It has had far-reaching consequences, few of which can have been foreseen by officials of the Protectorate government in 1910.

The origin of the epidemic

No medical officer was stationed in Busoga before 1901, but Christy noted that 'From 1898–1900 there seems to have been a good deal of distress in Busoga and Buvuma Island, due to famine . . . this may have masked a mortality due to disease.' It is in this paper that the suggestion was made that Emin's soldiers and their followers, brought down by Lugard between 1892 and 1895 from Emin's old headquarters on the Albert Nile, might have imported the infection. Christy also records the opinion of Dr. Hodges, the Chief Government Medical Officer, that the original focus of the epidemic was at Wakoli's in Busoga and that this was confirmed by local natives who said it had begun there six years before his inquiry, i.e. in 1896.† Evidently, to these contemporary observers, evidence about the date at which the disease began to be noticed by the natives themselves was not clear.

There is one other point. The Director of the Sleeping Sickness Bureau, commenting upon a progress report by the Principal Medical Officer in Uganda (Hodges 1908), remarked that 'What Dr. Hodges describes as an A case would not be regarded by the natives as sleeping sickness at all.' Evidently in Uganda cases could be classified in the same way that French doctors in West Africa were classifying patients seen in the Congo basin. Diagnosing by lumbar puncture on a small group of 105 people, Martin and Lebœuf (1908) obtained positive results in 83 per cent of patients showing definite clinical symptoms of sleeping sickness and in 53 per cent of those suspected of having the disease. But they also found 29 per cent in good

†Twenty years later Carpenter (1924) was told by a local African that the epidemic had begun in Busoga at Mukori. This was another way of saying Wakoli.

health, *cas en bon état*, who had trypanosomes already in the central nervous system. One of the more startling examples of healthy carriers was found in Uganda by the great German parasitologist Robert Koch who led an expedition to the Sesse islands. He examined 52 apparently healthy boatmen who had just paddled a dug-out canoe from Entebbe to the islands, a journey of perhaps 30 miles and of several hours' duration. Eleven of these men had enlarged cervical glands. Seven of the 52 showed trypanosomes on a single blood examination including 5 of those with enlarged glands and 2 without this symptom. Koch believed that a single blood examination would detect 50 per cent of infection and he therefore thought it probable that the crew of 52 paddlers included 14 carriers, 10 with and 4 without enlarged glands (Koch 1907). The importance of Koch's record consists in the fact that all these men were apparently healthy and doing hard work. Some of Koch's patients were taken to Kigarama near Bukoba in German East Africa. Five years later some were still alive and Steudel (1912) reported that many people who had been infected in Uganda had for long shown no symptoms and were probably recovered. There is no doubt about the violence and dreadful mortality of the Uganda epidemic. But there is at least a possibility that it grew out of a long-standing endemic condition not unlike that described by K. R. S. Morris (1960a) on the slopes of Mount Ruwenzori and mentioned at the end of Chapter 10.

It was always a favourite gambit of colonial servants connected with health, whether human or animal, to seek the origin of any epidemic or epizootic in neighbouring territories. Christy's idea about Lugard's Sudanese soon found almost universal acceptance. But it is quite possible that the epidemics at the end of the last century and the beginning of this were due merely to a change in the proportion of *cas cliniques* and *cas en bon état*, and the evidence for this is at least as good as the evidence of importation from outside. Recent expositions of the transcontinental theory of the origin of East African human trypanosomiasis are given by Morris (1963) and Willett (1965).

Other epidemics

In the interlake area and in Sukumaland the epidemics and epizootics followed upon changes in the distribution of the human population, either as a result of depopulation from various causes or, in the case of the Semliki river epidemic, of an official resettlement scheme. It is usually accepted that sleeping sickness and Hesketh Bell's prophylactic measures were the sole cause of the changes in the Busoga landscape. Nevertheless two causes of depopulation are known to have been present in Busoga before the appearance of sleeping sickness. Sir H. Johnston (1900) recorded in a despatch to the Marquis of Salisbury that in the Buganda houses there were bugs and lice, 'to say nothing of the jigger or boring flea, which has recently reached this unfortunate Protectorate from the Congo region'.

Contemporary records of Sukumaland and of the interlake countries of the depopulatory effect of this pest have been noted in Chapters 9 and 14. In Buganda and Busoga they were no less of a scourge, especially in the next few years in the camps set up to house the sleeping sickness patients. Gray (1908) reported, 'Chiggers are the pest of our camps. Every advanced case of sleeping sickness that is admitted swarms with them and they multiply with fearful rapidity. In a bad case of sleeping sickness the chiggers are not confined to the feet; the hands are often a mass of them, mouth, nose and ears get infected in turn and the result is a truly revolting spectacle.' At one camp 8 men were employed doing nothing else but extract jiggers (Wiggins 1960–1).

In another despatch Johnston (1901) reported to the Marquis of Lands-downe that smallpox, in the latter part of 1899, 'became epidemic on the coast line (of the Indian Ocean) and raged fiercely west over Kikuyu and the eastern frontier to the Uganda protectorate. It spread to the eastern shores of the lake but did not enter Uganda in epidemic form. On the other hand in 1891 and 1893 the disease became epidemic in Uganda and travelled eastwards towards the coast.'

There is thus some evidence of a condition predisposing to the spread of *Glossina*. Among the people other diseases and debilitating conditions must have provided unusually favourable conditions for infection.

The usual tales of inter-tribal warfare are to be found. Wallis (1920) says that Busoga originally consisted of a number of tribes all more or less in a state of war with one another. They were thus an easy prey to the depreda-tions of the Baganda, who were able to play off one Soga tribe against another. His next paragraph, however, suggests that this picture of per-petual strife is misleading, for it relates that at this time Busoga was thickly populated by a people singularly rich in food and cattle, so much so that Bukoli (Cook's 'Wakoli's' and Carpenter's 'Mukori'), one of the southern counties, was regarded as the promised land by caravans from the coast. A war-torn country and a promised land cannot both be right. In Busoga, as in many other parts of Africa, early visitors were often misled by tales of territorial aggression ceremonies embroidered by local poets with fictitious statistics of imaginary slaughter. This is borne out by Roscoe (1923).

Warfare on even a moderate scale was scarcely known, but some fighting took place, generally as a result of some man's encroaching on land of another clan. If he refused to retire the drums were beaten for war, but the chiefs would attempt to settle the affair without recourse to arms and a boundary might be arranged. If arbitration failed, the fighting might last from one day to two months.

Thomas and Scott (1935) refer to the famine in 1899–1900 that Christy (1903) had heard about and say that after the sleeping sickness epidemic had reached its peak there was another famine in 1908 that nearly completed the total depopulation of southern Busoga. This second famine almost certainly was a consequence of the epidemic; whether the first was a contributory cause or also a consequence of early unrecorded mortality, one cannot now know.

I have found no accounts of rinderpest that refer specifically to the epizootic in Busoga. It is a reasonable assumption that in 1890 and 1891 most of the cattle died as well as bushpigs, bushbuck, and buffalo.

Kavirondo before the epidemic

Glasgow, who worked in Samia and in Busoga, could not find written evidence about the nineteenth-century population of Samia. Like Carpenter, twenty-three years before him, he could still get verbal accounts of earlier occupation. Though convinced by this that half a century before coastal Samia had been densely populated, he sought more tangible evidence. It was not difficult to find.

A number of elderly natives, including Chief Mukudi, testify that there were many people there in their childhood, and that they kept cattle. Further, we are told in those days people lived in large villages. Huntingford† reproduces a picture of such a village [taken from Thomson's 'Through Masailand'] which is surrounded by a wall apparently of mud. A circular mud wall, with a ditch outside it, still exists about a mile from Mr. Wilson's house [at Port Victoria]. A number of other village sites have been discovered. In these the wall is represented only by a mound, but the combination of wall and ditch is unmistakable. Three such sites making, with the intact wall, four, have been found within two miles along the same ridge. There is also in the same area at least one stockade of *Euphorbia tirucalli*. As the greater part of the ridge is covered with impenetrable thicket, it is likely that more village sites exist undiscovered.

In Block E there are a number of ditches, now overgrown with lakeside forest. It is not certain whether these are village defences or ditches dug round shambas to keep out hippos, but in either case they indicate former human occupation, sufficiently close to suppress lakeside forest (Glasgow 1947).

Carpenter (1924) had seen similar relics.

We were able to see the remains of old bomas within a few hundred yards of the water, and found an old grindstone embedded in its original site. [Another curious piece of evidence was still alive.] All along the coast at intervals can be seen old fish traps of reed, which is now growing, but showing by its arrangement how it was originally put there.

Another find prompted a question relevant to this present inquiry:

Along the shore was a comparatively narrow belt of dense bush; behind was open country with scattered acacia trees. Immediately behind the belt of bush,

† Huntingford, G. W. B. *The people of Kenya, No. 14: The eastern tribes of Bantu Kavirondo*. Ndia Kuu Press, Nairobi.

and indeed partly among it (though this is probably due to recent overgrowth of the bush), was a wall built up of blocks of stone enclosing a space about forty yards in diameter and not more than that distance from the water (Carpenter 1924).

These dry stone circular walls had been built by people who had occupied the country before the arrival of the Luo. Carpenter's interpreter said they had been built by Masai, but this is unlikely. For the present it is sufficient that the evidences of Glasgow and Carpenter confirm the accounts of travellers at the beginning of the century of a dense population of Soga west of the Sio river, living on a diet of bananas, who looked across Berkeley Bay to populations of Luyia and Luo subsisting on cereals and sweet potatoes. These people were occupying country that at some earlier date had been inhabited by other people who built circular stonework walls of a size that suggested they enclosed the dwellings of a family group plus livestock.

The Yimbo story

Survivors from the first Kavirondo epidemic are still alive: fifteen old men from Yimbo, adjoining the Yala swamp, where the epidemic first reached the Kenya shore in 1901. Some of these men were babies at the time and must have got their information from relatives and friends, but one was 19, another 18, and a third 16 years old when the infection appeared in their villages. The account (Wijers 1969) is of great interest and bears out many ideas that suggest themselves from the Busoga record.

In 1900 Yimbo was densely populated and cultivated, with abundant cattle, but, as in Busoga, there were small patches of forest that harboured some bushpig, bushbuck, and other antelopes, but not in large numbers. Hyenas were also present. Shortly after the arrival of Europeans at Kisumu in 1901, some fishermen went by canoe to Sigulu island and the Uganda mainland in search of food. (Does this suggest that here too among the cereal-eating Luo there was a famine at about the same time as that which afflicted the banana-eating Soga on the other side of Berkeley Bay?) The travellers found, when they reached the mainland, many people suffering from a disease which made them fat and very sleepy. After their return some of the fishermen became drowsy, slept longer and longer, and died. The people of the islands became infected at this time (Map 14.1).

The spread of the infection throughout the Yimbo area was relatively slow and the last part of it, Ramogi, was not involved until 1908. By 1911 the worst of the epidemic was over. It seems clear that this was a consequence of reduction of the population, firstly by the disease itself and secondly by evacuation of their homes by survivors. In the densely populated Kanyathuon area:

The disease raged so terribly, particularly along the Yala River, that many families sent their young children to Goma to save their lives. At last the members of the unafflicted households in Kanyathuon broke up their homes and fled to Alego. In their attempt to shake off the disease, they took good care that no persons from compounds with one or more patients went along with them. Daniel was a member of such an afflicted household which was compelled to stay behind. Daniel, however, managed to escape to Nairobi where he became a house-boy. When he came back on leave in 1914, he found that every one of his relatives had died except one old man. Another family tried the method which was used with some success in Usigu: they gathered the survivors of several compounds and, together, they made new ones. They had to do this three times, however, before they had shaken off the disease and by that time most of them were dead (Wijers 1969).

Recollections of symptoms of the disease were accurate:

First a person started to complain of headache. Sometimes he had bouts of fever. Then he became more and more hungry and at the same time more and more drowsy. While he slept, saliva dribbled from his mouth and as soon as he awakened he asked for food. If he were not given food immediately, he was likely to start eating soil, or even his own excrement. To prevent this, and as death was inevitable anyhow, his family slaughtered their livestock one by one to provide food. The sufferers became very fat, sometimes too fat to walk, but they slept longer and longer and their eyes and mouth became very pale. Then they died.

The time it took for a patient to die, after he became drowsy, varied very much. It depended on the care his family could give him and the amount of meat they could put in front of him. In the chief's compound several people lived for nearly two years before they died, but generally it took nine to twelve months. It seems that the disease became more virulent as it moved inland. The Kanyathuon, people say that their patients died three to four months after becoming drowsy, whether they were given meat or not.

In the later years of the epidemic, when many people had already died, nobody could be sure how and when a patient would die. For by then the hyaenas, who had increased enormously in numbers, had become so bold that they entered the huts and ate the dead people who had nobody left to bury them. Often they ate sleeping persons too, not to mention the babies crying beside their sleeping mothers. The tendency of the survivors to concentrate themselves in new compounds was not only to escape the disease, but also to fend off this new menace.

Sometimes the main symptom of the disease was madness. Before they became hungry or drowsy, many people suddenly became aggressive, killing cattle, if not their fellow-men, with their spears. Such persons often ran away from home and started wandering through the bush, where they became an easy prey for the ever-present hyaenas. They had to be tied to the house or to a nearby tree. They died quickly, before they reached the sleeping stage. Others, but this was a rare symptom, just sat on a stool or a stone, not eating, not speaking, not moving. They died quickest of all.

The old men who were interviewed all agreed exactly about the symptoms of the disease. The most accurate description was given by the medicine-man. The Karodi people mentioned that women several months pregnant never produced a baby, but died many months later with the child still in the womb. The swollen neck glands, however, were noticed by nobody at that time.

Five of the old men, among them the medicine-man and the chief, said they had noticed that children contracted the disease slightly less often than adults. Some of them remarked that this did not help the children very much, for, if all the adults in such a household had died (and nobody from outside dared to visit an afflicted household), the children often died slowly from hunger and neglect if they were not dragged away by hyaenas before (Wijers 1969).

As a result of the depopulation the bush and forest invaded the deserted fields. Further inland the formerly cultivated lands reverted to grassland dotted with thickets. Here the surviving cattle multiplied, as well as the wild animals. 'Some game, which always had been present, increased rapidly in numbers and variety: all sorts of antelope grazed on the plains, bushbuck and bushpig were abundant everywhere and even elephant appeared in the new forests of Karodi' (Wijers 1969).

The decline of the Kavirondo epidemic

K. R. S. Morris's (1960b) explanation for the decline of the epidemic and then of the persistence of endemic foci on the Kavirondo coast since 1902 is so convincing that one asks why it is necessary to postulate a beginning for the disease at that time. Sir H. Hesketh Bell's policy of complete, compulsory evacuation was only applied in Busoga and not in Kavirondo (then included in the Uganda Protectorate). But it is clear from the Yimbo narrative that the people carried out their own policy of evacuation. When, towards the end of the epidemic phase, the medical authorities tried in some locations to persuade survivors to move, they were met with refusals.

The scheme was nearly wrecked by the refusal of the natives to quit their homes, which is not unnatural since they were asked to give up their favourite pursuit and livelihood of fishing and to come inland. It seems that few natives have in fact moved and that the alternatives are to acquiesce in their elimination by sleeping sickness or to bring them away by force. During the year twenty-three cases were treated with eleven deaths; six others were treated as out-patients (*Sleeping sickness bureau* 1909b).

The mortality rate is indeed high, but 29 cases in a year must mean a small population at risk. Most of the survivors of the epidemic had already gone. The same report adds that Dr. Bodeker found that 'almost all the huts and villages were outside the fly-belt. Villages which existed within the fly areas had been wiped out' (*Sleeping sickness bureau* 1909b). According to Morris (1960b) the epidemic by 1907–8 had decimated the population of the shores and islands down to the German border. More than one doctor dealing with these epidemics deplored the absence of quantitative data. The language difficulty still remains. Morris's use of the word 'decimated' may have been deliberately used to imply a 10 per cent death rate from the disease in the population at risk, but what was the size of that population and were the villages in the fly areas in fact wiped out or merely evacuated when the death rate became alarming?

Morris had no doubt about how control over the epidemic was achieved.

The people brought about their own control by moving away from infected places, often only a mile or so, just far enough to avoid the dangerous degree of man-fly contact. The effect in checking the epidemic was so rapid that the islands and shores of south Kavirondo, which had been severely depopulated by 1909, showed an increase of 820 huts, equal to 2360 people, by 1912. . . . This was, naturally, not a true population increase, but largely a movement of the people back to their abandoned homes. In consequence the disease did not disappear but remained at a low endemic level (Morris 1960b).

This persisted until 1920 when there was a small localized epidemic near Kisumu. In 1921 on the island of Mageta and the mainland opposite to it, at Kadimu, sleeping sickness again flared up. Mageta had been evacuated in 1907, but people gradually returned without experiencing any troubles and in 1918 large numbers of immigrants arrived. Soon afterwards infections began to appear and in 1922 the island was again abandoned. From that time onwards localized epidemics have occurred at various points along the north and south Kavirondo coasts, but have always been comparatively brief, while in the intervals a very low-level endemism has persisted. Medical surveillance was maintained and some bush clearing to control tsetse was intermittently available (Map 14.1).

The ideas of W. F. Fiske

Carpenter investigated the epidemiology of sleeping sickness on the Kavirondo coast in 1924. In this he tried to apply ideas worked out by W. F. Fiske, medical entomologist in Uganda, who had been studying the feeding habits of *Glossina fuscipes* (Chapter 2). Fiske had, at first, accepted unquestioningly that the measures adopted in Uganda in 1906–7 for the suppression of sleeping sickness were both wise and necessary. He recalled, in the introduction to his long report (Fiske 1920), that the original plans for severing connection between the population and the lake-shore tsetse had included provision for a study of the bionomics of *G. fuscipes fuscipes* ('*G. palpalis*') with a view to instituting measures for its extermination. These would, in due course, be put into effect and the people allowed to return to their homes. The results of the study were unexpected and he revised the ideas he had previously entertained about the wisdom of the policy of compulsory evacuation.

Fiske's disillusionment began when he visited the tsetse-infested island of Bukakata, the site (as it still is) of the steamer landing stage for Masaka. Here, 'the lands adjoining the lake in the depopulated or forbidden zone were valueless for agriculture. The fishing rights were valuable and would have been a considerable inducement to the natives to clear the shore of tsetse, except for the fact that the natives were already occupying them, openly, for the entire reach of six miles.' Infestation by tsetse was much heavier than in certain other districts, but still moderate, exceeding the average for the lake shore as a whole at only a few points, but about half the average of the region generally. 'Careful inquiry failed to elicit a particle of evidence that any of the native fisherman had suffered in the slightest degree from long-continued exposure to tsetse under these conditions.' Fiske found other similar situations and observed that at Entebbe, as at Jinja and Kampala, considerable portions of these townships were lightly but constantly infested by fly 'to an easily measurable degree'. He thought that under these conditions some infection must occur.

To my very great surprise I learned that . . . not a single case had been contracted within the Province of Buganda . . . since 1912 and that with the exception of two cases (one of them not surely trypanosomiasis, and the other possibly contracted in Busoga) among the men who accompanied Dr. G. D. H. Carpenter on his tour of the islands in 1911–12, no cases were known or suspected to have been contracted since the islands were depopulated in 1909.

Fiske abandoned his experiments and readjusted his ideas and preconceptions.

In theory it was necessary either to exterminate fly from populated districts or to make removal of inhabitants 'from the vicinity of tsetse complete and without exception'; but in practice it was proved sufficient to reduce the density of fly to within moderate limits in populated districts or to reduce density of population to within moderate limits in fly-infested territory. If this is really sufficient, knowledge concerning factors which control range of the insect is more or less superfluous, whereas knowledge of factors which operate to control breadth of contact between fly and population—equivalent to frequency of contact between hungry flies and men—is specifically required.

The intervention of the First World War prevented proper consideration being given to Fiske's ideas. In 1919 he was made Reclamation Officer, Sleeping Sickness, but by 1924 was involved in disputes with the administration (Carpenter 1925). It is evident from the *Annual Medical and Sanitary Report for 1926* (Uganda Medical 1927), that his attempts to modify the policy of evacuation were encountering difficulties. He left Uganda, and another opportunity for a logical entomological approach to the problem of sleeping sickness epidemics was lost until Nash and his followers took up the problem once more in Nigeria many years later (Nash 1948a, Page and Macdonald 1959).

Carpenter undertook his survey of the Kavirondo coast with Fiske's precepts in mind. His object was to carry out a survey that would provide data on local population density, on tsetse density, and on disease incidence. The first was measured by hut counts, the second by the numbers caught of male *G. fuscipes* 'per boy hour', and the third by gland palpation.

Morris (1960b), over-eager to find evidence to support his own thesis, states that Carpenter did not find a single positive case and saw only four suspects with enlarged glands. This is not true. Carpenter, who was accompanied by an official of the Kenya Medical Service, remarks that 'it was deemed inexpedient to puncture glands for the purpose of diagnosis, for reasons which need not be given here'.† He did, in fact, puncture glands in one patient, and obtained a positive slide. Having thus established beyond doubt the presence of trypanosomiasis, he 'made subsequent diagnoses by the nature of the enlarged glands in the neck and axillae, a matter in which (he) had acquired considerable experience'. This was a standard method and Carpenter recorded not 4 suspected cases only, but 14. In fact his work supports the ideas of Morris; or rather, one should say that Morris's study of the epidemiology of the disease in central Nyanza strongly supports the ideas of Fiske and Carpenter. A comparison of the maps of the Sakwa–Uyoma peninsula compiled by Carpenter and Morris shows that of the four foci of infection identified by Morris from Medical Department data collected over the years 1953–6 inclusive, two were located by Carpenter 30 years before. In Map 14.1 it may be seen that two of Carpenter's foci are included in one of Morris's, so that one may say that three foci identified by Carpenter existed 30 years later. Moreover, a focus indicated by Morris at Port Southby is an area in which Carpenter's data approach closely but do not quite meet the conditions which he subsequently decided were necessary to produce infection, namely a population in contact with tsetse of over 40 per mile² and a vector density of 15 or more male *G. fuscipes* per 'boy hour'.‡

Fiske's ideas found confirmation in the work of Carpenter and subsequently of Morris. They lead directly to the concepts associated with ideas of the 'nidality' of vector-borne diseases.

The distribution and behaviour of *Glossina fuscipes fuscipes* Newst. on the north-eastern shores of Lake Victoria

Carpenter and Fiske thought that the factors controlling the appearance of epidemics of gambian trypanosomiasis were (1) the density of the vector population and (2) the density of the human host population. This, although indeed a step in the right direction, was a gross oversimplification. Vector density may be broken down into (a) the population density, (b) the proportion of the vector population which attacks man for the purpose of feeding, (c) the proportion of the vector population infected with mature *Trypanosoma brucei gambiense* metacyclics, and (d) the proportion of bites given to human which inoculate dosages of metacyclics at or above the minimum infective dose. The density of the host population may be broken

---

† Presumably Carpenter had been asked not to do gland punctures or take blood slides because of the fear of witchcraft that such procedures engendered in local people. This, in turn, led to violence. As late as 1942, E. G. Gibbins of the Uganda Medical Entomology Section was speared to death when he halted his car outside a village during a survey of the Busoga *rhodesiense* epidemic area.

‡ The methods of measuring density of tsetse flies and also of diagnosis of trypanosome infections would be unacceptable today; but the principle is still sound.

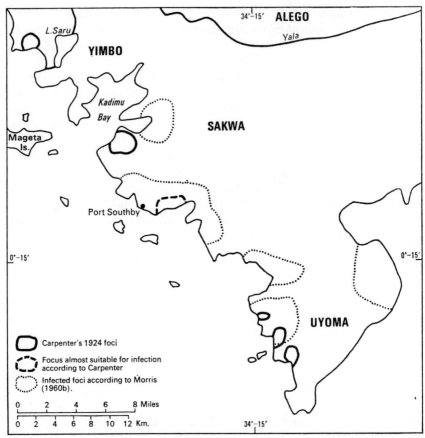

MAP 14.1. The Kavirondo coast, to show foci of infection observed by Carpenter in 1924 and Morris in 1960, together with sites of the Yimbo and Alego epidemics.

down into (a) the population density, (b) the frequency with which persons, separable into different sexes and age-groups as well as trades, come within range of infective vectors, and (c) the proportion of the host population already infected or in a state of premunity and not re-infectable by indigenous strains of trypanosomes. It is also necessary, in trying to assess the factors which give rise to epidemic conditions, to define the environmental circumstances in which they will attain their maximum interaction.

Glasgow (1954) investigated the biology of *G. f. fuscipes* (at the time known as *G. palpalis fuscipes* Newst.) as part of an attempt to eradicate this tsetse from various experimental blocks of lacustrine vegetation on the east shore of Berkeley Bay. He also carried out similar observations on the Kuja river which flows into Lake Victoria not far south of the Kavirondo gulf. He showed that on the lake shore the density of *G. f. fuscipes* is roughly correlated with the width of the lacustrine forest, being least where the forest is narrow. Where the depth of forest was about one hundred yards, a block 2200 yd long had an absolute population of 4600 non-teneral males indicating a density of 63 000 male tsetse per mile². One may suppose that non-teneral females were at least equal in numbers. The mean apparent density over the period in which the population size was measured was 357, so that an apparent density of 1·0 corresponds to a population of 176 non-teneral males per mile². This high figure implied a low availability which, in turn, indicated that only a small proportion of the population of *G. fuscipes* present responded to the presence of the catching teams. Glasgow noted that an observer stood outside a thicket in sunshine and saw tsetse inside it that displayed no interest in him while he remained outside; when he entered the thicket the flies attacked him. This suggested that the feeding response was inhibited by relatively high light intensity (cf. Chapter 2).

Comparing the behaviour of the lakeside and riverine populations, Glasgow found that the catches of the latter always yielded a much higher proportion of female and teneral flies than did the former. From this he deduced that the riverine populations were much hungrier than those beside the lake, a deduction supported by the parallel observation that the percentage of non-teneral males caught after having alighted on one or other of the catchers was much greater among the riverine than in the lacustrine flies. It is to be supposed, of course, that flies caught on a man rather than on the ground or on nearby vegetation are not members of the following swarm but are about to feed. From the months of September 1945 to June 1947, while 68·5 per cent of the non-teneral male catch was taken off one or other of the catching party on the Kuja river, only 44·0 per cent were taken thus in catches made on the lake shore at Port Victoria. In 1929–30 there was a widespread epidemic both north (lacustrine) and south (Kuja river) of the Kavirondo gulf. Of those at risk on the lake shore 37 023 people were examined among whom 213 or 0·575 per cent were infected. In the Kuja river basin, with about half the number of people at risk, 18 657 examined revealed 234 cases, an incidence of 1·254 per cent. These figures are at least in line with the results of Glasgow's entomological study of the tsetse populations of the two areas and with the hypothesis of Fiske and Carpenter. They should also be considered in relation to the data collected by Harley and his colleagues and described in Chapters 4 and 5.

15

RHODESIAN TRYPANOSOMIASIS IN BUSOGA

IN 1940, after seven years of freedom from infection apart from occasional cases attributed to contact with endemic foci on the Kenya coast on the other side of Berkeley Bay, trypanosomiasis again appeared at the western end of the Busoga fly-belt. From its first appearance the epidemic appeared to spread rapidly eastwards through the villages along the northern edge of the forests and reached, and crossed, the Sio river into Kenya by early 1942. By mid-1943, 2432 cases had been seen, of which 10 per cent were fatal. At the peak of the epidemic about 100 people were treated every week.

At first the epidemic was thought to be a resurgence of the old infection, but the clinical picture was not that of gambian sleeping sickness. The course of the disease was rapid and people died without intervention of the sleeping phase. Their blood, when inoculated into white rats, quickly produced a heavy parasitaemia and the trypanosomes showed abundant posteronuclear forms. The disease looked like rhodesian trypanosomiasis, but hitherto, apart from a very few isolated and forgotten cases, this had not been seen outside the semi-arid savanna and savanna woodland of eastern Africa south of the equator.

The Busoga epidemic was described by Mackichan (1944). The first case, in November 1940, was a schoolboy who had visited the lake between Iganga and Jinja and was taken ill on a visit to Kampala. Two more were discovered in Jinja hospital in the same month. Both were employees at the Kakira Sugar Estate on the western edge of the Busoga forests. They were Nyaruanda, two of the thousands of itinerant labourers that came into Uganda every year from the densely populated mandated territory of Ruanda-Urundi. In December another Nyaruanda was infected, as well as a local Soga living on the lake shore near Jinja town.

The first step was to repatriate Luo fishermen who might have had contact with the still smouldering gambian foci on the Samia shores across the Kenya border. The shore area was evacuated between Jinja and Kakira to a depth of 1–2 miles. Special clearings were made so that people could still go to the lake for water without encountering too many *Glossina fuscipes*. By March 1941 the shore area appeared to be safe and there were no more cases here. But on the Kakira Sugar Estate infection still persisted among the labourers. Then, in the same month a report was received of illness among inhabitants of Buluba, a leper colony at the head of Thruston Bay, 12 miles east of Kakira. In the next three months 20 cases were found here.

In April infection had spread further east among forestry workers at Kityerera (Map 15.1) and by June 1941 the total of cases since November 1940 had risen to 80. Surveys were now made among the people all around the edge of the forests. More cases were found at Kityerera and at Ikulwe. This was puzzling, since Ikulwe was 6 miles from the lake shore. A survey showed, however, that *G. fuscipes* was to be found in the Busoga forests some miles from open water (T. W. Chorley 1944) and this seemed to offer an explanation for the outbreak. Then, in November 1941 the infection flared up at Kyemeire, 20 miles further east and 12 miles from the lake. From there it spread eastwards into areas examined only two or three months before and found apparently free of infection. By January 1942 the epidemic had crossed the Sio river into Kenya and, incidentally, into a different ecological region.

Infections 12 miles from the lake cast more doubt on the hypothesis that *G. fuscipes* was the vector. Dr. H. Fairbairn from the Tinde Sleeping Sickness Research Laboratory and Dr. C. H. N. Jackson from the Shinyanga Tsetse Research Laboratory in Tanzania collected wild *G. pallidipes* from the Lugala area, at the eastern end of the Busoga forest, near the centre of heaviest infection and fed them, in batches of 50 or 100, on white rats (Jackson 1943). Five rats became positive with *Trypanosoma brucei*-type parasites in which posteronuclear forms were abundant. From each rat a man was inoculated with a dose of infected blood containing up to 100 000 000 trypanosomes. One of the five men became infected, with a large arm reaction at the site of the inoculation and an incubation period of six days. An assistant employed in catching tsetse in the same area where *G. pallidipes* formed 99 per cent of the catch also became infected. There was therefore no doubt that the disease was caused by a rhodesian strain of *T. brucei* and that *G. pallidipes* was a vector.

The same procedure was adopted in other collecting areas where *G. fuscipes* predominated. Again rats fed upon by flies of this species also became infected with pleomorphic trypanosomes showing many posteronuclear forms. However, no disease developed in an inoculated volunteer. This, of course, did not prove that *G. fuscipes* was not a vector. Indeed as it had already been demonstrated in the laboratory (Duke 1928) that *G. fuscipes* could transmit *T. brucei rhodesiense*, Fairbairn and Jackson concluded that this tsetse must also be a vector in Busoga. It was not until sixteen years later that proof was obtained that it, as well as *G. pallidipes*, was a natural vector in the area (Southon and Robertson 1961).

The Busoga epidemic of 1940 destroyed two ancient shibboleths: the first that rhodesian trypanosomiasis was confined to the *G. morsitans* fly-belts of eastern Africa, and the second that the disease transmitted by the *palpalis*-group tsetses was, of necessity, gambian sleeping sickness. Belgian workers in the Congo had clung tenaciously to this doctrine when they asserted that trypanosomes infecting inhabitants of Katanga and showing

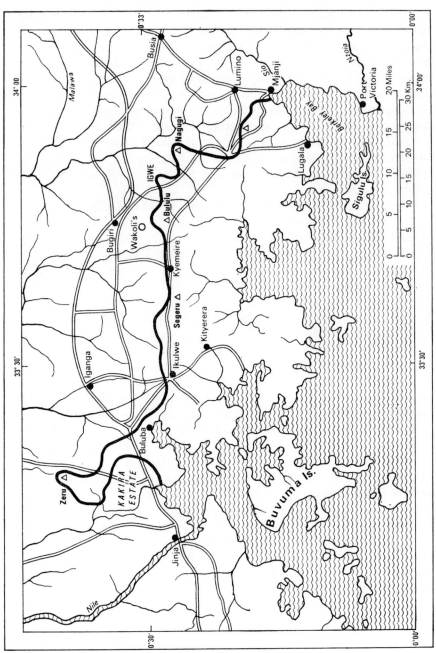

MAP 15.1. The Busoga tsetse belt in 1944.

all the characteristics of '*Trypanosoma rhodesiense*' must, nevertheless, be '*Trypanosoma gambiense*' because they were obviously transmitted by '*Glossina palpalis*' (e.g. van Hoof, Henrard, and Peel 1938).

From its first appearance in November 1940 the epidemic continued to grow, especially at the eastern end of the fly-belt. A temporary camp was built at Bugiri which, in March 1942, held over 1000 cases, with new patients coming in at the rate of over 100 a week. Then, quite suddenly, the infection rate declined and by the beginning of 1944 new cases were only appearing at a rate between 10 and 20 per month.

Mackichan (1944) could not explain the decline in the infection rate, but thought that recession of the tsetse at the end of abnormally heavy rains in that year, together with the rapid removal of infected persons into camp and away from contact with the vector, had contributed to this happy result.

Origin of the outbreak

The fact that the disease first appeared (apart from the schoolboy) among immigrant labourers at Kakira strongly suggested to Mackichan that one or more of these men had entered the country in an infected condition. The Kakira estates employed about 9000 labourers, most of whom were Rundi, Nyaryanda, or Ha from the Belgian territory of Ruanda-Urundi and adjacent parts of Tanzania. Moreover, early in the epidemic two cases were admitted to the Jinja hospital, both immigrant labourers of the same kind, who had fallen ill in Buganda while still on their way to Busoga to work. The evidence therefore was strong that the infection was introduced from this source.

These two men were not, in fact, the first sufferers from trypanosomiasis found among immigrant labourers from the interlake area. Two others had fallen sick on the long march near Masaka in 1932 and were found to harbour trypanosomes (Duke 1930, 1944, also Chapter 9). If Mackichan's hypothesis was correct the elaborate measures taken since that date, both in Uganda and in Tanzania, to prevent transport of infection across the border, had failed.

Condition of the Busoga fly-belt in 1944

For some years tsetse had been spreading rapidly in many parts of Uganda. At that time it was accepted doctrine that populations living in the path of the 'advancing' insects would sooner or later be driven from their homes. It seemed essential that vigorous measures should be taken to prevent further movement of the Busoga tsetse front, especially since this would be lethal not only to cattle, as were most of the other 'advances' in Uganda, but also to men, women, and children.

A survey of the limits of the Busoga fly-belt was made in May 1944. At that time standard procedure was to move from obviously tsetse-free land, with abundant settlements and healthy cattle, towards the uninhabited bush. When the first tsetse was caught, the place was recorded. In due course the series of spot records allowed the 'fly-line' to be drawn. In Busoga, earlier records of the Entomology Section of the Uganda Medical Department were available for incorporation in the map.

The 1944 survey established that the northern boundary of the *Glossina pallidipes* belt was associated with the watershed separating the short streams running south into Lake Victoria and the headwaters of longer northward running drainages that filled the swamps leading into Lake Kyoga. Along much of its length the watershed was marked by small, rocky hills, with summits 300–400 ft above the Lake Victoria level. At a number of places, northward-stretching outliers of these hills carried forest and thicket on their slopes in which the tsetse were also found. At its western end the Busoga fly-belt apparently came to an end at the Kakira Sugar Estate. From this estate, however, a line of hills culminating some seven miles to the north of it in a peak called Zeru on the map suggested that an extension of the infestation might be found there. On the first morning's visit one male and two females were taken in gardens adjoining the hillside thickets. This appeared to be an isolated population of tsetse. It was at the time thought to be living on waterbuck, as their spoor was plentiful. Today one would regard this conclusion with suspicion and look rather for signs of bushbuck and bushpig.

The significance of the association of *G. pallidipes* with these rocky hills was not appreciated in 1944. A specimen was captured at a water-hole just south of a hill called Nagugi in 1942 and more were taken in 1944 'in the fringing forest below the *Combretum* covered hilltop and above the settlement'. On the lower slopes of these hills are patches of treeless hardpan with much exposed flat, lateritic, ironstone. One noted that formerly settlement must have been much more abundant, for numerous *mweso* boards were carved in the ironstone. (*Mweso* is a game played with pebbles in lieu of counters which are moved from hole to hole.) It was this line of hills near the eastern border of Bukoli which Dr. Cook had crossed in 1897 and from which he had his first view of Lake Victoria.

The next northward-stretching line of hills reaches to within three miles of Bugiri, where Mackichan built his sleeping sickness camp. The previous most northerly record here had been on the eastern slopes of a hill called Bululu, where both *G. pallidipes* and *G. fuscipes* had been found, the latter apparently associated with the Nameseri river running north-east to join the Kyoga swamps. In 1944 *G. pallidipes* was again captured, 3 miles south of Bugiri in circumstances of some interest.

The approach was made from Bugiri and the first fly was taken within 700 yards of the rocky hill top. Altogether four males and one female were taken in shambas [*cultivation*] north of this hill which carried a certain amount of fringing thicket with riverine thicket on the streams leading from it. The sudden appearance of fly in the neighbourhood of the hill was striking. The same phenomenon was noticed even more markedly at Segeru, another hill further west. Here the approach ran parallel to and north of the watershed for a distance of some five miles, through shambas, forest and thicket, much of it suitable (apparently) for *G. pallidipes*. None, however, was taken during these five miles but, turning south to approach the eastern end of Segeru, several flies were taken all within 300 yards of the outlying rocks at the foot of the hill. On leaving the hill, the fly just as abruptly ceased to appear (Ford 1944*a*).

The point that escaped me at the time was that 'Wakoli's', the village of the chief of Bukoli that had so impressed Cook and Ternan and which was said by the Soga to have been the site of the original outbreak in 1896, had been situated just north of the watershed between the northern outliers of Bululu and Segeru. I have little doubt now that here, indeed, was the prime focus of infection not only of the 1896–1910 epidemic, but also of Mackichan's 1940 epidemic.† An incipient outbreak in 1957 and 1958 also began, if not precisely in the same geographical situation, in a focus only a short distance away and, ecologically and epidemiologically, in very similar circumstances.

The object of the 1944 survey was to provide a basis for planning a defence line. It was thought essential that contact should be broken between man on the one hand and the tsetse-infested forest on the other. This involved resettlement of people living in or along the northern edge of the forest. They were to be moved into a mile-wide corridor in which all trees and thickets would be felled. No houses would be allowed less than 400 yd from the edge of the cleared area and the intervening ground would be used for cultivation of low crops, such as sweet potatoes or eleusine, or else kept weeded to prevent regrowth of thicket. There was to be an absolutely sharp division between settlement and bush. When the 1944 survey had been completed it was estimated that this defence line, which would make as much use as possible of already open ground, would cost £60 000, in present-day values about £250 000. This was accepted by the Protectorate government, and officials of the Survey Department began marking out the boundaries. It soon became clear that no part of the scheme would be acceptable to the Soga who claimed that the lines being marked out had nothing to do with sleeping sickness but were, in reality, the boundaries of new farms to be handed over to European settlers. A discussion of this controversy by Fallers (1965) shows that not only was there a real fear of ultimate dispossession, but also that the proposals ignored customary laws of land tenure. While these arguments were developing the epidemic, as already described, had died down from a case rate of 100 per month to 10–20. The scheme lapsed, and apart from the supervision kept up by the Medical Service and the installation of de-flying posts on the

† Even at the end of the colonial period it was easy to overlook foci of infection. Nelson (1965) remarks, on grounds of personal experience, that this was not surprising in rural areas where the doctor : patient ratio was approximately 1 : 100 000.

three authorized routes to the lake shore, little more was done. The main residual focus of infection was around the road between Lunyo and Lugala at the eastern end of the fly-belt. A small hospital was built at the dispensary at Lumino and, at the time of a survey in 1952, held 5 trypanosomiasis patients.

The outbreak of 1957–8

In 1954, 1955, and 1956, cases for the whole area between the Nile and the Kenya border averaged 7 a month. In 1957 the incidence doubled. By this time the East African Trypanosomiasis Research Organization had built a laboratory at Sukulu, 30 miles north of the lake, and one wing was turned into a hospital. The *Annual reports* of this organization are a useful guide to research on human trypanosomiasis around the north-east corner of Lake Victoria (East African Trypanosomiasis 1956 onwards).

An analysis of the 1957–8 epidemic by Robertson (1963) shows that increase in infection rate may have been associated with changes in the activities of lake fishermen. The ordinance of 1908 for registration of canoes and control of landing places was still in force. The Medical Department maintained a cadre of sleeping sickness inspectors who collaborated with the Uganda police in detecting and prosecuting men who disobeyed the regulations. The difficulties of enforcing this system were sufficient evidence of its unpopularity.

After the war the fishing industry changed in character with the introduction of outboard motors and the replacement of flax nets by nylon nets. To build up the industry the government increased its issue of fishing licences. At the same time, to rationalize harvesting of the fish, a fisheries research organization was set up at Jinja. The fishermen with motorized canoes were now able to outstrip the inspection and police boats, and the new nylon nets, with a mesh smaller than the research team recommended, led to a temporary boom in the industry in 1957.

Robertson analysed the distributions, in respect of time, place, trade, and sex, of 864 cases of sleeping sickness recorded east of the Nile in Uganda and the two adjoining chiefdoms of Kenya, from 1954 to 1960 inclusive. The totals of the first three years show no change from the overall rate of 7 cases per month; but over this period the number of cases among fishermen rose from 23 in 1954 to 41 in 1956, and the even overall rate had been maintained by a decrease in the numbers of cases from persons in other occupations. In 1957 the increase in cases among fishermen continued but the decline among other occupations ceased and the infection rate more than doubled itself. The high level of infection among cultivators and others who were not fishermen continued into 1958 and 1959 but in the latter year infections among fishermen fell, to be followed in 1960 by a general decline, to about ten cases a month, a level that has since been maintained.

The seasonal distribution of infection among fishermen was different from that exhibited by inland cases. Among fishermen the peak month was in January and thereafter monthly cases at a somewhat lower rate occurred until July, when there was a marked fall in numbers of infections. This was explained by the reduction in fishing activity during the months of June to September associated with the thermally unstratified condition of the lake waters at this time. In these conditions fish disperse and their density in the fishing grounds is greatly reduced. With the reappearance of thermal stratification towards the end of the year, the fish population is confined to the better oxygenated waters near the coastline and more intensive fishing is again possible.

Among the farmers and others who do not fish the peak months are May and June. The build-up then is associated with a change in behaviour of *Glossina pallidipes* which, in the wet climate of Busoga, readily bites man during the rainy months of March, April, and May. During the drier parts of the year the attack is much less intense.

Robertson saw in the epidemic among persons on land the results also of changed conditions which predisposed the population to infection. One reason why the closely settled barrier suggested in 1943 failed to gain acceptance was that at that time the Soga had no urgent need of more land for cultivation. By 1957 the situation had changed. There was now a growing need to reclaim the land lost after the 1901–8 epidemic. The western end of the fly-belt, as defined in 1944, had already disappeared and no tsetse were to be found west of Thruston Bay. The main bulk of the Busoga forests, however, remained. Apart from satisfying the needs of land-hungry Soga, the obliteration of these forests by settlement would remove the main focus of endemic rhodesian trypanosomiasis from Uganda.

To co-ordinate the movement into the forest the government laid out two parallel roads, one mile apart, just inside the central third of the forest edge. This corridor was to be settled and when it was filled another would be opened so that eventually the forests would disappear. The road system southward through the forest station and saw mills at Kityerera to the lake shore at the western end of the fly-belt was improved as an aid to re-settlement. This was done in 1956 before the appearance of the incipient epidemic in 1957.

Robertson's analysis makes clear the different epidemiological circumstances of cultivators on the inland fringes of the fly-belt and of the fishermen working on the lake shores. It is now necessary to look more closely at the situation of these cultivators.

The cattle infections in Busoga

Wallis (1920) wrote that Busoga had once been 'singularly rich in food and cattle'. In 1921 the Veterinary Service estimated that there were only 44 170 head of cattle in the district. Eight years later the figure had more than doubled. The Busoga cattle, like all the rest in tropical Africa, were still recovering from the effects of the rinderpest panzootic. This recovery continued until 1935 when there were 157 902 head in the district. This was not maintained and in 1941 a rapid decline set in. The growing cattle population and the growing *Glossina pallidipes* and *G. brevipalpis* fly-belts had developed to the extent that mortality and morbidity due to try-panosomiasis were sufficient to halt and then reverse the trend of popula-tion growth. Evidently this began about 1936 (Fig. 15.1).

The reaction to infection was similar to that which has already been described in Ankole. The cattle moved north away from the fly-belt. In

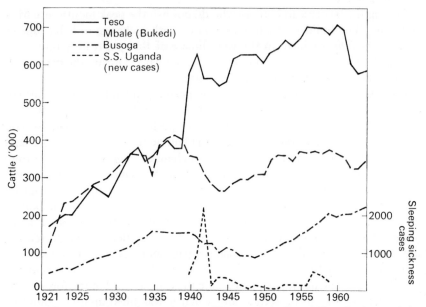

FIG. 15.1. Growth of the cattle populations of Busoga, Bukedi, and Teso districts, and the numbers of new cases of sleeping sickness in Uganda from 1940 onwards, nearly all of them from Busoga and Bukedi districts (from Ford 1969c).

Mbale (Bukedi) district which includes the eastern end of the Busoga belt, the cattle responded in the same way. One result of this movement was a sharp increase in the livestock returns for Teso district, around Lakes Kyoga and Salisbury, which reached a peak in 1941, a year before the peak of infection in the human epidemic. The treatment of the cattle epizootic has already been described in Chapter 5. The correlation between cattle population change brought about by *Trypanosoma congolense* and *T. vivax* infection with the appearance of an epidemic of *T. brucei rhodesiense* among the people is illustrated in Fig. 15.1.

What is the significance of these facts in relation to the origin of the 1940 *rhodesiense* epidemic? The strong presumption that the infection was brought in by immigrant labourers has been admitted. But these early cases were all among people (a schoolboy on a long journey and labourers subject to the health services of a large industry) with closer ties to the appurtenances of civilization than the peasants living in forests that were supposed to be closed to settlement. 'The people affected by this epidemic are all profoundly superstitious and distrustful of hospitals' (Mackichan 1944). It would be remarkable if the cases discovered in November 1940 were in fact the first in the epidemic.

The near coincidence of an epidemic among the people and an epizootic among their cattle, both due to trypanosomes transmitted by the same vector, has not before been considered. It is indeed possible that immigrant labourers introduced a new strain of *T. brucei*, but it is quite certain that they did not bring in *T. congolense* and *T. vivax*.

Growth of the human population in Busoga

It is more difficult, as always, to speak with confidence of the trend of the human than of the cattle population. In Busoga, as in all the high rainfall areas near the north shores of Lake Victoria, the early years of the Protectorate were years of population decline due to sleeping sickness and famine. Sir Albert Cook's view was that it was doubtful whether the ravages of the slave trade had been more disastrous than the epidemics of the first two decades of the century (Cook 1945).

The first reliable census in Uganda was carried out in 1948 and a second followed in 1959. During this interval the population of Uganda as a whole had increased at a rate of 2·5 per cent per annum. Somewhere between the downward trend of the last decade of the nineteenth and first two decades of the twentieth centuries and the strongly upward trend between 1948 and 1959 there had occurred a change. Goldthorpe (1955) suggests for Kenya and Uganda a turning point 'somewhere between 1920 and 1930'.

Changes in position of the tsetse front

The principal focus of infection in the Busoga fly-belt is now associated with the road that runs north to south through Bukoli chiefdom and leads to the fishing village at Lugala. This was surveyed for tsetse flies in 1944 and again in 1952. Since 1956 this portion of the fly-front has been under more or less continuous observation. There is little evidence for substantial change between 1944 and 1952. There was, however, a very considerable change in the distribution of cattle. The 1944 map does not show the whereabouts of cattle, though the accompanying report states that the cattle line was a good ten miles outside the fly-line. At the eastern end of the fly-belt, in Samia-Bugwe county, many deserted cattle kraals still showed how the herds had been driven away by the growth of the fly-belt. There were 71 head at Masaba, only 5 miles from the fly-line, but these were a special herd kept there for the use of the chief. By 1952, however, cattle now under drug protection were once more approaching the old pastures and the distance between them and the tsetse had been halved.

During the 1952 survey an inquiry among local people suggested that the old kraals, which could still be seen, had been abandoned in about 1928–9. In the absence of any other evidence one concluded that it had taken some twenty years from the evacuations of 1908 for the replacement of cultivation by secondary thicket to grow to an extent that enabled it to be invaded by an increasing bushpig, bushbuck, and buffalo population with their attendant parasites. This account put the collision between the fly-belt and the growing cattle population some eight years ahead of its reflection in the provincial veterinary statistics. In a country still very underpopulated by cattle the disease-free pastures further north were still understocked and cattle had no need to impinge upon the fly-belt. In 1952 the human population of Samia-Bugwe county was about 44 000 persons, giving a density of about 160 per mile^2.

In 1965 the fly-line at the eastern end of the belt had retreated westwards about 3 miles from the Mjanji inlet and southward on the Lugala road by the same distance. In 1959 the official census showed that Samia-Bugwe county had a mean population density of about 255 persons per mile^2 (*Uganda atlas* 1962). Robertson and Baker (1958) estimated that the population living within the area of G. *pallidipes* infestation in the Lugala neighbourhood had more than doubled itself between 1953 and 1957. It is clear that the retreat of the tsetse was a consequence of this population growth and its destructive effect upon the bush and its natural fauna. It may, however, be supposed that if the density of the human population in the county as a whole had increased 1·6 times between 1952 and 1959 then the opportunity and the need for tsetse to feed on man had also increased.

The Igwe focus

One section of the tsetse front that had attracted attention in 1944 was at Igwe, some seven miles south of Bugiri. A report written at the time ran as follows:

Between the Namaseri and Luvunya Rivers, which drain into the Kibimba Swamp, is a large tongue of forest of a width of some five miles, stretching across the road between the line of hills on the west and the swamp on the east. In such a block of forest G. *pallidipes* would only be expected to occur naturally around the edge or around islands of hardpan (laterite) if these occur. Mr Chorley (of the Entomology Section of the Uganda Medical Service) has demonstrated, however, that the breaking up of this type of forest by elephants is sufficient to allow fly to penetrate. At Igwe the forest has been broken up by settlers who came in some years ago, the area having been previously evacuated during the 1901–10 outbreak of sleeping sickness. Settlement is mainly on the west of the road and shambas are dotted about more or less haphazardly, separated from one another by blocks of forest through which they are connected by footpaths. The forest has thus been transformed into an ideal *G. pallidipes* habitat† and fly on the west of the road are numerous in the shambas. On the east of the road there is far less settlement and it is more recent. On a damp, cool evening a party on the east side failed to take any fly, while another party on the west took five. The next morning, in better weather, thirty-three flies (plus one *G. fuscipes*) were taken on the west during a walk of some six miles; on the east, in five miles the second party took five, none of them more than one and a half miles from the road. The settlers are now beginning to move to the east of the road because of sleeping sickness, there having been several cases on the west but only one on the east. The most westerly shamba belonged to a man who had already been infected. He had decided not to risk reinfection and had gone across the road to build a new house in the east. His family, at the moment of our visit, were just setting off with the last load of household goods to set up the new home (Ford 1944*b*).

In 1965 much but not all of the forest had disappeared and it was being felled and burned as people once more reclaimed it for agriculture. Mr. J. M. B. Harley, then Chief Entomologist of the East African Try-panosomiasis Research Organization, kindly arranged for another survey of the same area to be made in May 1966 (the former having been done in May 1944) using the same rather outmoded technique.‡ The fly-line had retreated by about $3\frac{1}{2}$ miles.

The Busakira settlement, 1956–7

The increasing numbers of sleeping sickness cases in 1957 and 1958 naturally attracted the attention not only of medical research workers but also of entomologists, especially K. R. S. Morris, who had had a long experience of entomological problems associated with sleeping sickness in Ghana. The piecemeal felling and burning of the forest that in 1944 had suggested that the people themselves were assisting the spread of *Glossina* was, in 1966, having the opposite effect, or seemed to be. It had been noted that, 'An abrupt change in the sex and age distribution of *T. rhodesiense* cases (from below five per cent female and nought per cent under 15, to 17 per cent female and 7·5 per cent under 15) took place in 1949 at a time when squatters' settlements were becoming common in the closed sleeping sickness area of south Busoga' (Morris 1958).

Morris studied the effect of settlement on the density of *G. pallidipes* at

† 'Ideal *G. pallidipes* habitat'. Today one might write with more accuracy that the transformation of the forest had produced conditions in which man was especially susceptible to attack; cf. Chapter 2 in which the notion of 'feeding grounds' is criticized. Intensified attack on man may indicate a habitat that is inadequate because natural hosts are less readily available.

‡ 'Outmoded technique'. A survey party walked through the bush carrying a black cloth screen to make them more attractive to *Glossina pallidipes*, a tsetse often reluctant to approach man. Use of traps or of bait cattle will reveal infestations not evident to moving parties of men and thus indicate larger areas for mapping as 'fly-belts'. Surveys by different techniques cannot easily be compared.

Busakira, 4 miles south of Ikulwe on the road to Kityerera on the lake shore. Of this settlement of about 400 people Morris wrote that it

is entirely surrounded by forests and, although compact, does not consist of continuous, open, farmed land. Only in the centre is there continuous clearing and cultivation. The greater part consists of groups of huts in a small island of cleared and cultivated land surrounded by uncleared forest, leaving bands of dense standing forest or thicket in between each family holding. Of the whole occupied area only about 50 per cent is cleared and cultivated.

Morris demonstrated that within this settlement *G. pallidipes* were caught at a rate of 0·6 per trap per week over a period of 64 weeks as compared with 25 per trap per week in the untouched forest. In a new settlement he measured the density of the tsetse in the cleared area before the people built their houses and moved in, and showed that when this happened the catch per trap per week fell from a mean of 11·7 to 1·5 (Morris 1958). His control traps, placed in undisturbed forest in October 1956, began to show falling catches after April 1957. This he attributed to the disturbances caused by more new settlers who had arrived in the control area.

The differences in the results obtained at Igwe in 1944 and at Busakira in 1956–7 can be attributed to the decline in human population density in progress during the first period and its increase in the second. As people moved away in 1944, the pigs and bushbuck moved, with their attendant tsetse, into the abandoned *shambas*. In 1957, as people moved into the forest, the pigs and bushbuck, again with their attendant tsetse, retreated further into its interior. Robertson (1963) published two aerial photographs of Busakira, taken in 1952 and 1960, that demonstrate clearly the erosion of the forest by the growing population. He estimated that in the 8-year period the area of forest canopy around Busakira had diminished by 29 per cent, a figure somewhat less than Morris's 50 per cent. This rate he regarded as too slow for safety. It is true that the incidence of infection rose sharply in 1957 and has remained well above the level to which it had fallen after the 1940 epidemic. On the other hand, during that interval the forest had been greatly reduced in area, almost entirely by the efforts of Soga cultivators.

The problem of human trypanosomiasis in Busoga illustrates very well one of the dilemmas that confront biologists concerned with zoonotic disease in underdeveloped countries. Development of the land, by bringing new populations into areas dominated by wildlife which includes the hosts of pathogenic organisms, must give rise, for a time, to conditions in which people suffer an increased risk of infection. In Busoga, Morris (1958, 1960b) advocated a development plan which he claimed would accelerate the disappearance of *G. pallidipes*. It gained the support of the Soga, but was opposed by Robertson (1963) on the grounds that it would increase the infection hazard. Both were right. The epidemic died down, but left an endemic condition with a higher incidence of infection than before; but on the other hand it became increasingly clear that the size of the fly-belt was diminishing under the pressure of population.

16

RESIDUAL FOCI OF ZOONOTIC INFECTION AROUND THE NORTH-EAST CORNER OF LAKE VICTORIA

THE explanation of the sequence of events that seemed to begin at the end of the last century in the countries adjoining the north-east corner of Lake Victoria encounters several difficulties. Some are historical: one cannot know what happened to the people involved except that very many of them died. This is one reason why it is valuable to write down, as Wijers has done, while people are still alive, their recollections of these times. In this chapter certain other aspects of the epidemic spread of gambian and then of rhodesian type infections in Kenya will be examined. The description of certain features of the geography and history of the progress of successive epidemics in Kenya will lead back to Busoga and to an examination of what happened on the northern or inland side of the epidemic area. This has hitherto been overlooked. Finally, the story will be brought up to date with a brief account of the Alego outbreak in central Nyanza in 1964.

The spread of infection into Kenya

In 1900–1 the epidemic condition spread around the lake in both directions and this spread was, without any doubt, associated with transmission by *Glossina fuscipes*. In Uganda the government ordered the evacuation of the lake shore. In German East Africa the epidemic was controlled by felling the fringe of lacustrine forest in which the tsetse were living (Steudel 1912). The 1940 epidemic only spread eastwards. By this time there was an appreciable gap in the distribution of *G. fuscipes* around the town of Jinja and although not a complete barrier, the great sugar estates at Kakira enlarged considerably the gap in vector distribution. And, of course, there was now a sleeping sickness control service to watch dangerous areas and to ensure that sporadically infected persons did not travel, untreated, about the country.

There was no evidence for the spread of the rhodesian disease beyond Samia until 1953. Although the Uganda medical authorities believed that the gambian disease had been eliminated in Busoga in 1933 it had certainly persisted along the Kenya shores. But in 1953, almost ten years after the rhodesian epidemic in Busoga had died down, it became apparent that some of the sleeping sickness patients in central Nyanza, the district immediately north of the Kavirondo gulf, were not responding to the standard treatment with the arsenical drug, tryparsamide. It will be recalled (Chapter 4) that failure to react to arsenical drugs was regarded as diagnostic of *Trypanosoma* '*rhodesiense*'. In the next year Willett (1955) isolated a '*Trypanosoma rhodesiense*' from a patient and in 1956 a similar trypanosome was obtained from a *G. pallidipes* caught on the Sakwa peninsula (see Map 14.1). Here, also, Heisch, McMahon, and Manson-Bahr (1958) made their notable isolation of this trypanosome from a bushbuck.

The antecedents of epidemics in south Nyanza

From 1953 onwards the rhodesian disease spread in central Nyanza and six or seven years later was identified south of the Kavirondo gulf in people living in the Lambwe valley in south Nyanza. This valley had been a centre of infestation by *G. pallidipes* and *G. brevipalpis* for many years. Where it ran out to the lake shore *G. fuscipes* was also present. The neighbouring valley to the south, the valley of the Kuja river, had been cleared of *G. fuscipes* between 1954 and 1958 and thus of the gambian disease which had been known there since the first decade of the century.

South of the Kuja, the next river of any size to enter Lake Victoria, is the Mori, site of the largest focus of infection encountered by the Germans in the first decade of the century. To deal with it they set up a hospital at Shirati. The next and much larger river, the Mara, runs through the northern portion of the *G. swynnertoni* and *G. pallidipes* fly-belt in which lie the sites of the Maswa and Ikoma epidemics mentioned in Chapter 13 as well as a recent outbreak of rhodesian trypanosomiasis in the Serengeti national park (Baker, Sachs, and Laufer 1967). All these rivers rise in the forests growing on the slopes leading off the south-west corner of the Kenya highlands. This forest separates the territories of three tribes: the Kipsigis in the north, the Masai in the east, and the Luo in the west. In the south lies the above-mentioned *G. swynnertoni* belt in the semi-arid *Acacia–Commiphora* thornbush of north central Tanzania.

A timetable of the successive appearances of the rhodesian infections north and south of the Kavirondo gulf has been very clearly set out by Willett (1965). The disease appeared in the Lambwe valley in 1960. This valley has been under observation as a centre of *G. pallidipes* infestation since the early 1930s. It was densely populated at the beginning of the century. The whole region about the Kavirondo gulf was involved in the slow movement in which 'the Bantu retreated before the rising tide of Nilotic conquest' (Owen 1932, and also Crazzolara 1950, 1951). The process involved local conflicts but to attribute the infestation of the Lambwe valley to tribal wars in about 1870, as did Swynnerton (1936), was clearly wrong.

Lewis (n.d.) explored the area very thoroughly in about 1935. His account which follows is confirmed in a short paper by Dobbs (1914). It had been customary for the natives to make enormous 'saucers' of mud and to fill these with water for calves and, in some cases, for larger cattle. Many of these 'saucers' and several small pits were still to be found in 1935. Derelict earth dams could be traced.

[There was] evidence that the inhabitants collected water from the mountain streams by means of deep channels and furrows that supplied fairly large surface reservoirs. . . . . It is fairly certain that the Lambwe Valley was densely populated and contained numerous herds of cattle in the early years of the present century. On the hills there are definite traces of habitation by an energetic tribe. Stone walls and terraces may still be seen on Kiangogo, Ugoro and the slopes of Ruri and Iringa. Disused water-holes and dams can be found in the valley and there is clear evidence of cultivated patches of land which has not long been abandoned. In the administrative records for 1908 it is stated that cattle were fairly plentiful in Kabwai, Kasigunga and numerous in Kaniamwa. . . . In Kisingiri . . . the report of the year 1911 states 'There has been a great deal of sickness among the livestock in recent years, which is now somewhat depleted' . . . Europeans speak of the numerous cattle in the valley in 1915. . . . . One gathers from the present native inhabitants that heavy mortality from malaria and human sleeping sickness among the tribes on the lake shore, especially in Kasigunga, gave rise to a fear that caused a steady evacuation of the area. As the people fell back the menace seemed to follow them. It extended and destroyed their cattle and the people were forced to retreat up the Lambwe. Disease then attacked the cattle from other directions also. . . . [Witchcraft was suspected and one ruling chief was murdered by the elders for poisoning the grass and water. This was a signal for people to leave the valley in large numbers to go to Tanzania.] The present chief and many elders state that only after most of the people had left did the bush become thick and beyond their control . . . (Lewis n.d.).

Glossina pallidipes was first recorded in this area in 1910 'probably in the lakeside section of Roo'. The Lambwe valley is bounded on its western face by two mountains, Gwembe and Gwasi, both rising to over 6000 ft. Roo is the pass between them. The forest patches on the more inaccessible slopes of these mountains are almost certainly to be regarded as having the same ecological ancestry as the forests around the highlands and to possess similar mammalian and insect faunas. Evacuation of the land from various causes, of which certainly human trypanosomiasis was one, was followed by a spread of *G. pallidipes* that, hitherto, had been confined to limited zones in forest or thicket patches above the level of human occupation. At whatever place one starts and wherever one goes, the same series of antecedent catastrophes are the prelude to epidemics, epizootics, and 'fly-advances'. Similar epidemiological sequences may be worked out everywhere.

Antecedents of epidemics in central Nyanza

Glasgow, whose account of former populations in Samia have already been noted, believed that *G. pallidipes* had invaded that portion of the Nyanza coast from the eastern end of the Busoga fly-belt in the 1920s. We have seen that it was towards the end of this decade that cattle moved away from this area on the Uganda side of the border. There were cattle at Port Victoria in 1924, but by 1935 they had disappeared.

The area, once so densely populated that it was kept very open, like a Sukuma cultivation steppe, but hilly, was partly depopulated because of sleeping sickness carried by lacustrine *G. palpalis* [= *G. fuscipes*]. Death was probably a less important cause of depopulation than evacuation, voluntary or forced. As a result of the partial depopulation thicket regenerated and produced conditions suitable for *G. pallidipes*. This tsetse spread from Uganda, exterminating the cattle and doubtless driving many people away, leading to a further regrowth of thicket and better conditions for *G. pallidipes* (Glasgow 1947).

This passage tells substantially the same story as that told by Lewis about the Lambwe valley. But its main interest is that when it was written the country south of Samia, of which the northernmost portion is Yimbo, seemed free of *G. pallidipes*.

There are other areas, notably Sakwa, where there are now large masses of thicket apparently suitable for *G. pallidipes*, and I believe that is only the fortunate chance, in the shape of the barrier afforded by the swamps of the Nzoia and Yala, which has prevented *G. pallidipes* from spreading further south. In other words, other conditions were probably equal, and the only reason that *pallidipes* is present in Samia and not in Sakwa is that it happened to gain access to Samia. If it happens to gain access to Sakwa that too will become a *G. pallidipes* belt (Glasgow 1947).

Glasgow did not know that a single *G. pallidipes* had been captured by a member of the Kenya Veterinary Service in Sakwa in January 1945 (Davidson 1945, quoted by Wijers 1969). Wijers, however, who did not see Glasgow's report, believes it possible that *G. pallidipes* only invaded Yimbo at the end of the war.

'After the second World War, but still before the reign of Blasio who became chief in July 1947, a disease broke out among the cattle in Yimbo. They became thinner and thinner and died in hundreds. Many goats and several dogs were also killed by the disease. By 1950 there was not a cow left on the mainland', except in a few small areas in isolated situations. In November 1948, while the epizootic was still killing cattle, a new disease appeared among the people of Ulungu in northern Yimbo. Ulungu adjoins the Yala swamp, but also abuts on two sides, on forested areas. Between 1948 and 1950 more than 50 people died. The disease was recognized as trypanosomiasis by the Kenya authorities, but this diagnosis surprised the local people because in the new disease, which they called *nyangona*, people did not become hungry or fat as in the earlier epidemic which they had called *nyalolwe*; they just wasted away, like the cattle. They tended to become mentally deranged and died in three to six months. These unusual symptoms, apparently, did not impress local doctors and it was not, as

Willett (1965) has recorded, until 1953 that failure of tryparsamide and the acute course of some cases suggested that the rhodesian infection was becoming a problem.

Occasionally, when listening to this sort of story from local people, one hears of events that seem extremely improbable. In Yimbo, according to Wijers' informants, 'The new cattle disease also seemed to affect the wild animals. Several times the hunters found dead bushpig in the forest, more often they found animals so weak that they could not run away and most of the wild animals trapped or shot were very thin, not fat and healthy as before (Wijers 1969). One cannot dismiss as idle rumour the notion that these animals were suffering from trypanosomiasis, for if the invasion by *G. pallidipes* was indeed new, then they were derived from populations that had been out of contact with infection for many generations (Chapter 4).†

The association between the spread of rhodesian infection in Nyanza and *Glossina pallidipes*

The rhodesian syndrome in sleeping sickness patients began to appear when local populations came into frequent contact with *G. pallidipes*. This may have happened in Samia because the tsetse had spread across the Sio valley via the thickets that had grown up where cultivation had been abandoned in the early years of the century. On the other hand *G. pallidipes* is a species able to persist in quite small foci. A classical example was observed in Dar-es-Salaam in 1934 (Swynnerton 1936) and around Lake Edward its presence in the Rift wall forests did not seriously hamper cattle raising in the valley floor (Chapter 10). It is possible that the growth of secondary thicket had enlarged the environment of bushpig and bushbuck and allowed long-established but hitherto small and confined fly-belts to expand. On the other hand, Wijers' account of Yimbo supports Glasgow's (1947) belief that spread into Sakwa had been delayed by the barrier of the Nzoia and Yala swamps. In any event the growing or recovering human population in due course came into close contact with the expanding populations of *G. pallidipes* and its hosts.

South of the Kavirondo gulf there can be no doubt that the forest fly-belts of the western scarp of the Kenya highlands form a focus of great antiquity. The presence in them of *G. fuscipleuris* is evidence of a former link between Pleistocene forests of East Africa and the forests around the rim of the Congo basin. The same may be said of its principal host animal, the giant forest hog (*Hylochoerus*), which has been found in a number of localities in the peripheral forests of the highlands and of Mount Elgon. The bushpig has a wider, but similar, distribution in the area (Stewart and

---

† If this is so, why were no deaths seen among game during the great 'tsetse advances' of the 1920s and 1930s in Tanzania, or in Uganda in the 1930s and 1940s? Partly because over wide areas animals were still dying in localized outbreaks of rinderpest; but partly also because local hunters kept quiet for fear of getting into trouble with game departments for poaching.

Stewart 1963). Between them they provide 72 per cent of the blood meals taken by this tsetse from wild hosts (Weitz 1963). The latter pig is, after the bushbuck, also the most important source of food for *G. pallidipes*. The third species of *Glossina* in these forests, *G. brevipalpis*, also depends largely on bushpig (40·7 per cent feeds) and on hippopotamus (31·1 per cent). The latter animal is present in the rivers of the Kuja–Migori river system and around the lake shore. Buffalo, the third important host of both these species, is also present in the area.

Finally, there is the lacustrine and riverine *G. fuscipes*. It does not often feed on hippopotamus because it is active during the day and the hippos come out at dusk, but apart from reptiles (43·3 per cent of feeds) *G. fuscipes* takes another 43·3 per cent of its food from man and bushbuck, in about equal quantities from each.

G. fuscipleuris and the giant forest hog demonstrate the antiquity of the southern Nyanza fly-belt. The other species, through the natural hosts they hold in common, provide the possibility of a continuous link between the trypanosome reservoirs of the forest and man. In normal times (which, from our present point of view, means before the European impact so violently disrupted human ecology in Africa) the forest complex of *G. fuscipleuris*, *G. brevipalpis*, and *G. pallidipes* was confined by surrounding human communities and kept very largely out of contact with the riverine and lake shore *G. fuscipes* which, in those circumstances, fed chiefly on man and reptiles (cf. the relationships of *G. palpalis* and man in Nigeria described in Chapter 24). With the collapse of the human population† the forest mammals enlarged their range and *G. fuscipes* then was able to bring man into direct association with the trypanosomes of the forest ecosystem. Is there any evidence to show the epidemiological consequences of these changes in transmission cycles?

Van Hoof in Busitema

In 1926 the League of Nations sent out a commission of experts to report on human trypanosomiasis. It was led by Dr. H. L. Duke and included Professor F. K. Kleine who had had a long experience of trypanosomiasis in the former German East Africa, Dr. L. van Hoof, in charge of sleeping sickness control in the then Belgian Congo, Professor G. Lavier of the University of Lille, Dr. M. N. Prates, Director of the Bacteriological Laboratory, Lourenco Marques, and Major M. Peruzzi of the University of Florence.

Van Hoof and Prates visited the Kavirondo–Budama area. Kavirondo, in this case, means the foci along the shores of Samia and Nyanza, including

† Mostly caused by deaths from trypanosomiasis or evacuation of infected areas, but also by administrative measures. The Kipsigis, one of the tribes whose activities confined the forests overlooking the infected area, said when shifted from part of their lands in 1903 in the interests of rural development, 'God has forsaken us and we are scattered' (Orchardson 1932).

the Mjanji neighbourhood in Uganda. Budama is a chiefdom which lies immediately north of Samia in the Uganda district of Bukedi. Immediately north of Budama is Bunyole. Both these chiefdoms are drained by rivers that run into Lake Kyoga. Not all arise on the south Busoga watershed. The largest, the Malaba or Malawa (see Map 15.1), flows southwards down the slopes of Mount Elgon in Kenya, turns west across the Uganda border, and finally runs north to join Lake Kyoga through the Mpologoma swamp.

People in Budama and Bunyole became infected quite early in the great epidemic, so severely that the Mpologoma country was voluntarily evacuated on the side adjoining Busoga in 1904 and, on the side adjoining Bukedi, compulsorily in 1908–9. In the south this infected area adjoined the *G. pallidipes*-infested hills in Bukoli at the eastern end of the Busoga watershed. One medical investigator, Dr. Collyns, reported in 1911 that

TABLE 16.1

Courses of infection in Samia and Busitema, 1926–7

Progress of patients	Samia (%)	Busitema (%)
Apparent cure . . .	31·3	33·3
Improvement . . .	19·3	61·1
Unchanged	2·4	0
Worse. . . .	8·4	5·5
Dead	21·7	0
No exact information . .	16·9	0

the people living around these hills had been killed off by sleeping sickness. The south-east portion of Budama was called Busitema. The Malawa runs through it. People living nearby became infected in 1906–7 and there was famine among them in 1908 (Carpenter 1925).

The Malawa runs through the most northerly tip of forest stretching down from the east Busoga hills, but, at least in recent times, no *G. pallidipes* or *G. brevipalpis* but only *G. fuscipes* has been found here. On the drainages in these northern infected areas the only vector was *G. fuscipes*.

Van Hoof's observations showed that the disease in Busitema was considerably 'less grave' than in Samia. One object of his visit was to test various drugs, including tryparsamide. Table 16.1 summarizes his findings (van Hoof 1928b).

Results of treatment were assessed by analysis of cerebro-spinal fluid and by observation of blood smears and clinical symptoms. The better condition of the Busitema patients was the more remarkable because 'The

Samia area was much better served as regards the treatment of patients than Busitema, chiefly on account of the proximity of the Lumino dispensary, where tryparsamide treatment had been regularly continued. . . . Mortality in the Mjanji [i.e. Samia] district is very high. . . . On the other hand, in the Busitema area, although treatment was often manifestly inadequate . . . mortality was nil.'

The mildness of the infection in Busitema in 1926–7 was apparently exceeded near the Namatala, a more distant branch of Lake Kyoga. 'Virulence varies greatly in different individuals in the same area and from one endemic area to the next. The two extremes may be met with together: intense virulence with rapid and fatal development (Samia and Kavirondo), and attenuation amounting to tolerance and possibly spontaneous cure (Namatala)' (van Hoof 1928b). The significance of the phrase 'the two extremes may be met with together' is clarified by remarking that the Namatala river is 50 miles north of Mjanji.

At that time it was considered that *G. fuscipes* was the only vector. Today it is evident that the foci of infections of greater virulence lay in the *G. pallidipes* belt in the south. As the infection spread further away into areas in which *G. fuscipes* only was present, so the disease became less severe.

Was there any evidence of involvement of *G. pallidipes* in the area of 'intense virulence' at the time that van Hoof was making his observations? In Carpenter's (1925) report we find that 'Facts submitted by Dr. Griffin and Mr. Fiske suggest that *Glossina* may not be the only vector at Mjanji, where the distribution of cases points to the possibility of house infection.' Unfortunately we are not told the precise nature of these facts. Presumably they refer to the sex ratio among patients showing a high ratio of female infections acquired away from the water's edge as shown in Robertson's (1963) map illustrating the endemic condition before the 1957 outbreak. In these areas people who stayed at home became infected by *G. pallidipes* that attacked them in their gardens in the way seen in the 1944 survey.

Recent cattle trypanosomiasis along the eastern Uganda border

It is a long interval between 1926 and 1966 but there is no reason to suppose that any fundamental changes have occurred in the ecology of the country drained by the Sio and Malawa rivers on the eastern end of the Busoga fly-belt. In Chapter 15 attention was drawn to a possible correlation in time between the rhodesian epidemic of 1940–3 and an epizootic in Busoga and Bukedi cattle. Recent studies suggest a special correlation between incidence of cattle trypanosomiasis and the character of the human infection at the end of the first great Uganda epidemic.

The Malawa river runs close to the farm belonging to the East African Trypanosomiasis Research Organization. The land it occupies was once part of a veterinary quarantine station and it was chosen as a site for a laboratory partly on the supposed grounds that there were no tsetse in its

T A E—T

vicinity. The rivers of the area had been cleared of fringing vegetation over much of their length in the 1920s, but in 1956 a flourishing *G. fuscipes* population was found on the Malawa river adjacent to the E.A.T.R.O. farm. However, no infections other than those created experimentally have been reported (Mwambu 1967). In 1956 the *Glossina* infestation was removed again by use of insecticide (Robertson 1957) from rather more than two hundred square miles of the Malawa basin around the E.A.T.R.O. land both in Uganda and across the Kenya border. Again the tsetse returned and in September 1966 an aggregation of high density was found a few hundred yards from the farm boundary. Five hundred and twenty-eight flies were dissected without revealing a single infection. This result was in sharp contrast to the infection rates of 10·1 per cent in males and 20·5 per cent in female *G. fuscipes* at Lugala, 45 miles away on the lake shore at the southern end of the main focus of infection of both bovine and human trypanosomiasis in the Busoga fly-belt (Harley 1967a and 1967b). The only wild mammals of any size seen in the vicinity of the E.A.T.R.O. farm were a few oribi (*Ourebia*).

These dissections of *G. fuscipes* give results that represent the two ends of a gradient which is revealed more fully in a survey of cattle infections between Mjanji (5½ miles north-east of Lugala) and the E.A.T.R.O. farm by Mwambu and Odhiambo (1967, see also Mwambu 1966). They took blood from samples each of 34 cattle at 25 places, plus three samples of larger numbers. One thick and one thin blood smear were examined from each beast and 0·5 ml of blood from each animal was inoculated into each of two mice. *Trypanosoma vivax* and *T. congolense* were found in cattle as far as 28 miles from the lake shore, but trypanosomes of the *T. brucei* subgroup were limited to the area within or contiguous with the fly-belt, by which is meant the lowland moist forest and thicket in South Busoga harbouring *G. pallidipes* and *G. brevipalpis* as well as *G. fuscipes*. Further analysis of the data shows that although, indeed, *T. congolense* was found 28 miles north of Mjanji, its contribution to total infection dropped abruptly at about 8 miles from the lake, beyond which distance *T. vivax* predominated (Table 16.2). Reference to the map (Mwambu and Odhiambo 1967) and a comparison with the fly-belt limits shown in the *Uganda atlas* (1962) suggests that the heavily infected herds lived mostly under 5 miles from the main *G. pallidipes* infested area.

The significance of these results in relation to the observations of van Hoof on the human infection in the same stretch of country 40 years earlier is that they demonstrate clearly that once the patient, whether man or beast, is out of range of *G. pallidipes* then, although still subject to bite by *G. fuscipes*, the epidemiological circumstances of the infection and its development are greatly changed. Beyond this crucial point the populations at risk cease to be subject to continual inoculation of trypanosomes obtained directly, via *G. pallidipes*, from the wild animal reservoir.

TABLE 16.2

Infection incidences (all trypanosomes) and T. congolense *and* T. vivax *infections at different distances from the eastern end of the Busoga fly-belt*†

Distance from lake	Cattle examined	% infected	T. congolense infections	T. vivax infections	Total of T. vivax and T. congolense infections
Less than 8 miles .	374	33·9	55	51	106
Over 8 miles . .	408	13·0	9	42	51
			64	93	157

$$\chi^2 = 15\cdot456$$
$$P < 0\cdot001$$

† From Mwambu and Odhiambo (1967).

The point has been reached, by a very different route, at which van Hoof's parasitological colleague, Prates (1928), ended his account of the strains of *brucei* group trypanosomes collected by the League of Nations' commission. It is true that he studied the transformations in trypanosome morphology that take place after numerous passages in laboratory animals. These effects, including loss of infectivity to man, have been recorded in Chapter 4. Nevertheless, Prates's conclusion is relevant to the argument. '*T. gambiense* behaves as if it had been separated longer than *T. rhodesiense* from its primary natural vertebrate host, probably the big game, the ordinary natural reservoir of *T. brucei* and *T. rhodesiense.*'

There is only one possible crucial experiment to decide how the virulent strains of Samia turned into the milder strains of Busitema and finally into the self-curing strains of the Namatala area. A *rhodesiense* type strain would be used to infect a man and from him a series of passages by cyclical transmission through *G. fuscipes* would be made in succession to other men in the same way that the Tinde strain was maintained by cyclical transmission by *G. morsitans* from sheep to sheep (page 73). It is an experiment obviously impossible to perform. It is known, however, that while the disease (by whatever name it may be called) persisted, and still persists, in Samia, it died out in the northern chiefdoms around the Mpologoma and Namatala swamps. The situation showed a close parallel to the gradual disappearance of infection in cattle, in spite of the presence of *G. fuscipes* on the rivers at which they drink.

But this must be a gross oversimplification, for in 1964 a severe epidemic broke out in central Nyanza which was clearly caused by a *rhodesiense* type trypanosome transmitted by *Glossina fuscipes.*

The Alego epidemic

The events leading up to and the character of the Alego epidemic have been described by Willett (1965). Although Mackichan (1944) had envisaged the possibility of *G. fuscipes* as a vector of *Trypanosoma brucei rhodesiense*, the line of spread of the 1940 epidemic along the northern edge of the Busoga belt, as well as the isolation of the trypanosome from *G. pallidipes*, tended to reinforce the view that the latter tsetse was the principal vector of this trypanosome. Later, Robertson and Baker (1958) brought forward further evidence in favour of this argument. However, at the southern end of the main focus of *rhodesiense* infections, *G. fuscipes* frequently fed on man and before long a *T. brucei rhodesiense* was obtained from a fly of this species collected at Lugala (Southon and Robertson 1961, see also Southon 1960). In none of this work was there any suggestion that the more virulent, *rhodesiense* type of disease was not caused by trypanosomes derived, in the beginning, from wild animals. Among these it seemed probable, after the isolation of Heisch, MacMahon, and Manson-Bahr (1958), that the bushbuck *Tragelaphus scriptus* was especially prominent.

The appearance of rhodesian trypanosomiasis in Yimbo between 1948 and 1950 and its confirmation by Willett in 1953 has been described. It continued to occur among people in central Nyanza at a generally low incidence, but with tendency towards periodical localized outbreaks in 1953–4, 1957–8, and 1961. In the eleven years 1953–63 there were 479 recorded cases, all of which could be attributed to an infective source in wild game, fed on by *G. pallidipes*. In some areas there was also the possibility of transmission by *G. fuscipes*. Odd cases in Alego and contiguous areas which lay inland behind the Yala swamp and north-east of Yimbo could be attributed to persons having acquired infection while visiting established endemic areas. These areas only yielded 21 cases in the 11-year period. Then, in 1964, an explosive epidemic of rhodesian infection flared up in Alego and 319 cases were recorded. An intensive epidemiological investigation was carried out and showed quite clearly that the only vector was *G. fuscipes* (Onyango, Southon, de Raadt, Cunningham, van Hoeve, Akolo, Grainge, and Kimber 1965).

This in itself was sufficiently interesting but even more so was the isolation of *Trypanosoma brucei rhodesiense* by Onyango, van Hoeve, and de Raadt (1966) from a cow. They obtained in all 43 stabilates of *brucei* group trypanosomes from Alego cattle. Of these they chose 6 and tested them for sensitivity to standard drugs. Two of the six were inoculated into volunteers, one of whom developed a typical *rhodesiense* type infection after an incubation period of 8 days.

The ecological situation of Alego at this particular time must be described. In 1961 unprecedentedly heavy rain fell in the Lake Victoria basin.

Its full effect took some time to manifest itself but by 1964 the level of the lake had risen 7 ft. Flying over the Nyanza coast in July 1963 one saw that the old shore line had disappeared and that many families had had to abandon their homes and move inland. The local base-levels of rivers had risen and their outlets into the lake were pushed back for considerable distances. Many years ago the suggestion had been made by Duke (1919) that by raising the level of Lake Victoria by damming the Nile it might be possible to eliminate the lacustrine habitat of *G. fuscipes* and hence the fly itself. A dam was constructed for other purposes but its effects on the lake level were smaller than the rise after the 1961 rains. The hosts and potential hosts of the tsetse moved with the shore line and the flies, wherever there was a suitable habitat, moved with them. One such habitat was found in the high hedges of *Euphorbia tirucalli* and other shrubs planted around the Luo homesteads in Alego. This vegetation has in recent years been greatly augmented by the exotic weed, *Lantana camara*, imported as an ornamental plant from India.

Alego is situated in the basin of the Nzoia river on the southern side of a tributary called the Wuoroya. The largest focus of infection was just north of the village of Ndere, in country drained by the Sese river running into the Wuoroya. There were abundant *G. fuscipes* but the tsetse were not confined to the rivers.

Ndere market and Ndere trading centre were found infested with *Glossina*. Contact between man and fly was partly domestic, partly in market places, but mainly on the rivers where there were numerous points at which contact seemed very close, e.g. where the population bathed and drew water, at posho mills on the banks of rivers where women and girls took cereals for grinding, at river crossings, and at fishing points where angling is a common practice (Onyango, van Hoeve, and de Raadt 1966).

It was also established that the infection rate in the Alego tsetse was high for *brucei* group trypanosomes as compared with Lugala: i.e. 1 : 321 at Alego as against 1 : 525 and 1 : 916 on two occasions at Lugala. (Unfortunately a different method was used in each of these surveys.) The domestic nature of this outbreak was confirmed by the sex ratio among patients. Willett (1965) found 72 infected males and 73 infected females. There were few cases among men between the ages of 20–29 and this could be attributed to the fact that many in this age-group are away at work elsewhere in Kenya. A peculiar feature was the relative absence of infection among children, there being only 5 cases in children under 10 years of age. A similar distribution was obtained a year later among patients in Yimbo where, in 1965–6, there was another epidemic flare-up. Bailey, de Raadt, and Krampitz (1967) suggested that the disease in the very young is frequently mistaken (presumably by their parents) for malaria which is hyperendemic.

The most interesting feature of the Alego epidemic was, of course, the isolation of *T. brucei rhodesiense* from cattle in the area. Alego is adjacent to locations in which sleeping sickness has been endemic for many years. It is possible that a movement of the *G. fuscipes* fly-belt, initiated by the rise in lake level, led to the introduction of trypanosomes derived, initially, from a wild animal reservoir in one or other of these places, into the Alego cattle. Like those 10–15 miles north of the Busoga belt, these animals may have been free of trypanosomes. One would then expect to see in them a temporary rapid proliferation of *brucei* type infections preceded, for a few days, by *T. vivax*, and followed by *T. congolense*. For a time the newly infected cattle serve in place of a wild animal reservoir in intimate contact with a vector well adapted to the human domestic environment. In due course one would expect the cattle would suffer the effects of an epizootic of *T. vivax* and *T. congolense*, but the *T. brucei* infections would tend to disappear from their peripheral circulations. This is supposition. Application of medical, veterinary, and entomological controls at Alego brought the process to an end before it could be further investigated.

A summary of the sequence of events preceding and following the 1900 epidemic

The infected areas of the Nyanza province in Kenya have been subjected to a variety of treatments in an attempt to eliminate tsetse flies over a period of many years. In Busoga little entomological control has been attempted. On both sides of the border the infection remains. This unfinished story can be summarized in its main points as follows:

Before 1890	Flourishing populations of people and cattle from the Nile around to the Kuja river. A *Grenzwildnis* in Bukoli separates the Soga and Kavirondo populations.
c. 1890	Rinderpest panzootic. Probable severe reduction of cattle population and of bushbuck, buffalo, and bushpig.
c. 1891–3	Smallpox epidemic; invasion of jigger fleas.
1896	Trypanosomiasis epidemic begins in Bukoli.
1898–1900	Severe famine.
1900	Trypanosomiasis well established.
1901	Epidemic spreads to north Kavirondo.
1903	Causal organism defined as *Trypanosoma gambiense* and vector *Glossina palpalis* (= *fuscipes*). *G. pallidipes* recorded in Busoga.
1904	Epidemic spreads north into Budama and Bunyoli.
1900–7	Probably 100 000 deaths. Disease spreads around lake. Voluntary evacuations in Bunyoli and in Kavirondo.
1908	Compulsory evacuation of surviving population from

2-mile strip of shore line in Buganda and Busoga, but not enforced in Kavirondo. Famine.

1910   The epidemic is over. (In Western Uganda the story begins to repeat itself, cf. Chapter 10.)

1918   Famine.

1919–20   Influenza pandemic.

1920   Able-bodied men in Bunyoli now total 105 as against a reputed 17 000 before the trypanosomiasis epidemic.

1912–33   Endemic trypanosomiasis persists, but with gradually falling incidence until apparently extinguished in Busoga, but not along Kenya lake shore.

1926–7   Van Hoof distinguishes between severe cases which are more frequent near the lake shore and mild cases, in Budama and Bunyoli, which in some cases may be self-curing.

1928–9   Cattle move away from pastures near to lake, both in Busoga and Samia.

1935   Busoga cattle, which have been increasing at least since 1920, reach maximum numbers and begin to decrease. Samia cattle have now disappeared.

1940   Second epidemic of trypanosomiasis (rhodesian) developing first along northern edge of Busoga forests. *G. pallidipes* transmission confirmed. Cattle population now leaving Busoga in large numbers.

1942   Peak of rhodesian epidemic with 100 cases a month. Spread into Samia. People move away from forest edge.

1943   Proposals for defence line.

1944   Busoga fly-belt mapped. Area about 600 mile^2. People still leaving forest edge. Epidemic over.

1945   Soga people refuse to collaborate in a resettlement programme.

1948   First Uganda census.

1949   Cattle population of Busoga at 88 531 head reaches lowest level since 1928. Among people at risk the proportion of women and children infected increases, indicating beginning of move back towards forest.

1950   Block treatment of Busoga cattle with antrycide produces marked decline of incidence of infection with *T. congolense* and *T. vivax*. Numbers begin to recover.

1950–6   Changing pattern of lake fishing industry. More licences issued; outboard motors replace paddles and nylon nets replace flax. Regulations regarding landing places now ignored. Incidence of human trypanosomiasis in Busoga stable at about seven cases a month.

1957   Incidence of trypanosomiasis doubles among cultivators.
1958   Incidence of trypanosomiasis doubles among fishermen. Second Uganda census shows, for the whole Protectorate, a 31 per cent increase on the 1948 total.
1959–66   Epidemic fails to develop, but endemic level now at about ten cases a month. Cattle population density higher than ever recorded and increase continuing. Fly-belt is reduced to about 400 mile^2 (as indicated by moving screen catches).
c. 1950 to present. Continued spread, with repeated outbreaks, of rhodesian trypanosomiasis, in Nyanza province (formerly Kavirondo) in Kenya, due to impact of expanding population on secondary vegetation populated by antelopes, wild pigs, and G. pallidipes.
1964   Abnormally heavy rains in 1961 alter distribution of G. fuscipes. Previously uninfected domestic cattle act as a temporary reservoir of T. brucei including strains infective to man. G. pallidipes as intermediary between the wild reservoir and the G. fuscipes–man cycle is no longer necessary.

In practice, of course, the first consequence of the appearance of the epidemic, was medical treatment of the infected population. The discovery that the cattle were acting as a reservoir of human infective trypanosomes was at once followed by their treatment too, and finally a massive attack on Glossina in and around Alego was mounted in a combined Kenya government and W.H.O. operation. Natural adjustment to the zoonosis was abruptly curtailed.

17

RHODESIA:
THE TSETSE-INFESTED *GRENZWILDNIS*

The situation between the tsetse belts

RHODESIA is itself a single natural system, centred upon the water-shed that separates the Zambezi from the Limpopo and Sabi–Lundi river systems before they descend from the African plateau into the Mozambique coastal plain. The Zambezi and the Limpopo form the northern and southern boundaries of Rhodesia. The eastern boundary, for the greater part, runs along the crest of the highlands that form the rim of the plateau. In the south-east, between the Sabi and the Limpopo, descent to the coastal plain is more gradual. Here an arid zone of low rainfall (200–400 mm yearly), centred over the Limpopo but extending chiefly north of it, with high temperatures and little ground water, provides a partial barrier both to man and tsetses. In the north-east the Inyanga mountains slope down to the Zambezi valley. In the west the boundary is also a natural one, for it follows approximately the eastern limit of the Kalahari along a line that had its starting point at the northern end of the route that circumvented the *Glossina morsitans* belt of the Limpopo valley before it disappeared in 1896. This same species of tsetse also infested the valley of the Zambezi river and continues to do so. At these latitudes *Glossina* finds its limits at about 3000 ft above sea level in the Limpopo valley and at about 4000 ft in the Zambezi valley. The politically effective portion of Rhodesia lies above these altitudes so that in the north and south it is held, as it were, between two *Grenzwildnisse* both of which, before the Great Rinderpest, were tsetse-infested. At the time of the pan-zootic the Limpopo basin lost its infestation of *G. morsitans* and, except on the Mozambique plain, its other tsetses as well. The Zambezi valley, at least in the Rhodesian sector, also lost most of its tsetse flies, but small foci of *G. morsitans* and *G. pallidipes* remained. The modern history of trypanosomiasis in this part of Africa is the history of the Rhodesian, South African, and Portuguese efforts to prevent the recovery of *G. morsitans* and its associated species.

Peculiarities of the Rhodesian situation

There are four features of special interest in the history of Rhodesian trypanosomiasis. The first is the character of the human infective strains of trypanosomes found in the Zambezi valley. They do not influence the pattern of human settlement today and are dealt with in Chapter 20. The second is the position of Rhodesia athwart the natural climatic limits of continental distribution of *Glossina*. This provides the opportunity for examining the control over tsetse distribution in man's absence. Thirdly, although in each of the other eastern African sample areas there are frequent references to tribal wars, these were seldom more than aggressive posturings often resulting in less violence than a contemporary British football match; but Rhodesia suffered, for three-quarters of a century, the full impact of the Zulu *mfecane* followed by the European invasion. All this was true warfare. Fourthly, Rhodesia provides the only example of a European society confronted by the threat of trypanosomiasis. In no other part of Africa south of the Sahara and north of the Limpopo are there any urban populations of which more than 25 per cent are of European origin. A European farming community established itself temporarily on a fairly large scale in Kenya, but its activities were almost entirely confined to country, the White Highlands, which lay above the altitude limits of *Glossina*. This is also the case with much of the European land in Rhodesia, but although little of the tsetse-infested land is European-owned, there are large areas in this category which were infested before the rinderpest. There is another important contrast between the responses of the pre-Independence European Kenya settler and the white Rhodesians to tsetse infestation. The Kenya settlers, for the most part, took over their lands after the railway from Mombasa to Nairobi had been built. They suffered no difficulties from trypanosomiasis in reaching their farms. When, in due course, they began to import exotic breeds of domestic livestock, these could be brought through the fly-belts in netted trucks. The Rhodesians, on the other hand, particularly those descended from pioneer families that came up from South Africa at the end of the last century, have an acute folk memory of the effects of tsetse fly. It derives from experiences of parents and grandparents and from the still older memories of Afrikaner Voortrekkers who were turned aside from their northward path when their oxen died at the encounter with the Limpopo fly-belts. The possibility of recovery of the fly-belts to their former extent in Rhodesia and via Rhodesia to the northern Transvaal is, therefore, a matter productive of acute political emotion. This emotion has been exacerbated because the principal technique used to control *Glossina* has been the slaughter of its natural hosts, the wild game. Among a community which regards hunting as a legitimate form of recreation and source of personal income, the large-scale destruction of wildlife by a government department has aroused strong feelings. Less vociferous, but better informed, opposition to animal slaughter based itself upon the more legitimate objections which can be adduced against destruction of a valuable natural resource. Recently less contentious methods of trypanosomiasis control have been introduced and facilities for hunting by white Rhodesians have been greatly improved.

These factors militate against a dispassionate appraisal of the role of the trypanosomiases in Rhodesian ecology. Another is 'land apportionment', as it is officially described, or possessory segregation or, in South African terminology, apartheid. This system has features which give the inter-actions of the wildlife ecosystems with those in which man dominates a character that is unique in Africa. It provides an experiment in human ecology that has much of interest. Whatever may be said about the political system in Rhodesia it has had one advantage for the student of trypano-somiasis. In order that the settler population should be able to develop the 'European' lands with the minimum of interference from the various fac-tors, including diseases, inherent in its African environment, strict controls were and are maintained over activities in the 'African' lands. Statistics are collected and published regularly and the population growth curve for African-owned cattle can be plotted from uninterrupted annual counts from 1897 onwards.

The situation in Rhodesia is therefore one which does not find any com-plete parallel in the countries from which other examples of the conflict between human society and the trypanosome ecosystems have been drawn. The nearest approach to the Rhodesian system was, perhaps, found in the interlake countries, Ankole, Karagwe, Rwanda, and others, up to the arrival of the colonial powers, where pastoral Nilo-hamite aristocracies maintained a more or less harsh rule over majority populations of agricul-tural serfs.† But in these countries the division of land between the two populations had a different basis and, whatever may have been the merits or otherwise of these pastoral aristocracies, they did not publish statistics.

Rhodesia has been more completely surveyed and 'planned' than any other country within the African tropics. It is therefore possible, to a greater degree than elsewhere, to relate areas of tsetse infestation to the economic potential of the land. Rhodesia also, because of the conspicuous richness of its archaeological sites, has had a comparatively thorough pre-historic exploration. It has had a long contact with the world outside Africa and almost matches the empires of West Africa in the length of its conven-tional or documentary history. This is due to the Portuguese who recorded their attempts to gain greater control over the gold export trade from the beginning of the sixteenth century until their expulsion by the Rozwi in about 1700. The confrontation of Afrikaner and British South African societies with the tsetse-borne diseases of the Limpopo basin is also fully documented.

Because of the peculiarities in the Rhodesian situation it is necessary to adopt an approach to its trypanosomiasis problems different from that

† In Rwanda, where the spread of *G. morsitans* has not yet demolished the bulk of the pastures, the principal effect of Independence was to permit a revolt of the Hutu culti-vators, so that the cattle aristocracy did not long survive the departure of the Belgians. In Ankole and Karagwe the deposition of the local kings after Independence was a peaceful act of administration, for cattle trypanosomiasis had already, some years before, eliminated the foundations of their rule.

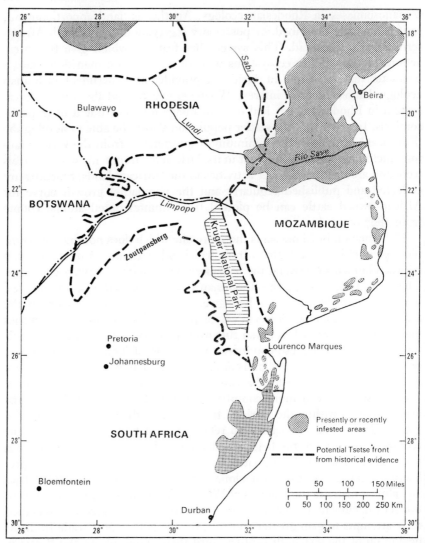

MAP 17.1. The distribution of *G. morsitans* in Rhodesia, southern Mozambique, and South Africa before the rinderpest panzootic in 1895 and in 1959. (The Zululand *G. pallidipes* fly-belt is shown but had been eliminated by insecticides by 1954.)

taken with the more northerly parts of eastern Africa. So much historical and prehistorical information exists about Rhodesia that to begin from these starting points would demand expert knowledge disproportionately large in relation to the uses to which it could be put. It therefore seems better to begin with a description of the *Glossina* systems of Rhodesia (and to some degree of its neighbours) and then work back from them to the more outstanding features of its history and prehistory. One archaeologist

(Summers 1960) has, indeed, done the reverse of this and, having described Rhodesian history from the earlier Stone Age to 1893, has invoked the tsetse-borne diseases to explain its principal trends. With some of his conclusions we shall agree; with others, not.

The Rhodesian tsetse belts: historical limits and subsequent recession

Map 17.1 shows the outline of the Limpopo fly-belt deduced by Fuller (1923), Jack (1914, 1933), and Curson (1932) from historical evidence for the years before the rinderpest panzootic. This outline is contrasted with that existing in 1959 (Ford 1960a, Sousa 1960). Much of the basic historical

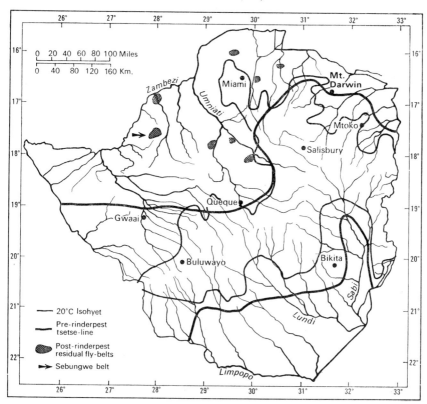

MAP 17.2. The *G. morsitans* fly-belts in Rhodesia before the rinderpest and after its passage in 1895. The Sebungwe belt is indicated (cf. Fig. 17.1).

data used by Fuller to reconstruct the outline of the Limpopo fly-belt was collated by Austen (1903). Map 17.2 shows pockets of tsetse known to have survived the rinderpest in Rhodesia (Jack 1933). Chorley (1947a) may also be consulted. Macaulay (1942) brought together a series of maps showing that the *G. morsitans* infestation of the Okovango swamps in Botswana underwent a similar contraction and expansion. His work has been brought up to date by Lewis (1963). Neave (1911) produced evidence for a similar recession and recovery of the *G. morsitans* belt of the Lwangwa valley in Zambia. His survey was supplemented by a report and map by Hall (1910).

These recessions, amounting in the Limpopo basin to complete disappearance of tsetse flies, followed rapidly upon the passage of the rinderpest panzootic which crossed the Zambezi in 1895. David and Charles Livingstone (1865) had already proclaimed that 'The destruction of all game by the advance of civilization is the only chance of getting rid of tsetse.' The Limpopo fly-belt was already much diminished before 1895 because of the large-scale slaughter carried out by Afrikaner settlers in the Transvaal.

Before considering the effects of these and other invasive societies upon the Rhodesian ecosystem it is necessary to describe the controls exerted over the distribution of tsetse flies by natural agencies other than man.

Climatic limits to tsetse dispersal

From the earliest days of research on tsetse, their restriction to forests, woodlands, and tree savanna has been regarded as an adaptation for escaping the ill effects of overheating and desiccation. 'Tsetse flies must have shade' is a statement to be found in almost every popular account of their habits. The glossinologist in Rhodesia has the advantage of working in climates that show wide variations, especially of temperature, not only seasonally, but also throughout the day. In addition, in the Zambezi valley, marked differences in climate due to abrupt altitude change can be measured over relatively small distances. Table 17.1 shows various mean temperatures measured at Chirundu, on the banks of the Zambezi, and at Gatooma which lies just within the limits that the fly-belt reached before its post-rinderpest recession. At the former place the average of monthly lowest screen temperatures recorded was 7·2°C and of the highest, 41·7°C. In the low-lying Sabi valley fly-belt in the south-east of Rhodesia it is not impossible, in the month of July, to find a ground frost at dawn and a midday temperature, six or seven hours later, rising to 32°C.

When it was realized, in about 1910, that *G. morsitans* was beginning to reoccupy the territory from which it had disappeared in 1896, it became a matter of some urgency to know how far it was likely to move. The collation of historical data led to the preparation of the maps already examined. The next step came during the 1930s. Under the leadership of P. A. Buxton, the physiological study of *Glossina* had begun at Gadau in Nigeria and in Uganda. These studies attempted to define, in terms of temperature and humidity, the environments in which *G. tachinoides* and *G. morsitans submorsitans* (Buxton and Lewis 1934) and *G. fuscipes fuscipes* (Mellanby 1936) could exist. Jack repeated the work on *G. morsitans* in Rhodesia (Jack 1939, 1941). One hour's exposure to a temperature of 40°C was

TABLE 17.1

Temperatures at the centre and on the edge of the Zambezi fly-belt†

	Mean maxima (°C)	Average highest maxima (°C)	Mean minima (°C)	Average lowest minima (°C)	Mean (°C)
Chirundu					
January .	32·1	36·6	22·0	20·0	26·6
July	28·6	32·7	11·7	7·2	19·8
October .	38·6	41·7	23·2	18·3	30·4
Gatooma					
January .	27·9	31·6	17·5	13·9	21·9
July	23·5	27·7	7·8	3·9	15·1
October .	31·9	35·6	16·4	12·2	24·0

† Recalculated from Phillips, Hammond, Samuels, and Swynnerton (1962).

sufficient to kill the majority of *G. morsitans* at any relative humidity. Three hours' exposure would kill all of them. The pupa could not survive three hours' exposure to a temperature of $-10°C$ or the adult the same period at $-5°C$. At $-10°C$ the adult flies were almost immobilized. (For a useful summary of this and other related studies see Glasgow 1963a.) Jack (1939) also noticed that the historical fly-line he had reconstructed followed fairly closely the 67°F (19·4°C) mean annual isotherm. He tentatively suggested that this isotherm marked the natural limit imposed by climate on dispersal of *G. morsitans*.

Bursell (1960) suggested that the controlling factor might be the length of time during the year at which mean temperature is below 16°C. During its development in the maternal uterus, the tsetse larva builds up reserves of 'fat' (chloroform-soluble lipids) which constitute the sole source of energy available for development of the pupa, for its metamorphosis into the pharate adult, for emergence, and for use in flight and other activities leading to the encounter with the first food host. Anything that affects the amount of fat used during development will influence the energy resources of the newly emerged insect and hence its chance of obtaining its first blood meal. The proportion of fat to other tissues (residual dry weight) in teneral flies that had emerged from puparia incubated at 24·9°C rose with increasing residual dry weight: the bigger the fly the higher the proportion of fat it contained. In addition, the mean size of *G. morsitans* and the proportion of fat in newly emerged flies was greatest when development had taken place at about 24°C. At temperatures lower, or higher, than this optimum, size and fat content diminished comparatively rapidly. It had been shown previously that when the fat content of teneral flies was reduced beyond 4·4 per cent of the total dry weight, survival was impossible and eclosion could not take place (Bursell 1959).

At 16°C the pupal period is just over three months. At this temperature some of the smallest pupae would have insufficient fat left to complete their development, and of those that did emerge the energy reserves left to them would be inadequate to ensure obtaining the first blood meal. Similarly, on the other side of the optimum for development, at about 32°C, when the pupal period is only just over 18 days, the same results will obtain because with a high metabolic rate fat is over-consumed. In areas where winters lasted for three months or more with mean temperatures below 16°C, *G. morsitans* could not survive in sufficient numbers to ensure their full replacement in the next generation. Similarly, a geographical limit would be imposed where continuous periods of about three weeks occurred with mean temperatures over 32°C.

Rajagopal and Bursell (1965) modified these conclusions. Bursell (1960) had supposed that the rate of fat consumption by the pupa was linearly related to temperature. Measurement of the rate of consumption of oxygen by the pupa during development, which also provides a measure of the rate at which fat is consumed, showed this to be untrue. The relationship between respiratory rate and development temperatures was not rectilinear and both at higher and at lower temperatures oxygen consumption tended to be slower than at the intermediate optimum. Extrapolations that assumed a rectilinear relationship therefore gave estimates of metabolic rate that were too great both at higher and lower temperatures. Nevertheless the principle established in the earlier paper, that the physiological basis of geographical limitation to dispersal of *Glossina* could be related to the rate of exhaustion of pupal nutrition reserves at low and at high temperatures, still remained unassailed.

The choice of sites by female tsetse in which to deposit their larvae varies from season to season and tends to ensure that the pupae are not subjected to extremes of temperature. The data provided by standard meteorological stations do not, therefore, necessarily show the conditions of climate experienced by the tsetse during this phase of its existence. It has recently been shown that temperatures in *G. morsitans* larviposition sites tend to be lower than screen temperatures, but the correlation values are high so that a good estimate of average pupal site temperature can be obtained from screen data. It appeared from the same study that in climates that showed mean monthly air temperatures ranging from 17°C to 35°C, female tsetse would be able to find a sufficient variety of larviposition sites to achieve tolerable conditions for their offspring (Jackson and Phelps 1967).

Table 17·2 was compiled from *Rhodesian climatological tables* (1952). It includes two places, Salisbury and Chipinga, that obviously have climates too cold to support tsetse and two, Triangle and Chirundu, that never approach even a marginally cold climate. Both lie within the historical fly-

TABLE 17.2

Critical winter temperature in Rhodesia for G. morsitans

Station	Mean annual temperature (°C)	Months in which means fall below:								No. of years recorded	No. of years in which 3 months were below 16°C mean
		16°C			17°C						
Salisbury . .	18·52	6	7	8	5	6	7	8		19	19
Chipinga . .	18·67	6	7	8	5	6	7	8		17	17
Mtoko . .	19·51	6	7			6	7	8		17	13
Miami† . .	19·52	6	7			6	7	8		17	14
Plumtree . .	19·65	6	7			6	7	8		16	12
Karoi† . .	19·67	6	7			6	7			9	3
Gatooma† .	19·71	6	7			6	7			18	7
Umtali . .	19·72	6	7			6	7			18	7
Gokwe† . .	19·72		7			6	7			17	1
Sinoia . .	19·75	6	7	8		6	7	8		19	18
Hartley† . .	19·79	6	7			6	7	8		17	14
Sipolilo† . .	19·83	6	7			6	7	8		17	12
Queque† . .	19·97	6	7			6	7	8		17	13
Bikita . .	20·05	6	7			6	7			15	8
New Year's Gift†	20·36	6	7			6	7			14	5
Mt. Darwin† .	20·58	6	7			6	7	8		17	13
Gwaai Siding .	21·09	6	7			6	7			14	11
Nuanetsi† .	22·02	6	7			6	7			17	4
Triangle† .	22·47	—			—					—	—
Chirundu† .	25·65	—			—					—	—

† Places on or within the historically known limits of *G. morsitans* distribution.

line. The remaining 16 stations have mean annual temperatures that are slightly above Jack's (1939) 19·4°C limit. All lie close to the historical line, and those that, before the rinderpest, lay within the tsetse belts are indicated. Of these 16 marginal stations only one, Sinoia, just outside the historically known limits of tsetse, has three consecutive months with mean temperature under 16°C. However, 8 of them show three-month winters with mean temperatures below 17°C. A safer index may be obtained by noting the number of years, out of the total for which records exist, that had three consecutive months showing mean temperatures of 16°C or less. Six stations showed fewer than half the years with three-month winter seasons under 16°C. Of these, 5, Karoi, Gatooma, Gokwe, New Year's Gift, and Nuanetsi lay within the old tsetse line. Bikita did not; but it will be observed in Chapter 19 that Bikita lies in a Shona refuge area and that during both the Ngoni and European invasions, human population here might have remained sufficiently dense to exclude tsetse. Of the remaining 10 stations, each with more than half its recorded years too cold, by Bursell's (1960) criterion, for *G. morsitans*, 5 lie outside and 5 within the historical line. Among the latter is Miami about which Jack (1939) remarked that although cattle were constantly infected there, it was probably too cold for tsetse breeding. Its altitude just lifts it above the surrounding tolerable environment (Map 17.2).

The historical tsetse line is an approximation only, so that there is little to be gained by discussion about individual marginal stations. In any event, the observations of Rajagopal and Bursell (1965) can be interpreted to mean that as environmental conditions move towards critical temperature thresholds a physiological adjustment of the metabolic rate takes place. This adjustment would have the effect of enlarging the area in which tsetse could survive. It is unlikely that this would be detectable within the limits of accuracy of the present inquiry. Three areas, however, deserve comment. Mtoko may have fallen into the same category as Bikita. It was a place that throughout the troubled second half of the last century maintained a sufficiently large human population to exclude *G. morsitans*.

There remains the third, and most striking, discrepancy between the historical line and the supposed critical annual isotherm, in the country north and west of Bulawayo. Agreement is good from Mt. Darwin southwest to Queque. Here the two lines diverge. The isotherm continues in a south-westerly direction along the northern face of the Rhodesian high veld to Plumtree, but the former tsetse boundary turns due west, more or less along the line of 19°S. The two divergent lines meet the western border of Rhodesia and with it form a triangle which coincides very well with the limits of distribution of the Kalahari sands in that country. Especially associated with these sands is a woodland locally known as *gusu*, dominated by the large tree, *Baikiaea plurijuga*. In some localities the Kalahari sands also support mopane, *Colophospermum mopane*, woodland. The *gusu* areas were recognized by Eminson (1915) and by Jack (1927) as unfavourable to *G. morsitans*. Buxton (1955) thought that possibly the limiting factor on the Kalahari sands was soil humidity. He found support for this view in the fact that in the centre of the main Kalahari sand area in these latitudes, the only area of tsetse infestation lay in the Okovango swamps of Botswana. It is more probable that the limiting factor is low winter temperature. Vincent, Thomas, Anderson, and Staples (n.d.) write that, 'In general sandy soils cool more rapidly than clayey soils. For this reason the incidence of frost is higher on the Kalahari sands which have the lowest clay content of all Rhodesian soils.' Temperature records are available only at Gwaai Siding where the mean annual temperature is 21·09°C. On Jack's criterion Gwaai Siding should be well inside the historical tsetse line. But in spite of its high mean annual temperature it nevertheless had 11 out of the 14 recorded years that showed a three-month winter with temperatures below 16°C. It is clear that an isopleth drawn to fit Bursell's definition would avoid the discrepancy in Jack's line caused by the Kalahari sands (Map 17.2; compare also Map 20.1).

One field experiment supports, if it does not prove, the hypothesis that cold, through its effect on pupal development, is the principal limiting factor in Rhodesian tsetse distribution. Goodier (1958) removed the trees from the banks of a stream draining a small valley with a high density of *G. morsitans* not many miles from its supposed climatic limit of distribution. This population of tsetse disappeared during the winter following the tree felling. The mean daily range of temperature during the winter in a nearby untouched area was 22°C, but where the trees had been removed the range was 27°C and brought night temperatures down to 0°C. An objection to the obvious conclusion was that disappearance of the tsetse population coincided also with the arrival of immigrant settlers into the valley.

Behavioural adjustment to hot climates

The mean October temperature at Chirundu in the floor of the Zambezi valley is 30·4°C (Table 17.1). Here the climate cannot be far removed from the critical condition in which a mean of 32°C for just under three weeks must lead to reproductive failure. Moreover, air shade temperatures exceeding 40°C are commonly recorded in standard meteorological screens so that the mature insects could hardly survive unless they could escape to cooler places. At Rekomitje, not far from Chirundu, *G. pallidipes*, during most of the year, rests after feeding on the undersides of branches of small trees and shrubs in riverine forests at heights between 3 and 9 ft. In the hot season, however, these sites are only occupied in the mornings and late afternoons. Towards midday, when the air temperature rises to 35°C and over, branch sites are evacuated. Flies can now be found at rest only on the boles of large trees, where they squeeze into the fissures of the bark, at heights generally less than one foot from the ground, or else hide in rot holes in big tree trunks, often quite high up. At these times they will not feed, even from a bait animal in the shade (Pilson and Leggate 1962a, b).

The mechanism of this behaviour was studied by Jack and Williams (1937). They kept *G. morsitans* in a cabinet, half of which was illuminated and half heavily shaded. When they heated the cabinet to 30°C the flies began to move into the darkened half and at 35°C were all in the dark. When temperature reached 40°C the flies moved into the corners of the dark part of the cabinet and crouched as close as they could to its walls. In doing this they were simulating the behaviour of wild flies that, on hot afternoons, creep into the deep crevices of the bark of big tree trunks. Professor E. B. Edney used small thermocouples to measure resting site temperatures. He showed that had the flies, in the afternoons of the hot season, used the branches that they rested on in the afternoons of cooler seasons and in the mornings and evenings of the hot, they would have exposed themselves, even though in the shade, to mean temperatures of 39·6°C between the hours of noon and 4.30 p.m. At this temperature the majority of them would have died. As it was, in the bark crevices mean temperatures did not go above 38·3°C, and in the rot hole 36·3°C (Ford 1962). Edney and Barrass (1962) also demonstrated the existence of a physiological escape mechanism which could come into play if the search for heavily shaded cool sites were to fail. When the circumambient temperature of the tsetse rises above 39°C they open all their spiracles and reduce their own body temperature by as much as 1·66°C when the air temperature has reached 45°C. Obviously, since flies die in one hour at 40°C, this device could not operate for long. The actual temperature that Edney measured in the refuge sites showed that their use evidently obviated the need for it to operate at Rekomitje.

Pilson and Pilson (1967) studied the resting behaviour of *G. morsitans* in another part of the Zambezi fly-belt. It had been an accepted doctrine that in very hot weather the leafless mopane woodlands were evacuated by the tsetse, which concentrated along the rivers where evergreen trees still provided shade. But when these workers took bait oxen into the mopane and watched throughout the day, they found that soon after dawn and also towards sunset flies came readily to feed, but ignored the bait ox during the hours of hot bright sunlight. This cessation of all activity is another protective device against the rigours of a climate that would otherwise be insupportable. Rajagopal and Bursell (1966) have shown that at Chirundu reserves of food that would allow a tsetse at rest to survive for 24 h in the cool season would suffice for less than 5 h in the hot. The need for immobility in adequately protected resting sites is evidently crucial. In the mopane woodlands, where there is little shade from vegetation save in bark crevices and rot holes, Pilson and Pilson (1967) found that much use was made of burrows used by warthogs. By placing nets over these holes during the day they were able to catch the tsetse as they emerged for the evening period of activity. The belief that the tsetse evacuated the mopane woodlands in the hot weather grew from the failure of survey parties to attract following swarms of males (Chapter 2) during normal working hours. In the Zambezi fly-belt, near Chirundu, in the early part of the dry season of 1964, when the rivers were dry but the weather was still cool, the puparia of *G. morsitans* could be sifted from the loose river-bed sand in large numbers. But in October, when the air temperature was high, riverine sites were no longer used and puparia were found under heavily shaded logs, in rot holes, and, especially, in burrows such as shelter antbears and warthogs. When the rains come and the trees burst into leaf and the grasses grow again, it becomes difficult to find puparia. They are much more randomly scattered because the females no longer are compelled to rest in places where they can escape the adverse effects of the sun (cf. Jackson and Phelps 1967).

Nature of the climatic limit

The limits imposed by climate upon dispersal of tsetse populations are evidently very complex. In the neighbourhood of the historical fly-line, the good fit with expectation derived from Bursell's 1960 paper suggests that even with the aid of physiological adjustment of metabolic rate to extremes of temperature (Rajagopal and Bursell 1965) life expectancy is shortened by the deaths of smaller flies that have emerged from the puparium insufficiently provided with energy reserves to enable them to obtain their first meal. It is probable that similar limitations are or were imposed in the hot seasons in parts of the Sabi and Limpopo valleys. At Beitbridge, on the Limpopo, at one time within the limits of *G. morsitans* distribution, the lowest minima in July are lower than at Gatooma, but in October highest maxima are almost as high as at Chirundu and the hot season persists longer. In such areas, where the search for the first blood meal is a critical event, the actual geographical limit of survival of tsetse must also be determined by the density of natural host populations. The bigger the populations of natural hosts, the greater the opportunity for feeding in the short interval available. But it is in the nature of a *Grenzwildnis* that confronting the fly-belt there is a human population and this, depending upon its density and social habits, affects the density of the host animals. In most of Rhodesia, therefore, where men are known to have produced a series of comparatively highly developed societies, tsetses may never have reached their natural limits during a thousand years up to the time of disaster in the nineteenth century.

Similar considerations must apply to subsequent blood meals. It is evident that hot season survival depends upon the discovery, in limited time, of adequately protective resting sites. The male fly that has burned up most of its available proline in a following swarm in the wake of a moving bait and, in doing so, has been carried into an area supporting vegetation in which protective resting sites are rare, may not survive the afternoon high temperature. If the habitat of an organism is the sum total of the places in which it actually lives then climate acts by reducing habitat size. As temperatures rise higher or sink lower, so the time available to find food or suitable parts of the habitat to carry out essential items of behaviour, like larviposition, becomes more and more restricted and life expectancy is reduced to the point at which the female no longer can achieve a reproductive rate high enough to ensure her own replacement.

Bursell (1969) has pointed out that if considerations of this kind are correct it should not be necessary to eliminate the whole population of natural hosts in order to achieve elimination of tsetse. But clearly, also, the level of reduction of host population density necessary to achieve elimination of tsetse will vary according to the potential of the latter to survive long enough to find the next meal. The rate of consumption of food reserves is balanced against the rate at which they must be replenished. As the habitat becomes more and more restricted, survival, firstly of the newly emerged teneral fly, and then of the mature adult, must depend upon a compensatory increase in host availability. It has, in fact, proved difficult to extend the Rhodesian game slaughter techniques into some warmer areas. The 10 000 mile^2 of the Zambezi valley that were reclaimed from tsetse between 1930 and 1950 lie along the cool, outer fringe of the fly-belt. In 1940 another section of the *G. morsitans* fly-belt, that had been expanding in Mozambique, overflowed the border into the Sabi river valley in the south-west of Rhodesia. The usual organization was set up to destroy the game animal population in the path of the spreading tsetse. It failed to halt it.

This failure was in part due to the fact that temperatures in the Sabi valley were, on the average, closer to optimal than were those in the areas of successful reclamation on the periphery of the Zambezi belt. More animals had to be destroyed to reduce the probability of host encounter to a critical level. However, another difficulty was that, because of the remoteness and generally inhospitable environment of the lower Sabi valley, it was much more difficult than in the north to recruit a force of hunters sufficient to produce an equivalent rate of animal destruction (Federal Ministry of Agriculture 1960). The boundary of tsetse distribution is determined by the intensity of the human attack. It is sometimes claimed by propagandists that this method of control of destruction of the fauna sometimes fails. The failure is solely due to the difficulties of destroying enough animals to prolong the period of search for a host beyond the critical level.

The Great Rinderpest

The rinderpest of 1889–96 was a far more efficient destroyer of tsetse hosts than the corps of hunters later recruited by the Rhodesian government to reproduce its effects. When intensive shooting of wildlife on a large scale began at least one contemporary observer of the panzootic argued ineffectively against it. Stevenson-Hamilton (1912) pointed out that the tsetse recession after the panzootic was not necessarily due to destruction of the wild game for, in fact, many animals had not been affected by it. If the removal of their natural hosts had caused tsetse to disappear it must be because they were dependent upon those species that died of rinderpest and that they were unable to survive on those species not affected by it. This argument failed to impress the advocates of game destruction, but it was correct.

The animals listed by Stevenson-Hamilton as having suffered most severely from rinderpest were buffalo, eland, kudu, bushbuck, reedbuck, duiker, and 'all the horned ruminants possessing a large moist rhinarium'. Warthogs and bushpigs also died in large numbers. Sable and roan antelope, wildebeest, impala, and 'others possessing a partially hairy rhinarium' appeared to have been much less affected.

Percival (1918), another contemporary observer, wrote that in the Transvaal the greater kudu were wiped out. He also described the disease in Kenya. Infection first appeared in domestic cattle but soon passed to buffalo and eland. Giraffe died in large numbers. Greater and lesser kudu, wildebeest, roan, and bushbuck suffered severely, but the gazelles (presumably Grant's and Thompson's), zebra, elephant, rhinoceros, and hippopotamus were immune. The remains of the carcasses of buffalo and wildebeest were still to be seen along the river banks on the Athi plains near Nairobi in 1902.

All sorts of pigs suffered from rinderpest.

In South Africa I saw my first bushpig, dead—not one but many; and in B.E.A. [Kenya] the outbreaks among warthog have been numerous. In fact it is almost certain that if rinderpest breaks out, the warthog will get it—even when there are no records of the disease amongst other game—and I look upon them as a distinct cause in spreading the disease. Without doubt the game, and also the local cattle, have developed to some extent an immunity against the disease; yet the warthog does not appear to have done so (Percival 1918).

Carmichael (1938) reviewed current knowledge of rinderpest in African game animals. Buffalo, giraffe, eland, bushpig, and warthog were listed as highly susceptible. Reedbuck, wildebeest, kudu, and giant forest hog were also susceptible. Bushbuck and situtunga were generally highly susceptible, but in some outbreaks only slightly so. Kob were similarly classified. The response of impala, oribi, and duiker was variable. Roan, waterbuck, hartebeest, and topi were either not susceptible, or only slightly so. Elephant, rhinoceros, and hippopotamus were never affected. Simmons and Carmichael (1940) noted that buffalo, warthog, bushpig, and bushbuck were the species most commonly implicated in the spread of rinderpest, but that situtunga, eland, reedbuck, giant forest hog, and kob all, on occasion, played a part in outbreaks. As an example of the varied response to presence of the virus they note that kob died in large numbers in Buganda in 1915–16, but did not suffer during an epizootic in the West Nile district of Uganda in 1925.

There is not always complete agreement, but all three authorities include the favoured hosts of *Glossina* among the animals that suffered severely from rinderpest.

The three groups of highly susceptible, variably susceptible, and non-susceptible species, as they appear from these early observations, and the host preferences of the savanna-dwelling tsetse flies revealed by Weitz's analyses (1963), are compared in Table 17.3. *G. fuscipleuris* is included with the east and southern group because there is evidence that before the rinderpest it was to be found south of the Zambezi river (Santos Dias, 1962).

Table 17.3 is condensed in Table 17.4. Animals highly susceptible to

TABLE 17.3

Positive blood meals analysed by Weitz (1963) arranged according to susceptibility to rinderpest in early epizootics

Host	Susceptibility to rinderpest†			East and southern							West		
	H	V	N	G. swynnertoni	G. austeni	G. fuscipleuris	G. morsitans	G. morsitans 'orientalis'	G. pallidipes	Totals	G. m. sub-morsitans	G. longipalpis	Totals
Suidae													
warthog	3			3179	—	2	929	487	430	5027	493	1	494
bushpig	3			52	188	175	78	77	305	875	7	33	40
giant forest hog	1			—	—	90	—	—	—	90	—	—	—
Giraffidae													
giraffe	2			417	—	—	46	15	10	488	4	—	4
Bovidae													
buffalo	3			386	4	12	318	39	180	939	53	142	195
kudu	3			2	6	—	139	413	9	569	5	—	5
eland	3			67	1	—	77	46	4	195	3	—	3
bushbuck	3	1		5	4	9	87	25	1099	1229	51	649	700
reedbuck	2	1		1	—	—	81	15	10	107	1	—	1
duiker	1	1		9	29	—	32	8	2	80	5	10	15
oribi	1	1	2	—	—	—	—	—	—	—	12	—	12
roan/sable	1		1	34	—	—	35	3	18	90	38	—	38
impala		1	1	25	—	—	9	2	—	36	1	—	1
waterbuck			2	1	—	—	14	1	1	17	—	—	—
hartebeest		1	1	9	—	—	—	—	1	10	21	—	21
gazelle			1	1	—	—	1	—	1	3	—	—	—
Other mammals													
elephant	1		1	45	1	—	32	219	28	325	2	2	4
rhinoceros			1	140	—	—	43	46	13	242	20	—	20
hippopotamus			1	—	—	79	41	—	14	134	—	—	—
miscellaneous spp.	—	?	—	50	1	1	65	52	5	174	74	4	78
Reptiles	—	—	—	9	—	—	10	1	5	25	8	—	8
Birds	—	—	—	64	—	—	26	23	7	120	69	2	71
Domestic livestock	—	—	—	40	56	55	369	83	38	641	18	15	33
Man	—	—	—	162	18	2	305	95	62	644	198	14	212
Totals				4698	308	425	2737	1650	2242	12060	1083	872	1955

TABLE 17.4

Susceptibility to rinderpest of the hosts of East and West African tsetse flies

Susceptibility to rinderpest	East African species		West African species	
	Total blood meals	%	Total blood meals	%
Highly susceptible				
Suids	5992	49·68	534	27·31
Bovids	3527	29·25	908	46·44
Variable susceptibility				
Bovids	206	1·71	66	3·38
Non-susceptible				
Bovids	30	0·25	21	1·07
Other mammals . .	875	7·26	102	5·22
Reptiles	25	0·21	8	0·41
Birds	120	0·99	71	3·63
Man and domestic stock .	1285	10·66	245	12·52
Total	12060	100·01	1955	99·99

rinderpest account for 78–93 per cent of tsetse feeds among the East African species listed, and 73–75 per cent in the two West African species. Wild bovids of variable susceptibility (duiker, oribi, roan, sable, and impala) are of trivial importance, and species not affected, waterbuck, hartebeest, and the gazelles (to which may be added zebra which have never appeared among tsetse blood meals) of none at all. Elephants, rhinoceros, and hippopotamus are not susceptible to rinderpest and are fed on readily by *Glossina*. However, elephants living in savanna vegetation are too mobile to support permanent populations of tsetse, or, alternatively, if confined, tend to destroy their habitat, which is also the habitat of *Glossina*. Rhinoceros may indeed have been important hosts in the years immediately after the panzootic and conceivably may have contributed greatly to survival of small fly-belts such as Jack (1914) described on the Manzituba *vlei*. Hippopotamus may have performed a similar function along parts of the Zambezi, for around the lakes of south-east Ankole they displace warthog as the favoured host, although the latter prevailed outside the grazing limits of the hippos (Glasgow, Isherwood, Lee-Jones, and Weitz 1958). But these large animals, because of their localized habits or because of their mobility, could not have supported *G. morsitans* or *G. pallidipes* over wide areas. When, therefore, Stevenson-Hamilton asked whether the fly disappeared because of the practical extinction of the animals which suffered most from the rinderpest, the answer is quite evidently 'Yes'. Of course, they did not cease to exist everywhere. In some places they never recovered (e.g. giraffe north of Lake George in Uganda or buffalo in the Shinyanga and Nindo bush in Sukumaland) but in most of the savanna country they did so remarkably rapidly.

Recovery of the Rhodesian fly-belts

Glossina morsitans disappeared from the Limpopo valley and from much of the Zambezi valley in 1895–6. Within Rhodesia it was known to have survived in five foci which were studied between 1910 and 1913. By 1913 the largest of these fly-belts had been surveyed on various occasions and Jack was able to reconstruct its growth from the small focus in which it had remained around a small *vlei* at Manzituba. In this work he was helped by an administrative officer whose station, Kariangwe, became engulfed in the

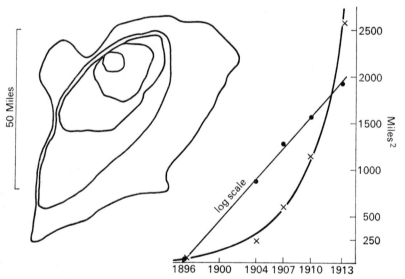

FIG. 17.1. Outlines of the Sebungwe *G. morsitans* belt between 1896 and 1913 from Jack (1914). The area increased geometrically over the 17-year period. (cf. Map 17.2).

fly-belt between 1907 and 1910. The successive outlines for 1904, 1907, 1910, and 1913, with a hypothetical outline around the *vlei* for 1896, were published by Jack (1914) and are reproduced in Fig. 17.1 in which the growth rate of the fly-belt is also plotted. The increase in area of the belt was virtually a geometric one at 28·2 per cent per annum. This rapid expansion reflects the unimpeded growth of the recovering host populations with unlimited fodder and largely free of their normal parasite burden.

Although Jack's 1913 map of the various fly-belts by then located in the Zambezi valley may have been incomplete, and some small foci remained unidentified, he was able to point to a good deal of negative evidence for the absence of *G. morsitans* over large areas that later became infested and which were known to have been infested before the rinderpest. Police patrols in the Zambezi valley habitually were mounted on horseback while cattle were imported from areas north of the Zambezi to replenish stock lost during the rinderpest. This traffic continued until 1914. Chorley (1947*a*) summarized Jack's work and published a map in which the limits reached by the expanding *G. morsitans* belt in 1930 are compared with Jack's 1913 map. By this time the infestation within the Southern Rhodesian portion of the Zambezi valley occupied 21 000 mile^2 and the residual belts originally surveyed by Jack had all coalesced. By 1930 the fly-belt was expanding at a rate of 1000 mile^2 a year.

18

CATTLE TRYPANOSOMIASIS IN RHODESIA

THE first veterinary surgeon to enter Rhodesia came with the pioneer column sent by Cecil Rhodes in 1890. In 1893 legislation was enacted for the registration of livestock and a cadre of inspectors was engaged. The rinderpest panzootic led to the appointment of a controller of stock and establishment of a small veterinary staff which was enlarged as epizootics of glanders in 1898, contagious bovine pleuropneumonia and ulcerative lymphaginitis in 1900, East coast fever in 1901, and foot and mouth disease in 1903 appeared in succession (Phillips, Hammond, Samuels, and Swynnerton 1962). East coast fever was controlled and eventually was eliminated by a vigorously applied programme of dipping. But there were other tick-borne piroplasms and compulsory dipping continued. All African-owned cattle are dipped twice a month. Herds from a number of neighbouring kraals, usually between one and two thousand head, meet at the dip on an appointed day and on these occasions are seen by a government veterinarian or an animal health inspector.

Each stock owner has a registration card which records the size of his herd and the village to which he belongs. Failure to produce cattle may result in prosecution. A count of all animals is made and reasons for change are noted, i.e. deaths, losses, sales, etc. Appropriate diagnostic material is collected from any animal showing obvious clinical signs of disease. If trypanosomiasis is suspected, blood slides (thin and thick films) are taken from about 10 per cent of the herd, although if clinical illness is widespread smears may be taken from the whole herd.

Slides are returned to the district veterinary laboratory where, according to the results of the examination, an appropriate treatment is decided upon. Drugs are administered usually within the next two weeks. If infection is not heavy treatment is confined to those herds in which it is seen. If it is widespread then a block inoculation of all animals attending the dip may be undertaken.

The Sabi epizootics

Trypanosome infections were found in May 1952 at the dipping inspection centre of Mwangazi (Map 18.1) in the centre of the Chipinga district on the eastern border of Rhodesia. Along the northern portion of the Chipinga border, cattle trypanosomiasis had been known for many years. There the disease is controlled by a large clearing that prevents the spread of tsetse into the Chipinga highlands, an area for the most part near the altitude limit of tsetse survival, between 3000 and 4000 ft above sea level. Tsetses present are *Glossina pallidipes*, *G. brevipalpis*, *G. austeni*, and, very occasionally, *G. morsitans*. The fly-belt from which they are derived was described by Swynnerton (1921) and by Pires, Marques da Silva, and Teles e Cunha (1950).

Mwangazi lies at the northern end of the semi-arid southern half of Chipinga district, below 2000 ft above sea level. Rainfall in the highlands is over 40 in per annum. Less than 10 miles away, in the Sabi valley floor, it averages 12–16 in only (Vincent, Thomas, Anderson, and Staples n.d.). In the highlands temperatures average about 18·5°C, with October mean maxima rising to 27°C and July mean minima falling to 12°C. In the Sabi valley mean annual temperatures may reach 25°C, with mean maxima rising to 35°C in October but in July occasional ground frosts occur.

Twenty miles to the south of Mwangazi and 10 years earlier cattle had suffered severely from trypanosomiasis in the remote and scarcely administered neighbourhood of the junction of the Sabi and Lundi rivers. The survivors were moved into tsetse-free areas further north (Chorley 1943–7). *G. morsitans* was found on the Portuguese side within 10 miles of the border and a protective shooting operation was started in 1940. It was quite ineffective (Federal Ministry of Agriculture 1960).

The infections at Mwangazi in May and at a neighbouring centre, Muumbe, in August 1952 were also due to the spread and closer approach of *G. morsitans* and *G. pallidipes* from another sector of the Mozambique fly-front. Map 18.1 shows several centres on the Sabi river, some of which receive infection from the southern area of tsetse encroachment. Infected centres in the highlands are also included. Some of these acquired their trypanosomiases from the high-level fly-belts as well as from the new focus near Mwangazi. For five of them, Upper and Lower Umsilizwe, Lettie Swan, Busi, and Nyamadzi, data are given by Cockbill (1960a). These five centres were not involved in the Sabi epizootics.

In 1952 and 1953 no specific diagnoses were made and a co-ordinated plan of control had still to be developed. The numbers of the infected herds at Mwangazi and Muumbe were reduced, in these two years, by 325 head. In 1955 there was a spread of infection to ten more centres. Over 20 000 head of African-owned cattle were now at risk of infection in the low-level pastures of the Sabi. Trypanosomes were found for the first time in livestock on the European-owned Humani ranch on the west bank of the river. But by now diagnostic procedures had been greatly improved and 20 667 doses of dimidium bromide were administered in June 1955. In October the majority of these same cattle received 15 878 injections of the new prophylactic drug, antrycide pro-salt.

During the period of the Sabi epizootics the drug manufacturers marketed an increasing number of powerful and sometimes dangerous drugs which veterinarians all over Africa had to learn how to administer.

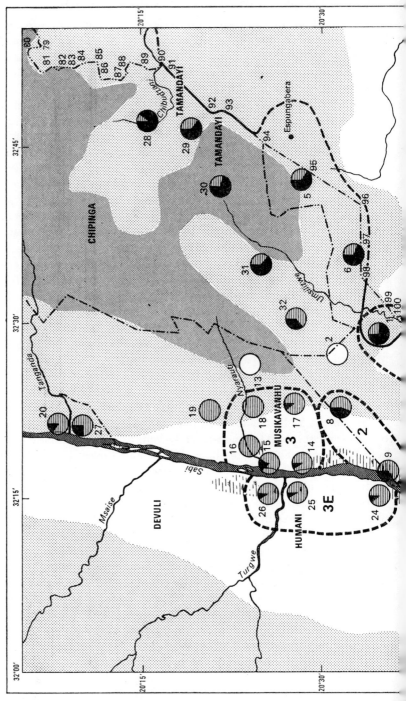

MAP 18.1. Cattle inspection centres in the Sabi river valley, Rhodesia, pr

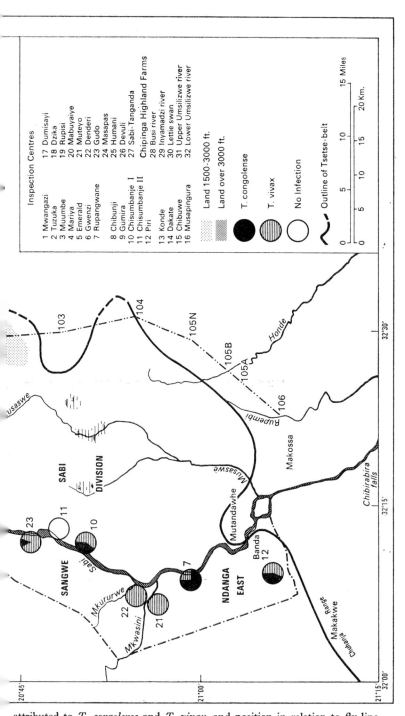

attributed to *T. congolense* and *T. vivax*, and position in relation to fly-line.

After the first massive administration of antrycide pro-salt in the Sabi valley in 1955 many cattle died from its toxic effects. This was due to failure to rest them after the injection before beginning the walk home. Such events led to the extension of recording systems, so that in areas where it became necessary to maintain an intensive drug administration service, stock owners' registration cards carried details of deaths (both by slaughter and other causes), removals by sale, etc., births and additions by other means, as well as blood smears examined, diagnoses, and treatments given.

The patterns of infection

The use of the *vivax* ratio was described in Chapter 5. Its significance in the Sabi epizootics is clarified if the inspection centres are divided into three groups. Group (1) includes the centres Mwangazi, Muumbe, and Mariya; from 1954 to 1962 these centres gave 30·8 per cent of *Trypanosoma vivax* infections, the remaining 69·2 per cent diagnosed specifically being attributed to *T. congolense*. Group (2) yielded 59·6 per cent *T. vivax*, and Group (3) 91·8 per cent in African cattle east of the Sabi, and 92·5 per cent in European ranch cattle on the other side of the river, Group (3E). The locations of these groups are shown on Map 18.1. Other centres either showed transient infections or were clearly associated with other foci of infection.

The infections recorded every two months in each of the three groups are shown in Fig. 18.1. In 1954–5, before administration of dimidium, Group (1) centres showed 38·9 per cent of *T. vivax*, Group (2) showed 53·4 and Group (3) only 20 per cent. The inoculations halted the epizootic, and the continuation of two- or three-monthly treatments of the Group (1) cattle with the prophylactic antrycide pro-salt not only suppressed infection in those cattle grazing close to the fly-belts, but also, apparently, stopped spread of trypanosomes into the more distant Group (2) and Group (3) cattle. The latter received no treatment in 1956 and 1957 and showed no signs of disease, except for a single *T. congolense* infection in the European ranch cattle west of the Sabi in May 1956.

Because of this freedom from infection it was judged that whatever agent had conveyed trypanosomes to the Groups (2) and (3) cattle in 1954–5, it was no longer active and after September 1957 the prophylactic treatments in Group (1) cattle were stopped. Nothing happened until March 1958 when one *T. congolense* infection was found at Muumbe; but in April trypanosomes were found in herds at various centres in all three groups. For the remainder of 1958, during the latter half of which the cattle west of the Sabi also became infected (though no specific diagnoses were made), treatments in Groups (1) and (2) were on a herd basis. Herds in which one or more infections were found received treatment, others did not. This was not effective in controlling the epizootic in the Group (1)

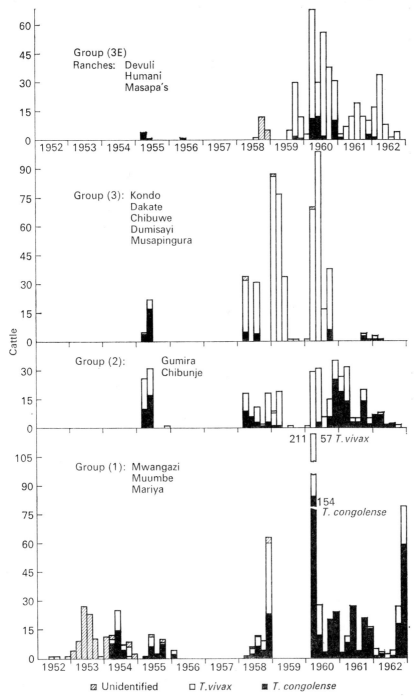

FIG. 18.1. Bi-monthly infection totals in cattle in the Sabi river valley.

herds and the number of infections of both *T. congolense* and *T. vivax* continued to rise until December when block treatments were resumed. In April and again in August 1958 there were two heavy outbreaks in Group (3) cattle, with *T. congolense* in only 14 per cent of cases, the remainder all being attributed to *T. vivax*. The second outbreak was suppressed by two block treatments with antrycide methyl sulphate. In January 1959 Group (3) cattle again suffered widespread infection but now with *T. vivax* alone. This was extinguished by the same means in April. Meanwhile the Group (1) centres adjacent to the fly-belt were kept free of patent infection throughout 1959 by block treatments with the same drug every two months.

In the second half of 1959, throughout the 15 000 cattle involved east of the Sabi only 4 infections were seen; but among the European cattle west of the river, infection continued to spread in spite of close supervision and continued herd treatments.

One obvious explanation was that tsetse were filtering across the Sabi valley from the fly-belts along the Mozambique border, their passage masked by the protective effects of the block inoculations. To test this, injections were stopped after the treatments in December 1959. The response, in March 1960, was startling. Six hundred and fifty-two cattle among the total of 5478 at the Group (1) centres were smeared and yielded 156 *T. congolense* and 55 *T. vivax* infections. In the next month widespread infection, all of *T. vivax* appeared among the Group (3) cattle and continued to increase in May and June, while in April the highest incidence so far seen was recorded on the European ranches. Finally, 17 miles north of the infected area, cattle at Mabuyaiye showed 1 *T. congolense* and 5 *T vivax* infections in February and March.

No tsetse flies could be found except in the Group (1) area close to the Mozambique border. The entomologist-in-charge reported that some indication of the laborious nature of survey work in the area was given by the fact that about 750 patrols with bait cattle were carried out before both *G. morsitans* and *G. pallidipes* were found near Mwangazi in 1960 (Goodier 1961a). In this year also it was decided to assume that *Glossina* had, indeed, crossed the Sabi. In August and September6 225 gal of 3·6 per cent dieldrin were sprayed on 13 700 acres of presumed tsetse habitat on the Humani and Devuli ranches. Infections declined, but did not disappear.

This attack on an unseen vector was of necessity empirical. The drug campaign, too, was carried out without full knowledge of what might be its consequences. One of the earliest experiments on the field use of antrycide was that of Fiennes (1953) who demonstrated that if the drug was administered in dosages that were too small, strains of trypanosomes developed that were no longer responsive to it. The same effect, of course, might be obtained when treatments to cattle in high risk areas were stopped. They would continue to be subject to repeated inoculation by tsetse bite of new strains of trypanosomes which would find themselves in a blood environment with diminishing concentrations of the drug. By this time another drug, berenil, had become available. It was supposed to have no residual prophylactic effect, but possessed the valuable property of being able to kill trypanosomes that had ceased to respond to antrycide.

Group (1) cattle, after a preliminary inoculation with berenil to eliminate drug-resistant trypanosomes, were put back on prophylactic treatment with antrycide pro-salt. Elsewhere berenil was used for treatment of infected herds, except that in June 1960 and in May 1961 block treatments with antrycide methyl sulphate were given to the Group (2) cattle at Chibunje and Gumira.

In one respect these empirical treatments were very successful. Mortality from trypanosomiasis had been relatively heavy in the Mwangazi and Muumbe cattle in the first three years of the epizootic, when infection

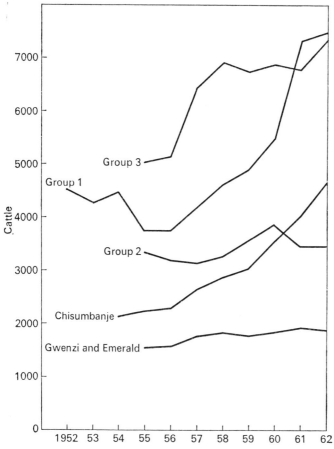

FIG. 18.2. Growth of populations of different infection groups of cattle involved in the Sabi river valley epizootic, 1952–62.

incidence, by comparison with later years, was still quite low; but once the drug regime had started cattle numbers increased (Fig. 18.2) and continued to do so. It was still not known what might happen if the intensive inspection and treatment routines were to be discontinued. To discover this would have involved an experiment that the Rhodesian Veterinary Service would not itself have initiated. Instead the cattle owners themselves began one. In August 1960 those who sent their cattle to the Kondo and Chibuwe centres refused to allow them to be treated. This was a political protest which was joined, in October, by all owners in the Musikuvanthu reserve, thus involving all the cattle of the Group (3) centres. Rejection of treatment continued until September 1961.

It was confidently expected that many deaths would ensue, but although the cattle owners did not readily impart information, mortality was certainly far less than was expected. In December 1960, 71 deaths were known to have occurred among the 7000-odd cattle involved and deaths at the same level continued in January and February 1961. But from March onwards the death rate fell and by the second half of the year, at about 0·2 per cent per month, was not greater than might be expected in cattle not subject to trypanosomiasis.

In July 1961 stock owners at two of the three Group (1) centres, Mwangazi and Mariya, also refused treatment and inspection. After legal action had been taken against some of them, inspections and treatments were resumed throughout the whole area in October 1961. There had been no significant rise in the infection rate among the cattle that had not received treatment. During this period, cattle at three centres, Muumbe (Group (1)) and Chibunje and Gumira (Group (2)) and, of course, the European-owned cattle west of the Sabi, had continued to receive injections but there was no indication at either of those places that the trypanosome risk was as high as it seemed to have been early in 1960. These results, especially the failure of cattle to die when treatment was refused, seemed to the entomologists to provide evidence for the success of the anti-tsetse operations they were undertaking near the Mozambique border.

The need to use whatever means are available to control diseases of which neither the epidemiology nor the aetiology is fully understood leads to the unsatisfactory situation that successes and failures may be in reality due to factors of which the existence is hardly appreciated. Throughout the decade since the Sabi epizootic began, the record-keeping procedure of the Rhodesian Veterinary Service had continued to improve so that at many of the inspection centres, by 1962, case histories were being kept individually for each animal.

The stock owners who refused treatment for their sick animals continued to present them at the inspection centres. It was observed, in 1964, that of 280 newly infected animals that received no drug treatment 137 (73 *T. vivax* and 64 *T. congolense*) recovered spontaneously. Most of these recoveries took place in the area of most frequent contact with the vectors, *G. pallidipes* and *G. morsitans*, around Mwangazi. These cattle seemed to have developed a resistance to infection (Cockbill 1964) and the improvement was therefore not necessarily due to the intervention of the entomologists. Field observation in the Sabi had reached a point at which further understanding could only come from research at a different level of investigation.

The empirical nature of the treatments, although successful in preventing heavy mortality and possibly assisting the emergence of physiological defence mechanisms in some of the cattle, did not provide a basis of knowledge upon which to obtain a repetition of the same favourable result. At the northern end of the Rhodesia–Mozambique boundary *G. morsitans* (but not *G. pallidipes*) had also been spreading towards the border of the Inyanga and Mtoko districts since the early 1940s, although no tsetse were found on the Rhodesian side until 1950. The succession of events was, at least superficially, much the same as in the Sabi valley, but the consequence of politically inspired refusal of treatment was what had been expected. If there were any spontaneous recoveries from infection they were masked by very numerous deaths, amounting to over 4800 in 1964 (Cockbill 1964).

The concept of the natural focus of infection applied to the Sabi epizootics

Pavlowsky (1963) regarded a natural focus of infection as a biogeocoenosis: that is, a linking together at a single locus, defined in terms of the inanimate environment ('landscape ecology') and the vegetation (basic food and shelter) of the parasite, its natural hosts, the vectors, and the adventitious hosts, in circumstances favouring maximum circulation of the parasite. In the Sabi valley the appearance and development of several foci of infection can be studied. So far we have looked at the structure of the Mwangazi focus described in terms of the geographical pattern of its two principal infections. A historical background is implied, for the spread of the Mozambique fly-belt was part of the recovery from the recession initiated by rinderpest among warthogs, kudu, and other favoured natural hosts of the tsetse in 1895.

Other historical factors are to be found in the subsequent political and administrative activities of the colonial governments. The first of these was the definition of the boundary between Rhodesia and Mozambique. It cut through the kingdom (or empire) of Gazaland which had been set up by Soshangane, another leader who had brought his people north from Natal in the *mfecane* and defeated the Portuguese in 1836. He was succeeded by his sons, Mzila and Gungunyana.† The latter was finally overcome by the

---

† These names have a peculiar niche in the history of the trypanosomiasis problem. They were used respectively by G. A. K. Marshall (later Sir Guy Marshall, Director of

Portuguese and exiled to the Canaries in 1895. It was Swynnerton's study of the methods of Mzila that provided the foundation for the Shinyanga anti-tsetse campaigns in 1923–30 (Chapter 11). The different policies of the Portuguese and Rhodesian governments led to the land owned by the former remaining very largely undeveloped, except in the small enclave around the district station of Espungabera. On the Rhodesian side, however, Gazaland was occupied in the late 1890s by pioneer families from South Africa and its economy has continued to expand ever since. But because of the lack of development in Mozambique no action was or could be taken against the spread of tsetse into the lands formerly cleared of it by the Ngoni. Not until tsetse reached the border and began to infect cattle on the Rhodesian side could it be studied and measures taken for its control.

The direction of spread of trypanosomes in the cattle populations and, as it subsequently was confirmed, of the tsetse also, followed the pattern of the natural vegetation which, in turn, is closely correlated with soils, geology, and topography. These relationships were worked out in some detail by Farrell (1961) whose vegetation outlines are reproduced in Map 18.2.

The first crossing of the Rhodesian border by *G. morsitans* occurred at about 21° 15′S., where they became established in the *Brachystegia tamarindoides* woodlands on the post-Karoo granites of the Makossa hills. This woodland, over most of its extent, has a thicket layer of deciduous shrubs including *Gardenia* sp. (? *resiniflua*), *Grewia monticola*, *Bauhinnia petersiana*, *Capparis kirkii*, and *Croton pseudopulchellus*.

Intermingled with this woodland is another dominated by *Terminalia sericea*, *Combretum apiculatum*, *Kirkii acuminata*, *Lonchocarpus capassa*, *Acacia nigrescens*, and *Sclerocarya caffra*. Elsewhere on the hills are patches of *Julbernardia globiflora* and *Colophospermum mopane* woodland.

The Sabi river cuts through the granites in a deep narrow gorge. This was no impediment to the spread of *Glossina*. Tsetse were first found west of the river at this latitude in 1944 (Chorley 1945). The infections shown at the inspection centres along the Sabi river as far north as Gudo (No. 23 on Map 18.1) were probably all derived from this southern extension of the fly-belt.

The larger mammal population of the granite hill woodlands included elephant (in large numbers west of the Sabi), buffalo, eland, kudu, nyala, bushbuck, impala, duiker, Sharpe's grysbok, bushpig, warthog, zebra, baboon. Hippopotamus and crocodile are abundant in suitable stretches of the Sabi and Lundi rivers.

To the north the Makossa hills and their *Brachystegia* woodlands overlook the broad basin of the Musaswe river, covered either with open treeless grassland or with a scanty growth of *Combretum ghazalense*. The black,

the Imperial Institute of Entomology) and by C. F. M. Swynnerton for the farms they bought early in the century on Mount Selinda, some 18 miles north-east of Mwangazi.

badly drained soils overlie a band of Karoo basalt and their comparatively treeless state prevents their infestation by tsetse. Along the Sabi itself and on the upper reaches of the Musaswe tributary a variety of woodland, wooded savannas, and thickets provide environments for natural hosts and for tsetse.

The Chipinga highlands terminate somewhat abruptly in a deep narrow valley running WNW.–ESE. which receives the Msilizwe river (Swynnerton's Mossurise) which drains westwards into Mozambique. This steep-sided valley is the Mwangazi gap and in it lies the cattle inspection centre of the same name. The gap cuts through the uplifted block of so-called Umkondo sediments that form the Chipinga highlands. The walls of the Mwangazi gap and also the steeper upper portions of the highlands escarpment overlooking the Sabi are covered with *Brachystegia tamarindoides* woodlands with an under-storey of *Diplorrhynchus condylocarpon*, *Combretum microphylla*, and *Hippocratea* sp. Termitaria are common and carry a thicket which includes *Boscia hildebrandtii*, *Dalbergia arbutifolia*, *Acacia ataxacantha*, and *Gardenia resiniflua*.

Between the Mwangazi gap and the open grasslands of the Musaswe basin lie the Massosote hills composed, like the highlands to their north, of Umkondo sediments, but of considerably lower altitude. These hills are drained by the Namagamba river which joins the Msilizwe near the Mozambique border. Except on their steeper outer slopes, where they carry *Brachystegia tamarindoides*, they are clothed with *Julbernardia globiflora* woodland in which are also found *Pterocarpus angolensis*, *Pseudolachnostylis maprouneaefolia*, *Terminalia sericea*, and *Ochna stuhlmannii*.

Within this woodland, south of the Mwangazi gap and west of the Namagamba river are some separate stands of *B. tamarindoides* woodland, with termitaria thickets of the kind already described. It was in these that the first *Glossina pallidipes* were taken in the Mwangazi region in August 1960.

As one moves south away from the highlands the country becomes drier. At Mount Selinda, rainfall is over 48 in a year. At Mwangazi, 18 miles away, it is between 32 and 36 in and in the centre of the Musaswe basin it has fallen to between 12 and 16 in. The vegetation catena that may be observed in the descent from the highlands is, in part, a response to edaphic change, in part to an increasingly drier climate.

The *Julbernardia* woodlands give way, in the south, to *Albizia–Acacia* parkland where the headwaters of the Musaswe rise on a belt of Karoo conglomerate. Farrell has recorded parkland of *Albizia harveyi–Acacia* ? *nilotica* and *Acacia nigrescens* woodland with a thicket, more or less impenetrable, of *Zyzyphus mucronata*, *Strychnos innocua*, *Gardenia resiniflua*, *Millettia usaramensis*, and *Vitex amboniensis*.

The conglomerate zone separates the southern slopes of the Umkondo sediment hills from a zone of Karoo sandstones. On this are found

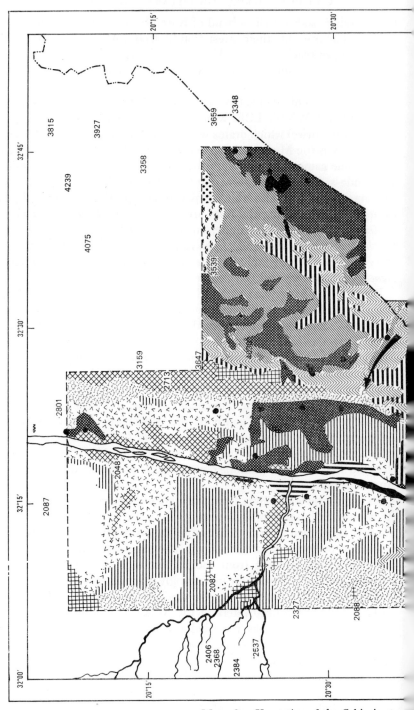

MAP 18.2. Vegetation of the Sabi river v[...]

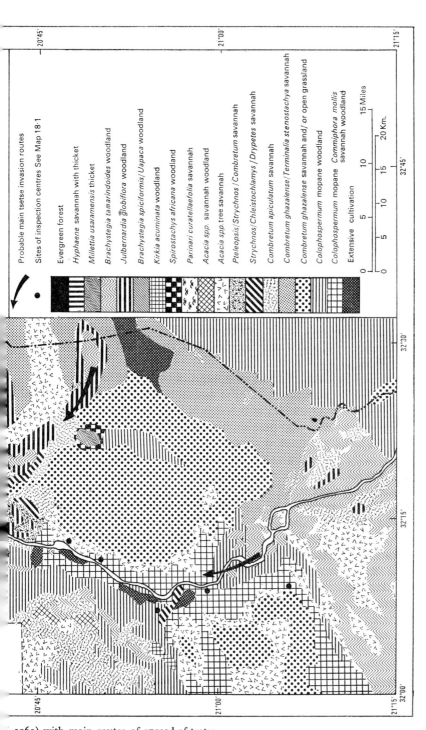

Legend:

- Probable main tsetse invasion routes
- Sites of inspection centres See Map 18·1

- Evergreen forest
- *Hyphaene* savannah with thicket
- *Milletia usaramensis* thicket
- *Brachystegia tamarindoides* woodland
- *Julbernardia globiflora* woodland
- *Brachystegia spiciformis*/*Uapaca* woodland
- *Kirkia acuminata* woodland
- *Spirostachys africana* woodland
- *Parinari curatellaefolia* savannah
- *Acacia* spp. savannah woodland
- *Acacia* spp. tree savannah
- *Pteleopsis*/*Strychnos*/*Combretum* savannah
- *Strychnos*/*Cleistochlamys*/*Drypetes* savannah
- *Combretum apiculatum* savannah
- *Combretum ghazalense*/*Terminalia stenostachya* savannah
- *Combretum ghazalense* savannah and/ or open grassland
- *Colophospermum mopane* woodland
- *Colophospermum mopane   Commiphora mollis*
  savannah woodland
- Extensive cultivation

0   5   10   15 Miles
0   5   10   15   20 Km.

1961) with main routes of spread of tsetse.

complexes of (1) *Albizia anthelmintica–Strychnos stuhlmannii–Drypetes mossambicense*, (2) *Combretum ghazalense* with *Acacia* ? *nilotica, Lannea kirkii, Lonchocarpus capassa*, and *Combretum imberbe*, and (3) a woodland of *Spirostachys africana* fringed on its outer margin by a thicket that includes *Capparis corymbosa, Cleistochlamys kirkii, Lecaniodiscus fraxinifolius, Albizia anthelmintica*, and *Millettia usaramensis*.

These various communities are associated with different combinations of soils derived from Umkondo sediments, conglomerate, sandstone, and, at the bottom of the catena, from the basalt. They are also influenced by the rapidly changing climate and topography.

In particular the belt of sandstone that separates the conglomerates from the basalt seems to be associated with the spread of infection. Near to the border, 10 miles due south of the Muumbe centre (No. 3, Map 18.1) is the Lusongo ridge, marked with a row of sandstone kopjes. The kopjes, like most places where the parent rock breaks through, carry woodland of *Brachystegia tamarindoides*. This woodland gives way to *Julbernardia globiflora* which may be replaced in some situations by woodlands dominated either by *Terminalia sericea* or by *Pterocarpus angolensis*. The latter, on its lower borders, may give way to an ecotonal zone of *Pteleopsis myrtifolia, Millettia stuhlmannii, Strychnos innocua*, and *Combretum apiculatum* and *C. methowianum*.

The interrelationships of these communities associated with the belt of sandstone is further complicated by the drainages which either rise in it or, like the Musaswe river itself, cut through it. The Lusongo ridge is much used as a pasture and it also provides a route by which *Glossina morsitans*, as well as *G. pallidipes*, crossed the border from Mozambique.

Away from the big rivers or other conspicuous features of the landscape, great areas of relatively featureless land are covered by mopane (*Colophospermum mopane*) woodland. In some situations this woodland and its associated fauna may serve as a complete environment for *G. morsitans* throughout the year (Pilson and Pilson 1967). But in much of the arid country of the Sabi basin it appears that at the height of the dry season, when temperatures are maximal, the tsetse are, at least in part, dependent upon the shelter provided for them and their host animals by the more mesophytic vegetation found along river banks and in hills.

G. morsitans approached the Makossa area in the south via the drainages of the Rupembe and Honde rivers (Map 18.1) and the felling of trees on alluvial soils associated with them was used as a protective measure in 1956–8. When the tsetse reached the *Brachystegia* woodlands, populations of relatively high density developed. It seems probable, therefore, that the spread of this species and of *G. pallidipes* across the border at Lusongo and further north at Mwangazi was due to the favourable environment provided for it by the *Brachystegia* woodlands in those places. The line of the Mwangazi gap, as well as the line of the sandstones north-west from

Lusongo, both lead across from the Group (1) area of high infection to the Group (2) centres of intermediate infection incidences. But, while these natural features of geology, topography, and vegetation may indeed have provided routes for spread of tsetse, they also provided the most practicable lines for road construction.

The spread of infection westwards was primarily a phenomenon of *Glossina* population growth. It is not possible to say to what extent road traffic assists movement, but there is no doubt that tsetse carried out of the fly-belts on road traffic can cause outbreaks of infection in cattle with which they come into contact. Cockbill (1958*a*, *b*) showed that there was a positive correlation between infection incidence in donkeys in villages around the periphery of the Musaswe basin and the numbers of tsetse collected from road traffic. The data are given in Table 18.1. The tsetse involved had been

TABLE 18.1

Correlation between infection rate in donkeys and numbers of tsetse caught on traffic entering each area

Area	No. of smears	Infection rate (%)	T. brucei	T. congo- lense	T. vivax	T. congolense- T. vivax	T. brucei- T. vivax	Tsetse taken at control points G. morsitans	G. pallidipes
Makoho	18	39	5	—	1	—	1	106	30
Mabee	76	21	6	7	2	1	—	42	51
Chisuma	108	5	2	3	—	—	—	4	—
Iurongwezi	108	5	2	3	—	—	—	7	—
Mariya– Zamchiya	238	—	—	—	—	—	—	—	—

carried out of the Makossa hills and the Honde and Rupembe river basins. The preponderance of *Trypanosoma brucei*, a trypanosome only rarely recorded in cattle in the area, is due to the survey having been carried out in donkeys.

It is difficult to locate foci of infection when the density of the tsetse population is low. The assumption that *Glossina* had, in fact, crossed the Sabi river has been mentioned. The reduction of infection incidence in Humani cattle after the suspected areas of tsetse habitat had been treated with insecticide has also been noted. No live *Glossina* could be caught on this ranch but in 1962, because infection still persisted, another intensive survey was carried out from March to September. Traps and bait oxen were used in the hope of finding adult insects and searches were made for puparia. None was found but, most remarkably, three wings of *Glossina*, two evidently of *G. morsitans* and one of *G. pallidipes* (judged by measurements of wing veins) and the wingless thorax and abdomen of a female

G. morsitans were sifted from rubble thrown out by bees from a hollow tree (*Trichilia emetica*) in which they had made their nest. Eventually, in 1967 one male *G. pallidipes* was found in riverine thicket on the Sabi river which forms the eastern ranch boundary (Lovemore 1967).

The use of bait cattle to demonstrate the presence of tsetse in areas where cattle are infected but the insects are so rare that they are never caught by normal survey methods was first described by Bedford (1927). On the Lundi river (Map 17.2) the spread of *G. morsitans* and *G. pallidipes* across the *Brachystegia*-covered granites led to the appearance, in 1958, of fulminating and rapidly fatal strains of *Trypanosoma vivax* in cattle pastured 10 miles away from the nearest tsetse located by normal survey methods (Phelps 1959). Goodier (1961*b*) laid out a 'fly-round' in an area

TABLE 18.2

Tabanids and tsetse caught on an ox at Chipinda Pools, Lundi river, Rhodesia

Philoliche medialis Oldroyd	109
P. silverlocki Austen	823
P. zonata Walker	3
P. fodiens Austen	16
Tabanus gratus Loew	657
T. pertinens Austen	95
T. atrimanus Loew	2
T. distinctus Ricardo	147
T. unilineatus Loew	11
T. copemani Austen	7
Mesomyia decora Macquart	17
Haematopota albihirta Karsch . . .	633
H. vittata Loew	234
Glossina morsitans Westwood . . .	1
Total	2755

between the known fly-front and the infected area. A bait ox was used on this round, which was worked 191 times between May 1960 and March 1961. The biting flies captured, other than Stomoxydinae, are listed in Table 18.2.

To catch these 2755 flies the catching team and their bait ox walked over 86 miles. Although they demonstrated that *Glossina* could be found outside the fly-belt as normally defined, it was still thought that the spread of epizootic trypanosomiasis, especially of *T. vivax*, must be greatly helped by mechanical transmission. Goodier (1962) thought that *Philoliche silverlocki* Austen, with its very large proboscis and hovering habit while sucking blood, might be an especially effective agent for transmission.

An experimental herd of 10 clean animals was established in the Sabi valley outside the known epizootic area. Artificially infected animals were then introduced. The experiment ran for 755 days during which at least one animal infected with *T. congolense* was present for 724 days, two animals on 152 days, and three on 19 days. *T. vivax* was present in one artificially infected animal on 469 days, in two animals on 179 days, and in three on 32 days. Only one case of trypanosomiasis among the originally clean animals was seen, but this occurred at a time when naturally occurring infection had appeared in herds pastured in land contiguous with the experimental paddock.

Regular periodical catches of haematophagous Diptera were made from the animals in the herd and over the two years 63 503 Stomoxydinae and 6205 Tabanidae were captured, the latter including 1442 representatives of the genus *Philoliche*. In spite of the one doubtful infection, it seemed safe to conclude that mechanical transmission was playing little part in the maintenance of the epizootic, even in the Group (3) areas where *T. vivax* caused 90 per cent of infections (Cockbill 1966).

One may sum up the history of the Sabi epizootics, so far as it goes, as follows:

(1) High infection incidence is associated with a high proportion of *T. congolense* infections (Group (1) area, *vivax* ratio about 30 per cent).

(2) *T. congolense* infections in turn are associated with proximity to the main tsetse belts.

(3) The areas of intermediate frequency of *T. congolense* infection (Group (2) area, *vivax* ratio about 60 per cent) are associated with vegetation which appears suited to the rapid extension of the fly-belt, but if infection is indeed due to the spread of tsetse this might be an effect of road traffic in those areas favourable to *Glossina*.

(4) The periodical appearance of *T. congolense* infections in Group (3) areas far from the main fly-belts suggests that fluctuations in the epizootic in these peripheral areas may be caused by the occasional appearance in them of *G. morsitans* or *G. pallidipes*. This conclusion is supported by evidence of extremely low sporadic tsetse infestation.

(5) The preponderance of *T. vivax* infections on the periphery of the epizootic area may be due to any or all of the factors evoked to explain the same phenomenon in other parts of Africa. The Sabi experience, however, does not support the view that it is due to its greater facility for mechanical transmission.

Cattle infections around the Zambezi valley fly-belt

The Sabi epizootics developed in response to invasion by tsetse of land which had been free of the insects for half a century. They were dealt with empirically as they developed by drug treatments and by control of the vector. The Sebungwe fly-belt is that portion of the Zambezi valley infestation now lying immediately south of Lake Kariba, which bounds it in the north. Its growth from the residual foci remaining after the passage of the rinderpest panzootic first made itself acutely felt in 1918 on the Gwaai river, where cattle belonging to a European farmer contracted trypanosomiasis, and during the next few years native-owned cattle died freely from the disease along a section of this river. Shooting to drive back the tsetse began in 1919 and continued for three years. 'The results of these operations were (1) the advance of the fly was immediately checked, (2) the surviving cattle along the Gwaai River became free from fly disease by 1922, and (3) fly in the area of operations was greatly diminished and to all appearance entirely eliminated between the Gwaai and Shangani Rivers' (Jack 1933).

The organized shooting was halted in 1922 and it was hoped to hold the position by encouraging settlers to intensify hunting in this neighbourhood for sport. This was ineffective as a control measure and by 1927 the same area was being re-invaded rapidly. In 1930 a policy of maintaining a cordon of hunters all around the periphery of the Zambezi tsetse belt was adopted with the intention of creating a protective zone in which the host populations would be reduced to a level too low to support a population of *Glossina*. Where it was necessary to push back the tsetse, hunting was intensified. By 1950 *G. morsitans* had been removed, together with an unknown proportion of its natural host population, from 10 000 mile^2 around the periphery of the Zambezi tsetse belt. Most of this 'reclaimed' area was not occupied but lay within the defensive corridor.

During the next few years tsetse control in Rhodesia became a matter of political dispute to such an extent that an official commission was appointed to inquire into the possiblities of using methods other than game destruction. The commission recommended that while alternative methods were being explored, slaughter at the rate then prevailing (about 40 000 head per annum) could be reduced by confining shooting to corridors that would be fenced to prevent animals within the fly-belt from moving into the shooting area. On the outer edge of the corridor cattle fences would keep domestic stock out of the 'game-free–cattle-free' zone (Thomas, Davey, and Potts 1955).

The fencing of the corridor on the southern edge of the Sebungwe belt was finished in 1957 and shooting which had been stopped during its construction was resumed. The Sebungwe corridor was 96 miles long and varied from 10 to 20 miles in width. Its area was approximately 1200 mile^2. From December 1957 to October 1961, 21 669 animals were destroyed of which 223 were elephants, and 10 836 were duiker (*Sylvicapra grimmia*). There was some evidence that the latter increased during the period of shooting, perhaps because relieved of competition with other species, while the pigs, warthog and bushpig, after an initial drop, seemed to maintain their numbers (Lovemore 1963).

Child and Wilson (1964), who analysed *Sylvicapra* material collected in the Sebungwe corridor, showed that continuous hunting had altered the age structure of the population so that mortality due to shooting was compensated for by early maturation and increased reproduction rate. Wilson and Roth (1967), observing a similar failure to reduce a duiker population in Zambia, found that hunting had a marked effect on behaviour and the peak of maximum activity shifted from the morning to the afternoon and evening. Duiker are seldom fed upon by *G. morsitans* (Weitz 1963) but the demonstration that they and probably other animals reached equilibrium with the hunters was evidence that a corridor, free of game and of cattle, had not been achieved.

Infections in cattle south of the defence zone began to appear early in 1959 and continued, apart from seasonal fluctuations, to increase. The defence zone between the fences, although more heavily hunted than any area of similar magnitude in earlier operations, had not proved effective. During the last month of shooting the first *G. morsitans* was taken near the most heavily infected centre at Maganganga.

The distribution of infection incidence and its relationship to the *vivax* ratio at the peak of the epizootic in 1961-2 is shown in Maps 18.3*a* and *b*. The highest infection incidences at Maganganga (E) and Silumbani (Y), 12·0 and 6·4 per cent per annum respectively, were associated with the appearance of a new focus of *G. morsitans* and also with a higher incidence of *T. congolense* and therefore a low *vivax* ratio (Ford 1964).

There are three points of interest about the spread of these infections. The first is that they occurred in approximately the same area that Jack (1933) had already twice reclaimed by shooting in 1919-20 and in 1928-32. It is a reasonable assumption that this third epizootic was a manifestation of activity in the same natural focus of infection as the two earlier epizootics. The second point is that the fenced corridor had failed as a barrier to tsetse. This was demonstrated by Pilson (1961) who marked and released 1467 *G. morsitans* in an area of high tsetse population density north of the corridor. Two were recaptured on its southern edge and had probably been carried in motor traffic. Six others had penetrated into the corridor perhaps by natural means. Map 18.3 shows that the foci of high infection incidence and low *vivax* ratio lie due south of rivers that cross the defensive corridor from north to south.

North of the Maganganga focus of infection lies the Dongamusi river that runs south into the Mzola which in turn joins the Shangani. Some miles to the east another area of high infection incidence, but less precisely defined, is associated with the headwaters of the Lutope river. The weak points in the defence zone were those in which the natural vegetation associated with drainage lines appeared to provide links with the fly-belts to the north.

The third point of interest is that here it is possible to carry the concept of the development of the natural focus of infection to its origin in the wild

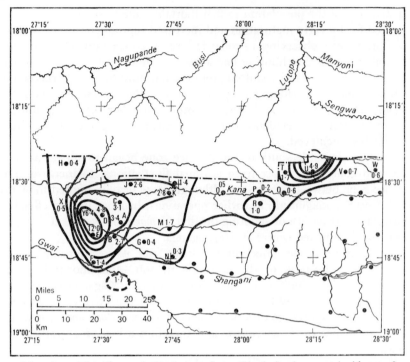

MAP 18.3*a*. The Shangani–Gwai tsetse front, Rhodesia. Apparent incidence of infection 1961–2.

game. The failure of glossinologists generally to study the relationships between tsetse and their natural hosts has already been noted. Although when the massive Rhodesian shooting campaign was stopped in 1961 some 750 000 animals had been killed, very little was understood about the biology of the method. One basic principle, however, was stated in a semi-popular memorandum in these words: 'Every hunter knows favoured localities where he can *depend* on finding game, whatever the season; these are the places that, within certain climatic and vegetative limits, are the true haunts of *G. morsitans*. Eliminate tsetse from these areas, and the remainder of the flies cannot maintain themselves throughout the vastly larger areas where game are scattered and seasonal in distribution; they cannot survive permanently on chance encounters with food hosts' (Trypanosomiasis committee 1945). This statement is more or less accurate. It states a principle that was overlooked when the alternative method of setting up game-free and cattle-free corridors was devised in 1954, for the corridors were planned to avoid the areas with dense game populations. As a consequence the hunters were withdrawn from the places in which *G. morsitans* flourished and were concentrated where they did not. It became clear, when the growth of the Maganganga focus was studied, that

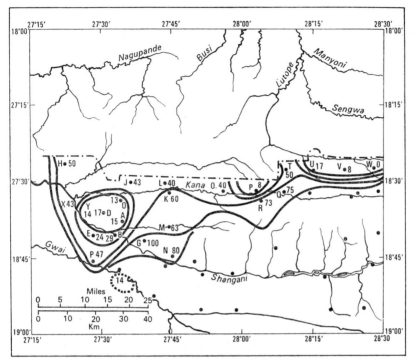

MAP 18.3*b*. The Shangani–Gwai tsetse front, Rhodesia. Proportions of positive slides diagnosed as *T. vivax*, 1961–2.

it had its origin in the *Glossina* population of the headwaters of the Nagupande river, 20 miles to the north on the other side of the game-free–cattle-free zone. Under the earlier regime, terminated in 1956, the Nagupande basin had been a principal focus of hunting activity. Doubtless the Rhodesian government's African hunters had been directed into the Nagupande area, but had they merely been told to go out and bring in as many trophies as possible, the Nagupande was one of the areas into which they would have gone.

Of 351 fully identified blood meals from *G. morsitans* collected in the Sebungwe fly-belt 45·0 per cent were from warthog and 21·9 per cent were made up by kudu, buffalo, bushbuck, and bushpig. Insecticides had failed at Nagupande in 1961 and it was decided to eliminate these five host animals.

The Nagupande headwaters, an area of about 200 mile^2, was fenced in after 45 elephants and 21 buffalo had been driven out or killed. Four rhinoceroses left the area at this time. Intensive hunting of warthog, bushpig, kudu, and bushbuck was begun in October 1962. The principal results are shown in Fig. 18.3. In five years 1922 warthogs, 176 bushpigs, 289 kudu, and 80 bushbuck were killed. The mean apparent density of the

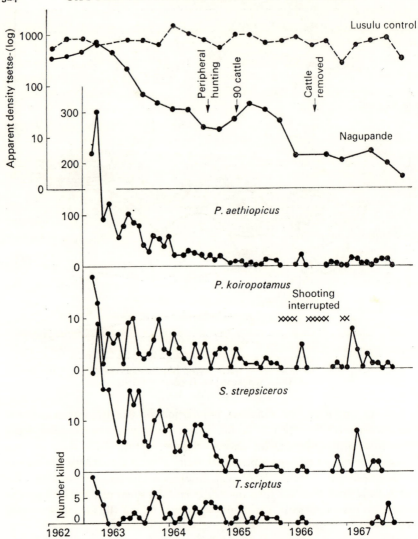

FIG. 18.3. The Nagupande experiment. Kills of warthog (*Phacochoerus aethiopicus*), bush-pig (*Potamochoerus koiropotamus*), kudu (*Strepsiceros strepsiceros*), and bushbuck (*Tragelaphus scriptus*), with mean quarterly apparent densities of *G. morsitans* in the experimental and control areas.

G. morsitans population was reduced from 732 per 10 000 yd of traverse with a bait ox in the last quarter of 1962 to 1·7 in the last quarter of 1967. (It is usual to express apparent density as the number of non-teneral males per 10 000 yd but these figures include males, females, and tenerals.) The reduction of 99·77 per cent shown by these figures is an exaggeration. It will be observed that the quarterly mean of the Nagupande fly-rounds reached a peak coinciding with the start of hunting. Apart from reducing the natural host population, hunting disturbs animals and affects their normal behaviour. They become less available to tsetse which tend to turn their attentions to other potential hosts including man. A temporary rise in the catch above the normal level is commonly observed whenever the natural ecosystem is violently disturbed. A safer estimate of the fall in tsetse density is made by comparing the mean figure of 481 flies per 10 000 yd for the third quarter of 1962, before shooting began, with the mean of 2·3 for the third quarter of 1967. The reduction is still considerable, amounting to 99·3 per cent. The control fly-rounds at Lusulu, some 15 miles away, showed mean apparent densities of 854 and 824 for the same two periods (Robertson 1968).

Sixty hunters were used in the 200 mile² area from October 1962 to September 1964 when their numbers were reduced and other procedural modifications were made. In these two years the reduction of apparent density was 96·7 per cent and the bulk of the host population had already been destroyed.

Operations of this kind are experimental. The Nagupande work was the first attempt to apply the knowledge gained by the Weitz analyses to the problem of tsetse control. As an experiment it had several faults. A preliminary census of all larger mammals would have been an advantage, but census techniques for large animals living in densely wooded areas have not yet been developed. In any case, the experiment was primarily an attempt to achieve control over trypanosomiasis in cattle 20 miles away and the need for speed was over-riding. Towards the end of the five-year period the area still supported impala, zebra, reedbuck, eland, roan, sable, duiker, grysbok, baboons, and hyenas (Cockbill 1967). It was an improvement on earlier Rhodesian techniques. However, although only the four species were shot, after elephant, buffalo, and rhinoceros had been driven out, it seems very likely that populations of species that were not molested also fell, if only because they now had to share their environment with 60 hunters and ancillary staff, perhaps amounting in all to about 100 persons.

Infection at Maganganga and neighbouring centres was extinguished by the middle of 1964 (Cockbill 1967); but here also the experiment was inconclusive, for around the infected centres extensive bush clearing and insecticide spraying had been undertaken. From the viewpoint of the relationship between the tsetse-borne trypanosomiases and African ecology, the importance of Nagupande lies in its demonstration that hunting animals where they are most abundant can bring about a significant decline in the tsetse population without completely exterminating them. A relaxation of hunting pressure is followed very rapidly by recovery of the animal population by immigration from other areas. Game fences are a hindrance but not a complete barrier and, when shooting is in progress on one side and not the other, they act rather as indicators of danger than as true barriers. It is also possible that in a hunting area animals change their habits and revert to normal when the menace is withdrawn. In Chapter 2 it was noted that some of the animals in the Wankie national park changed their habits to avoid tourists. Fig. 18.3 shows that when the Rhodesian government, in November 1965, withdrew the hunters' firearms, the population of the four hunted species began to recover. There was no shooting for 4 months. It was resumed for 1 month in March 1966 and then stopped again for 5 months. During that one month 22 warthogs were killed as against an average of 9·8 per month in the 12 months before the shooting was stopped. Five bushpigs were killed compared with an average of 2·1 per month in the previous year. There was hunting in September and October 1966 and then after another halt it was resumed from January to August 1967. The high kills of both kudu and bushpig at the beginning of this period are clearly shown on the graphs.

Bursell (1969) finished his paper on the relationship between frequency of host encounter and density of the tsetse population by looking forward to control of the fly-belts not by game destruction but by game cropping. When we look back at the successful control exercised by the Rhodesian authorities from 1931 to 1950 and the great rapidity with which game and tsetse recovered when hunting was relaxed, it is evident that this is what they were doing, although perhaps doing it wastefully. Except in two important respects Chorley's methods were essentially an exercise in man/game animal predation of the same kind that had been used, perhaps unwittingly, perhaps not, to control the spread of infection in the centuries before the arrival of the Europeans.

19

TSETSE FLIES IN THE RHODESIAN PAST

Monomotapa

ALMOST certainly the first recorded attempt of Western civilization to come to grips with the African trypanosomiasis problem was made in 1569. In that year the Portuguese soldier Francisco Barreto led an expedition up the Zambezi valley to establish contact with a country that spread its name across almost every early map of Africa, the empire of Monomotapa. Barreto was accompanied by and perhaps took his orders from the Jesuit Father Monclaro. When they reached Sena, 120 miles up-river, horses, cattle, and men began to die. This, said the Jesuit, was because their Moorish guides had poisoned the grass. He compelled Barreto to put some of them to death in case they should next poison the waters (Walker 1957). The horses may have died of *Trypanosoma brucei* infections or, as Henning (1956) thinks, of African horse sickness, a virus infection transmitted by various species of the biting midges, *Culicoides*. The cattle probably died of *T. congolense* and *T. vivax* infections and the men of malaria. Soon afterwards Barreto died, of a broken heart, some said, brought on by the harassments of Father Monclaro. The Moors were murdered in vain and the infections and their vectors stayed in the Zambezi valley. The Portuguese did not penetrate effectively into central Rhodesia for another fifty years and then did not remain for long, for from 1696 to 1835 their contact with that country was restricted to African or half-caste agents (Abraham 1966). To ensure access for these men, mostly gold buyers, the Portuguese paid an annual tribute to Monomotapa of cloth and beads to the value of 3000 *crusados* (£600). The Portuguese were not allowed to climb Mount Fura 'because from its crest a great proportion of the lands of Monomotapa could be seen and he [Monomotapa] feared lest their extent and beauty excite the covetousness of the Europeans' (Axelson 1960).

Mount Fura, now Mount Darwin, lies on the edge of the historical tsetse belt (Map 17.2). Monomotapa, a westernization of the praise name of one of its kings, Nyatsimba, known as Mutoka Churuchamutapa or Mutapa, was a long-lived state with connections to the orient, the western world and the tropical African north.

The Mutapa empire was founded by people called Karanga who came from the neighbourhood of Lake Tanganyika and settled near the modern Sinoia. This was about 1325 and the Karanga, under their leader Mbire, practised hoe agriculture, were cattle keepers, and skilled iron-workers and masons. On their arrival on the central plateau of Rhodesia they are said to have encountered people who were Muslims (Abraham 1966). Possibly these were Arab predecessors of the Portuguese, also come to buy gold. Mbire and his followers found a well-developed mining and trading society already in occupation of the Rhodesian plateau.

During the fifteenth century Matope, the son of Nyatsimba, extended the Karanga dominion so that by the time of his death in about 1480 the empire of the Mutapa stretched from the Kalahari to the Indian Ocean, as far south as the Sabi estuary. This can only mean that the Karanga sent out war parties that bullied or cajoled other tribes throughout this vast area to acknowledge the suzerainty of the Mutapa and to pay tribute. The whole great area eventually became the territory of Shona-speaking tribes, each with its own chief but each owing allegiance to Mutapa (Ranger 1968). Although it seems likely that in the heartland of the empire the fly-belt of the Zambezi valley was extinguished over large areas that later became reinfested, much of what became Mozambique must have been, as it is now, occupied by *Glossina morsitans* and the coastal forests and some highland forests too, also supported *G. pallidipes*, *G. brevipalpis*, and *G. austeni*.

The Karanga dynasty of Mutapa remained in power for two hundred years. On the southern border of their empire, in the Limpopo valley, in the fourteenth century, were a small clan, the Rozwi. They were governed by a branch of the Mutapa family, the chief of whom, at the end of the fifteenth century, declared himself the independent ruler of the central Rhodesian plateau. The coastal Arabs called him the Amir Changa, a title that was soon changed to Changamire. Mutapa continued in charge of the Zambezi valley, but by the end of the sixteenth century had ceded great estates to the Portuguese especially around Quilimane, Sena, and Tete. However, by the end of the seventeenth century Changamire had extended the Rozwi rule and in 1693–5 drove the Portuguese from most of their country west of Tete. The Mutapa dynasty now was relegated to a small chiefdom near the Zambezi. Its last titular representative, Chioko, was involved in an insurrection against the Portuguese in 1902 (Abraham 1966). Alpers (1968) gives an account of the Mutapa and Rozwi empires that differs much in detail from that of Abraham; but there is no doubt in either account that this society was long-lived, stable, and relatively well organized. The Rozwi lasted until about 1830 when they began to be submerged in successive waves of the Ngoni explosion.

The Karanga empire of Mutapa and its continuation under the Rozwi was one of the great states of the African Middle Age, contemporary with the kingdom of Kongo and with many of the empires of West Africa. It had a riverine route to the sea, down the Sabi river (Rio Save) from its confluence with the Lundi, where there is still the remains of an artificial lake (Summers 1960). This was perhaps the chief route by which gold was conveyed to the Arab port of Sofala, established in the tenth century. Clark

(1959), however, says that gold was already being exported to Sofala in A.D. 600. The trade was certainly flourishing by the fourteenth century when the Karanga arrived to take over an already existing mining industry on the central plateau. Monomotapa was, therefore, not the creation, except politically, of the Karanga. The country already had a widespread and well-developed culture. Early attempts at African history, based on unskilled interpretation of native legend and myths, gave the impression of great hordes of people continually roaming about the continent and driving each other out of the lands they temporarily occupied. Hordes there were on occasion and Zwangendaba's Ngoni, operating in the same century, travelled further than Napoleon between Paris and Moscow, but the movement of the great mass of the people was a slower process; sometimes it involved racial extermination as when the Bantu on the one hand and the Boers on the other reduced the last Bushmen to the status of ethnological relics, but more often it was a matter of genetic and cultural drift that resulted from comparatively peaceful contacts between ordinary people.

The ecological situation of successive societies in Rhodesia

According to Clark (1959), cattle and other livestock probably entered southern Africa during the first half of the first millennium A.D. They were introduced by Iron Age people. The earliest cattle came into tropical Africa from the north. This introduces one of the most interesting of the problems of the human ecological relationships of trypanosomiasis. Clark remarks that the earliest Bantu groups entering southern Africa were stock owners and therefore kept to more open country where grazing was plentiful and the tsetse fly would not destroy their herds. Country of this sort may have been easy to find near the climatic limit of tsetse distribution, but further north the penetration of the equatorial *Glossina* belts was a remarkable achievement. It will be mentioned further in Chapter 25.

In Rhodesia itself, as in the rest of Africa, the succession of human cultures must be considered against the background of climatic fluctuation. Summers (1960) considered what might have been the changes in distribution of vegetation in Rhodesia when rainfall had been either wetter or drier than at present. He distinguished six periods of increased rainfall during the Pleistocene, but pointed out that a comparatively small change in precipitation may have had a marked effect upon the geological record of heavier average rainfall, and that a more even distribution of rainfall could have a greater effect on vegetation than would a moderate increase of average rainfall where the annual fall is erratic as it is in parts of Rhodesia today. One source of absolute comparison is provided by the degree of wearing of feldspar grains on successive horizons at the Khami ruins near Bulawayo. This technique, developed by the Rhodesian geologist, Bond, indicates that the Still Bay culture of the Middle Stone Age flourished in a climate with a rainfall 140 per cent of that of the present, that is to say, about 36 in annually.

Summers's (1960) discussion of the ecological relationships of successive societies on and around the Rhodesian high veld compels attention since he invokes trypanosomiasis as a principal factor in controlling their distribution. That one cannot accept his conclusion in this respect does not greatly detract from the value of his study for whether or not it is correct in detail, the succession of climates must be considered (and has been in Chapter 3) if the role of the tsetse flies in African ecology is to be understood.

Summers's main conclusion was that successive inhabitants of the country avoided areas clothed with mopane (*Colophospermum mopane*) woodlands. In wetter periods these woodlands were replaced by *Brachystegia* and the areas which had supported *Brachystegia* were invaded by closed forest. In drier periods the forest retreated to the mountains, mopane invaded the former *Brachystegia* areas, and was itself replaced with grassland (steppe) or, in the driest areas, by windblown Kalahari desert sands. The reconstructed rainfall maps and the vegetation distributions they are held to indicate show a negative correlation to exist between the distributions of various cultures and the supposed distribution of mopane. Mopane is held to be an indicator of the presence of *G. morsitans* and Summers suggests that the Stone Age hunters avoided the mopane because they realized that any hunting party venturing into them was liable to contract sleeping sickness. This avoidance of the tsetse-infested mopane persisted in later times when Iron Age invaders brought cattle into the country.

The argument must be rejected on many grounds. It is based upon the supposition that tsetse distribution is directly correlated with vegetation. This is an argument taken from the glossinologists. It is valid only in so far as tsetse are not found in open, treeless grassland. *G. morsitans*, in Africa as a whole, is associated with *Brachystegia* woodland rather than with mopane. Much of the area which mopane occupies in southern Africa today lies outside the climatic limits that tsetse can tolerate. In Rhodesia itself *G. morsitans* in some parts of its range infests the *Brachystegia* woodlands. In respect of the disease itself it has been argued that the indigenous populations of the Zambezi tsetse belts have developed some degree of physiological adjustment to infection. This could not have taken place before the end of the Stone Age, for a sparse population of mobile hunters and gatherers could not have provided the epidemiological circumstances necessary for adjustment to be achieved. One may therefore suppose that when a Stone Age hunter was infected in due course he died; but it seems very unlikely that the course of the disease was so different from its course today that it was in most cases, as Summers suggests, 'crippling within a few hours in most cases', and not, as now, within a few weeks. Glasgow (1963*b*) argues that sleeping sickness does not exclude modern hunters.

It seems probable that the drier areas were more inhospitable to hunters than the less dry and that they were avoided by Stone Age man for the same reason that they were avoided by his technically more able successors, namely, that they were more uncomfortable to live in. In present-day Rhodesia there is an abundance of river water throughout the year. Under a drier climate rivers such as the Limpopo and the Sabi–Lundi, or the larger tributaries of the Zambezi, may well have been waterless through much of the year as are rivers of similar size in countries further north today. According to Summers's maps the archaeological evidence shows that cultures of wetter epochs were much more widely spread than were those of the dry. Man's distribution was and still is far more closely related to distribution of water and fertile soil than to tsetse fly.

Mapumgubwe in the Limpopo valley lies in the middle of what was the pre-rinderpest fly-belt. The earliest occupation of Mapumgubwe has been given a C^{14} date of A.D. 1058 ± 65 years (Clark 1959). Its founders may have been pastoralists of a 'Bush-Boskopoid' physical type similar to people who had lived on the plains of northern Tanzania, and Clark suggests that the change from a Stone Age to an Iron Age economy may have resulted in the breaking away of some bands in search of new pastures and it may be that one such group settled at Mapumgubwe. Around this site are signs of extensive occupation and the recovery of golden ornaments, some worked with great artistic skill, shows that its later occupants can hardly have been a small community struggling for survival in tsetse-infested bush. Mapumgubwe is now well inside the mopane area of the Limpopo valley. Summers (1960) claims that it flourished under a some-what wetter climate than the present and therefore lay in a *Brachystegia* area. Unless the temperatures experienced by the Mapumgubwe peoples were appreciably colder than they are now, then *Brachystegia* woodlands might well have provided a more favourable environment for *Glossina* than does the Limpopo valley today. A more likely explanation is that Summers is indeed correct in postulating a wetter climate for the heyday of Mapum-gubwe and that this enabled a society to develop in the Limpopo valley that was numerous enough and sufficiently well organized to substitute its own ecosystems for a natural one of *Brachystegia*, game animals, tsetse, and trypanosomes. In any case it was eventually incorporated into Mutapa's empire.

One connection between that empire and the north must be mentioned. Among the objects found at Zimbabwe and in other Rhodesian ruins were soapstone bowls ornamented with beautifully executed carvings of animals including, especially, cattle with the large lyre-shaped horns charac-teristic of several types of Sanga cattle and particularly reminiscent of the cattle of the Hima–Tusi pastoralists of the interlake zone. Another object found at Zimbabwe is a 'rosette cylinder'. Its function is unknown but the only other rosette cylinder so far found was dug up from the Bigo fortifications in the Katonga valley just outside the modern boundary of Ankole in Uganda. Most prehistorians now agree that a connection exists between the founders of the Mutapa empire and the pastoral rulers of the interlake countries (see, for example, Walton 1957, Clark 1959, and Cole 1964).

The terraced ruins of Inyanga on the eastern border of Rhodesia have been described in great detail by Summers (1958). This immense complex of terraced walls, forts, and stone-lined pits covers the Inyanga mountains at altitudes from 3000 to 7000 ft above sea level. The dry-stone walling was used to support cultivation terraces and the pits may have housed small livestock. Carbonized grains of millet, sorghum, and pulses have been found. Summers who listed other sites in Africa where terracing and irrigation have been practised, suggests that these laborious techniques are only developed under pressure created by the threat of 'enslavement'. The most recent example that he gives was in Rwanda-Urundi, dated 1920. Contoured terraced agriculture is still being practised in Kigezi in Western Uganda. Here the 'threat' is over-population. But as Scaëtta (1932) saw, the population pressures developed in Rwanda because of the Tusi demand for the grasslands created by Hutu cultivation. Summers (1958 and 1960) suggested that the Inyanga terraces, built during the latter half of the sixteenth century (Clark 1959), were made by peoples from the south of Lake Nyasa who had fled from the attacks of cannibalistic 'Zimbas'. But the main Zimba thrust was to the north and Alpers (1968) believes that they moved away from Malawi because of intensification of Portuguese intervention between 1570 and 1580. A more likely explanation is that the terraces were made by former inhabitants of the Zambezi valley who had become subject to the Karanga in the same way that the Hutu, Iru, and Nyambo ancestors had become subject to the Tusi and Hima in Rwanda, Nkore, and Karagwe. The Karanga found, on their arrival in the Zambezi valley in the fourteenth century, pastures that had been created under a somewhat less arid climate than that of today by cultivators who had felled the woodlands, tilled the land, and, by burning, established a grassland sub-climax. These people they made their serfs when they needed servants or pushed further into the forest edges into land as yet unfitted for pasture, just as their Tusi and Hima cousins were starting to do, at about the same time, in the interlake region. There, however, the displaced cultivators had the whole ecotone of the Congo forests at their disposal. The makers of Inyanga had only one small mountain range from which, as its soils became exhausted, they moved, family by family, and were absorbed by other tribes. In due course, too, their pastoral dispossessors succumbed to other pressures and the fine lands that Mutapa had kept from the eyes of the covetous Portuguese reverted to bush, wildlife, and *G. morsitans*, as did the Hima and Tusi pastures in the interlake area.

The Ngoni in Rhodesia

The most far-flung of the Ngoni peoples who spread out from Zululand and became the Tuta have already been encountered in the description of the events that preceded the spread of *Glossina* around Sukumaland at the end of the nineteenth century. Under their leader Zwangendaba they entered what had been Mutapa's empire, now ruled by the Rozwi Mambo, in about 1831. Another Ngoni horde under Nxaba invaded at about the same time. The two armies fought and Zwangendaba was defeated. He moved away towards the Rozwi heartland and sacked Zimbabwe, Khami, and other Rozwi strongholds. The Mambo dramatically flung himself from a great granite inselberg. Nxaba meanwhile went further west and crossed into Barotseland when he came up against another migrant group from the *mfecane*, led by Sebetwane, whose allies drowned Nxaba in the Zambezi (Omer Cooper 1966).

Zwangendaba enlarged his forces with his captives that escaped slaughter when he defeated the Rozwi and moved on to cross the Zambezi near Zumbo on 19 November 1835, a date marked by a solar eclipse. One account of the crossing says that a number of cattle were drowned (Barnes 1951) but they may have lost their cattle while crossing the Zambezi fly-belt (Epstein 1955). They went north to replenish their herds in the Songea area of Tanzania and a branch that turned back to Malawi under Zwangendaba's son Mpezeni in 1865 introduced the East African zebu to that country.

Soshangane, like Zwangendaba, had been a general in the army of Shaka's main opponent, Zwide of the Ndandwe. After the latter's defeat in 1819 Soshangane led his followers to Delagoa Bay. In 1828, to get further out of reach of Shaka's regiments, he moved north to the Sabi river. Here he encountered Zwangendaba and defeated him in battle but left his rival to devastate the Rozwi empire, while he himself founded his own empire of Gazaland. It was the methods of Soshangane's son Mzila that inspired Swynnerton (1921)† in his attempt to work out techniques of tsetse control that did not involve wholesale slaughter of the wild game.

Swynnerton's study of the methods of Mzila

Soshangane had travelled north to attack the Portuguese settlements in Manicaland and the Zambezi valley leaving the usual devastation in his wake. One area that had already been depopulated by Zwangendaba in 1831 was the valley of the Msilizwe or Mossurisse river (on which lies the cattle inspection centre of Mwangazi described in Chapter 18). Mzila came back to the Msilizwe valley in 1861 to find that what had been a country occupied by a cattle-keeping agricultural community before the Ngoni invasion in 1831 was now covered with tsetse-infested woodlands.

† In Swynnerton's account Soshangane is given one of his other names, Manikusa. Gaza was yet another of his names.

At this time Mzila was raiding for cattle among the survivors of the Rozwi empire. The captured animals were brought into the mountain grasslands north of Chipinga, but this country was not to Mzila's liking. Although the Ngoni were aware of trypanosomiasis, which they called *nagana*, and its association with tsetse and regarded proximity to game as dangerous, Mzila had made several attempts to introduce them to the lowland woodlands. Why, asked Swynnerton, if they knew about tsetse, did they do this? 'They said "this whole country is full of it—where *shall* we put our cattle?" ' Finally Mzila 'sent an order to *sondela enkosini* (draw near to the king). Thereupon an immense compulsory movement of the population took place. . . . Everyone of my informants has described graphically the result of this concentration. The bush simply disappeared and the country became bare, except for the numberless native villages and a continuity of native gardens' (Swynnerton 1921).

An interesting feature of the resettlement of the Msilizwe valley by Mzila was that certain areas were left unsettled and remained as game reserves, in particular a large area between the Sitatonga hills and the Buzi river which Swynnerton called 'the Oblong'. Outside this area all wild animals were hunted.

Drives with nets were organized across the entire country, and game, pigs and baboons were thus killed wholesale. If a herd of buffaloes was reported subsequently anywhere west of the Sitatongas it was at once hunted; if pigs appeared in a garden, they were at once tracked down to their retreat and, the people round having been called out, were surrounded and killed. Except on its fringes the 'Oblong', then as now, was a great uninhabited game reserve.

And, of course, also a tsetse reserve. Mzila maintained a force of some 30 000 men at his capital in the Msilizwe valley (Omer Cooper 1966). During his lifetime the Portuguese began to recover their power. He died in 1885 and was succeeded by his son Gungunyana whose capital was Manhlagazi (Mwangazi?) where he was visited by a Portuguese expedition. Both he and Mzila tried to play off the British and the Portuguese against one another, but unsuccessfully. In 1889 Gungunyana evacuated Gazaland and returned to his grandfather's old headquarters at Bileni by Delagoa bay where he tried, but failed, to get help from the British. The Portuguese found a pretext for attacking him in 1895 and he was defeated and exiled to the Canary islands, having held out for two years longer against the European invasion than had his father-in-law, Lobengula, in Rhodesia. When Gungunyana left Gazaland, taking his followers with him on the long march to the coast, control over the wildlife was withdrawn.

Before Gungunyana carried off the population to Bileni (near Lourenco Marques) in about 1889, he had already commenced to protect the game. He had decreed *azi-zale* (let them multiply), and the game had become more abundant both outside and inside the cattle keeping areas. The guard areas still opposed its passage into and out of these areas and no harm resulted to the cattle. When the population left the game (in the words of my native informants) just 'burst forth' (*zadabuka*). At the same time the wooding was let loose and soon re-established itself throughout the previously settled country (Swynnerton 1921).

One can sum up the recent history of the Mwangazi focus of infection by noting that before 1830 it was suppressed by settlement that was part of the Rozwi empire. Between 1830 and 1861 it recovered, but was again suppressed by Mzila. Gungunyana's flight to the coast allowed it once more to recover. The existence of a modern international boundary on one side of which no development is taking place suggests that it may continue to exist for many years to come.

The Kololo and the dwarf Tonga cattle

Another outpouring from the *mfecane* was composed of a group of Sotho people who after various vicissitudes took the name of Kololo and under their chief Sebetwane moved westwards around the Limpopo head-waters and into what is now Botswana, where they defeated the Ngwato, captured their cattle, and went on to Lake Ngami. Here they lost their cattle again, of thirst, according to Omer Cooper (1966), although one may suppose that *Glossina morsitans* accounted for some, for they took a route to the Zambezi via the western end of the Okovango delta and thence along the Chobe river. Eventually they crossed the Zambezi, defeating the Lozi and the Tonga (Toka) from whom they replenished their herds.

Livingstone met Sebetwane near the Victoria Falls:

> They have two breeds of cattle among them. One called the Batoka, because captured from that tribe, is of diminutive size but very beautiful, and closely resembles the shorthorns of our country. The little pair presented by the King of Portugal to H.R.H. The Prince Consort is of this breed. They are very tame and remarkably playful; they may be seen lying on their sides by the fires in the evening; and when the herd goes out, the herdsman often precedes them and has only to commence capering to set them all a-gambolling. The other, or Barotse ox, is much larger and comes from the fertile Barotse valley. They stand high on their legs, often nearly six feet at the withers and they have large horns. Those of one of a similar breed that we brought from the lake, measured tip to tip, eight and a half feet (Livingstone 1857).

It seems more likely that the cattle given to the Prince Consort were West African Muturu which are also dwarfed humpless shorthorns. There still remain, though much crossed with Matabele cattle, a small population of dwarf Tonga cattle in the western Sebungwe tsetse belt. Although now involved in the prophylactic drug programmes of the Rhodesian Veterinary Service these cattle, like their owners, the Tonga or Toka of the Zambezi valley, had adapted themselves to the difficulties of life in the *morsitans*-infected bush of the Sebungwe fly-belt long before the arrival of the

Kololo. The Barotse oxen, like the similar animals with 8½-ft horns that formerly had been kept by the peoples of Botswana, were Sanga types that had developed in tsetse-free pastures. The Kololo were finally extinguished by the Lozi (Barotse). Their importance in this narrative is that they enabled Livingstone to see and record the dwarf Tonga cattle.

The Ndebele, the Shona, and the Rhodesians

The most important group of people coming to Rhodesia as a result of the Zulu explosion were the Ndebele under Mzilikazi. They have been so much written about that there is no need to give them special attention here, especially as they have little to contribute to the history of Rhodesian trypanosomiasis. Like the Kololo they went from Natal across the Transvaal where they tried to settle, but were driven on by the Afrikaner Boers. They circumvented the Limpopo tsetse belt by the western route that was later taken by the missionaries and hunters who followed them. They occupied the western part of the Rhodesian high veld and began to assert their authority over the Shona whose Rozwi rulers had recently been destroyed. In the task they were interrupted by the Europeans. White Rhodesians are not unique in maintaining that their rule is beneficial to the conquered peoples. The Ngoni were notorious for their savagery in battle, nevertheless they represented the nature of their rule over the conquered tribes as enlightened and beneficial (Rennie 1966). Ranger (1968) shows that at least some of the earlier inhabitants of Central Africa preferred Lobengula to the British South Africa Company.

There is no need to summarize the Rhodesian conquest for it has been fully explored by European historians to whom it tends to be either the record of a noble and civilizing mission or else of a sordid confidence trick. When its history is eventually written by African historians it will no doubt wear yet another aspect. In addition to the sources quoted Gann (1965) and Wills (1964) are useful general histories. Many Rhodesians found it difficult to believe that Africans can have built the stone ruins, especially Zimbabwe itself. For an account of their numerous theories by a Rhodesian who typically believes that 'the black man's past is speechless, and the words of the present-day Bantu valueless' reference may be made to Paver (1957). A modern and acceptable account is given by Summers (1963).

The ecological condition of Rhodesia in 1890–1900

Modern Rhodesian statistics can be used to give a quantitative expression to the idea of the *Grenzwildnis* in the ecology of African trypanosomiasis. Before this can be done it is necessary to obtain some idea of the ecological state of Rhodesia at the time of the occupation by Rhodes's pioneer column. Ranger (1968), a historian not sympathetic to the Rhodesian viewpoint, chooses an impeccable source (one that the most ardent imperialist would hardly question) to give an eye-witness account of the Rhodesian plateau during the last century.

In 1893 the famous hunter, F. C. Selous, drew a picture of Mashonaland as it must have been 'some fifty years ago. The peaceful people inhabiting this part of Africa must then have been at the zenith of their prosperity. Herds of their small but beautiful cattle lowed in every valley and their rich and fertile country doubtless afforded them an abundance of vegetable food.' [The paramount chiefs were then] 'rulers of large and prosperous tribes . . . whose towns were for the most part surrounded by well built and loop-holed stone walls. . . . Hundreds of thousands of acres which now lie fallow must then have been under cultivation . . . while the sites of ancient villages are very numerous all over the open downs'.

Selous, who had walked and ridden over much of Rhodesia in the 1870s, believed that this emptiness had been caused by the Ndebele, but it is now clear that these people were still in process of asserting their rule and that the depopulation had come from other causes. If it was due to warfare it was the expeditions of Zwangendaba, Nxaba, and Soshangane that had prepared the way for the Ndebele.

By Selous's evidence as well as the more recent archaeological data, there must have been vast depopulation. We have already seen the effect of the European impact further north. The epidemics and epizootics that followed the Ngoni invasions have not yet been investigated; but there is evidence of the same sort of sequence as that which happened in the inter-lake region, in Sukumaland, and in Busoga. A bad smallpox epidemic that began in the Cape in 1858 reached Matabeleland in 1862 and was accompanied by an epidemic of measles, a disease that, we tend to forget in modern Europe, brings heavy infant mortality. In 1863 there was a major epizootic due to a new disease which, like the later rinderpest, came from Europe. Contagious bovine pleuropneumonia, a bacterial disease, reached the U.S.A. in 1843, Australia in 1858, and South Africa in a Friesland bull from Holland landed at Mossel bay in 1854. In two years 200 000 animals are known to have died in South Africa. In 1861 a European trader brought it in his oxen from South Africa into Matabeleland (Henning 1956). By the 1880s it had reached the pastoral societies north of the equator. If not quite so devastating as the rinderpest, it was very severe and was remembered for many years all over Africa. In Chad it was the major preoccupation of the first French military veterinarians and Lugard heard of it as a predecessor of rinderpest in Ankole. It is at least probable that pleuropneumonia was a depopulating agency of Shona livestock more powerful than either the Ngoni or the Ndebele.

These diseases were in part themselves invasive, but in part also were consequences of weakened resistance to infection caused by famine. In 1968, at the time of writing, we see in Nigeria the consequences of war in a land inhabited by peasant cultivators practising subsistence agriculture.

Because of the disorganization caused by the fighting cultivation cannot be carried out and there is no harvest. The seed corn and tubers must then be eaten and after that nothing is left. The deaths caused by military action become trivial in comparison with the mortality, especially among the children, that is caused by starvation. And because it is the young who chiefly suffer there is a failure of the next generation. There can be little doubt that these were the principal consequences of the Ngoni invasions of the Rozwi empire. The entry for 6 April 1863 in Livingstone's journal is significant. He was then at a mission on the lower Zambezi and was reporting a conversation with one of the missionaries. 'The country has been devastated by the Makololo—the people of Chibisa—the famine and the slave dealers. Waller says that the famine caused 99 out of the hundred deaths that happened' (Livingstone 1956).

When Rhodes's pioneers arrived in 1890 they took over a country emptied by famine and disease and shortly after their arrival the rinderpest (another European or Euro-Asian invasion) came in from the north to complete, or nearly complete, the devastation. Yet enough was left of the Shona and Ndebele societies to reproduce yet again the same consequences of war on a peasant society. This time the evidence is in writing, in the annual reports to the shareholders of the British South Africa Company. In 1897 the Chief Native Commissioner, Mashonaland, reported: 'Owing to the harassing received at the hands of our troops, the natives in these districts are not too well off for grain and it will take two or three years before they can thoroughly recover themselves in this respect. Where it has been absolutely necessary, grain has been provided to ex-rebels on promise of payment as soon as the harvest is gathered.' Where there was no 'rebellion' the natives 'are naturally far better off in every respect'.

In Matabeleland in the same year the Chief Native Commissioner wrote: 'The Indunas reported great want of food and actual starvation amongst the people.' Nearly a million pounds of grain were distributed. 'The rebellion upset the whole country and prevented that nursing of their stores which was imperative after three bad harvests in succession.' One may suppose that these bad harvests were very largely a consequence of the war.

Evidence of disease in the wake of the famines is not lacking. The Matabele report continues: 'Hundreds of natives fell victims to a peculiar disease which, I believe, is still unknown to the medical men in the country and which was, I think, attributable to the combined effects of starvation and the eating of the remains of cattle which had died of rinderpest. Already this season numbers of them are starving.' In 1898 the same official wrote 'Deaths are of frequent occurrence amongst the natives. . . . At one period of the year an unusual number of deaths seemed to take place, in some instances several people dying at one kraal, from which it would appear that some epidemic or contagious disease was prevalent at the time.' There was also smallpox about, from the note on which we find that there had been an epidemic shortly after the arrival of the pioneer column. 'Vaccination is well known to them, and the majority of natives show marks on various parts of the body, principally the arms, where they were vaccinated on the last outbreak of smallpox some six years ago' (British South Africa Company, 1896, 1898).

Since, at this time, almost all the medical services available were devoted to preserving the health of the invaders, less can be gathered about the health of local populations than is the case in countries further north, but it seems clear that they underwent the same sort of sequence of famine and disease that afflicted the whole continent. Also, as in the rest of the continent, the same pattern of self-congratulation on the beneficial effects of colonial rule began to appear in official records. 'Pacification' and an end to 'tribal warfare' soon, in the eyes of the new rulers, began to result in multiplication of the native populations. In fact the colonial impact had been so violent that the populations can scarcely have failed to multiply once the epidemics had spent themselves and the surviving people were again able to resume their cultivation. The colonial governments were witnessing not the results of their own beneficent rule but only the re-establishment of ecological equilibrium. Everywhere this was happening in the context of new social and political environments. In Rhodesia these had a unique character which must now be examined.

20

LAND APPORTIONMENT AND
THE RHODESIAN *GRENZWILDNIS*

Recapitulation

So far Rhodesia has been treated as a geographical unit more or less isolated between a northern and southern *Grenzwildnis*, both, in the past, infested by tsetse. Archaeological evidence makes it virtually certain that before the Ngoni invasions of the early nineteenth century, these fly-belts were much smaller than they had become by about 1870. Their expansion between 1830 and 1870 had been a response to depopulation brought about by famine and disease that followed the social disorganization produced by the Ngoni impact.

The researches of Jack (1914 et seq.) and more recently of Bursell (1960, 1966, 1969) have shown that at these latitudes and altitudes *Glossina* has reached the geographical limits which its physiology and ethology will permit. In these marginal regions the insects maintain a tenuous hold upon life. In the hot seasons in the south-east of the country and, in the north, in the Zambezi valley floor, physiologically life is lived so rapidly and the size of the habitat is so reduced by adverse climate that the problem of host encounter and hence of obtaining food sufficiently frequently can hardly be overcome. In the winter, on the outer fringes of the fly-belts, where they begin to impinge upon higher ground, pupal life is so prolonged by cold that the smaller flies have not sufficient nutrient reserves to supply the energy necessary for finding the first meal. Host encounter is again a limiting factor. In these conditions reduction in density of the larger mammal fauna, especially of the preferred hosts of *Glossina*, has a rapid effect in reducing the tsetse population. Energetic settlers like Mzila and his people in Gazaland were quickly able to create conditions in which cattle keeping was possible where, a few years before, the land had been full of tsetse. Here also, around the Rhodesian periphery, the rinderpest was followed by far more extensive recessions of the fly-belts than in countries nearer the equator.

It was shown, in chapters on the interlake region and Sukumaland, that the essential character of the *Grenzwildnis* is not that it is tsetse-infested, but that it consists of land that is inherently poor or else difficult to exploit. In Rhodesia the western frontier region, or a substantial part of it, is not infested by *Glossina*. Earlier European hunters and prospectors were able to enter what they called Matabeleland by a route that circumvented the fly-belts of the Limpopo. The western limits of the country were created by the sub-desert climate of the Kalahari and the poor foundation that its sands provided for agriculture and pasture.

It is useful, as a preliminary to discussing the role of the *Grenzwildnis* in modern Rhodesian society, to look again at the paper in which Summers (1960) attempted to show how past changes in Pleistocene rainfall had altered the distribution of the major vegetation communities of pre-historic Rhodesia. His speculations on the effects of human trypanosomiasis on prehistoric communities have been rejected, but there can be no doubt that extensive shifts in the distributions of different vegetations took place and that these must have influenced the lives of those animals which lived in them, including man.

The Later Stone Age occupants of Rhodesia practised a Wilton culture and in their later period were responsible for many of the rock paintings that are found so abundantly on suitable granite outcrops. The climate of the Later Stone Age was much the same as it is today. Clark (1959) gives a number of C^{14} dates which suggest that it began in southern Africa 7000–8000 years ago. It endured until the first Iron Age people appeared near the beginning of the first millennium A.D. These people cultivated, made Channelled Ware pottery, and may have owned cattle. At the time that they began to flourish rainfall, although not greatly in excess of that of the Later Stone Age or of today (perhaps 120 per cent), was better distributed so that the dry mopane woodlands were smaller and the *Brachystegia* woodlands were larger than they are now.

Under these conditions agriculture could flourish and whether or not *Glossina morsitans* found a congenial climate in respect of temperature, it must have been pushed further and further from its natural limits by cultivators who also became miners and traders in gold and copper. No doubt, also, they were hunters.

Summers's maps show how closely the distribution of the archaeological remains of these people, whose successive cultures lasted until the beginning of the nineteenth century, coincided with the areas now occupied by European settlers, except that they had a wider distribution. The heartland of the Mutapa empire certainly overlapped widely parts of the Zambezi valley that, after its collapse, became infested with tsetse. In the tsetse-infested Dande area, north of that Mount Fura up which the Portuguese were not allowed to climb, it is possible to find dry-stone ruins that greatly resemble similar structures used elsewhere in Africa as cattle kraals. No ruins or other Iron Age remains have been found in the Sebungwe area and perhaps this was always as unfavourable for agriculture as it is today. What the subjects of Mutapa and the Rozwi certainly avoided was the Kalahari sand. This was scarcely surprising in a mixed farming community. 'Inherent fertility is very low and moisture retention in the rooting zone of field crops and grasses is poor. . . . Beef production is not considered possible on holdings confined to this Area. The grasses are extremely poor

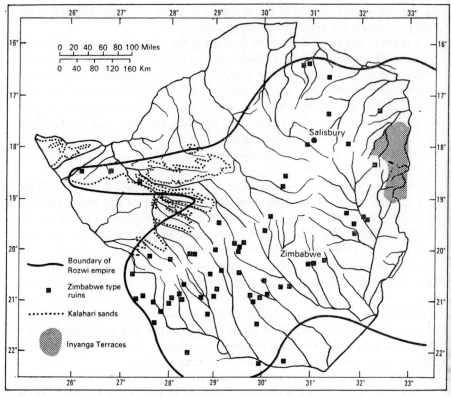

MAP 20.1. 'Boundary' of the Rozwi empire in 1700 (from Ranger 1968), with distribution of Zimbabwe type ruins and the Inyanga terraced area (after Summers 1960). The dotted outline shows the limits of Kalahari sand.

and the veld can only be considered as summer grazing.' This verdict of Vincent, Thomas, Anderson, and Staples (n.d.), who were judging the Kalahari sands chiefly from the viewpoint of the European farmer, expressed also the verdict of their Iron Age predecessors. Into this western frontier wilderness the Shona group of tribes pushed the less technically and militarily able people they supplanted. Well into this century the only inhabitants of what became the Wankie national park were the Bushmen (Davison 1967) who were, perhaps, descendants of the people who made the Rhodesian rock paintings. Into the Kalahari sands also the Europeans in their turn pushed the Ndebele. The first native reserves were created in land of which it might be said that some of it was too inhospitable even for tsetse flies. The largest of the reserves allotted to the Ndebele after the 'rebellion' were Nyamandhlovu, Lupani, and Nkai, which, together with the Wankie park, occupy most of the Kalahari sands area of Rhodesia. Ranger (1968) gives a rough outline of the boundary of the Rozwi empire in 1700. Part of this outline is included in Map 20.1 which also shows the distribution of Zimbabwe type ruins from Summers (1960). The indentation made by the Kalahari sands on the western frontier is very clear. How have the Rhodesians handled the problem of the *Grenzwildnis*?

The land apportionment map

An interesting document for students of the African *Grenzwildnis* was the Rhodesian land apportionment map (Surveyor General, Salisbury 1963), now out of print. It showed a patchwork of colours which indicated seven different land categories. In 1959 they were arranged as follows:

European area	48 062 000 acres
Native reserves	21 020 000 acres
Native purchase areas	8 052 000 acres
Special native areas	12 878 000 acres
Wankie game reserve	4 000 000 acres
Forest area	3 190 000 acres
Undetermined	57 000 acres
Total	97 259 000 acres

The three categories of native areas together totalled 41 950 000 acres. These figures are taken from a Southern Rhodesian government report (Quinton 1960) which proposed to abolish land apportionment, and, as an interim measure, intended to deduct 10 million acres from land set aside from European use, add 2 million acres to African land, and create a new category of 10 million acres of National land which was to include the Wankie game reserve and a much modified Forest area. Eventually all except the 10 million acres of National land were to become Common land, open to purchase by persons of any race. Much of the 2 million acres added to the native land came from the former forest area, while of the 10 million acres to be deducted from land originally scheduled for European use, a half went into the new category of Common land (and was therefore still available for purchase by Europeans) while of the remainder 3 645 851 acres were either inside the 1960 fly-line or within the area of earlier tsetse infestation. Of this, over one-third was given to the Africans, while the largest single parcel of 1 613 000 acres became National land and was developed as a resort for sportsmen.

Although the Quinton report took away very little from the European minority and gave very little to the African majority, its slightly more liberal outlook was one factor leading to the Rhodesian 'rebellion' five years later. Another report that also failed to find favour with some of the Rhodesian oligarchy was that of Phillips, Hammond, Samuels, and Swynnerton (1962) which discussed the economic resources of Rhodesia with particular reference to the role of African agriculture. A complementary work concerned chiefly with the potentialities for European farming had been issued two years earlier (Vincent, Thomas, Anderson, and Staples n.d.). These three reports, together with the annual reports of the Chief Native Commissioner, provide most of the data on which the remainder of this chapter is based.

Possessory segregation and the fly-belts

Map 20.2 is a simplified version of the Land apportionment map on which are superimposed four outlines of the *G. morsitans* belts: (1) the maximum extension shortly before the Great Rinderpest; (2) the limits reached by the recovering fly-belts when intensive wild host slaughter was begun about 1932 (from Jack 1933); (3) the outline towards the end of the intensive slaughter period in 1949 (Whellan 1950); and (4) that of 1961 (Phillips, Hammond, Samuels, and Swynnerton 1962).

In 1894 an Order in Council of the British government required that the British South Africa Company should 'from time to time assign to the native inhabitants of Southern Rhodesia land sufficient for their occupation'. No limit was placed upon the land which might then be allocated. The African population of Rhodesia was thought to amount to about 500 000 at the time of the occupation by Rhodes's pioneers in 1890. By 1913 Africans were estimated to number 712 000 of whom 400 000 were living on the reserves and 312 000 on lands outside the reserves. At this time Africans owned 377 000 head of cattle and 895 000 sheep and goats. By 1914 the area of the reserves had risen to 21 million acres and a Native reserves commission felt that this should be sufficient for all time since there still remained 78 million acres open to purchase by Africans or Europeans. Mineral rights in the reserves belonged to the British South Africa Company. Africans could be dispossessed to allow mining development, provided 'just and liberal compensation in land' was given elsewhere.

Although it was and still is maintained that the establishment of reserves was necessary to protect Africans from the predatory acquisitiveness of white Rhodesians, by 1921 the latter were sufficiently apprehensive of future competition to press for more legislation. In 1925 another land commission, the Carter commission, 'advanced many social, economic and psychological reasons for advocating possessory segregation' (Quinton 1960). Its recommendations were embodied in the Land Apportionment Act 1930 which created another category of land, the Native purchase area, of 7 500 000 acres. By this time Europeans owned 49 million acres, and there remained, apart from less than a million acres of forest land, 18 million of Unassigned land. Implementation of the Land Apportionment Act began in 1932. At the time the Zambezi fly-belt was still in process of recovery from the effects of the post-rinderpest recession and covered some 24 000 mile^2. Over half of this area was included in the Native reserves. Of the 28 million acres allotted to Africans under the Act of 1930, one-third was inside the Zambezi fly-belt.

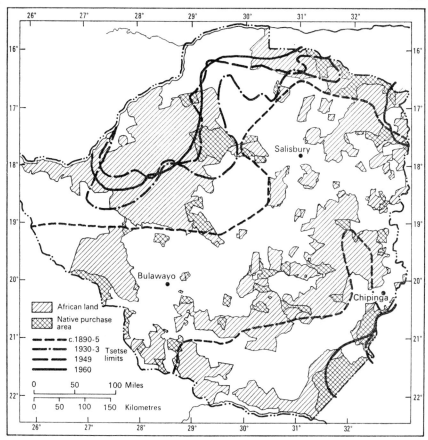

MAP 20.2. Land apportionment and tsetse infestation in Rhodesia.

At that time it might have been argued that these tsetse-infested lands would, in due course, be freed of infection and, as we have seen, by 1950 some 10 000 mile² had, in fact, been reclaimed. If one accepts the conventional judgement on the 'tsetse problem' that the presence of the insect deprives the African population of vast areas of land which could otherwise be put to useful purposes, it might seem that the apparent injustice of allocating so much tsetse-infested land to the indigenous people was illusory. The application of simple entomological techniques would soon rectify matters. But this did not happen. The combined effects of the shooting operations and the reallocation of land in the Quinton report (1960) greatly improved the relative position of European landowners *vis-à-vis* the Africans within the tsetse-infested areas. Table 20.1 shows the land apportionment categories within the tsetse-infested country before the shooting campaigns began and in 1961 when they were finally closed. The Quinton report (1960) in fact gives a table showing 2 355 000 acres

TABLE 20.1

Land infested with tsetse in Rhodesia and its allocation to African and European ownership

Land apportionment	1931		1961	
	Mile²	%	Mile²	%
African land . .	13 496	57·51	11 912	71·53
European land . .	7 848	33·45	1 633	9·81
Forest or national land	2 121	9·04	3 107	18·66
Total . . .	23 465	100·00	16 652	100·00

(3679 mile²) of European land within the tsetse-infested areas. However, this was before the adjustment made by the transfer of 1 613 000 acres (2520 mile²) from land allocated for European occupation to form the Urungwe hunting area already referred to, plus other smaller similar transfers from European to National land. It will also be noted in Table 20.1 that the reduction in area of the fly-belts by 1961 is less than the 10 000 mile² achieved by 1950. This is because shortly after that year substantial invasions of *Glossina* from Mozambique entered Rhodesia in the Sabi–Lundi basin and in the Mtoko area in the north-east of the country.

Natural resource potential and the fly-belts

Cockbill (1967) has recently referred briefly to the relationship of tsetse infestation to the natural resource potential of the fly-belts and it is useful to carry his analysis further. Vincent, Thomas, Anderson, and Staples (n.d.) divided Rhodesia into five natural regions based upon climate, soils, topography, and vegetation. Regions I, II, and III comprise land adaptable to various types of intensive mixed farming. Region IV is suited to extensive cattle rearing with a small amount of arable for raising supplementary fodder crops. Region V should be used only for extensive ranching, with a carrying capacity of between one beast to 20 acres and one to 50 acres, or as wildlife reserves. Much of Region V is waterless through most of the year. Vincent, Thomas, Anderson, and Staples (n.d.) estimated that in Region V 'an African beef producer with a herd of about twenty animals could, under good management, produce on an average four animals for sale yearly and that his net income from these, after deducting dipping costs and marketing and development charges and making allowance for the interest on the capital value of his herd, would be about £45 per annum'. To achieve this he requires 600 acres of land. The European rancher in similar country needs between 50 and 100 mile² (*c.* 50 000

acres) to support himself in reasonable comfort (i.e. to gain a net income
of perhaps £2500 a year). A sixth category (XX) includes land in any
region, but mostly in Region V, that is unexploitable, usually because of
its violent topography.

The areas occupied by these various regions as estimated for the country
as a whole by Phillips, Hammond, Samuels, and Swynnerton (1962) are
set out in the second column of Table 20.2. In the third column are the
areas of the different regions allocated to Africans. They obtained less than
one-fifth of the top grade of Region I, less than a quarter of Region II, and
just over one-third of Region III. Of the lower categories, unfit for arable
farming, they obtained almost half of Region IV and well over half of
Region V. They had a two-thirds share of the completely useless XX land.
Within the limits of the actual and potential fly-belts we may observe the
following points. In Rhodesia as a whole the less productive regions
(IV, V, and XX) cover 62·3 per cent of the land's surface, but in the area of
maximum tsetse spread which was close to the natural limitation imposed
by climate (including both the Zambezi and Sabi–Limpopo belts) these
poorer land categories occupied 83·6 per cent of the land's surface. When
the phase of reclamation came to an end in the Zambezi belt (Column 5),
these three categories totalled 94·3 per cent of the land still left un-
reclaimed. Over half of the country's unusable XX land still remained in
the reduced fly-belt (Ford 1969c).

The Zambezi fly-belt provides an admirable illustration of the ideas of
Gillman (1936) that it is not the tsetse that keeps out man, but that the
tsetse flourishes where man cannot. The point was well made in a conversation I overheard between two Rhodesian members of Parliament, one white
and one black, while flying over the Zambezi fly-belt. The rains had just
begun and one looked down upon a smiling landscape of fresh green foliage.
The Rhodesian said, 'Look at that. You are always grumbling because you
haven't enough land. Why don't you come and take this?' The African
answered, 'If it had been any use at all, you people would have had it long
ago.'

Land-use techniques and the *Grenzwildnis*

The Rhodesian shooting campaigns of 1930–50 came to a halt when it
was obviously uneconomic to go further. In fact the campaign had already
overshot its mark and freed more country than could be safeguarded from
re-invasion with the resources available. In 1950 tsetse began to spread
again into the Urungwe native reserve where some 8000 cattle had become
established following successes achieved by game destruction in that area
by 1944. By 1952 trypanosomiasis had killed about 2800 animals. Another
2300 were slaughtered because unfit to walk, and the survivors were
evacuated (Chorley 1954). The rapid response of the wildlife to cessation of
hunting in the Nagupande area has already been described. The Urungwe

TABLE 20.2

Natural regions of Rhodesia (1) in whole country, (2) in African areas, (3) in Zambezi fly-belt at period of maximum extension, (4) in Zambezi fly-belt in 1949, and (5) in Sabi–Limpopo fly-belt at period of maximum extension

Natural region	In all Rhodesia†		In African land‡		Maximum extension of Zambezi fly-belt§		Zambezi tsetse belt in 1949¶		Maximum extension of Sabi–Limpopo belt§	
	Mile²	%	Mile²	%	Mile²	%	Mile²	%	Mile²	%
I	2 368	1·6	438	0·7	Nil	0	Nil	0	Nil	0
II	28 351	18·7	6 496	9·9	595	1·2	Nil	0	Nil	0
III	26 467	17·4	9 209	14·1	11 166	22·2	892	5·7	Nil	0
IV	50 231	33·1	23 821	36·3	27 017	53·7	7 268	46·8	1 610	7·5
V	39 723	26·1	22 481	34·3	6 969	13·8	4 545	29·2	19 956	92·5
XX	4 711	3·1	3 101	4·7	4 566	9·1	2 847	18·3	Nil	0
Totals	151 851	100·0	65 546	100·0	50 313	100·0	15 542	100·0	21 566	100·0

† Phillips, Hammond, Samuels, and Swynnerton (1962).
‡ Vincent, Thomas, Anderson, and Staples (n.d.).
§ Jack (1933).
¶ Whellan (1950).

epizootic evidently followed a similar recovery of the wild animal populations as soon as hunters were withdrawn.

Unusable land becomes usable when appropriate techniques are invented and applied and, in fact, the Zambezi *Grenzwildnis* is used by the Tonga, most of whom live in Zambia, who have survived in small communities by developing quite complicated agricultural practices described in detail by Scudder (1962). But their hold upon the land is tenuous and their numbers too small to affect the populations of tsetse hosts to a sufficient degree to limit the size of the fly-belts. On the whole the Zambezi fly-belt fulfils the conditions required for the *Grenzwildnis*. It is avoided by the majority of the people, especially the ruling caste who tend to drive unwanted members of subject races into it, it serves as a wildlife reserve and reservoir of zoonotic infection, and also as a base of operations for dissident political groups. The Rhodesian political detainees as well as the freedom-fighter groups may be compared with the followers of the surviving brothers of interlake divine kings.

As soon, however, as techniques are developed for its full exploitation, the *Grenzwildnis* loses its status. In Rhodesia the greater part of the Sabi–Limpopo potential tsetse area is occupied by European-owned ranches. The attraction of the area is not, indeed, its low carrying capacity pasture, but the fact that a very large part of it is irrigable. This is illustrated by Map 20.2. The southern *Grenzwildnis*, formerly tsetse-infested, contains a large area of European land. In the Sabi and Limpopo basins some 4750 mile^2 are irrigable (Phillips, Hammond, Samuels, and Swynnerton 1962). Two-thirds of this potentially valuable land lies in the European area. The only substantial portion of the Zambezi fly-belt still retained for European occupation in the Quinton report (1960) contains a large irrigable area, much of which had been already planted with sugar by 1965. In Rhodesia as a whole, at the end of 1961, some 90 000 acres of land were under irrigation from rivers and dams and of this area only 10 per cent was on African land. As the technical ability of a people develops in ways that permit exploitation of formerly waste land, so the *Grenzwildnis* disappears. With it go the zoonoses. The full development of the irrigable lands of south-eastern Rhodesia will greatly reduce the magnitude of the problem of trypanosomiasis control. Vast acreages of sugar, citrus, and cereals will support neither tsetse nor their natural hosts, for crop-raiding animals on big estates are ruthlessly killed off.

Before leaving the subject of the Rhodesian *Grenzwildnis* it is worth while to glance at a curious attempt to codify an appearance of liberal intention in the 1932 Land Apportionment Act. The so-called Native purchase area created by this Act amounted, by 1960, to 8 052 261 acres (Quinton 1960). This area was, of course, divided into numerous, often small, parcels of land. Within them sufficiently wealthy Africans could acquire a legal (though strictly limited) title to their own farms. The

Quinton report does not specify how much of the N.P.A. had been sold, but 6257 plots had been made available by 1960. However, in that year 6 500 000 acres out of the original 8 million still remained unsurveyed. This was not surprising as 54 per cent of the total Native purchase area adjoined the borders of the territory and its largest component parts lay in tsetse-infested land or in land in course of invasion by tsetse. The N.P.A., often referred to as land in which Africans could acquire their own farms on terms equivalent to those enjoyed by their masters, was, for the most part, carefully sited within the *Grenzwildnis* and therefore was virtually useless.

The Rhodesian cattle population

Whether the expansion of the Sebungwe fly-belt at a rate of 28 per cent per annum (Fig. 17.1) was a reflection of the unimpeded growth at the same rate of warthog, kudu, and buffalo populations may be a matter for speculation. But there is little doubt about the recovery of the cattle after the rinderpest had spent its first fury.

Every year from 1897 onwards the total of African-owned cattle has been published in the annual reports of the Chief Native Commissioner. The records of the first few years, at least up to 1901, refer only to the cattle of the Ndebele. Thereafter for some years more and more small herds must have been brought within the administrative orbit. When Lobengula was dead and the Ndebele uprising was finally suppressed the British South Africa Company took over the titular ownership of the indigenous cattle and through its Native Department assumed a protective role to prevent the animals that survived the panzootic being completely appropriated by white Rhodesians whose stock had, of course, also been reduced to a fraction of what it had been. In his account of this Ranger (1967) is misleading. He states that before the 'rebellion' the Ndebele owned about 250 000 animals and implies that the difference between this figure and the total of about 40 000 registered in 1900 was largely due to misappropriation by settlers. If informed opinion and the slight quantitative evidence available elsewhere of the effects of the rinderpest is correct, then we should expect to find that a population of 250 000 cattle in February 1895 would have been reduced to about 13 000 by the end of that year. Rhodesian pioneers did commandeer the cattle of the defeated natives, but the panzootic can have left very few for them to take.

Fig. 20.1 shows the population growth curve of the African-owned cattle population of Rhodesia and the changes, from year to year, in its growth rate. This fluctuated violently up to about 1912. In part this may have reflected an increasing efficiency of censuses, but in part it was due to disease. The rinderpest virus was soon eliminated by a vigorous isolation and vaccination campaign, but between 1900 and 1903 contagious bovine pleuropneumonia, ulcerative lymphaginitis, East coast fever, and foot and

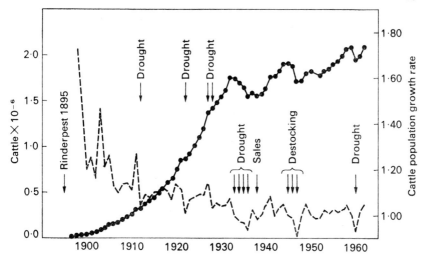

FIG. 20.1. The growth of the Rhodesian (African-owned) cattle population, with the curve of growth rate, and events observed to have controlled it.

mouth disease infected the Rhodesian cattle in rapid succession. In spite of these successive epizootics the cattle population continued its rapid increase and one is reminded again of Hornby's (1938) comment on Sukumaland, that it is not disease that controls the cattle, but starvation. While the pastures were still understocked, the birth rate far outstripped the death rate, even as one disease after another re-invaded the country. But in 1912 the first heavy losses of cattle due to drought were recorded. From 1897 to 1911 the mean increase rate shown by the figures available was 26·2 per cent per annum. A second severe drought occurred in 1922. Between the 1912 and 1922 droughts increase had slowed to a rate of 9·6 per cent per annum. In the next decade the mean annual increase rate fell to 6·8 per cent. There were droughts in 1927 and 1928. From 1932 to 1962 the mean annual increase rate was only 0·6 per cent per annum. This 30-year period began with severe droughts in four successive years. The Southern Rhodesian government then began to put pressure on owners to sell their stock and the decrease in numbers observed between the 1937 and 1938 cattle counts was attributed to the effectiveness of this measure. But sales for cash did not have a continuing popularity and cattle numbers again began to rise. To counteract this, for it could only bring about more deaths from starvation and thirst, the government introduced compulsory destocking. This lasted over three years, 1945–7, and again slowed down the growth rate. But in the era of political liberalism that followed the end of the war the government was reluctant to use compulsion. Propaganda in favour of cattle sales, with government guaranteeing a minimum price, was to some extent successful, but the cattle population continued to grow, with the expected result of sharp losses from starvation in 1960.

The growth of the cattle population of Sukumaland is controlled by the availability of pasture. There, however, because Sukumaland is surrounded on three sides by tsetse-infested bush, it is possible to argue that trypanosomiasis does exert a control by preventing cattle from occupying more land. This is not the case in Rhodesia, for from 1930 to 1950, when growth of the cattle population had virtually ceased, trypanosomiasis was negligible in its effects even on the borders of the *Grenzwildnis* because the zone in which shooting took place was closed to cattle. Only where, from 1938 onwards, the Sabi–Lundi basin began to be re-invaded, or from the early 1940s the Mtoko area in north-east Rhodesia also began to feel the effects of the still expanding fly-belts in Mozambique, did the African cattle of Rhodesia suffer severely from trypanosome infection. The limitation on expansion for the majority of these cattle was exerted not by the fly-belts but by the artificial boundaries of the Land Apportionment Act. But the effect was the same. As the capacity of the pastures was reached and then exceeded, cattle population density became increasingly controlled by thirst and starvation (Engledow 1958).

Starvation not only controls numbers of cattle; it also limits their size. Selous, quoted in Chapter 19, remarked that the Shona cattle of the 1870s were 'small but beautiful'. Today the descendants of those that survived the rinderpest are much crossed with other types and breeds, so that comparisons cannot be made; but it is appropriate to close this account of the African cattle population of Rhodesia by giving the latest instalment of the story of the Sabi valley cattle related in Chapter 18. The series of epizootics that beset them after 1950 were successfully controlled by drug administration, by bush clearing, and by use of insecticides. The consequences of this success are described in a local veterinary report quoted by Lovemore (1967):

Cattle populations . . . continue to increase relentlessly in Sabi East and this must in part reflect the minimal disease position. In the case of Mariya the removal of the trypanosomiases threat has resulted in a census increase of 52 per cent in only three years. . . . Although not directly a veterinary problem this population growth could easily become one unless something is done about it. There could be a natural decline in the size and quality of the cattle, as it appears has taken place in the small stock.

If one looks again at Fig. 18.2 one might suggest that not only will size and quality decline, but that the rapid multiplication will, in Sabi East as elsewhere in Rhodesia, be brought before long to a sudden halt by heavy mortality due to starvation.

European-owned cattle are less liable to this catastrophic form of population limitation. There are fewer of them than of African cattle;† they are raised not as direct pecuniary assets but for sale, so that carcass weight or

† 1 650 948 European and 2 082 515 African-owned cattle in 1962 (Federal Ministry of Agriculture 1963).

milk yield is of more importance than population density; they are pastured on better land which is by no means cultivated to full capacity; and reserve grazing and crops of various kinds for winter or dry-season fodder offset periodical natural poverty. In short, an agriculture managed with different objectives in view provides population control with monetary profit instead of one which only results in periodical loss. It is fair to add that it has been the professed aim of the Rhodesian government to achieve this form of control for all cattle, regardless of ownership, and further to note that some progress has been made in this direction.

European responses to *Glossina*

If it were true that vast areas of eastern Africa have been closed to human occupation because of the presence of *Glossina* and the disease it transmits, then the sudden removal of the pest coincidentally with the arrival of the Rhodesian pioneers should have permitted them to take up and develop land denied to their predecessors. This did not happen. The Rhodesians occupied the best lands, the lands that for a thousand years had been worked over, mined, and cultivated by their Bantu forerunners. Like them too, they drove the defeated survivors of their invasion into the *Grenzwildnis* and into the granite hills.

It was estimated that rather less than 500 000 Africans had survived the catastrophes of the nineteenth century. For a long time, therefore, there was ample room for them as well as for the vast estates given by Rhodes to his pioneers. But when it was realized that much of the still empty land in the Sabi–Lundi basin that had once harboured tsetse was irrigable, this section of the *Grenzwildnis* was declared to be European land. The development of irrigation did not, however, move fast enough to provide a barrier to the re-invading tsetse. At present this spread of *Glossina morsitans* into its former habitat, which threatens also to re-invade the Limpopo basin, is being contained by annual insecticide campaigns (Robertson and Kluge 1968). Applied entomology provides other devices for overcoming the disadvantages of the frontier wilderness. In the Sabi–Lundi basin, it enables landowners to ranch cattle while they await the completion of a hydrological programme that will allow them to turn to far more productive agricultural activities.

In addition to new techniques of land management and pest control, the Rhodesian invasion introduced a quite new factor into the African trypanosomiasis problem. This was private ownership of land.† The great estates were marked out, fenced (especially where they adjoined native reserves), and registered with all the legal paraphernalia of a fully developed European society. Associated with this process was, of course, political power; overwhelming on the European side of the fences, negligible on the African.

† The *Mailo* lands given to loyal chiefs by the first Protectorate governments in Uganda were small by comparison and hardly influenced policies of trypanosomiasis control.

This situation has had advantages as well as disadvantages in respect of control of zoonoses. The pushing of the African population outward from the central, mainly European occupied high veld, towards or into the *Grenzwildnis* has meant that between the white farmer and the sources of infection is a zone populated with people and with cattle. The latter are subject to strict and very thorough inspection systems and the epizootiological data thus recorded are superior to any yet available in countries nearer the equator. These cattle also provide an invaluable buffer against spread of infection to the European farms. Between the reserves which support cattle and the tsetse-infested bush was further interposed the zone in which destruction of the natural hosts of the tsetse, supplemented in recent years by insecticides and bush clearing, provided yet another line of defence. In recent years the pattern has been modified, in some sectors, by use of mass drug treatments which have allowed cattle to penetrate further towards the tsetse-infested bush.

The effects of isolation

Workers on tsetse flies, in English-speaking parts of Africa, only became involved with cattle trypanosomiasis after the introduction of large-scale drug therapy and prophylaxis between 1950 and 1955; nevertheless they heard of and had opportunities to see the effects of infection in cattle. I began work on *Glossina* in 1938 and although I often saw infected cattle and even, very occasionally, a corpse and although, also, most of my work has been concerned with the control of tsetse in order to control cattle trypanosomiasis I have never, in thirty years, been directly involved in an epizootic in which large numbers of cattle have died. I have, indeed, witnessed the evacuation of country by cattle because of infection, but there was never any mortality on a scale large enough to have a spectacular and immediate effect on the lives of local people. The only places where I have been aware of recent disruptive epizootics causing very large numbers of deaths have been in Rhodesia. One of these has been mentioned and took place in the Urungwe reserve in 1951–2. The other was in the northeast corner of Rhodesia in 1964.

In Ankole, in Sukumaland, and in Eastern Uganda the spread of tsetse fly resulted in changes in cattle distribution but did not halt the increase in their numbers. In Rhodesia the majority of African-owned cattle were confined by the boundaries created by Land apportionment. Where they became exposed to spreading tsetse these boundaries prevented them and their owners from moving away. In 1918 native-owned cattle died freely from the disease on the Gwaai river when the expanding Sebungwe fly-belt reached them. Near the confluence of the Sabi and Lundi rivers, when the Mozambique fly-belt spread across the border, the majority of cattle also died. In neither case were the owners able to move away from the sources of infection because of the restrictions of possessory segregation. In both cases the cattle involved had been out of contact with *Glossina* at least since the post-rinderpest recession in 1896. The Urungwe epizootic of 1951–2 took place in similar circumstances. These cattle and their parent generations had also been out of contact with trypanosomiasis for half a century. The only drug available, dimidium bromide, was ineffective in controlling the disease and the mortality (including slaughter of animals too weak to move) was over 50 per cent before the survivors were brought out.

The outcome of the Sabi epizootics described in Chapter 18 has been very different. The cattle around Mwangazi and Muumbe also began to die in fairly large numbers when infection first reached them from the spreading Mozambique fly-belt. But here after eight years of control of infection by drugs and exposure to continuously spreading, though partly controlled, tsetse invasion, a condition was created in which withdrawal of the drugs produced almost no ill effects. Moreover towards the end of the period, cattle that had received no drug treatment and had become infected with either *Trypanosoma congolense* or *T. vivax* succeeded in throwing off the infections. These cattle are now multiplying at a rate that threatens their survival (page 352).

In contrast to this situation an apparently similar withholding of drug treatments in the north-east of Rhodesia was followed by over 4800 deaths in a relatively circumscribed area in 1964. In what way did events prior to this disaster differ from those that have been described in the Sabi valley?

In 1943 Portuguese officials reported the presence of tsetse near Villa Gouveia just below the eastern slopes of Inyanga mountain. In 1944 there were heavy losses of cattle in Mozambique just opposite the Mtoko district in the north-east corner of Rhodesia. The Rhodesians began to think about building a fenced corridor along their border from which all potential hosts of tsetse would be removed or killed (Chorley 1944, 1945). In 1946 a European farmer claimed his cattle were becoming infected and moved his herd to another estate in a different part of the country. No infections were seen in cattle in adjacent native reserves, but in 1947 8 positives were seen among several hundred blood slides. No tsetse were found (Chorley 1947b, Mossop 1948). In 1948, however, there were rather over 100 deaths among nearly 5000 cattle in the Mkota Reserve, adjoining the international border, and it was estimated that the infection incidence was about 5 per cent. All cattle in affected kraals were treated with dimidium. After exhaustive searches no tsetse were found except on the Portuguese side of the border, 13 miles from the Mkota outbreak area. In 1949 the Portuguese *Missao de Combate as Tripanossomiases* installed a de-flying chamber on the road that crossed the border and began a campaign of game destruction (Whellan 1949, 1950). In 1951 the Rhodesians also erected a chamber and prepared to put their own shooting scheme into operation. Meanwhile, in November 1951, an outbreak of infection in Rhodesian native reserves near the border failed to respond to dimidium and cattle began to die at a rate of over 100 a month and continued to do so throughout 1952. The first *G. morsitans* on the Rhodesian side of the border were captured in 1950, and in 1951 the shooting began in a 10-mile-wide belt between game fences although it was not until 1955 that the programme was in full operation. Meanwhile all cattle had died in Mkota and in another reserve, Chikwizo, also adjacent to the border, a cattle population which had totalled over 2000 in 1948 was now reduced to under 300 (Chorley 1956).

By 1956 the shooting programme seemed to be taking effect; the area of detectable tsetse infestation was reduced and cattle began to recover in Chikwizo, where antrycide had replaced dimidium as the drug of choice. On the Rhodesian side of the border the position continued to improve until 1959, although on the Portuguese side the density of *G. morsitans* was still rising. In 1960 it was realized that rapid deterioration was taking place in a reserve, Inyanga North, immediately south of the shooting zone, where a single tsetse had been taken in 1958. This was a densely populated area and only along river banks or in clefts in the hills, where the natural vegetation persisted, did it seem possible that tsetse might establish itself. Drug treatment in Inyanga North now began to fail and trypanosomes became resistant to antrycide. The drugs were changed but in 1961 some owners refused to accept treatment for their animals and there were about 200 deaths. In the adjacent Chikwizo reserve, however, in five years cattle had increased under the influence of antrycide from under 300 to over 1000. Bush clearing was begun along the rivers and shooting was stopped. In the areas which the shooting had been designed to protect the situation continued under control, but in Inyanga North more stock owners refused treatment. Game destruction here would hardly have been possible, for cattle were present in such numbers that they alone could suffice to feed the tsetse and, indeed, in 1964 *G. morsitans* were caught in cattle kraals 20 miles from the nearest bush where they could be captured by using a slowly moving Land Rover as a bait. In this year the continued refusal of cattle owners to accept treatment resulted in 4800 deaths out of some 12 000 cattle considered to be at risk of infection (Cockbill 1965). (Control over the epizootic was finally achieved by use of insecticides and has been described by Casewell 1968.)

What are the similarities in the antecedents of the epizootics at Gwaai in 1918, at the Sabi–Lundi confluence in the early 1940s, in the Urungwe reserve in 1951–2, and in Inyanga North in 1964, in all of which mortality of cattle was very heavy? And in what way do they all differ from the Sabi epizootic, which was equally severe in terms of infection incidence, but which ended not with massive deaths but with self-curing cases in a rapidly multiplying population? In the first three epizootics there were no drugs or else they were ineffectual, and all cattle involved and their parent generations had been out of contact with trypanosome infection for many years. In the case of the Sabi and Inyanga epizootics, however, the same drugs were used although in the latter drug-resistant strains of trypanosomes were detected. It is probable, also, that in the earlier years of the Inyanga epizootic, recording and drug administration were less efficient, largely because of the inaccessibility of the area.

The outstanding difference between the Sabi epizootic and that at Inyanga (as well as the earlier Gwaai, Sabi–Lundi, and Urungwe outbreaks) is that the drugs were used over a long period during which tsetse control was partial and inefficient; cattle were held under drugs for almost a decade during which they were subjected to a relatively low or gradually developing risk of infection. At Gwaai and at the Sabi–Lundi confluence, cattle that had been for many generations out of reach of infection were suddenly exposed to a rapidly expanding spread of tsetse. At Urungwe this was also the case, for the cattle admitted to the reserve after tsetse had been cleared from it were also animals whose ancestors had not been exposed to infection since the rinderpest of 1896.

In the Sabi epizootic cattle were subjected to 8 years of drug treatment before their owners began to refuse treatment. In Inyanga North full-scale drug control had only been in operation for 1 year before treatment was refused. One of the earliest results obtained by experiments with antrycide injected into cattle pastured in tsetse-infested bush was that of Soltys (1955) who showed that in this way it was possible for the animals exposed to infection to build up a high degree of immunity (see also Soltys 1963). Had the people of Inyanga North waited another five years or so before making their political gesture of refusing government veterinary aid, they might, perhaps, have done so with impunity.

Disruptive epizootics with rapidly occurring and heavy mortality appear when cattle which have had no opportunity to build up resistance are exposed to infection. When, whether under drug protection or merely by selection under a trypanosome risk that is not too severe, they are subjected to continuous inoculation of trypanosomes, they adjust themselves to infection. This had happened naturally in the Tonga cattle that Livingstone saw near the Zambezi and it happened, with the aid of drugs, among the Sabi valley cattle. It also happens among human populations in similar circumstances.

The Rhodesian system of dealing with the tsetse-infested *Grenzwildnis* by isolation has been very successful, especially for the European cattle owner, but this success has been achieved by sacrifice of physiological adjustment to trypanosomiasis, so that livestock are exceedingly vulnerable to trypanosome infection. It has also meant the abandonment, inevitable under possessory segregation in land ownership, of that ecological flexibility which has enabled the countries further north to adjust themselves to the presence of an infested *Grenzwildnis*. In underdeveloped countries this is a great advantage.

In tropical Africa, as in the rest of the world, man has achieved his present control over zoonotic infection chiefly by substituting for the natural ecosystems artificial ones which he manages for his own purposes. Rhodesia, because of the peculiarities of its politics, is a patchwork of land-use patterns none of which are reproduced on a comparable scale elsewhere inside the tsetse zone. Rhodesian African peasant populations are prevented by land apportionment from making the traditional adjustments to population growth, that is, expansion into unused land; they are also prevented from making a natural adjustment to the presence of heavy infection by withdrawing to other areas where the risk is not so high. Behind this protective barrier are European-owned ranches, in most of which carefully managed herds of fat cattle range over vast areas where they provide yet another potential tsetse host among the wild animals already there. The European low-veld ranches are extremely vulnerable to tsetse infestation, in spite of the protection given by interposition of native reserves between them and the fly-belts. Finally, a third item in the patchwork and, again, mostly on European land, is the growing area of irrigation which will, especially in the south, eventually so raise the economic level of the *Grenzwildnis* that it will cease to exist.

Human trypanosomiasis in the Zambezi valley

In opening this account of the trypanosomiases in Rhodesia it was remarked that the human disease does not influence the pattern of settlement in the country today. It is, however, present in the Zambezi valley and a consideration of some of its characteristics follows appropriately upon the discussion of adjustment to infection in cattle. Three features of the disease are particularly striking. It has never produced a disruptive epidemic, it is confined to well-marked foci, and a high proportion of so-called 'healthy carriers' has always characterized the infections among the indigenous people of the valley. This endemic situation has been the subject of a number of papers beginning with that of Fleming (1913) and ending, at present, with that of Blair, Burnett Smith, and Gelfand (1968). The most important review between these two is that of Blair (1939), while the subject has also been discussed by Morris (1956) and Ross and Blair (1956). The relationship of the infection in Rhodesia to that also attributed to *Trypanosoma 'rhodesiense'* in other parts of Africa has been examined by Ormerod (1961) and by Apted, Ormerod, Smyly, Stronach, and Szlamp (1963). Ormerod (1963, 1967) has produced evidence that the strains in the Zambezi valley as well as in the fly-belt of the Okovango delta in Botswana are typologically distinct from the causal organisms of rhodesian trypanosomiasis further north in Africa. For this reason he distinguishes them as Zambezi strains (Ormerod 1967).

The numbers of cases of human trypanosomiasis recorded annually in Southern Rhodesia are shown in Fig. 20.2. The first two cases, found in 1909, were a European who had been on a hunting trip in 1908 in Northern

Rhodesia (Zambia) and an African who had also travelled elsewhere in Central Africa. The former, William Armstrong, who died six months after being sent back to England, was the source of the strain described by Stephens and Fantham (1910) as *Trypanosoma rhodesiense*. The acute infection in rats and the posteronuclear forms of trypanosomes, then seen for the first time, were thought to distinguish it from *T. gambiense*, named nine years before as the causal organism of West African sleeping sickness and, shortly afterwards, of the Uganda epidemic.

The presence of sleeping sickness in the Katanga region of the Congo and the discovery of cases among people living near the Lualaba river where it forms the boundary with Zambia, at that time also administered, like

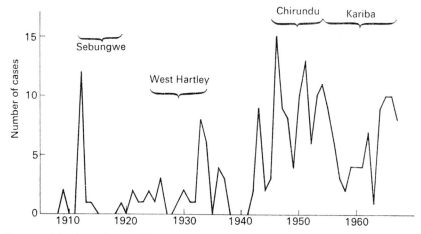

FIG. 20.2. Numbers of cases of human trypanosomiasis diagnosed in Rhodesia from 1909 to 1955. The figures include a small number of infections acquired outside the country. These include the two in 1909.

Rhodesia, by the British South Africa Company, had already led to extended searches for *G. palpalis* in the Zambezi basin. The absence of this tsetse, except on the north-west corner of British Central Africa, had hardly been established long enough to allay the anxieties of the Company's directors when the case of William Armstrong, soon followed by others in Zambia and Malawi in areas where there were no *palpalis*-group tsetses on the rivers, caused much alarm. The early investigations have been vividly described by Gelfand (1961). A suggestion by one worker that the disease might be transmitted not only cyclically by *G. morsitans* but also mechanically by the almost universal cattle pest, *Stomoxys*, provoked fears that it might spread throughout the whole of South Africa.

In 1912 another European became infected, this time undoubtedly within Southern Rhodesia. This was an official stationed in the neighbourhood of the Sengwa river. A survey was at once begun and was carried out by Drs. Stohr and Fleming. Eleven more cases were found, all of them

Africans living near the Busi river, a tributary of the Sengwa, itself a tributary of the Zambezi. The Sengwa basin had lain within the tsetse belt before 1896. After the passage of the rinderpest it was free of tsetse for some years, until the spread of the Sebungwe fly-belt once more engulfed it between 1904 and 1910. The 11 indigenous Africans and the 1 European case make up the peak that appears in 1912 in Fig. 20.2. Obviously one factor contributing to the appearance of the peak in that year was the survey by Drs. Stohr and Fleming. Had they gone earlier the peak in this figure might have shifted to the left. Some 6000 Africans were evacuated in 1913 and the peak collapsed. The doctors questioned the people about the infection and all stated that it was a new disease, except the chief, an old man, whose assertion that it had long been known was discounted as worthless (Fleming 1913). As had been the case in Uganda, local officials were anxious to prove that the infection had entered their territory from outside and again the Congo was blamed. The case for a Congo origin of the rhodesian infection was last argued by Willett (1965).

The entomological counterpart of the medical survey was carried out by Jack (1914) and resulted in the description of the expansion of the Sebungwe fly-belt already illustrated in Fig. 17.1. This work provides a second and more fundamental reason for the appearance of a peak of infection around 1911–12. The Busi people had evidently been out of continuous contact with *G. morsitans* (and, almost certainly, *G. pallidipes*) between 1896 and 1907 or thereabouts. The 1912 peak was evidence of their renewed encounter, after a decade of freedom, with the insect vector and the natural hosts of the trypanosomes. The chief had probably spoken the truth.

The stresses of the time also predisposed people to infection. Medical authorities were more concerned with the productivity of mine and other labour than in native health *per se*.

The effects of the drought, which was general over the sub-continent, were felt not only in Southern but also in Northern Rhodesia, our chief recruiting centre for native mine labourers, and more especially affected natives coming to work, in that there being a shortage of fresh food stuffs, they arrived on the mine in a lowered condition and unsuited for the arduous labour they had contracted to perform. On the mines themselves fresh vegetables were, in many instances, unprocurable, whilst meal and meat were enhanced in price. Further, slaughter stock suffered from drought and lack of pasturage, and the meat in consequence was not as good as usual. All this combined to increase the cost of labour and lower its general efficiency and rendered the labourers less capable of resisting disease. In other words the evil effects on the mortality rates of a famine year were particularly marked in the case of native mine labourers (Southern Rhodesia 1912).

Two years later another official reported that because of the long-protracted drought, children suffered considerably from various forms of diarrhoea and infant mortality was high (Chief Native Commissioner 1914).

As elsewhere the early epidemics of sleeping sickness coincided with periods of famine, with epidemics of other diseases and with the manifold stresses of violent political events.

Support for the antiquity of human trypanosomiasis in these latitudes has recently come from Botswana. It was not, indeed, diagnosed in that country until 1935, but there was a tradition of the existence of a disease, *gotsello* or *kotsela*, meaning 'slumbering'. A recent study by Heinz (1968) of the *kotsela* tradition strongly supports the view that the disease is an ancient one and is associated with residual foci of infection that, periodically, have expanded and contracted. There are aspects of the disease in Rhodesia that suggest a long history. They emerge from a study of papers by Apted, Ormerod, Smyly, Stronach, and Szlamp (1963) and Blair, Burnett Smith, and Gelfand (1968).

Four foci of infection have been mapped by the latter authors. Three of these foci coincide with three of the seven residual fly-belts mapped in 1913 by Jack (1914). The fourth is a new development since the construction of the Kariba dam. Possibly a fifth should be added to cover the Mvurandura focus, south-west of Kariba.

It is convenient to begin with the latter, because its history as given by Apted, Ormerod, Smyly, Stronach, and Szlamp (1963) admirably illustrates the difficulty of attaching any weight to evidence for the absence of the infection based upon negative medical data for remote areas. It is not referred to in the later paper of Blair, Burnett Smith, and Gelfand (1968). The inhabitants of the Zambezi valley between Kariba and the Victoria Falls are Tonga. In 1956–7 some 1500 of them were moved from the floor of the valley out of reach of the rising waters of Kariba, to a site where their traditional methods of obtaining food could not be used. A grain store was set up from which rations were issued but they suffered severely from malnutrition. The store was sited in the steep-sided gorge of the Bumi river at Mvurandura. *G. morsitans* and *G. pallidipes* were present. In July 1958 a man employed by the Rhodesian Game Department, who lived in a hut near the grain store, was discharged from work for laziness. In September he became ill. In December, by which time other definite cases of trypanosomiasis had been diagnosed, he was treated for the disease, although no trypanosomes had been found in him. A caretaker at the grain store was first seen on 14 October, when he had fever and was thin and emaciated. He said he had been ill for several months. Trypanosomes were found in his blood and he recovered after treatment. Another caretaker, admitted on 9 September to the local hospital (96 miles distant over a very rough road) was treated with penicillin for a lung complaint and then discharged himself from hospital. Later his blood slide was examined and found to contain trypanosomes, but before he could be found he had died in his village by about mid-October. His successor as caretaker at the store became ill in the same month and received no treatment, but regarded himself as having been infected with the same disease that had killed his predecessor. Yet another fifth employee at the store became ill at the same time and went to the hospital, but his blood was not examined and he recovered. Of these five men who became ill at the store in the second half of 1958 only two were confirmed as cases of trypanosomiasis. The area was cut off by flooding during the rains and was not visited until March 1960 by boat across the newly formed Lake Kariba. At this time the local chief said that 20 people had died during the interval, with symptoms resembling those of the earlier cases. This was confirmed by the game ranger, the only official in the neighbourhood. Two more cases were diagnosed in 1961 on visits made by boat.

Mvurandura, the site of the grain store, lies below the western end of the Matusadona mountains. In 1956 a single case had been diagnosed from Sampakaruma in the Sanyati river valley at the eastern end of the same range. It had been higher up the valley of the same river that the second focus to be discovered in Southern Rhodesia was located in 1923 when a wood-cutter died of the infection. The area was surveyed in 1924 by a doctor who had also conducted a survey there at the time of the Busi outbreak in 1911, but without finding any cases. Later in 1924 two more cases, also African and one of them fatal, appeared. There were two more in 1930 and in 1933 two Europeans, one of whom died, and six Africans, of whom two died, were found. In 1934 there was another African case and an intensive survey was then undertaken by Blair who reported on his results and those of other doctors, and, in particular drew attention to the high proportion of infected Africans who were 'healthy carriers'. One of these men, named Kahondera, was chief of the small village of Gowe on the Sanyati river, which lay at the centre of this focus of infection.

Kahondera was infected with malaria, *Plasmodium falciparum*, and with microfilariae, the organisms seen by Cook in the first cases from the Uganda epidemic (Chapter 14). Kahondera also showed abundant *Trypanosoma brucei* in his blood. (If Ormerod 1967 is followed it is likely that these were one of his Zambezi strains and not what, in his terminology, are called rhodesian strains.) He was, so he thought, in good health. Ross and Blair (1956) describe seven such cases and Blair, Burnett Smith, and Gelfand (1968) give details of another seven (of whom two were among those people diagnosed in 1911). One of these seven was a child of 11 years.

The latter authors remark that the term 'healthy carrier' is not, perhaps, a good clinical description, but it is a convenient one. They note that all so far observed have been Africans who

give a history of having lived in tsetse fly-infested areas for a considerable period and generally have been inhabitants of small villages of fifty persons or less. They are rarely women or small children and most commonly are people who are hunters, fishermen, honey-gatherers, woodcutters, etc. who spend considerable time away from their village homes. . . . The 'healthy carrier' case gives a consistent history, commencing with a febrile illness which is generally of little consequence and from which a full recovery is made. The patient returns to his normal occupation and probably remains in this state . . . until accidentally discovered. These cases are generally discovered by the finding of trypanosomes in a blood smear in a routine survey of the human population of an area, and the patients deny feeling ill and are generally apyrexial (Blair, Burnett Smith, and Gelfand 1968).

Blair's two first 'healthy carriers', Kahondera and Zariro, also provided evidence that they were able to endure considerable physical strain without deterioration of their condition. Kahondera, whose infection was first recorded on 21 May 1934, walked 22 miles to pay his respects to Dr. Blair during July. He still had trypanosomes in his blood and was suffering from bronchitis. Presumably he also still retained his malaria and microfilariae. Zariro, also from Gowe village, was diagnosed in July 1934 and was seen again in September immediately after completing a walk of 40 miles in two days. He still had trypanosomes in his blood. He was only with difficulty persuaded to go to hospital, but eventually did so, making the 70-mile journey on foot. His blood was still positive on arrival there. (One is reminded of Koch's canoemen on Lake Victoria, with trypanosomes in the blood, but quite fit after paddling for 30 miles.)

The third focus of infection mapped by Blair, Burnett Smith, and Gelfand (1968) is the North Lomagundi focus and from here also healthy carriers, including the above-mentioned child of 11 years, were discovered. This focus extends eastwards down the Zambezi valley and is centred around Zumbo in Mozambique (Sousa 1947).

The majority of cases observed among indigenous Africans in these foci are not 'healthy carriers'. For the most part they develop a sub-acute disease, lasting for several months, and are often too ill to leave the villages.

In a third category, sometimes seen among the inhabitants of tsetse areas, but also and especially among people infected during short visits to the bush, are the cases 'who become ill with an acute pyrexial illness within some days after the introduction of the infection; they progress rapidly to a fatal issue if diagnosis is not promptly made and specific therapy given' (Blair, Burnett Smith, and Gelfand 1968). European cases fall into this category as well as Africans who have not previously lived in tsetse-infested bush. Of 185 cases of human trypanosomiasis known to have been contracted south of the Zambezi river since 1911, 17·3 per cent were Europeans.

No indigenous cases of sleeping sickness were reported in Rhodesia between 1935 and 1944. Blair, Burnett Smith, and Gelfand (1968) say that 7 African cases seen during this decade originated outside the territory. However, Fig. 20.2 shows 9 in 1943 from Morris (1956). Discrepancies of this nature tend to arise from confusion between the year in which an infection was diagnosed and the year in which it was published in an official report. From 1944 onwards the general level of incidence of the disease appears to have increased, although there are considerable fluctuations.

Between 1911 and 1934 only 39 cases were diagnosed in the Zambezi valley of which 17·9 per cent were European. When the North Lomagundi focus became active between 1945 and 1953, 64 cases were discovered, of which 7·8 per cent were European. It seems not unlikely that the higher incidence of infection among Europeans in the first period was, in part, accounted for by the relatively neglected state of indigenous Africans in the Zambezi valley as compared with Europeans, and this state of affairs certainly characterized treatment of the Mvurandura outbreak as described by Apted, Ormerod, Smyly, Stronach, and Szlamp (1963). But there can be little doubt that the contribution of 25·3 per cent by Europeans to the total of 79 infections observed around the eastern end of Lake Kariba between 1953 and 1967 represented a true increase in relative incidence of such cases. The construction of the dam itself and, after its completion, the development of sections of its shore as a holiday resort resulted in a large increase in the numbers of European visitors to the area.

In the description of the Mvurandura focus around the grain store it was emphasized that it lay in a gorge with steep sides, covered with a thick canopy of vegetation in which ran the Bumi river, and where *G. morsitans* and *G. pallidipes* were abundant. Spoor of bushbuck (*Tragelaphus scriptus*) was seen. In Chapter 23 it will be observed that one specialist in Nigeria listed, among the causes of epidemics in that country, the African's habit of seeking shade and water, 'as do the tsetse'. Gelfand (1966) has described the circumstances in which three European brothers were infected between 7 and 15 September 1964. During this period they were camped, with their father, on the banks of the Zambezi, 20 miles below the Kariba gorge. They slept in the open. The banks of the Zambezi are lined with discontinuous patches of riverine thicket, often better described as gallery forest.

Many of the thicket and gallery forest trees and shrubs are evergreen and provide the habitat of *G. pallidipes*. The four men were heavily bitten by tsetses, probably mostly *G. morsitans*. Their environment was not described, but they were fishing, so that it is likely that their behaviour was much the same as that of the majority of such holidaymakers and that they chose to remain, for much of their time, in the dense shade of the riverine vegetation. It is possible that the same infected tsetse attempted to feed from all three of the infected brothers. Equally, it is possible that the tsetse in the circumscribed area in which they were fishing showed a high rate of infection because all were essentially dependent upon one or two natural hosts living nearby, which carried an abundant population of human infective *T. brucei* in their bloodstreams. It is not difficult to envisage a much-localized population of *G. pallidipes* living in one of these thickets and feeding on a family of bushpigs or a pair of bushbuck, and that when the father and his sons established themselves in the shade of the same vegetation, the animals moved away and the tsetse that had hitherto fed upon them now turned their attention to their human supplanters.

The family left the Zambezi on 15 September. One brother became acutely ill on 22 September, the next on the 25th, and the third on the 27th. Each showed a trypanosome chancre on the legs—one on the right ankle, the second on the back of the right knee, and the third on the right kneecap. The position of all these infective bites is not inconsistent with the biting habits of *G. pallidipes*. A tendency for chancres to be found on the lower limbs during the 1957 rhodesian epidemic in Busoga was thought to be suggestive of *G. pallidipes* (Robertson and Baker 1958).

The majority of the Kariba cases appear to have acquired their infection near the eastern shores of the lake around the entry of the Charara river. This area is heavily infested with *G. morsitans* and *G. pallidipes*. Between December 1961 and April 1962 8 cases were thought to have originated here. A study of infections in the tsetses showed that 0·95 per cent of the latter species carried *brucei* type infections, but a sample of *G. moritsans* showed none (Federal Ministry of Agriculture 1963). The general picture yielded by the unavoidably imprecise information as to where the infections were acquired suggests that certain quite restricted localities were more dangerous than others and that they tended to be associated with areas of riverine thicket. This in turn suggests the involvement of *G. pallidipes* and a thicket-haunting natural host and, at the same time, the entry into such places by persons who later became ill.

In Chapter 17 it was stated that small foci of *G. morsitans* and *G. pallidipes* remained in the Zambezi valley after the passage of the Great Rinderpest. It is an assumption that *G. pallidipes* was present in these residual foci. This tsetse was not discovered in the Zambezi valley fly-belt until 1942 (Lovemore 1958). A number of entomological studies had been carried out by R. W. Jack and J. K. Chorley in various parts of the fly-belt before that date and the shooting campaign, during which field staff, some of long experience, collected *Glossina*, had been in operation since 1930. It is difficult to believe that *G. pallidipes* had invaded the Zambezi fly-belts shortly before 1942 but it is also difficult to suppose that it would not have been noticed earlier had it then been as widespread as it later became. The conclusion must be that its recovery after the post-rinderpest recession had been much slower than had that of *G. morsitans*. Therefore, although undoubtedly the increase in cases of human trypanosomiasis after the construction of the Kariba dam was due to the increase in numbers of persons being bitten, particularly the susceptible visitors from outside the fly-belt, it seems not impossible that the earlier increase, beginning in 1945 according to Blair, Burnett Smith, and Gelfand (1968), was a consequence of the spread and regrowth of the *G. pallidipes* population and thus of the increased involvement of the highly favourable natural reservoir animal, the bushbuck, in the circulation of *brucei*-group trypanosomes.

Human trypanosomiasis and the *Grenzwildnis*

The effective country of Rhodesia, like its predecessors, the empire of Mutapa and the Rozwi confederation, lies between the Zambezi and Limpopo *Grenzwildnisse*. Although modern boundaries follow the beds of these rivers and the bush is apportioned out between black and white, the bulk of the population still lives on the high and middle veld. The indigenous people of the Zambezi valley lived, for all practical purposes, outside the central states. The greater part of the Tonga people live in Zambia and one may suppose that the southern Tonga derived from family or kinship groups that had pressed southwards until they were stopped by the dwellers on the middle and high veld. The people of the eastern part of the fly-belt, in the north Lomagundi focus, belong to various small tribal groups. Some of them are called Korekore, a nickname given to the Karanga followers of the Mutapa, and may therefore be descendants of these earlier rulers of Rhodesia. Both they and the valley Tonga have been living in the fly-bush for many generations. It is they who produce the 'healthy carriers' as well as sub-acute and acute cases. The Tonga own the descendants of dwarf humpless cattle, seen by Livingstone, which are also 'healthy carriers'. These remote peoples and their livestock have survived in part because they have been able to achieve some degree of physiological adjustment with infection. Those other tribes, Shona, Ndebele, Europeans, who by their military and technical skills have been able to seize and retain the more fertile areas, have destroyed the bush and freed themselves from the danger of infection, but have done this at the cost of losing their ability to adjust to trypanosomiasis and, when by accident they become infected, they die quickly unless modern medical aid is easily available.

21

BACKGROUND TO TRYPANOSOMIASIS
IN NIGERIA

NIGERIA is used as an example of West Africa as a whole. The intention is to examine the differences and similarities that exist between the epidemiology and epizootiology of these infections in countries where tsetse of the *palpalis* group predominate and those where, as in East Africa, they are comparatively unimportant.

West Africa, defined here as the countries west of the Cameroon Republic, lies between the Sahara desert, the shores of the Bight of Benin, and the Atlantic coast as far as Senegal. Mean annual rainfall at Port Harcourt just east of the Niger delta is 2497 mm or about 100 in per annum, and a few miles nearer to the sea rises to over 4000 mm. Some 1400 miles further west, Freetown in Sierra Leone has a mean of 3587 mm annual rain. The latitude of Port Harcourt is slightly below 5°N and of Freetown about 8°N. The southern limit of the true desert lies roughly between 16° and 18°N. The Niger bend in Mali at 17° is a convenient topographical mark of the northern edge of the West African region and is about 800 miles north of Accra. Between these limits the rainfall diminishes northwards from about 2500 mm (100 in) to less than 200 mm (8 in) per annum and the living organisms of the region tend to arrange themselves in parallel zones appropriate to the succession of climates. There are interruptions and irregularities in this general pattern produced in part by topography, where highlands like the Bauchi Plateau in Nigeria, the Adamawa massif on the Cameroon border, or the Fouta Djallon and other mountains of Guinea and Sierra Leone draw, as it were, the damper climates inland. Conversely, in the savanna gap between Lagos and Accra, especially in Dahomey and Togo, a drier climate with between 1000 and 1400 mm (40–55 in) of annual rain reaches south to the sea coast. Here the tropical moist forest is broken by woodlands and savanna that elsewhere in Africa are encountered 200–300 miles inland. The trypanosomiases of south-western Nigeria are influenced by the savanna gap.

The great volcanic mass of Cameroon Mountain (13 350 ft) conveniently marks the eastern limit of West Africa near the Atlantic coast, and Lake Chad serves the same purpose on the southern border of the Sahara. The Republics of Cameroon and of Gabon occupy an intermediate position between West Africa and the vast area of the Congo basin and this position is, to some extent, reflected in the unique abundance of different *Glossina* species. They cover the common dispersal centre, defined in Chapter 3, of both the *fusca* and *palpalis* groups.

Because of the zonation of climates and biota in West Africa, the pattern of tsetse and trypanosome distribution is easier to see than it is in the eastern half of the continent or the Congo basin. This is one reason why a discussion of trypanosomiases in West Africa illuminates the problem over much of the rest of the continent. Some of their basic pattern has already been described in Chapter 5.

Glossinologists in West Africa were emphatic that their problems were quite different from those encountered by their colleagues in East Africa. 'It is essential for the reader to forget the East African picture of tsetse occurring throughout hundreds of square miles of wooded savanna, attacking all pedestrians, motorists and cyclists. In Nigeria tsetse tend to be confined to the streams and rivers, the country in between being fly-free except in the *morsitans* belts' (Nash 1948a).

The contrast with East Africa is chiefly due to the presence of the *palpalis* group flies on river systems draining into the Atlantic ocean and the Mediterranean and their absence from Indian ocean drainage systems. This in itself would not necessarily create epidemiological and epizootiological differences. The essential factor is the ability of *palpalis*-group tsetse to live on reptiles and to turn their attention from them to other animals, including man, that make use of the rivers. They are indeed closely confined to their riverine and lacustrine habitats by well-defined climatic limitations, but this confinement has allowed them, provided water remains throughout the year in river beds, to penetrate much further towards the deserts than any other group and also to survive where human populations are so dense that all other tsetses are eliminated. Man does not generally totally destroy riverine vegetation. It grows on river banks that are often too steep for cultivation or are seasonally apt to be flooded. He may indeed destroy the natural fauna of this vegetation, but only does this when he himself is present, with or without his domestic animals, in sufficient numbers to provide an alternative food supply for riverine tsetses.

Another object of study in Nigeria is the cattle population and the contrast it provides, in its responses to trypanosome infection, to cattle populations on the other side of the continent. In eastern Africa the Sukuma or the Masai will, when hard pressed in years of severe drought and pasture famine, take their animals deliberately into the fly-bush, if there is any near enough, knowing that many will die of the infection but that some will survive, whereas if all were to be kept on the impoverished disease-free pastures, all might die of starvation. In West Africa Fulani cattle are driven, every year, south from the semi-arid, sub-desert pastures of the Sahel and Sudan zones into the rich grazing of the tsetse-infested Guinea zones. There are some losses and it is certain that, as yet, these cattle could not survive exposure to continuous frequent reinfection by tsetse bite. The wet season return to the northern tsetse-free pastures is essential to their well-being. One says 'as yet' because earlier invaders of the northern borders of the tsetse-infested savanna had, on at least two occasions, brought other races of cattle from the Mediterranean lands and these have become adjusted to infection, at least by strains of trypanosomes prevalent in their own localities. The N'Dama and Muturu cattle of West Africa have, by the process of natural selection, achieved the goal now being sought in several European and American as well as African laboratories, of immunity to trypanosome infection.

Again it will be the object to set the discussion in historical perspective; not so much locally as in relation to the major trends of West African history as a whole. The difficulty lies in the abundance of material and its lack, so far, of accepted historical co-ordination. One cannot yet refer to historical events, as one could in a discussion of European disease, with the assurance that they will be generally comprehended and accepted. Part of this difficulty comes from the absorbing interest of the subject. 'La problème de l'origine des Peuls' remarks one historian 'passionne les Africanistes' (Cornevin 1963) and it is not only the Peuls or Fulani that arouse scholarly passions. The centuries-long trans-Saharan commerce between the Mediterranean lands and the great emporia of towns such as Timbuctoo and Kano, and the contacts between the Moors and Berbers and the sub-Saharan empires are of great interest and importance to the student of the effects of trypanosomiasis in African society. They lead back inevitably to speculation about the rock paintings of longhorn cattle and Fulani-like herdsman at Tassili and other mountain sites now in the middle of the great desert. These in turn prompt questions about the wild fauna that at one time occupied the Sahara and about the vegetation relics on these desert mountains that show both African and European affinities. From this remoteness one passes to the sort of speculations already made about the origins of tsetse and pathogenic trypanosomiasis in Chapter 3.

From another starting point, the slave trade to the Americas, trypanosomiasis is soon encountered for it was known to the traders as the negro lethargy and the first description of it, by a ship's surgeon John Atkins, was published in his book, *The navy surgeon*, in 1734. The symptom which had long been associated with it by West African peoples, the enlargement of the neck glands, was described by Winterbottom in 1803 and became known as Winterbottom's sign. Shippers of slaves would not accept people with swollen cervical glands. Nevertheless sleeping sickness had reached the Antilles by the beginning of the nineteenth century although it never became established there. European contact with the West African coast had begun in the fifteenth century but it was not until colonial occupation began in the middle of the nineteenth century that the outside world gradually came to recognize that inland from the coast, on the forest savanna interzone, lay another series of kingdoms. In Nigeria, Benin and

Oyo were examples that showed, chiefly through their impressive works of art and in spite of some customs of extreme barbarity, that here also were societies showing a high level of political organization. There is an increasing number of sources easily available to which one can turn for further study of Nigerian and West African history, but as yet none that is fully acceptable to African as well as to European scholars. However, these sources are sufficient to supply much of the historical background that will be required in the next chapter. This background of history provides a fourth reason for examining the trypanosomiases in Nigeria. In West Africa there is an opportunity of studying the responses of the outside world to tsetse-borne trypanosomiasis which is not provided by the history of the sea-borne impact.

Glover's (1965) report on *The tsetse problem in Northern Nigeria* is a most useful source book, while Nash's (1948a) shorter monograph *Tsetse flies in British West Africa* although in some respects out of date is still very valuable. A useful starting point for study of the historical and ethnological associations of human trypanosomiasis in West Africa is provided by Hoeppli and Lucasse (1964) or Hoeppli (1969).

The West African ecosystems

Before turning specifically to trypanosomiasis it is necessary to recall, in slightly more detail, the biotic zones already referred to in the analysis of cattle infections in Chapter 5. There it was shown that in moving south from the tsetse-free steppes of the Sahel and Sudan zones to the rain forests of the coast, the *vivax* ratio diminished steadily: in the north cattle infections were predominantly of that trypanosome, in the south *Trypanosoma congolense* was more frequently seen. It was also shown that as cattle moved from the fly-free pastures into the *Glossina morsitans* belts of central Nigeria they first displayed *T. vivax* parasitaemias. A few days later *T. brucei* appeared in the blood, followed by *T. congolense*. Finally, as that trypanosome became more evident, *T. brucei* disappeared, leaving *T. congolense* and *T. vivax* as the two principal causal organisms of bovine trypanosomiasis as elsewhere in Africa.

The modern classification of West African vegetation is chiefly due to the French botanist, Chevalier (1900). A successor, Aubréville (1949), classified the vegetation of Africa on a basis of interaction between climate and the process of '*désertification*', that is, the destructive activities of man. This word echoed the title of a contemporary work by a Belgian ecologist, Harroy (1949), whose *Afrique, terre qui meurt* expressed a view prevalent among biologists and agronomists during the colonial period. It is not one with which I find myself still in sympathy. These works describe processes of which the historical context is not yet fully understood. In Nigeria a local adaptation of the classification of Chevalier was made by Keay (1949) who, with Aubréville and others, was responsible for the production of a widely used vegetation map of Africa (Keay, Aubréville, Duvigneaud, Hoyle, Mendonca, and Pichi-Sermolli 1958).

The West African coastline carries a belt of mangrove forest that may be 50 miles in width. Over much of their length the mangroves merge, inland, with a zone of freshwater swamp forest. Although some mangrove forests lie in very humid climates, as in the Niger delta, they are edaphically controlled and may be found, even under quite dry climates, where tidal and river waters maintain a suitable environment, for example, at the mouth of the Gambia river or in places along the East African coast. The coastal mangroves in West Africa form a habitat for some of the *palpalis* group tsetse (Roubaud and Maillot 1952). Machado (1954) thinks that they may have provided the route by which this group of tsetse spread westwards from the area that now forms the Congo basin (Map 21.1).

Inland from the freshwater swamps lies the lowland rain forest of Keay (1953), or tropical moist forest or closed forest of Richards (1952). In the Congo basin it stretches more than half-way across the continent, but in West Africa is seldom more than 250 miles wide. As one moves towards the northern edge of the lowland rain forest, changes take place in the species composition of its flora associated with a gradual decrease in rainfall.

Top-storey trees of the Nigerian forests reach a height of 150 ft and there are a number of lower storeys, with an under-storey of evergreen shrubs and climbers. It is known that the *fusca*-group tsetse spend much of their time at rest on tree trunks (Nash and Davey 1950, Nash 1952) but, except in general terms, a description of vegetation structure cannot yet illuminate our knowledge of *fusca* group biology. The dense lower-storey vegetation of some secondary forests obstructs vision, and Chapman (1961) has shown that G. *medicorum* does not respond to baits at distances greater than 25 yd, in marked contrast to species of the open savanna which will react to a moving bait 150 or more yards away.

There is little of the Nigerian forests that has not, at one time or another, been felled and cultivated. Few forest trees are tolerant of fire and use of natural forest areas for agriculture is preceded by under-storey felling and burning. Where these activities are abandoned for a sufficient length of time the forest regenerates. Tropical moist forest established in an optimum environment is not easily destroyed and regeneration of secondary forest may be very rapid. Towards the climatic limits of its habitat it is less secure, so that the central forest areas tend to be surrounded by zones in which regeneration is permanently suppressed.

Nigerian botanists speak of this zone of suppressed forest as derived savanna. It is also called the forest–savanna mosaic. It forms the second major vegetation zone met when moving inland in West Africa, and runs along the whole length of the northern edge of the moist forests in a band varying from less than 50 to over 150 miles wide. Forest elements that can tolerate fire persist in it and trees such as *Chlorophora excelsa*, *Dialium guineense*, and

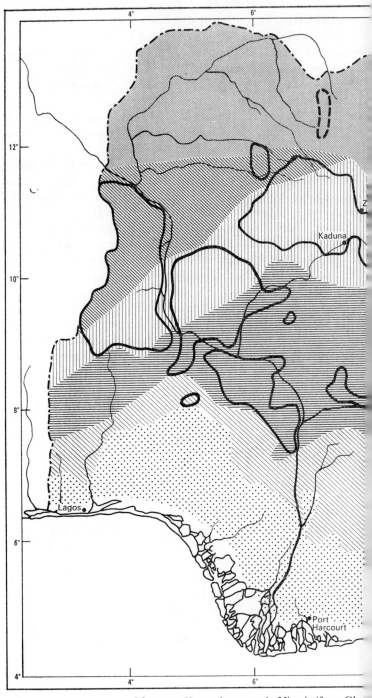

MAP 21.1. Vegetation zones in Nigeria (from Glo

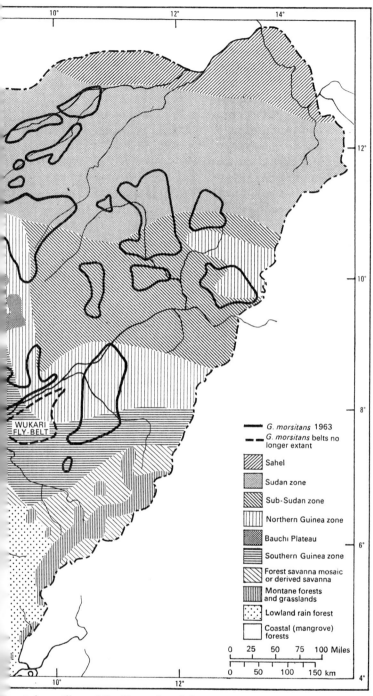

WUKARI FLY-BELT

sent-day outlines of the *G. morsitans* belts.

Phyllanthus discoideus are conspicuous in the derived savanna across Africa from Guinea to Uganda. But the derived savanna is, indeed, savanna and not forest. Where the forest has been destroyed by felling, burning, and prolonged cultivation, the surface of the land is invaded by grasses and by fire-tolerant savanna trees. Only where topographically inaccessible sites such as steep hillsides, gullies, crevices between rock outcrops, and so on, or, as on river banks, steep surfaces or zones liable to flooding, protect the vegetation from the cultivator, does the natural vegetation survive and provide habitats for forest-edge species of tsetse as well as for the riverine species. Over the greater part of the surface of the derived savanna, where population is abundant and active there is, in general, freedom from tsetse infestation. Cassava, yams, sweet potatoes, maize, plantains, and cocoyams are cultivated. Propagation of the indigenous oil palm, *Elaeis guineensis*, is a major item in agricultural industry and plantations may form an artificial *Glossina* habitat. More important, epidemiologically, is the fact that in some parts of the derived savanna, the villages themselves, especially where domestic pigs are maintained, become a habitat for *G. tachinoides*. It is important, however, to note that while the land is under human occupation neither the field crops themselves nor the fallows provide a *Glossina* habitat.

The fate of the fallow lands depends on the quality of the soil and the social economy of the region. Near towns the fallow period is short, but elsewhere, on good soil, cessation of cultivation may be followed by comparatively rapid forest regeneration at least to secondary forest which is likely to be worked over again long before the climax forest is restored. However, where cultivation has been prolonged and the soils impoverished or where soil is naturally poor, grasses invade the fallows. The common species are widespread across Africa to Uganda, wherever forest is replaced in this way, and they include *Imperata cylindrica, Ctenium elegans, Pennisetum purpureum, Loudetia* and *Andropogon* spp. Their presence ensures that grass fires become a regular feature of the passage of the seasons and this, in turn, encourages the invasion of fire-tolerant savanna trees (Keay 1953). The derived savanna thus formed permits the penetration of a savanna fauna which may include the hosts of *G. morsitans* and then, following them, the flies themselves.

The derived savanna or forest–savanna mosaic gives way northwards to a savanna called, by Chevalier, the Guinea zone. This is conveniently divided into the Northern and Southern Guinea zones, the latter adjoining the forest–savanna mosaic. One speaks of these vegetation zones and they are shown in maps as if they pass abruptly one into another. In the middle of any one of them one has little difficulty in assigning to it its proper name, but there is much overlapping and interpenetration. The Southern Guinea zone, in so far as it is a savanna vegetation subject to annual burning, is dominated by trees like *Daniellia oliveri, Lophira alata*, and *Terminalia glaucescens* standing among relatively tall grasses; but the rivers that run through it may be bordered by wide fringing or gallery forests and certain localities, presumably favoured edaphically or in aspect, carry islands of forest. Keay (1953) recalls Chevalier's opinion that because many of the trees of the Southern Guinea zone are closely related to some of the forest species they may therefore be recently evolved from them. Richards (1952) has noted that where outliers of forest vegetation occur, the component trees are usually less tall than they are in the main forest area and there is commonly only a two- rather than a three-storeyed structure.

Before passing on to the Northern Guinea zone one must draw attention to the Bauchi or Jos Plateau which almost divides it into separate eastern and western halves and interrupts the continuity of its junction with the Southern Guinea zone. For the most part the whole of Nigeria except the Adamawa highlands on the Cameroon border rises very gradually from sea level to about 1500 ft 100–150 miles inland except where the Niger and Cross rivers break through. Another 50–100 miles northward a shallow depression across this gently rising surface contains the Niger–Benue trough in which the rivers run at about 800 ft above sea level. Between the arms of the trough the land surface continues its gentle rise to reach 3000 ft above sea level. Here it forms the watershed between the Niger–Benue system and the rivers running north-east to Lake Chad. The Northern Guinea zone runs centrally across this watershed, but it is broken, or nearly so, by the Bauchi Plateau. This plateau rises abruptly on its western and southern sides for 1500–2000 ft above the surrounding country. For the most part it is covered by short, treeless grassland or bare granite outcrops. It is free of tsetse and is shown clearly on Map 21.1. Less obvious, though of great epidemiological significance, is the narrow zone of derived savanna with relict forest vegetation that lies in the shelter of the west and southern scarps where they abut upon the Southern Guinea zone.

If one may regard the Southern Guinea vegetation as to some degree evolved from the forests, this is not the case with the Northern Guinea zone. It is the western extension of the great *miombo* (*Isoberlinia–Brachystegia*) woodlands of eastern Africa. There are grass fires every year but it is probable that protection from fire would not greatly alter either the floral composition nor the appearance of the *miombo*. Forest trees and shrubs invade or persist along river margins and the *palpalis* group tsetse are found among them. But the *fusca* group tsetse have disappeared and *G. longipalpis* as well. This is the principal habitat of *G. morsitans*. It is difficult to avoid the conclusion that the evolution of this species and its various subspecies has been intimately bound up with the evolution of the *miombo*. In West Africa the dominants include *Isoberlinia doka, I. tomentosa, Monotes kerstingii*, and *Uapaca somon*.

The Northern Guinea zone gives way, on its northern borders, to the Sudan zone. Much of this zone is densely inhabited in Nigeria and of the natural vegetation only a few economically valuable trees remain standing over large areas of cultivation. Among them the Shea butternut, *Butyrospermum parkii*, is conspicuous and with one or two other species gives the cultivated areas a park-like appearance. If one sought for an East African equivalent of the densely populated Sudan zone emirates of Northern Nigeria one might point to Sukumaland. Both are densely populated, both are flat, both overlie or adjoin Pleistocene lake sediments, and both lie between the *miombo* and the thornbush. There are several differences. One is due to the presence of *Butyrospermum* and other useful farm trees such as *Tamarindus indica*, *Balanites aegyptiaca*, *Acacia albida*, and *Adansonia digitata*. The last four are also locally common in East Africa, but none has the economic value of the butternut. *Adansonia* is abundant in some small, localized areas of Sukumaland, because it is difficult to destroy; but as Glasgow (1961b) has pointed out, the value of any local tree to the Sukuma farmer is outweighed by its tendency to act as a focus for grain-eating birds such as the *Quelea*. Sukumaland is therefore treeless, for neither the *miombo* nor the thornbush contains any trees worth preserving, while all over the cultivation of the Nigerian Sudan zone are scattered these large economically valuable shade trees.

Where there is no population the Sudan zone bush is often dominated by *Anogeissus leiocarpa*, *Sclerocarya birrea*, *Lannea microcarpa*, and *Prosopis africana*. Various Combretaceae are common and there are several acacias, but it is, in general, still a broad-leaved vegetation in contrast to the Sahel where thorny trees with finely divided leaves predominate. Fringing or gallery forest, often locally very dense, still occurs in the Sudan zone. *Mitragyna inermis*, *Diospyros mespiliformis*, and *Khaya senegalensis* are common in the top storey and they shelter a dense lower-storey thicket. The role of these riverine vegetations in providing a hot-season habitat for *G. morsitans* was first studied in detail by Nash (1939, 1942). The disappearance of tsetse from the intervening bush and their survival in the hot weather only in the riverine vegetation has enabled control teams to use insecticides and very economically to eliminate tsetse from the rivers draining into Lake Chad (Davies 1964).

It is sometimes said that latitude 14°N. marks the limit of the *Glossina*-infested portion of Africa. This is roughly the northern limit also of the Sudan vegetation and its contact with the Sahel. The Sahel must, however, receive some notice, for trypanosomiasis does not disappear with the disappearance of *Glossina*. The Sahel is a wooded steppe dominated by *Acacia*, *Commiphora*, and other spiny or thorny and generally small trees, with scattered shrubs, often belonging to the Capparidaceae. The grass cover is sparse but provides nutriment for the herds of nomadic cattle. Except south of Lake Chad, where the Sahel makes a deep salient into the northern quarter of Cameroon, *Glossina* are usually absent. In this salient, however, *G. tachinoides* penetrates the Sahel along the banks of the

Logone–Shari river where it finds an adequate habitat in thickets of *Mimosa pigra* and a narrow, low, gallery thicket dominated by *Morellia senegalensis* (Gruvel 1966). In Chapter 5 it was noted that the nomadic herds carry *Trypanosoma vivax* infections for 500 km north of the fly-belts, where they overlap with infections of *T. evansi* transmitted by Tabanidae particularly among camels.

The 'middle belt'

One is not long in Nigeria without encountering the geographical concept of the 'middle belt'. The valleys of the Niger and Benue, down to their confluence at Lokoja, form a broadly V-shaped trough that divides the country into two northern and southern parts, which, however, do not correspond either to present or to past political divisions. The 'middle belt' indicates another division which does not correspond with the Niger–Benue trough. In the west it is crossed by the Niger valley and in the east is partly crossed by the Benue. In the centre of the country the middle belt is an area of varied indigenous peoples brought under the administrative control of the Emirs after the Fulani conquest. Its population density is often low and it lies between a northern area dominated by Hausas dependent on a basic cereal crop economy with cash crops of groundnuts and cotton and a southern area with a basic root crop economy of yams, cocoyams, and sweet potatoes with oil palm and cocoa cash crops, which supports a number of peoples among whom the Yoruba and Ibo are the most numerous. It is, in short, the gap between the zone of the sub-Saharan civilizations and those of the forest, and it stretches across West Africa to Senegal and can be traced on a population map of the continent eastwards to the watershed between the Oubangi–Bomu and Bahr-el-Ghazal basins which forms the boundary between the Sudan and Central African Republics. Pullan (1962) was concerned to find a climatic definition for the middle belt which he arrived at as follows: 'The Middle Belt is that area in Nigeria in which, over a period of years, 50 per cent or more of all the years have a dry season of four or five months duration.' This is a comparatively precise definition of a geographical region which is perhaps chiefly perceptible by the general sparsity of its population and therefore the comparative abundance of its natural savanna-type vegetation. In terms of the ecological zones of Chevalier and Keay it corresponds most nearly to the two Guinea zones. For the glossinologist it contains most of the *G. morsitans* fly-belts.

One other point needs to be made about the middle belt. Immediately to the south of the very densely populated countryside around the Sudan zone cities of Katsina, Kano, and Zaria lies the largest *G. morsitans* fly-belt in Nigeria. In part the emptiness of this countryside is still, perhaps, to be attributed to the northern slave trade. 'Southern Zaria was for long regarded as the source of slaves by the northern states and its population suffered accordingly' (Grove 1961). But that the middle belt was raided both by the northern Emirs and by those who traded towards the coast must have been because of inherent weaknesses in its populations. Grove also says, 'In southern Zaria and the southern fringe of Kano Emirate dense woodland heavily infested with tsetse fly and soils derived in part from laterized crystalline rocks provide a less congenial environment than further north.' One often finds sentences of this sort describing the *morsitans* belts. Nothing is incorrect in them save the order of their clauses. We ought to say that in southern Zaria soils derived in part from laterized crystalline rocks provide a less congenial environment so that human societies do not entirely suppress the natural fauna and flora and so suffer from the disadvantages conferred by the presence of tsetse and trypanosomiasis. It is clear that the Nigerian middle belt is a West African example of a *Grenzwildnis*.

The distribution of *Glossina*

The distribution of tsetse is related to the zonation in the climate and vegetation. This is most apparent in the *fusca* and *morsitans* groups. Their more or less parallel, but overlapping, distributions are, however, overlain by the ramifications of the *palpalis* group along rivers and streams. They too show some zonation, but it is less clear since the predominating influence is the presence of permanent water surfaces. All species are influenced by the activities of man. The influence may be restrictive, where the natural vegetation is destroyed and the natural hosts are driven out by tree felling and burning or by intensive hunting. On the other hand men may modify the environment so that some species can extend their range. When primary forest is destroyed forest-edge species find their habitats enlarged. A special case is the adaptation of a tsetse to a peri-domestic habitat. It seems likely that *G. tachinoides* was originally a riverine species of the savanna zones and that its present southward extension into the derived savanna could not have occurred before pig-keeping villagers made a new environment for it (Baldry 1964). In the following paragraphs the distributions of the six *fusca* species and two *morsitans* group species are briefly described. The overlying network of the *palpalis* group, ramifying through and uniting all zones from the coastal mangroves to the edge of and even into the otherwise tsetse-free Sahel, is described last.

The fusca *group*

The *fusca* group tsetses can be divided into three categories: those found only in the lowland rain forests; those that occur around the periphery of these forests and may penetrate, in relict forest islands or along gallery forests, into the derived savanna; and last those that, chiefly in East Africa, carry this habit to the extent that they may be found wherever suitable thickets or forests survive throughout the savanna vegetations.

There are three true lowland rain forest species in Nigeria. G. *tabaniformis* readily attacks man and it is perhaps because of this habit that it is, as yet, the only *fusca*-group fly to have been found throughout the Congo basin. It extends as far west as the Ivory Coast, but its continuity is broken by the savanna gap in Dahomey and Togo and also in south-eastern Nigeria where the dense population of Ibo peoples has eliminated the forest.

G. *haningtoni* and G. *nashi* have a more limited distribution. The latter was first described from five specimens among a collection of about 500 *fusca*-group tsetse collected in the rain forest of southern Cameroon (Potts 1955).† Since that time other specimens have been found and it seems that both G. *haningtoni* and G. *nashi* inhabit an inverted triangle with its apex near the Congo mouth (Cabinda) and its base extending from the south-western corner of the Central African Republic to the region of the Niger delta. These two species therefore are only known, so far, from Evens's (1953) dispersal centre of the *fusca* group.

G. *nigrofusca* is associated with the periphery of the lowland rain forests. Jordan (1963) regards it as a rare but widely spread species, never captured in large numbers. It may be found in the heart of forests as well as on their their edges. It stretches west to Liberia and eastwards to Uganda.

G. *fusca* is the most widely spread of the peripheral forest tsetse, reaching from Sierra Leone eastwards to Uganda. In Nigeria there is one record well to the north of the derived savanna, in a forest island in the Southern Guinea zone.

G. *fusca* was separated by Newstead and Evans (1921) into two varieties, G. *fusca fusca* and G. *fusca congolensis*. The subject has been reviewed by Jordan (1965d). The distinction between the two varieties is based upon the size and form of both male and female genitalia. Machado (1959) suggested that G. *fusca fusca* was confined to the forests stretching from Ghana westwards through the Ivory Coast and Liberia, and that the form G. *fusca congolensis* was found in Southern Nigeria and thence extended eastwards into the Congo basin and so to Uganda. According to him, therefore, the two varieties were separated by the Togo–Dahomey savanna gap. These conclusions were supported by Le Berre and Itard (1960). Jordan (1965d) however measured five specimens from Ghana and found that four of them undoubtedly fell into the category of G. *fusca congolensis*. He therefore thought that although the two varieties had arisen because of the isolation created by the savanna gap and that this separation was of considerable antiquity, nevertheless in comparatively recent times the gap had been penetrated, from the east, by the *congolensis* form. It is, indeed, probable that during the last century the fly-belts on either side of the savanna gap have expanded. Finelle, Desrotour, Yvore, and Renner (1962)

† And hence not inside modern Nigeria. However, Baldry (1967) considers that it will be found in due course on the Nigerian side of the border.

have described the expansion of the area of distribution of *G. fusca congolensis* in the Central African Republic, one of the few cases in which a *fusca* group tsetse has been implicated in an epizootic of cattle trypanosomiasis.

Finally, the sixth of the Nigerian *fusca*-group flies, *G. medicorum*, seems to avoid the moister portions of the lowland rain forests and frequents the forest edge or forest islands and gallery forests in the derived savanna. In Ghana, Chapman (1960) has found it in secondary thicket no more than 15 ft high.

Keay (1959) discussed the derived savanna and asked, 'Derived from what?' Looking back to an era before the development of agriculture led to the replacement of the forest edges by cultivation and fallow, he suggested that at one time a true ecotonal vegetation occupied the interzone between the lowland rain forest and the Guinea savanna and perhaps included the Southern Guinea zone which is also 'derived'. This is an interesting idea for the student of tsetse evolution. It is difficult to believe that the forest-edge species, *G. medicorum. G. fusca*, *G. nigrofusca*, and, outside West Africa, *G. schwetzi*, *G. fuscipleuris*, and *G. brevipalpis*, all of which tend to be associated with secondary forest, could have evolved in response to the pressures developed by cultivation. Rather it may be supposed that they belong to a natural vegetation association that has disappeared in most places to be replaced by cultivation with forest regeneration, relict forest islands, or gallery forests. The true lowland forest species, *G. nashi*, *G. haningtoni*, and *G. tabaniformis*, will, perhaps, become more and more restricted as the closed rain forest is replaced by seral vegetations.

The morsitans *group*

In Chapter 3 it was suggested that *G. pallidipes* and *G. longipalpis* were savanna flies that had secondarily adapted themselves to a forest-edge habitat. They tend to occur in the same areas as those *fusca*-group species that belong to the forest edges or interzones. *G. longipalpis* has been regarded by some authors as the West African variety of *G. pallidipes*, but it is more usual to treat them as two closely related species. In some respects their habits are similar, but the East African species is ecologically much more plastic than *G. longipalpis*. The latter is confined almost entirely to the derived savanna and Southern Guinea zones whereas *G. pallidipes* is found throughout a wide variety of environments from high rainfall forest types to semi-arid thickets. Both require a thicket or forest-edge habitat and both are usually reluctant to come to the human bait. Both feed largely on bushbuck (*Tragelaphus scriptus*) and bushpig (*Potamochoerus porcus*, called red river hog in West Africa). Page (1959c) studied *G. longipalpis* in a forest island in derived savanna in Nigeria, where it was found in company with *G. palpalis*, *G. tachinoides*, *G. fusca*, and *G. medicorum*. The only other full-length study is that of Morris (1934) who investigated its habits in derived savanna near the coast at Takoradi, Ghana, at the western end of the savanna gap.

Moving north from the forests and derived savanna one enters the zone dominated by *G. morsitans submorsitans*. This tsetse was first described as a separate species, *G. submorsitans*, but was later relegated to subspecific rank (Newstead, Evans, and Potts 1924). There seems no special reason for insisting, as most authors do, on using the subspecific name and we shall here refer to it as *G. morsitans*, thus following Nash (1948*a*) whose account of the factors controlling its distribution is still illuminating. In terms of rainfall it has as great a range as in eastern Africa, being found in country with as little as 20 in and as much as 55 in† annually. The heart of the *morsitans*-infested country is the *Isoberlinia doka* woodland of the Northern Guinea zone, but the species flourishes in neighbouring vegetation communities, both drier (Sudan zone) and wetter (Southern Guinea and even derived savanna zones). The factors controlling distribution of *G. morsitans* in Nigeria will occupy much of Chapter 22.

The palpalis *group*

Two members of this group, *G. caliginea* and *G. pallicera*, are especially associated with the zones of mangrove, swamp forest, and lowland rain forests. Two short papers by French workers summarize most that is known of *G. caliginea* and its role as a vector of trypanosomes (Roubaud, Maillot, and Rageau 1951, Roubaud and Maillot 1952). One may, perhaps, conceive of *G. pallicera* as a forest *G. palpalis* that does not attack man. *G. palpalis* itself has been much studied, for with *G. tachinoides* and *G. fuscipes* (long regarded as a subspecies of *G. palpalis*) it is responsible for nearly all transmission of human trypanosomiasis. (*Rhodesiense* type infections transmitted by *morsitans* group tsetse, in Africa as a whole, form only a very small proportion of the recorded total of cases of sleeping sickness.) *G. palpalis* finds its southern limit in West Africa along the coastline from Douala in Cameroon to Dakar in Senegal. Its northern limit closely follows the 34-in isohyet, but in places can penetrate drier country where rivers contain permanent water.

A detailed study of the ecology of *G. palpalis* was made by Nash and Page (1953) in Northern Nigeria, and this was followed by a paper by the second of these authors (Page 1959*b*) on its ecology in Southern Nigeria. In the first investigation at Katabu (10° 42′N., 7° 31′E.) measurements of climate (temperature, rainfall, relative humidity, evaporation rate, saturation deficit) were made in three stations at 4 ft and at 4 in above ground level. Two were set up inside the riverine habitat of *G. palpalis*, the third was in open savanna just outside it. Katabu is in the *Isoberlinia doka* woodland of Keay's Northern Guinea zone. *G. palpalis* and *G. tachinoides* live

† But up to 90 in a year in Guinea, although there this heavy rainfall is associated with a dry season of 5–6 months (Nash 1948*a*).

here along streams fringed with gallery forest with an evergreen under-storey of forest shrubs and climbers. These streams and the forest vegeta-tion on their banks may be only a few yards wide. The rains reach their peak in August, and the months November to April are virtually rainless. During the six years of the Katabu investigation mean annual rainfall was 46·6 in. In the dry season the streams cease to flow and water remains only in disconnected pools. One of the two meteorological stations in the riverine habitat was set up in a place where the stream always dried up, the other was beside a permanent pool. In the rains there was little difference in the climates registered at 4 in and at 4 ft in either site. In dry seasons, in mild years, there was also little difference between the two levels; but in severe years, when temperatures elsewhere reached critical levels, only the climate at 4 in remained tolerable. Here the highest temperature recorded was 32·2°C, although at 4 ft above the water it reached 36·2°, and in the woodland just outside 39·4°C. *G. palpalis*, during the dry season, therefore tends to concentrate wherever standing pools provide a microclimate in which it avoids the extremes of temperatures and humidity to be found elsewhere. In severe years the flies survive only in places where pools never dry up. During the rains, however, when water is continuous in the stream bed and the general climate is more humid and temperatures lower, the flies spread along the whole length.

At Ugbobigha on the northern edge of the forest belt of Southern Nigeria, Page (1959*b*) found, in complete contrast to the situation at Katabu, no significant seasonal concentrations of the flies on the stream beds, which never dried up, for the mean rainfall was about 70 in annually and temperatures nowhere rose so high nor fell so low as at the northern station. Nor were the flies confined to the river bed. Odd specimens were found near the camp built half a mile away from the nearest stream and on a fly-round used to catch *G. longipalpis* in the savanna woodland, a half to one and a half miles away. These captures were made throughout the year, although mostly in the middle rains. 'This is a very different picture to that found in Northern Nigeria, where this species is entirely riverine in habit, specimens being rarely encountered in the savanna and then only during the period of heaviest rainfall' (Page 1959*b*). These two studies so briefly summarized are among the most illuminating made on the epidemi-ology of trypanosomiasis since the work of Fiske (1920) and Carpenter (1924) so many years before in Uganda.

One other Nigerian *Glossina* remains to be noticed. This is *G. tachinoides*. In some ways it is the most remarkable and, perhaps, the most important tsetse in West Africa. For long regarded as essentially a species belonging to dry climates, it reaches further north than any other tsetse. Its penetra-tion of the Sahel zone along the banks of the Logone–Shari has already been noticed. In these arid areas it can survive in riverine thickets of low bush without many of the upper-storey trees that seem essential elements in the environment of *G. palpalis*. At Geidam, on the Yobe river in the western drainage of Lake Chad, rainfall is only 15 in per annum. There is a seven-months dry season (Nash 1948a) and hot season maximum temperatures rise to 43·3°C (Davies 1964).† But just west of the mouth of the Cross river the same tsetse is found in country where the average rainfall is about 130 in. Nash's earlier studies (Nash 1939, 1942) suggest strongly that in the dry months *G. tachinoides* survives the hot weather by confining itself to small microclimates in much the same way as he and Page later demonstrated in *G. palpalis* at Katabu; at the other end of its range he thought it as capable of withstanding a very high humidity as *G. palpalis* but limited by unsuitable vegetation. He observed that whereas 60·6 per cent of attacks on a man by *G. palpalis* in the dry season were made above his waist (40–56 in above ground), 79·1 per cent of *G. tachinoides* attacks, at the same place, were made below the knee (0–22 in above ground). In the rains, in cooler weather the same trend was observed, but was somewhat less marked.

The layer of shrubs in the bottom storey of the lowland forest vegetation offered no impediment to the high flying *G. palpalis* but were a barrier to the low flying *G. tachinoides* except where dense populations of Ibo and associated peoples had destroyed the forests east of the Niger delta. Baldry (1966) reached a similar conclusion: 'The species is physically prevented by marginal evergreen thickets from entering the forest belt.' He also showed that the southern limit of distribution of *G. tachinoides*, even outside the Cross river salient, was much further south elsewhere in Nigeria than had appeared from the surveys of earlier workers. Nash (1948a) estimated that *G. tachinoides* was to be found throughout an area of 187 000 mile² in Nigeria. Baldry (1966) now supposes it to cover an area of 208 000 mile². Its limit is indeed the northern edge of the lowland rain forest except where Ibo cultivators have replaced that forest with cultivated oil palms. It had not been recorded throughout its more southerly range because in much of the derived savanna it ceases to be a riverine tsetse and has lost its propensity for attacking man. Instead it has become an inhabitant of villages where it feeds on domestic pigs (Baldry 1964). A few miles from Ilorin on the northern edge of the derived savanna it is uncomfortable to stand on the banks of the Oyun river (unless one has a bait ox to draw off the attack) because of the avidity with which *G. tachinoides* bites the ankles. Here there is no doubt about its presence. Its willingness to attack man has always been regarded throughout West Africa as characteristic of its behaviour, but in the villages around Nsukka, where man is far more numerous than his pigs, he is rarely fed upon. Elsewhere in the same ecological zone cattle may replace pigs but again man is neglected. The ecology of *G. tachinoides* in these regions is 'so different from the classical concept, that one might be dealing with a different species' (Baldry 1966).

† *G. tachinoides* and *G. morsitans* were exterminated here between 1955 and 1964 (Davies 1964).

The *palpalis* group tsetses were described after the *fusca* and *morsitans* groups to emphasize the way in which they ramify through and unite the whole West African and Congo basin areas. The *fusca* group belong essentially to the forest and the *morsitans* group to the savannas; the *palpalis* group joins all together and, especially in the savanna ecosystems, does so parasitologically as well as geographically. They are the principal vehicles whereby trypanosomes that have leaked, as it were, out of the transmission cycles maintained within the wildlife reservoirs by *morsitans* and *fusca* group tsetses, are circulated and re-circulated within human societies. The presence of *palpalis* group tsetses enables massive epidemics to develop in a way that is impossible where they are absent. The epidemic that reached a peak in Tanzania in 1928, although sufficiently alarming, was numerically trivial in comparison with that which, soon afterwards, devastated parts of Northern Nigeria.

Trypanosome infection rates in Nigerian tsetse

The movements of the fly-belts and their significance in causing epidemics and epizootics will be considered in the next two chapters. The importance, in this context, of the flies themselves is directly due to two factors: (1) the nature and intensity of their own infections with trypanosomes, and (2) their behaviour towards man and his domestic livestock considered as natural or adventitious food hosts and hence as recipients of trypanosomes.

The significance of different tsetse as vectors of human trypanosomiasis has for long been a preoccupation of West African workers, both British and French. In particular the researches of Nash and his successors have been illuminating. Our knowledge of tsetse infection rates owes much to the work of Jordan (1961, 1964, 1965*a*) who collated his own results with those of Nash and Page (1953), and Page (1959*a, b, c*), as well as of the earlier workers, Johnson and Lloyd (1923 and other papers). Two summaries of mean infection rates of the commoner tsetses in Nigeria are given in Table 21.1.

Jordan (1961) compiled a table summarizing infection rates obtained by various workers for nine species of *Glossina* in southern Nigeria and Cameroon and showed that mean infection rates obtained by combining results from different places and at different times could be misleading. Jordan's summaries are used here, supplemented by other data (Table 21.2), but omitting data from Johnson and his team in the 1920s, as they require separate treatment.

Two points emerge from Table 21.2. The gross infection rates (that is percentage of flies infected by any trypanosome) vary considerably between species. The contrast between the infection rates of *G. tabaniformis* and *G. fusca* is striking. Of the former all but 29 of the flies were collected at Ugbobigha in the mid-western region of Nigeria some 50 miles north of

TABLE 21.1

Summaries of mean infection rates in commoner Nigerian Glossina

	Infection rates (all trypanosomes) according to:	
Species	Nash (1948) (%)	Davies (1962) (%)
G. longipalpis .	24–35	25
G. morsitans .	23–8	20
G. tachinoides .	6–11	6
G. palpalis .	6–10	5

† After Nash (1948a), and Davies (1962).

TABLE 21.2

Trypanosome infection rates: combined data from various sources from Nigeria and Cameroon

Species	Total dissected	Total positive	% positive	% analysis of infections		
				T. vivax	T. congolense	T. brucei
G. haningtoni .	59	5	8·5	(5)	(0)	(0)
G. tabaniformis .	3389	110	3·2	60·9	38·2	0·9
G. nigrofusca .	182	44	24·2	88·6	11·4	0
G. fusca . .	1301	206	15·8	88·8	10·7	0·5
G. medicorum .	252	39	15·5	87·2	12·8	0
G. longipalpis .	4360	939	21·5	82·0	18·1	0·1
G. morsitans (1) .	1669	113	6·8	54·9	45·1	0
G. morsitans (2) .	341	99	29·0	72·7	27·3	0
G. caliginea .	230	84	36·5	84·5	14·3	1·2
G. pallicera .	119	3	2·5	(3)	(0)	(0)
G. palpalis (3) .	2497	45	1·8	75·6	24·4	0
G. palpalis (4) .	3382	101	3·3	90·0	9·0	1·0
G. tachinoides .	274	18	6·6	61·1	16·7	22·2

Benin. Of the latter nearly half were dissected at the same place. Jordan showed that:

The proportion of G. fusca infected at Ugbobigha was significantly higher than the proportion of G. tabaniformis infected ($\chi^2 = 135\cdot55$; $P < 0\cdot001$), both species having been collected in the same area of rain forest. This may suggest that G. fusca is more readily infected than G. tabaniformis, a possibility that requires investigation, but it is more likely to be a result of differences in the feeding habits of the two species. In the same area of forest both tsetse fed mainly on red river hog (*G. tabaniformis*, 72 per cent of meals, *G. fusca* 73 per cent), but, whereas 21 per cent of the meals of *G. tabaniformis* were from porcupine (*Atherurus africanus*), 21 per cent of those of *G. fusca* were from Bovidae (Jordan, Lee-Jones, and Weitz 1961).

Evidently it is the Bovidae that are important as the source of infection and not the preferred host, the red river hog.

The argument that the infection rate in tsetse flies primarily depends upon the food host has been well developed by Jordan, but it was a line of thought first elaborated by Johnson and his colleagues in Northern Nigeria between 1922 and 1927. To their work we must now turn.

The investigations of Johnson and Lloyd on the food of Nigerian tsetse

Johnson and Lloyd (1923) produced data for *G. tachinoides* that contrasted the infection rates in flies found where 'large game' was present and in those where it was absent (Table 21.3). The significance of the presence or absence of large game is clear from a passage in another paper:

There are many areas in Northern Nigeria, mainly in the drier northern parts, in which the larger wild fauna has been practically exterminated. In these there is little evidence of the existence of the smaller antelopes or wild pig and the larger antelopes have entirely gone. Monkeys and sometimes baboons remain plentiful and from this one may judge there is a considerable fauna of small mammals. Where there is suitable water *Varanus* always persists and in some cases crocodiles also. The birds are not greatly affected, except where farms have entirely replaced the forests. Cattle, horses, asses, sheep and goats generally abound in them (Lloyd and Johnson 1924).

The 'gut only' infections in Table 21.3 are immature and not transmissible to vertebrate hosts. If they are omitted and the other two categories, 'gut and proboscis' which are likely to have been *congolense*-type and 'proboscis only', *vivax*-type infections, it is evident that where 'large game' were present, the numbers of mature *congolense* and *vivax* type infections were much greater than where they were absent. Johnson and Lloyd also showed that *G. morsitans* (only found in the presence of 'large game') developed much higher infection rates (21.2 per cent mature infections) than did *G. tachinoides* in the same situation (8·1 per cent).

Lloyd, Johnson, and Rawson (1927) summing up the work of this early Nigerian research team showed that in *G. tachinoides* the infection rate begins to rise about the middle of the dry season and continues to do so until the middle of the rains when it falls to a low level again. They demonstrated this in three successive years and concluded that as the weather got hotter in the second half of the dry season, both flies and large game concentrated 'in the more secluded bush'. The flies therefore became increasingly dependent upon the principal trypanosome reservoirs for

TABLE 21.3

Prevalence of flagellates in G. tachinoides *in areas where large game is absent or present*

Large game	Number dissected	% showing flagellates in:			Total % infected
		gut only	gut and proboscis	proboscis only	
Absent .	407	9·3	0·5	1·7	11·5
Present .	1093	3·1	1·3	6·8	11·2

their food. In the wet season, a large proportion of the flies fed on reptiles and this caused the infection rate to fall. The infection rate tended to be negatively correlated with the proportion of gorged flies showing nucleated (i.e. reptilian or avian) blood cells in their crops.

The seasonal variation in infection rates of G. *morsitans* were less easily explained, for the proportion of antelope blood 'from which the vast majority of infection is certainly derived' showed only a slight seasonal change. They suggested that the fluctuations observed might be associated with changes in the age structure of the populations, so that a low infection rate would be correlated with a high proportion of flies too young to have acquired infections.

Johnson's team used a crude method of blood meal analysis based upon the size of erythrocytes and the separation of nucleated from non-nucleated cells (Lloyd, Johnson, Young, and Morrison 1924). Jordan (1965a) has summarized their results. Of 215 specimens of G. *morsitans* from which they were able to identify the blood meals, 74·3 per cent showed corpuscles indicating that they had fed on 'various antelopes, cattle (or buffalo), bats or rodents'. The infection rate (all trypanosomes) obtained by dissecting nearly 6000 flies was 18·8 per cent. Among 550 G. *tachinoides*, 40·8 per cent had fed on reptiles (and, perhaps, frogs) while the two categories in which antelopes were included only amounted to 21·6 per cent of feeds. The gross infection rate of G. *tachinoides* found by dissection of nearly 11 000 flies was only 5·4 per cent.

It is of considerable interest that the proportion of feeds from Bovidae in this early work (we can safely ignore possible feeds on bats, although perhaps not on rodents) is higher than Jordan himself found in the game reserve at Yankari (in Table 5.7), and very much higher than in his two localities at Gamagira and Mando. Bovidae were undoubtedly plentiful in the Sherifuri area, where the Johnson team operated in 1923, for hunting was limited because the human population had been depleted by sleeping sickness. On the other hand 19·6 per cent of blood meals taken by

G. tachinoides were derived from primates. *G. morsitans* only took 4·2 per cent of meals from this source. Use of the precipitin test showed that these primate meals in *G. tachinoides* were from man (Lloyd, Johnson, and Rawson 1927). This was important for it indicated that sleeping sickness epidemics in the Sherifuri area must have been transmitted by *G. tachinoides*.

The species of *Glossina*, their diet, and their infections

Jordan (1965a) applied these ideas to the study of the host relationships of different species of tsetse and summarized his results in correlation diagrams. Within the genus as a whole and with a single species (*G. morsitans*) the incidence of infection with trypanosomes (regardless of species) is positively correlated with the proportion of blood meals taken from

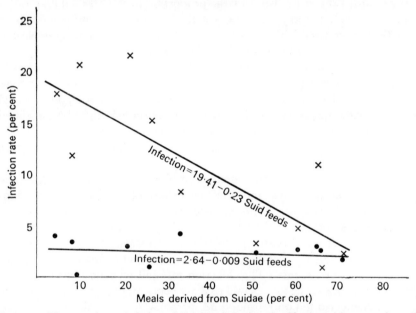

FIG. 21.1. The negative correlation of *T. vivax* infections in *Glossina* with proportions of feeds from Suidae. This implies a positive correlation with proportions of feeds from Bovidae There is no significant correlation between *T. congolense* and diet (after Jordan 1965).

× *T. vivax*;   ● *T. congolense*

Bovidae. Jordan's data also yielded a correlation which may have some bearing upon the zonation of the *vivax* ratio in cattle. He showed that as the proportion of feeds taken from Suidae increased, so the proportion of *T. vivax* infections in the tsetses declined. There was no such negative correlation with *T. congolense* (Fig. 21.1). The most likely explanation for this is that, 'Whereas *T. vivax* is *par excellence* a trypanosome of Bovidae and probably seldom, if ever, occurs naturally in Suidae, *T. congolense* occurs in both Bovidae and Suidae.' As the number of meals derived from Suidae increase and those from Bovidae decrease, so the chances of *Glossina* acquiring infections by *T. vivax* also decrease, although there is little change in the chances of infection with *T. congolense*.

22

ANTECEDENTS OF EPIDEMICS AND EPIZOOTICS IN NIGERIA

ONCE more it is necessary to leave *Glossina* and *Trypanosoma* in order to give an account of events that involved people in a massive epidemic of sleeping sickness and their cattle in a novel epizootio-logical situation the outcome of which is not clear. It was possible to deal with the trypanosomiases of Rhodesia as one problem because the country itself could be looked upon as a single ecosystem occupied for a thousand years or more by a succession of societies half surrounded by a *Grenzwildnis* infested with *Glossina morsitans*. Nigeria is a recent political creation, with no inherent biological unity. Its people have, indeed, an ancient history, but modern boundaries cut across and divide the political units in the same way that they divide the natural ones. It is therefore not possible in a short space to describe the trypanosomiases in Nigeria as the development of a single process.

In particular Nigeria, especially Northern Nigeria, has served to illustrate what may be called the *Pax Britannica* theory of origin of African epidemics, although it was not a particularly British conception. All colonial powers believed that by 'pacifying' the warring tribes they had enabled people, for the first time in their history, to move safely about the country and, in so doing, to carry with them the infecting trypanosomes. To proclaim that this was not so is not to deny that population movements were never involved in production of epidemics. Locally they were and still are often of extreme importance; but they were not a consequence of pacification nor do they explain why it was that during the first forty years of this century hundreds of thousands, perhaps millions, of people died of sleeping sickness. The 'pacification' theory still survives because no alternative has yet been given careful attention. A study of the antecedents of the great epidemic of sleeping sickness that spread through Northern Nigeria in the 1920s and 1930s should provide at least the outline of another hypothesis.

When these antecedents have been examined and discovered to be essentially the same as those that preceded the epidemics and epizootics in East Africa it will be necessary to show that the *Grenzwildnis* in Nigeria also provides the basis for persistence of foci of infection. As an adjunct to this concept in West Africa it will be found that here, too, human societies have by their growth and activity in cultivating and hunting eliminated large fly-belts and are still doing so.

Similarities with East Africa having been noted, the contrasts must be described. It has already been recorded that they are a consequence of the presence of the *palpalis*-group tsetses and their peculiar ability to adapt themselves to living in areas where wild hosts have been eliminated and man himself and his domestic livestock are the only sources of food. This habit has had an effect upon the evolution of the trypanosomiases of cattle as profound as upon that of the disease in man.

Population trends in Northern Nigeria

Because some West African people had a rather more sophisticated social organization than their contemporaries in East Africa, some quantitative data are of less value than is the case in the sample areas already studied. Cattle population estimates have large errors that have their origin in a well-organized system of tax-dodging dating from pre-colonial days. The most recent estimates of human population density in Nigeria are suspect because the census results provided, according to the post-colonial constitution, the basis for political division of the country between tribal groups (Okonjo 1968, Udo 1968).

In the three areas examined in the Victoria basin it appeared that human population density began to fall at about the time of arrival of the colonial powers and did not begin to recover until between 1930 and 1940. In Rhodesia a major collapse initiated by the Ngoni invasion during the first half of the nineteenth century was prolonged by events associated with the take-over by Rhodes's British South Africa Company. None of the East African areas fell within the zone of influence of the slave trade, but in Nigeria this factor cannot be ignored.

Kuczynski (1948), in his great demographic survey, saw little evidence for change in the size of the population of Northern Nigeria either before or after 1900. 'I doubt whether in any earlier period the population of Northern Nigeria had been very much greater than in 1900.' But Kuczynski was obviously influenced by his desire to demonstrate the inadequacy of colonial demography and at the same time to demolish a view widely held after about 1930 that the colonial administration had had, necessarily, an immediately beneficial effect upon population growth. Heinrich Barth in 1854 had put the population of Northern Nigeria at 30–40 million. In 1904 Lugard estimated it to be around 9 million. Barth's figure was dismissed by Kuczynski as not worth consideration; nevertheless, it is difficult to believe that events after about 1840 did not affect population density from the Niger–Benue valley northwards.

Kuczynski's view of the population of Nigeria as a whole was that it increased very little, if at all, in the first quarter of the twentieth century and that it increased somewhat, but probably less than 10 per cent, in the following fifteen years. The figures that he reproduces (p. 392) for Northern Nigeria suggest indeed that a marked decline was in progress until 1907.

1904	9 161 700	1907	5 935 000	1910	7 811 309
1905	8 782 183	1908	—	1911	8 110 631
1906	7 164 751	1909	6 714 038	1921	9 994 515

Lugard's view of the first decade of the century was that 'There seems to be little doubt that since the partition of tropical Africa between the European Powers the native populations in most territories have not increased and have probably decreased' (Kuczynski 1948).

There were severe famines in 1904, 1914, and 1927. In 1899 smallpox was 'a terrible scourge throughout the territories and when epidemics occur the natives die by thousands'. In 1918 the influenza pandemic 'caused probably many more deaths in Southern Nigeria than any other catastrophe that has ever befallen the country'. 'Nearly 3 per cent of the population of the Southern Provinces of Nigeria, that is at least 250 000 individuals, died from influenza during the epidemic.' In Northern Nigeria 'the native population was universally affected and a very large number of deaths occurred' (Kuczynski 1948).

In the first quarter, and perhaps longer, of the present century demographic evidence, poor though it may be, points to the conclusion already arrived at for East Africa. The population first declined and then made a recovery leading to the increases finally demonstrated in the last decade of colonial rule. Kuczynski's interpretation of Nigerian history before 1900 would not allow him to admit any significant change from the figure (for Northern Nigeria) of 9 million. He held that although Northern Nigeria had suffered much from slave raiding by the Fulani emirs, this did not cause much depopulation because the slaves remained in the country. This internal slave raiding, he suggested, 'probably caused less depopulation than the raids which, before 1860, had furnished slaves for export to America'. But in a peasant society living on a subsistence economy, the main depopulating effect of slave raids, or any other form of large-scale disorganization, acts through failures of cultivation and harvest and the impact of this, in turn, upon infant survival. The history of Northern Nigeria does indeed suggest that from about 1840 onwards social disorganization was unusually widespread.

The Jihad

The beginnings of modern Northern Nigerian history are to be found in the Jihad or Holy War begun by the Fulani Shehu, Usuman dan Fodio, in 1804. The reader who wishes to learn more of the Jihad can consult Stenning (1959), Crowder (1962), or Hogben and Kirke-Green (1966), either of whom will serve as starting points for further study. The Jihad was essentially a war of ruling castes employing quasi-professional armies. It lasted until 1809 and, apart from Bornu in the region of Lake Chad and Bauchi in the sub-Sudan Zone just east of the Jos Plateau, resulted in the union of the emirates of Northern Nigeria under the hegemony of Sokoto, where Usuman's son Bello was ruler. 'The period of Sultan Bello's reign must be regarded as the great period of the Fulani empire in Hausaland' (Northern Nigeria region 1955). Bello died in 1837 and with his death the empire, which had been governed according to the strict Muslim ethic which had been Usuman's inspiration in raising the Jihad, fell apart. 'It was found more profitable to leave the pagans in a condition in which it was lawful to enslave them. Cruelty, venality, nepotism, avarice, all enhanced the decadence and degradation which marred the Fulani rule of the latter half of the century' (Northern Nigeria region 1955). This quotation from an official propaganda document of the last decade of British rule in Nigeria summarizes a situation in which the majority of historians seem to agree. They do not support Kuczynski. The decline in population that Lugard observed in the first decade of this century was the continuation of a process begun sixty years earlier with the death of Sultan Bello.

In the southern regions of Nigeria disorganization caused by the Atlantic slave trade had been growing since the sixteenth century. Barth (1857) thought the main cause for the increase in Fulani slave raiding after Bello's death was their perception of the commercial advantages of exploiting their subjects as merchandise for the American market. Trypanosomiasis in the forest regions has been little studied and the possible influences on it of the Atlantic trade will not be discussed further. In Northern Nigeria the contrast between the estimates of Barth in the middle of the nineteenth and of Lugard at the beginning of the twentieth century almost certainly grossly exaggerates the demographic picture. But political and administrative conditions during this interval were such that populations seem more likely to have decreased than to have increased. Some communities certainly underwent a marked redistribution. Because of the widespread insecurity in and around Hausaland after the death of Sultan Bello people stayed within or as close as possible to their walled towns and cities. One consequence of this immobility was that Fulani cattle were unable to go on their usual seasonal migrations in search of new pasture. 'For many years cattle were emaciated owing to confinement within walls and precincts of villages and, finally, according to modern accounts, the majority of the bovine population died in the great rinderpest epidemic of 1887–91' (Hopen 1958). To this tremendous panzootic, already described in Uganda, in Tanzania, and in Rhodesia, it is necessary to turn once more.

Rinderpest and pleuropneumonia

The Fulani (Peul, Fula, Felaata, Fulbe) are not basically of negro stock. They are for the most part nomadic cattle keepers, the pastoral Fulani or Bororo, but others have become settled, the Fulanin Gida or Town Fulani. Although they have provided the rulers of Northern Nigeria since the Jihad, their relationship, especially that of the pastoral Fulani, with the

Hausa peasants differs very much from that of the Hima and Tusi to the former serf tribes of the interlake region; but their cattle were afflicted with the same devastating epizootics.

St. Croix (1945) gives an account of the effect of the rinderpest panzootic that recalls East Africa.

In the years 1887 to 1891 a great outbreak of rinderpest decimated the herds of cattle owners. Starting apparently about Darfur, the disease reached what is now the French *Colonie du Tchad* in 1886, spreading straight from East to West. In the greater part of present day Nigeria the disease wiped out the great majority of cattle. The outbreak was commonly known in Hausa as '*sannu*' from the Hausa greeting used as an expression of sympathy. The older men tell terrible stories of those days. Attempts were made, by some, to fly from the disease and preserve their cattle. Fulani, having lost all, or nearly all their cattle, became demented: many are said to have done away with themselves. Some roamed the bush calling imaginary cattle: assaults on persons for imagined provocation or suspected derisive remarks as to the loss of cattle were common. [When the outbreak had spent itself] so great was the demand for cattle that, locally, it was common in many places to offer large prices for the unborn calf.

Stenning (1959) records that 'Fulani cattle-owners were said to have left their families and wandered unclothed in the bush, eating dust, looking for their dead livestock and, we may infer, their sanity'.

There was another catastrophic epizootic in 1913–14 and yet another in 1919–20, so devastating 'that even the hyaenas did not eat the bodies of the dead cattle' (St. Croix 1945). The disease was never eliminated, as it was in most of East Africa, but strains of the virus became attenuated and vaccination campaigns kept it more or less under control.

No information seems to be available about the effects of the rinderpest on West African wildlife, but it must be supposed that the same genera suffered as in eastern Africa and a recession of *G. morsitans* fly-belts must be borne in mind, as well as diminution of populations of the hosts of *G. longipalpis*.

A study of rinderpest in the former French colonies has been made by Thomé (1964). Rinderpest appeared between 1884 and 1891 and may have entered Africa in Russian cattle from the Black Sea region. These animals were used as rations by troops ascending the Nile in 1884 in the abortive attempt to relieve General Gordon in Khartoum. (This is an alternative to Lugard's hypothesis which blamed the Italians in Eritrea.) In Cameroon in 1891 and in French West Africa in 1892 there was a terrible epizootic in which losses, in some regions, amounted to 98 per cent of the cattle population. In 1914 losses in another epizootic were estimated at 10 per cent, and ten years later this epizootic was said to have cost Chad 400 000–500 000 head of cattle. Another report, of local relevance, suggested loss of no more than 2–4 per cent. Also in Chad the epizootic of 1918–19 caused losses of up to 70 per cent among herds not protected by antibodies acquired in the 1913–14 outbreak. Total losses were evaluated at 200 000 head out of a population of about 1 million. Since 1919 the disease has persisted in enzootic form as it has through the whole African Sudan zone.

When French veterinarians arrived in Chad in 1900 they were not aware of the existence there of rinderpest, for their attention was chiefly directed towards an outbreak of contagious bovine pleuropneumonia. This had been recorded in Chad in 1870. There is evidence that pleuropneumonia entered the interlake region in East Africa sometime before the rinderpest and, in Chapter 19, Henning's (1956) view that this disease was first imported into South Africa at Mossel Bay in 1854 has been recorded. Perhaps there is no need to attribute the 1870 infection in Chad to this source, for cattle may have been imported into Africa at many places at the outset of the 'scramble'.

The cattle that suffered these devastating epizootics find their main pastures in the grass steppe of the Sahel and the more northerly, tsetse-free, portion of the Sudan zone. In eastern Africa the Sukuma cattle populations graze in similar types of vegetation. Their pastures are limited by the fly-belts and their numbers are controlled by starvation aided by periodical epizootics of East coast fever (Chapter 12). The West African pastures are limited in the south by tsetse but in the north by the Sahara desert which contains no pasture. There is no East coast fever. Nor does it appear that massive mortality from starvation unaccompanied by disease exerts a major control over numbers. The principal control is exerted by trypanosomiasis. In East Africa the Sukuma or Masai may, in bad years, take their cattle into the fly-bush. Many die but a proportion escape the death by starvation that would otherwise have been their lot had they remained in the exhausted pastures. In West Africa, every dry season, hundreds of thousands of cattle leave the northern pastures and are driven south to graze in the tsetse-infested country of the Sudan or Guinea zones. They pass through but do not remain in the G. morsitans belts, but even if their owners are able to avoid the latter they still come into contact with G. tachinoides and G. palpalis on the rivers where they are watered.

The annual exposure to infection is the price that must be paid for the extra dry-season pasture and for the rest that this gives to the grasses in the tsetse-free north. Some deaths, more morbidity, a constant proportion of abortions result from the infections but the catastrophic periodical mass mortality from starvation is avoided. There are bad years when losses from hunger and thirst are appreciable, but generally their effects are indirect. It is in the lean years that trypanosome infections, tolerable when pasture is abundant, take their greatest toll. But the risk is spread and one does not find, as happened in 1949–50 in the disease-free cattle of Sukumaland, that nearly one quarter of the stock population died of starvation in a single season.

For the present, however, it is only required to point out that for some years after the passage of the rinderpest there can have been no need for the depleted remnants of the cattle population to seek additional grazing in the south. There was plenty of room and to spare in the north. Moreover, if from long usage the Fulani who still owned cattle now resumed the habitual transhumance they must have found the fly-belts of *G. morsitans* and of *G. longipalpis* greatly shrunk, for in Nigeria one must suppose that the favoured hosts of these flies were much reduced by the infection just as they had been elsewhere in Africa.

The Nigerian middle belt and the 'great forest'

The usefulness of the Nigerian middle belt as a pasture reserve derives from its situation as a *Grenzwildnis*. In some parts its soils lack fertility and there may be large areas badly supplied with water. Elsewhere it is densely populated. The *G. morsitans* belts of West Africa are fragmented: there is no vast continuity of infestation as there is in Tanzania, Zambia, or the Central African Republic. The approximate area of the Guinea and sub-Sudan zones in Nigeria is 165 000 mile². This may be regarded as the potential size of the habitat of *G. morsitans* (although there are local extensions along rivers in the Sudan zone as well). The fly-belts of this tsetse were estimated in 1963 to occupy 58 700 mile² (MacLennan 1963*a*). Two-thirds at least of the population potential of *G. morsitans* in Nigeria is suppressed by human activity. What are the origins of this activity? To answer this question one must look again at the earlier historical background.

The 'middle belt' of Nigeria is, in fact, only a section of a much greater *Grenzwildnis* that stretches across West Africa from the Cameroon to Senegal. To its north lie the populations whose forefathers dwelt in the successive empires of the Sudan. Ghana flourished from A.D. 800 to 1100. Mali or Melli, which absorbed Ghana after 1100, remained as a powerful empire until after 1400. One of its kings, whose reign heralded its decline, Mansa Mari Diata II, died of sleeping sickness in 1373 or 1374. The Songhay Empire, at the period of its greatest growth under Askia the Great (*c*. 1493–1528), stretched from its capital at Gao on the Niger westwards to the Gambia and eastwards as far as Agades and Kano. Further east still was the long-lived empire of Bornu, centred around Lake Chad. It came into history with a dynasty that began to reign in about A.D. 850 (Davidson 1965). When the Songhay Empire collapsed under a trans-Saharan attack from Morocco, it lost its hold on the Hausa peoples of Northern Nigeria who already possessed a long history and began to develop their cities as commercial centres of long-distance trade. It was these Hausa city states that were taken over and welded into the Fulani Empire by Usuman dan Fodio at the beginning of the nineteenth century. This empire was halted in its eastward expansion by Bornu.

There were two reasons for thus briefly condensing a millennium of history into a paragraph. One has been mentioned: the position of the Sudan empires in relation to the *G. morsitans* belts of the Guinea zones. The other was to lead up to the confrontation of Sokoto and Bornu across a *Grenzwildnis* that branches north from the middle belt between longitudes 10° and 12°E. Within these limits a dozen small emirates stretch along the western boundary of Bornu from Gumel and Hadejia in the north to form a chain that runs south-eastwards towards the Benue river. They are clearly shown in a map provided by Hogben and Kirke-Greene (1968). They are supported on their eastern flank by a large area of savanna woodland of the Sudan type, for the most part waterless. This is the 'Great Forest of Bornu', so named by Heinrich Barth who crossed it from Kano into Bornu in 1851 and came back by the same route five years later (Barth 1857).

The situation of the 'great forest' is shown by Stenning (1959) as a great rectangle bounded on the north by the Yobi river, draining eastwards into Lake Chad. In the south the 'great forest' reaches almost to the Gongola river, a large tributary of the Benue. It is almost 60 miles from west to east and 100 from north to south. It is crossed in a north-easterly direction by four tributaries of the Yobe, the Hadejia, Katagum, Jamaari, and Gana rivers.

The nature of the 'great forest' was quite clear to Barth. 'Predatory incursions are nothing new in these quarters, where several provinces and entirely distinct empires have a common frontier.' Between the rivers the 'great forest' is free of *Glossina* and Barth had nothing to say of tsetse. However, on one occasion he had passed through a village lying on a ridge between two water courses. 'Descending immediately from this considerable ridge, we entered a dale very thickly overgrown with trees, where I was greatly astonished to see a herd of cattle watered from the wells, while the river was close at hand; but on addressing the neat-herds, I was informed by them that the stagnant water of the Komadugu [*meaning river*] at this season is very unwholesome for cattle' (Barth 1857). Many years later Nash (1939) was to demonstrate, on the Katagum river, that in the hot season, when the rivers cease to flow, large numbers of puparia of *G. tachinoides* are to be found below the river banks around the residual pools. This tsetse and *G. morsitans* were recorded in the region in the first decade of this century.

Factors limiting expansion of *G. morsitans* fly-belts in Nigeria

In an arid climate where no rain falls at all during the five months November–March, and October and April each yield less than one inch of rain, intensive agriculture is only possible where use can be made of the wet-season floods for irrigation. In the 'great forest' area where circumstances were propitious dense populations had, from time to time, developed in the borderland emirates, but in places agriculture must have been difficult and not only *G. tachinoides* but also *G. morsitans* survived. Here, especially, Duggan (1962a) has suggested that sleeping sickness had a zoonotic origin, via *G. morsitans* directly to man. Whenever, in times of stress, villages were evacuated because of border warfare, the opportunities for spread of infection must have increased. The fly-belts of the 'great forest' of Bornu had to be eliminated by insecticides in a series of operations described by Davies (1964).

Further south the case is different. The *G. morsitans* fly-belts of the Northern Guinea and sub-Sudan Zones have expanded since 1950 for reasons that will be considered below, but which did not operate in the years that led up to the Nigerian sleeping sickness epidemic that reached its peak in 1935.

It has been suggested above that two-thirds of the potential *G. morsitans* population of Nigeria has been suppressed by human activity. This activity controls density of wildlife and hence of the tsetse that feed on it. 'Generally speaking *G. morsitans* occurs in areas with population densities ranging from 0 to 40 per square mile; occasional flies of this species are found in areas of 40–100, but never when the population exceeds 100, to the square mile' (Nash 1948a). In 1945 the *G. morsitans* belts were tentatively estimated to cover about 33 350 mile^2. The estimate of 58 700 in 1963 suggests an expansion of 25 000 mile^2 in 18 years. On the other hand it is quite certain that the Wukari fly-belt (see Map 21.1), that once covered an area of about 2000 mile^2 had disappeared by 1956. People moving into a new area have a direct and an indirect effect upon its wildlife populations. Animals are destroyed by hunting and some, under these pressures, move away to find new territory. Others disappear, or fail to reproduce themselves, because man destroys their habitat. Both of these effects were perhaps operative in 1966 in the Mando Road section of the largest Northern Guinea fly-belt some 30 miles west of Kaduna.

The biology of *G. morsitans* in this area had been studied by Jordan (1965b) for five years. Twice a month, throughout this period, tsetse were caught along a fly-round 1300 yd long, between the hours of 08.30 and 10.30. Two men caught and one recorded. In all they caught 7412 flies of which 15·2 per cent were females. This means that the average catch was approximately 52 males and 9 females. The maximum monthly means reached almost double this number of males in the late rains or early dry season in two years and fell to about 15 at the end of the dry season or beginning of the rains also in two years. These catches suggest a high absolute population density. Blood meal analysis showed that 51 per cent of feeds were taken from warthog and that man supplied 16 per cent. The fly-round ran along a path leading from a main road to a village 8 miles away. Man, therefore, was a relatively abundant potential host. The spoor of at least seventeen other potential host animals was observed with varying frequencies, and between them they contributed 16 per cent of blood meals.

Another 4·5 per cent came from birds, reptiles, and rodents, and the remainder from various unidentified sources. It is clear that warthogs were of overwhelming importance.

Jordan's work ended in April 1964. Just over two years later, in June 1966, I wished to collect large numbers of *G. morsitans* and went to the Mando Road area because Jordan's data suggested that they should be easily obtainable. Six visits, totalling some fifteen hours of observation along Jordan's fly-round and in its surroundings, yielded 29 flies, an average of about 2 per hour. Jordan's data enable his mean catching rate in June, over five years, to be calculated. It amounted to a mean of 29·5 flies per hour. It therefore appeared that in the two years' interval the density of *G. morsitans* had dropped by about 93 per cent. It was clear that this change was associated with human use of the area. Whereas in 1955–64 man had been a regular passenger through it, in 1966 he had become a settler. Adjoining the main road, opposite the beginning of the fly-round path a small hamlet had appeared, consisting of three or four family groups who had, between them, cleared and planted perhaps 20 acres of former woodland. This was not the only change. During five years of observation Jordan and his assistants had seen cattle spoor on 3 of the 120 occasions on which they visited the round. These were spoor of trade cattle being driven to the markets of the south. During the week of fruitless endeavour in 1966 cattle on at least three occasions had used the path and were moving northwards. They were therefore not trade cattle, but were herds returning to the northern home pastures at the end of a dry season spent in transhumance to the Southern Guinea zone. It was clear that the whole ecological pattern of the area had changed and that this change was reflected in the density of the *G. morsitans* population. One may guess that among these changes had been the killing off, or moving away, of two or three families of warthogs. It is the sort of situation that is fundamental in the problem of trypanosomiasis but is neglected because it demands the exploration of fields of knowledge not within the usual purviews of entomologists or parasitologists.

The Wukari fly-belt

It is possible to describe the disappearance of the Wukari fly-belt (shown in Map 21.1) in different terms. Its outline, as of others shown in Nash (1948a), was derived from specific catches made by different persons at different times and recorded on a large-scale map now in the Northern Nigerian headquarters of the Medical Service. The earliest records in the Wukari belt are from Pollard (1912). The most recent were inserted on the map after the publication of Nash's 1948 version in 1949 and 1950. According to Wilson (1958) the 2000 mile^2 Wukari fly-belt had disappeared by 1956.

There is no doubt as to the cause of this disappearance. It is entirely attributable to rapid growth of population of the Tiv people. The Tiv appear in earlier records under the name of Munshi (or variants thereof) and were present in the Benue valley in 1854 and were described, wrongly, as a group of people escaped from slavery. 'The Mitshi were originally a set of slaves who had rebelled and, settling in part of Akpoto, had greatly increased in numbers, had become independent, were spread over an extensive territory and were very troublesome neighbours. Their language was quite peculiar' (Baikie 1856). Almost uniquely in West Africa the Tiv, according to most authors, speak a Bantu language (Bohannan and Bohannan 1953).

At the time of Baikie's visit the Benue valley was suffering severely from the Fulani slave raiding that had escalated so much after the death of Sultan Bello. Baikie saw some of these people who operated on horseback.

Hearing that there were horses we asked to see them and were accordingly shown several fine Arabs, nicely groomed and cared for and in fine condition. . . . The possession of horses is one of the distinguishing marks of the Pulo [*Fulani*] tribes, one, too, which adds greatly to their power and the terror of their name. . . . Annual excursions for the purpose of collecting slaves are made from their towns, chiefly against the Mitshis, which may account for the suspicions they entertained of us, especially as many of the Pulo people are light coloured (Baikie 1856).

An earlier expedition to the Benue in 1841 noted 'A very small portion of its course only is known, and that has been almost depopulated by the frequent slave catching expeditions' (Allen and Thomson 1848).

Three points are to be observed: (1) the Tiv were already established in the Benue valley and had been multiplying; (2) in the middle of the nineteenth century they were harassed, along with other tribes, by slave raiders from the north; and (3) the latter were using horses, some of which, at any rate, were in good condition. These observations suggest that at the time of maximum slave raiding into the Benue valley, *G. morsitans* must have been confined to relatively small foci and that the growth of the fly-belts followed upon depopulation.

The Tiv country was not taken over by the Nigerian administration until 1909. Their expansion had been resumed and was the cause of boundary conflicts. Up to 1925, along some sections of their periphery, it was taking place at a rate of 3–4 miles a year. It was halted in the south where administrative action prevented incursion on the Southern region of Nigeria. One response to this was a reduction in area of cultivation per family which was offset by shortening the period of fallow. 'The Europeans have spoiled the land' they said, but against this, in areas where administrative divisions did not prevent expansion, European law enabled them to move without conflict and without the necessity of maintaining kinship links when moving into lands 'not their own' because they no longer feared marauders or slavers (Bohannan 1954b).

The present condition and known history of the Tiv has been described in various works by P. and L. Bohannan (Bohannan 1954*a*, *b*, Bohannan and Bohannan 1953). The Tiv are subsistence farmers living chiefly on yams (*Dioscorea* spp.), millet (*Pennisetum* spp.), and Guinea corn (*Sorghum* spp.). Their country can be described, in an older terminology, as cultivation steppe. It is treeless cultivation and fallow, except around the houses of family groups, where mango trees provide fruit and shade.

The southern marches of Tiv country form the boundary between what are today the Northern and Eastern Provinces of Nigeria. In some places this boundary can actually be seen: the fertile soil of Ugi and Udam country, in the south, supports a dense bush vegetation of high grass and small trees between the larger trees. But on the Tiv side, the grass is short and all the smaller trees have been cut down to make room for the fields in which a population which rises to a density of over 550 per square mile struggles for food against constantly deteriorating soil, due in large part to over-cultivation and insufficient periods of fallow (Bohannan 1954*a*).

The rainfall, at 50–65 in per annum, makes the Tiv country, which is also varied by granite inselbergs, look rather like a wet Sukumaland (Chapter 11). There were some 800 000 Tiv in 1954. Their expansion was 'one of the most notable features of Tiv society' (Bohannan 1954*a*). Like the Sukuma the Tiv have eliminated a very large infestation of *G. morsitans* during the last 20–30 years. This expansion has been discussed by Bohannan (1954*b*) who remarks that one of its most puzzling aspects is that it is most rapid in those areas in which land shortage is least severe and he used the useful phrase 'centrifugal expansion' to describe it.

The first epidemiological description of the Tiv country comes from Pollard (1912). He found *G. palpalis* and *G. tachinoides* on the rivers and *G. morsitans* in the hinterland where the town of Wukari formed 'an island of fly-free land in a sea of tsetse'. A well-remembered epidemic of sleeping sickness had happened some twenty years before his visit, that is in about 1891, that fatal year. The victims were not Tiv but Jukun living in villages along the Benue. In 1911 case incidence in these settlements indicated an endemic condition of chronic trypanosomiasis. The tsetse most evident along the Benue was *G. tachinoides* which, in spite of much clearing, continued to be found in bungalows and offices. Imported Fulani cattle all died and no horses could live. Small black cattle belonging to the Tiv were 'apparently immune to tsetse'. 'The Munshi are great hunters and have practically destroyed all the wild game in their district, and yet, in spite of this, the trypanosomiasis of cattle and horses is rampant' (Pollard 1912).

Although it may not have been until 1941 that the expansion of the Tiv population began to emerge as an administrative problem, it is clear from the above account that their activities which were to lead to the eventual elimination of the Wukari fly-belt were already in operation. The wild hosts of *G. morsitans* were being killed off in 1911. Early observers of *G. mor-sitans* thought of the insect as being dependent on game; that is, animals that one killed for sport. In this case they had in mind antelopes and buffaloes. Warthog and bushpig hardly fell into the same category so that although Pollard remarked that the wild game was practically all destroyed in 1911, a wide margin of error must be allowed for the wild pigs and the bushbuck. The black dwarf or Muturu cattle might also provide acceptable food for *Glossina* for long after the more spectacular wildlife had become very shy and scarce. In fact the wildlife had not been destroyed. Lester (1930) found that 10·4 per cent of the dwarf cattle and 12·8 per cent of the wild game were infected with *T. brucei*. His diagnostic methods were of doubtful value, but the important point is that wild animals still existed. In

TABLE 22.1

Growth rate of population of Tiv division compared with neighbouring areas†

Division	Populations		% increase	Annual growth %
	1952	1963		
Shendam . .	194 194	359 193	85·0	5·4
Lafia . . .	131 556	289 659	120·2	7·0
Wukari . . .	136 673	285 646	109·0	6·5
Tiv . . .	718 619	1 244 185	73·1	4·8
	1952	1962 projection		
Shendam . .	194 194	259 596	33·7	3·0
Lafia . . .	131 556	198 822	51·1	4·1
Wukari . . .	123 876	189 654	53·1	4·2
Tiv . . .	718 619	869 871	21·0	1·8

† After Okonjo (1968).

the end, however, not only were the wild hosts of *G. morsitans* destroyed but the bush also disappeared from the heart of the Tiv country.

The process of centrifugal expansion began when the heart of Tiv had been turned into 'cultivation steppe'. This is precisely the condition de-scribed in Sukumaland in Chapter 13. The centre of that country main-tained a steady density of human population throughout the period for which figures are available. Population fluctuation took place on the peri-phery.

According to Bohannan and Bohannan (1953) the main expansion areas of the Tiv are northward into the Lafia and Shendam (or Lowland) divi-sions and westwards into Wukari. Okonjo's (1968) data for these areas are compared, in Table 22.1, with those for Tiv division. Whichever of the two sets of data are chosen it appears that the fully populated Tiv division is now growing slowly in density compared with the peripheral areas. Tiv division, therefore, and its neighbours is exactly paralleled by Kwimba and the peripheral districts of Sukumaland. 'Centrifugal expansion' is not puzzling, as Bohannan and Bohannan (1953) thought. It is the inevitable result of population growth in an environment not fully occupied.

During a visit in 1963 one learned that up to 1952 the only cattle in the Tiv country were the dwarf black Muturu. In 1962 there were 13 061 of these in Tiv itself, plus 4883 northern zebus. In Lafia there were 13 217 of the latter, while Wukari division had 9779. This rapid growth of the zebu population had been to some degree assisted by drug treatments, but the latter were not administered frequently and the main effect was due to reduction in the population of *G. morsitans*. It is dangerous to generalize. At Gboko, some 60 miles south-west of Wukari, Fulani cattle did not penetrate until the Sleeping Sickness Service had eliminated riverine infestations of *G. palpalis* and *G. tachinoides*. Here, perhaps, was a parallel to the Zonkwa situation to be described in Chapter 23.

Factors leading to expansion of the *G. morsitans* belts in Nigeria

The reduction of tsetse density following the establishment of a small agricultural community near the Mando Road fly-round, and the elimination of a whole fly-belt by the expansion of the Tiv population are examples that illustrate the operation of competition for habitat in which man-dominated ecosystems overcome, at least temporarily, those dominated by wildlife. However, a review of the literature and an examination of available maps shows that the rate of recession of the *G. morsitans* belts has by no means exceeded or even equalled the rate at which they have expanded during the last half-century. The evidence also points to a marked acceleration in their growth rate since about 1950. To a considerable extent this has been offset by the work of control services, but important as that work may be, it is with the factors affecting natural control of *G. morsitans* that this account is concerned.

1900–50

It is assumed that the rinderpest panzootic in the last decade of the nineteenth century and the subsequent periodical epizootics up to about 1930 reduced the populations of host animals of the *morsitans* group tsetses in the same way as it did in the savanna ecosystems on the eastern side of the continent and with the same effects on the fly-belts. In regard to the human population the views of Kuczynski may be accepted, namely that in the first two decades of the century the Nigerian population did not increase significantly and for the second two decades the increase, if any, was slow. The Nigerian population 'may have increased between 1926 and 1940 by something like 10 per cent, but one cannot rule out the possibility that it did not increase at all' (Kuczynski 1948). The official figures support this conclusion: 1921, 18 624 690; 1931, 19 922 729; and 1941, 21 040 566.

Growth of the human population, therefore, cannot seriously have impeded the recovery of the *Glossina* hosts after the rinderpest. At the same time the cattle population was overcoming, in part naturally but largely assisted by veterinary inoculation campaigns, the effects of the same disease. In these circumstances of slow recovery of the cattle population and slow growth of the *G. morsitans* belts, cattle trypanosomiasis might be expected also to grow slowly in importance as a veterinary problem. It is necessary, however, to remember that the *palpalis* group tsetses which could maintain themselves on a reptile, human, and domestic animal diet presumably were not seriously affected by rinderpest save locally where cattle provided the greater part of their blood meals. They may also have been affected by localized depopulations during the second half of the nineteenth century in places where men and women provided their basic diet. It is certain, however, that *G. palpalis* and *G. tachinoides* were not eliminated from large areas as was *G. morsitans* in Rhodesia and, as we have assumed, in Nigeria. The recovering cattle populations were always, to some degree, subject to infection from riverine tsetse, although the rate of inoculation of infective trypanosomes per fly-bite was much lower than that associated with the *morsitans* group tsetses (cf. Tables 21.1 and 21.2). This continued subjection to a low trypanosome risk from *G. palpalis* and *G. tachinoides* has conferred great advantages upon West African cattle not enjoyed by their eastern African relatives.

Trypanosomiasis in cattle received little attention from government veterinary surgeons in the first quarter of the century. They were more concerned with the disease in horses,† while in cattle rinderpest claimed most of their attention. In 1924, however, cattle trypanosomiasis was said to be increasing. 'In the absence of systematic investigation by means of an adequate field staff it is impossible to estimate the prevalence of the disease or the annual losses caused by it, but it is certainly on the increase and will be a serious drawback to cattle raising in the future. . . . Trypanosomiasis is slowly but surely spreading northwards up the river systems' (Nigeria Veterinary Service 1925). Three years later a net decrease in the cattle census of 186 276 head was attributed to rinderpest. It was very difficult to estimate the numbers that died of trypanosomiasis. 'There is no doubt, however, that this disease is responsible for a mortality only second in severity to rinderpest, but that owing to its insidious and chronic nature, its ravages are not so apparent. It is frequently made apparent by rinderpest inoculations' (Nigeria Veterinary Service 1928). The same report recorded

† Because government officials used horses for transport and drew an allowance for their upkeep. Horse-racing and polo became favourite sports for officials in Northern Nigeria.

that animals born and reared in tsetse areas acquire a tolerance or resistance to infection. Trypanosomiasis came more into prominence in 1930, in which year curative treatments by intravenous injection of tartar emetic were made available to stock owners. Diagnosis also became easier, for it was recognized that the habit of earth-eating, known to local people as *modu*, was due to trypanosome infection. In 1931 nearly 9000 tartar emetic treatments were administered and the number had risen to almost 29 000 in 1947 (Glover 1965, Nigeria Veterinary Service).

The *Nigerian veterinary reports* repeated themselves on the seriousness and widespread distribution of cattle trypanosomiasis with monotonous regularity until 1939, when it was noted that from all provinces the incidence of the disease was on the increase. Many more cases were being reported but it was thought that 'this may be the result of closer contact between the Veterinary Staff and the Fulani who are gaining confidence in our methods of treatment' (Nigeria Veterinary Service 1940). In 1942 'disturbing reports about the increased incidence of trypanosomiasis in cattle have come from nearly every province' in Northern Nigeria (Nigeria Veterinary Service 1945). The explanation offered was that there had been a rapid increase in the area of land under cultivation which restricted pasture and so, especially at the end of the dry seasons, obliged the Fulani, in search of food and water for their herds, to enter tsetse areas that previously had been avoidable. Curiously there was no suggestion that the cattle population had increased, although by this time massive annual immunization programmes had put an end to periodically disruptive epizootics of rinderpest.

Part of the difficulty in assessing progress came from the use of the *jangali* or cattle tax count as a measure of the stock population. These figures, from 1930 to 1958, have been collated by Glover (1965). Up to 1941 they fluctuated around 2 750 000. No records were published from 1942 to 1947 inclusive, but in 1948 the *jangali* count was just over 4 million and it remained at about this level until after 1960.

It was customary for officials to assert that these figures represented about half the true total of cattle. The arguments have been set out by Shaw and Colville (1950) who showed that although the tax count for 1947 was somewhat under 4 million, a total export of 700 000 hides in that year could only be explained if the true cattle population was in the neighbourhood of 7–8 million. Shaw and Colville (1950) believed that the increase of about 1 250 000 in the *jangali* figures between 1942 and 1947 was attributable to more efficient tax assessment. It is difficult, however, to believe that the success achieved by the Nigerian Veterinary Service in its immunization campaigns against rinderpest, which by 1930 had eliminated the enormous mortalities of earlier years, could have had no effect upon cattle population growth. Moreover, this was not its only achievement and control had become increasingly efficient over other epizootic

diseases such as anthrax, blackquarter, and contagious bovine pleuropneumonia.

The widespread trypanosomiasis that attracted veterinary attention in
1939 and 1942 was the manifestation of the meeting, over wide fronts, of the
expanding *G. morsitans* fly-belts and of the growing cattle population. It
had probably already been in progress for some years. The numbers of
treatments with tartar emetic from 1930 to 1950 are shown in Fig. 22.1.
The rapid rise to 1933 suggests that the Fulani were not slow to appreciate
their value, but thereafter there is a fall in numbers treated until 1937 and
then a very marked increase in 1938 and 1939. Many possible explanations
might be adduced for the decline in treatments between 1933 and 1937.

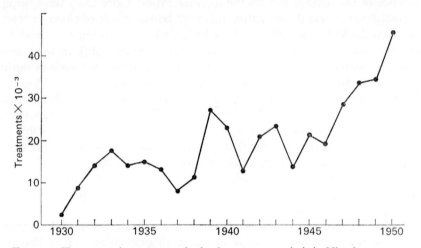

FIG. 22.1. Tartar emetic treatments for bovine trypanosomiasis in Nigeria, 1930–50.

All that need be done here is to note that this was the period of maximum
incidence of human trypanosomiasis (see Chapter 23).

During the 1940s various phenanthridinium compounds were tried out
experimentally, but tartar emetic remained the drug of choice in the field.
In 1950 over 45 000 treatments were given, no mean achievement when one
treatment involved four to six intravenous injections each requiring the
patient to be thrown and tied. In 1945 the Director of Veterinary Services
had noted the widespread distribution of *G. tachinoides* and *G. palpalis* but
added that, 'Fortunately *Glossina morsitans* is not so commonly encountered as the other two species' (Nigeria Veterinary Service 1947).

The first comprehensive map of *G. morsitans* distribution in Nigeria was
published by Nash (1948a) and represented the condition as known in
1945. Two earlier maps, by Simpson (1912) and Johnson and Lloyd (1923),
are very valuable but obviously incomplete. Up to 1950 only two instances
of the spread or 'advance' of *G. morsitans* had been described. The first was
observed by Nash whose map shows six comparatively small fly-belts

within the area now occupied by the single great central fly-belt which stretches from longitude 5° 45′ to 10° 30′E. and almost engulfs the two large towns of Zaria and Kaduna (Map 21.1). Two of these smaller belts Nash described as follows:

Since 1933 I have known of a G. *morsitans* belt on the Kaduna–Jos road which extends for eight miles through an uninhabited stretch of *Isoberlinia doka* woodland, but ends when cultivation starts. In 1944 I discovered G. *morsitans* 32 miles further down the road at Pambeguwa Rest House, where I had never seen them before. It seems likely that cars may have carried this species from the old belt to Pambeguwa, where people often spend the night. A recent fly survey has shown no trace of this species for thirty miles between the two belts (Nash 1948a).

The increasing use of motor transport was certainly a factor assisting the spread of tsetse, but it must be remembered always that tsetse, however introduced into a new area, can only survive if suitable host animals are already there. Johnson and Lloyd (1923) recorded G. *morsitans* just west of Kaduna, but none east of that town, perhaps because the area was still unexplored.

Wilson (1958) described another 'advance' of G. *morsitans* which took place in the Song area of Adamawa province, near the eastern border of Nigeria, between 1940 and 1955. This fly-belt had been extant in 1922 as shown by a single record on the map of Johnson and Lloyd (1923). The Song area covers about 2500 mile² and is drained by the Kilangi river, a tributary of the Benue. Except around the main villages the area is hilly and relatively unfertile. Most of the rivers dry up in March and April. Ecologically the Kilangi basin lies for the most part in a salient of the Northern Guinea zone from across the Cameroon border. Around this salient the vegetation is of the sub-Sudan type.

Local evidence suggested that in 1940 the boundary of the Kilangi fly-belt included an area of 910 mile². In the next ten years this expanded by 333 mile² and finally, between 1950 and 1955, by another 906 mile². Two villages engulfed by this spread together possessed 3014, 1344, and 572 head of cattle in the periods respectively 1940–4, 1945–9, and 1950–5. Wilson adds that 'Human population figures show a very similar downward trend.'

The causes of the spread of tsetse were evacuation of the area by the human population

due both to the high incidence of human diseases such as onchocerciasis and sleeping sickness and to shifting cultivation on this relatively infertile soil which necessitated long periods of fallow. The incidence of onchocerciasis is high especially along the Loko River where 24% of all persons over thirty years were afflicted with blindness in some form and many villages are now completely evacuated. Also in the absence of tribal war, the local pagan cultivators who are responsible for most of the bush destruction are tending to move away from the hills to the more fertile riverine plains near the Benue (Wilson 1958).

In 1955 it was noted that 'game had greatly decreased throughout the area and chiefly consisted of warthogs and baboons and small numbers of bushbuck, duiker and oribi'.

After 1950

Up to about 1940 government veterinarians were not seriously worried about *G. morsitans*, probably because its fly-belts were very much smaller than they became after 1950. In 1949 Curd and Davey (1949) announced their discovery of antrycide, the first of a series of efficient drugs, some of them, like antrycide itself, possessing marked prophylactic properties. In Nigeria, as elsewhere in Africa, possession of these drugs encouraged the veterinary services to take a greater part than hitherto in the control of cattle trypanosomiasis. A Veterinary Tsetse Control Unit was established in 1954. Its findings in the first four years of its existence are described by Wilson (1958) and MacLennan (1958). The former drew attention to excessive demands by Fulani cattle owners for treatment of their herds by modern drugs, 'during the past five years', that is since 1953. From this time onwards the tartar emetic treatment was no longer used and a number of other drugs appeared in fairly quick succession. The numbers of treatments rose from 45 000 in 1950 to about 750 000 in 1957 (Fig. 22.2).

The greater demand for treatment had two sources. Compared with tartar emetic the new drugs were easy to use and involved the stock owners in far less trouble, and they were obviously effective. Secondly, spread of *G. morsitans*, especially in the Northern Guinea and Sudan zones, was accelerating. In particular the union of the small fly-belts to form the great central belt and, after this union, the further expansion of the whole belt continued at a faster rate than could be dealt with by the newly formed Veterinary Tsetse Section.

One 'advance' that attracted particular attention was in the Anchau area, some 30 miles east of Zaria. Anchau had been under observation by the Sleeping Sickness Service since 1934 and became the site for a large rural development and settlement scheme for the control of human trypanosomiasis. *G. tachinoides* and *G. palpalis* were eliminated and *G. morsitans* was absent, the nearest belts lying some 50 miles to the south, east and west of Kaduna (Nash 1948a, b). In 1950 it had become clear that the spread to Pambeguwa that Nash had first seen in 1944, and had attributed to carriage of tsetse by motor traffic, was increasing, and that his focus was the northern extremity of an eastward extension of the fly-belts which had existed for many years in the neighbourhood of Kaduna. Nash's original observation indicated that it had begun before 1944. A description of the subsequent spread is given by Wilson (1958) who showed

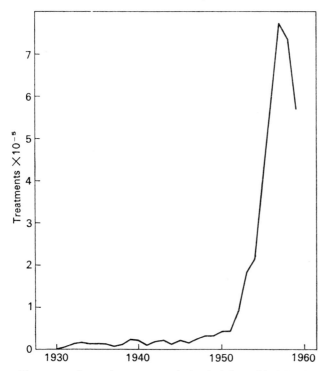

FIG. 22.2. Treatments for cattle trypanosomiasis administered in Nigeria, 1930–59.

that it cut across a number of routes used by Fulani cattle during the annual dry-season transhumance to the southern pastures. From 1950 onwards *G. morsitans* spread along the cattle routes, particularly in a northerly direction from the neighbourhood of Pambeguwa. This spread was recorded by successive surveys and regular patrols were used to measure changes in apparent density. On the Malamawa–Katini cattle route, apparent density of *G. morsitans* multiplied 24-fold between June 1955 and June 1957. Wilson's account suggests that the eastward spread of *G. morsitans* had moved relatively slowly until about 1950, after which it spread very rapidly, especially along routes on which passing herds of cattle provided a constant food supply (Map 22.1).

Another spread of *G. morsitans* observed closely by veterinarians took place near the government stock farm at Shika, 10 miles west of Zaria. Again the rate of spread seems to have accelerated greatly after 1950. In the previous decade country was being occupied by *G. morsitans* at a rate of about 110 mile² per year. From 1950 to 1957 the rate had more than doubled to about 240 mile² annually.

Wilson's last example was taken from the Kontagora fly-belt. This fly-belt is said to have come into existence as a result of the activities of the

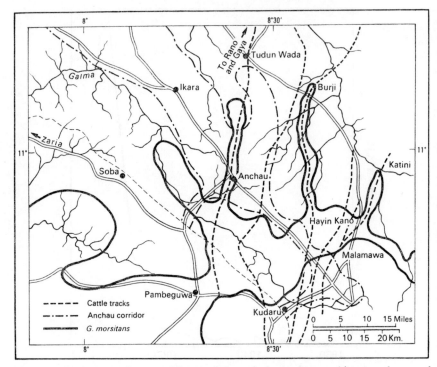

MAP 22.1. Cattle routes (compare Map 23.4) through the Anchau corridor area, the spread of *G. morsitans* (1944–56), and residual foci of infection. Cattle routes and spread of tsetse from Wilson (1958) (see page 433).

last independent Emir of Kontagora, who is reputed to have replied to Lugard's message ordering him to cease raiding for slaves, 'Can a cat cease from mousing? When I die I shall have a slave between my teeth.' A recent history (Hogben and Kirke-Green 1966) appends a footnote suggesting that the Emir's reputation may be undeserved.

The northern boundary of the Kontagora fly-belt was surveyed in July and August 1946 by an entomological team belonging to the Medical Department and in February 1947 by another team sent by the Veterinary Department. They agreed in their assessment of the position. In 1948 plans were made for a settlement scheme immediately north of the *G. morsitans* infested area. Again the two teams surveyed the area. *G. palpalis* and *G. tachinoides* were both found (as on the earlier occasions) along the rivers, but there was no *G. morsitans* north of its previously defined boundary.

Occupation began in 1949 and in order that settlers could keep cattle in good health the riverine vegetation was cleared and the area rendered almost free of *G. palpalis* and *G. tachinoides*. Some infections among the first cattle to be introduced in 1949 were not unexpected, as the riverine tsetse were not yet eliminated. Cattle continued to be brought into the area, but infection incidence, instead of declining with the continuing reduction of the *G. palpalis* and *G. tachinoides* populations, increased. In 1949 6·5 per cent of the introduced cattle died of trypanosomiasis. In 1951 deaths amounted to 13·8 per cent of a much greater population of cattle. The increasing mortality suggested that *G. morsitans* was invading the area and in 1952 this was confirmed and it became obvious that the whole *G. morsitans* front had moved northward to the edge of the settlement. Cattle continued to be brought in but were now placed on a regime of prophylactic injections every two or three months. By 1954 the tsetse had penetrated the settlement area and in 1956 it was found that cattle were infected with a strain of *Trypanosoma congolense* no longer sensitive to the drug. The scheme was closed down in 1957 and the cattle sold for slaughter.

The interest of the Kontagora failure lies in the evidence that *G. morsitans* moved into an area at the same time as a human community. It will have been observed in various earlier chapters that an increase in human population is normally followed by a decrease in the density of adjacent *G. morsitans*. At Kontagora both increased together in the same area. Wilson (1958) discussed the spread of this tsetse in Nigeria at some length and remarked that, 'The factors which influenced the advance of *G. morsitans submorsitans* into the Kontagora settlement area from 1951 onwards would, if properly understood, yield valuable information on the behaviour of this tsetse.' Ten years later the explanation seems much more clear.

The change in the rate of expansion of the *G. morsitans* fly-belts between 1945 and 1955

The restoration of equilibrium between the wildlife ecosystems and the man–cattle–cultivation ecosystems had been in progress in the Guinea and Sudan zones, as elsewhere in Africa, since the beginning of the century. The great cattle epizootics were subsiding and the human infections became gradually less disruptive. There had been a widespread epidemic of cerebro-spinal meningitis in 1905 and of smallpox in 1906. The 1918–19 influenza was almost the last; only human trypanosomiasis remained and this, in due course, took its toll and the resulting depopulations assisted the spread of the large wild mammals and their attendant parasites. In general, however, the recovery was slow and gradual. There was no indication from veterinary sources of any major spread of trypanosomiasis such as must have become evident if any rapid and large-scale spread of *G. morsitans* had taken place.

A dependent limiting factor in constant operation was human predation of game animals. Local hunters, using home-made weapons called 'Dane guns', operated mainly at night with the aid of acetylene-burning lanterns. During the war years gunpowder and carbide were scarce and hunting pressure on wildlife was much reduced. The immediate response of the wild mammal population in Rhodesia to temporary cessation of hunting has been remarked in Chapter 18, and Nash (1968) believes that the relaxation of hunting may have been a major contributory cause of acceleration of rate of spread of *G. morsitans* in Nigeria.

After the war this form of hunting might have been expected to stabilize the position once more; but new factors now emerged to accompany the constitution-making through which the administration hoped to guide the movement towards independence. There was a great increase of expenditure on roads. Large-scale commercial hunting began. Ibo merchants went out in motor lorries to buy 'bush-beef' for export to the meat-hungry areas of the south. This commercialization of hunting, by non-Muslims to whom the Suidae were acceptable, should in due course have led to further retreats of tsetse and, indeed, it was encouraged by the control services (e.g. see Davies 1964.)

'The 1940s were a period of peace for fly and game and the 1950s a period of biological chaos' (Nash 1968). From the viewpoint of control of the *G. morsitans* population the principal contribution to this chaos was made by the introduction of the new drugs for cattle. The protection given by antrycide, and later by homidium, enabled cattle to remain in areas from which, before 1950, they would have been forced to retreat. One effect of the injections, quickly noticed by pastoralists all over Africa, was the marked reduction in the number of abortions from cows that otherwise displayed little indication of trypanosome infection. In the space of a few years a vast new supply of blood in highly acceptable host animals was made available. The best estimate available, though with an admitted wide margin of error, for the cattle population of 1953 was 4 830 000 (International Bank 1955). Ten years later the best available estimate was in the neighbourhood of 10 million (Oyenuga 1967).

Wilson (1958) discussed a number of possible causes for the spread of *G. morsitans* that accompanied the settlement scheme west of Kontagora. Up to 1949 the activities of the peoples of that emirate must certainly have kept the wild hosts of this tsetse at a distance. The introduction of cattle in large numbers was all that was needed to offset their absence.

The Kontagora scheme was closed down principally because of the appearance of trypanosome strains insensitive to antrycide. Drug-resistance was regarded as highly dangerous, as it was supposed that the insensitive strains might spread and render the drugs useless. The importance of this problem is still not defined. At Kontagora continuation of the scheme and intensification of cultivation leading to complete elimination of woodland might have led in time to the disappearance, once more, of tsetse.

Since that time a number of examples of recent spread of *G. morsitans* associated with presence of cattle have been described. The eastward extension of the central Zaria–Kaduna fly-belt has been attributed to this factor by Tarry (1967) who observed that it had been expanding at a rate of 10 miles per year in several places. He worked near the Bunga river, which is the headwater portion of the Jamaari and runs into Lake Chad. The area had been a pasture for many years but in 1959 was invaded by *G. morsitans* from what was then the eastern extremity of the central fly-belt. Within a year riverine habitats, previously supporting only *G. tachinoides*, were found to be generally occupied by *G. morsitans*. Tsetse patrols in the Gau river basin showed, as on at least four occasions during earlier work in the vicinity, that extension of the fly-belt was preceded by the sudden appearance and build-up of numbers of *G. morsitans* on cattle migration routes outside their former area of distribution, especially where these routes ran along drainage lines (Tarry 1967). The case seems to be precisely matched by the spread of the same fly-belt in the Anchau area, 70 miles to the west, described some ten years earlier by Wilson (1958).

It is difficult to devise experiments to test hypotheses when of necessity they must be conducted in very large areas of land and take many years to produce a result. As has so often been the case, one has to look for and assess by hindsight the results of 'experiments' devised and implemented with quite different objectives. The end result of one of these has quite recently been announced by Baldry (1969).

The first relevant observations were made well over fifty years ago in the province of Ilorin which lies south of the River Niger. The town of that name is situated approximately upon the junction of the forest–savanna mosaic and the Southern Guinea zone. Fifty miles north of Ilorin a road and rail bridge crosses the Niger at Jebba. Macfie (1913a) carried out a survey of tsetse distribution and trypanosomiasis incidence in the Ilorin province. Fulani cattle were only found in the western half, which is traversed by the Jebba–Ilorin road. These cattle were in good health in spite of the presence of *G. palpalis* and *G. tachinoides* on most of the rivers. In the less densely populated eastern half of the district *G. morsitans* and *G. longipalpis* were found, and here the only cattle seen were small numbers of the dwarf Muturu.

In addition to the cattle living in the district, a supplement to the diet of *Glossina* is provided by the daily passage of herds of slaughter cattle trekking, via the Jebba bridge, to the markets of the south. In 1912 this movement ceased during the rains, but 'During the dry season, herds of cattle pass, day after day, in an almost continuous stream, along the high roads on their way to Lagos from the north. How many die on the journey no one can tell, for the fate of those that sicken is to be butchered on the way, and it is a common experience to come across a carcass hewn up and laid out for sale by the road side' (Macfie 1913a).

In Chapter 5 the succession of infections that appeared in these cattle after their passage through the *G. morsitans* fly-belts of the Guinea zone was described from two surveys, by Unsworth and Birkett (1952) and

Godfrey, Killick-Kendrick, and Ferguson (1965). Associated with the second survey was an entomological investigation by Jordan (1965c) who found G. *morsitans* distributed down the cattle route from Jebba almost to Ilorin. Early in 1967 tsetse of the same species were found at Oyo, 68 miles south-west of Ilorin and also, of course, on the trade cattle route. Baldry (1969), in discussing this discovery, suggests that the presence of G. *morsitans* at Oyo has resulted from a steady population advance over the last fifty years. A study of various maps shows that whatever may have been the actual successive limits of a number of G. *morsitans* fly-belts in the Niger Valley over the half-century since Macfie (1913a) failed to find this tsetse on the Jebba–Ilorin road, the story is a complex one. For the purposes of this account what is certain is that G. *morsitans* along the cattle track from Jebba to Oyo owes its existence to the continuous passage of trade cattle. As G. *morsitans* must feed roughly once every three days if it is to maintain its population, the crucial events which allowed the spread to take place was the improvement in communications, especially the bridging of rivers other than the Niger, allowing the road to remain open throughout the year. A second event was the introduction of efficient drugs and the consequent rapid increase of the cattle population. The spread of G. *morsitans* down this route gives further evidence in support of the argument developed from Wilson's study of the Kontagora spread in 1950–4, of the same author's account of the Anchau advance, and finally Tarry's conclusions about the eastward movement of G. *morsitans* to the headwaters of the Bunga river, that the primary cause of the very rapid general spread of this tsetse since 1950 has been the great increase in available blood due to growth of the cattle population greatly accelerated by the widespread use of drugs giving temporary protection against infection. But it is only temporary. Where the spread of tsetse through the agency of cattle brings the flies into areas in which natural hosts still survive, the use of drugs rapidly becomes uneconomic. The cattle and their owners depart and the wildlife ecosystems take over again. On the Oyo road, however, an interruption of cattle movement for, say, one month should eliminate G. *morsitans*.

23

FOCI OF INFECTION OF
HUMAN TRYPANOSOMIASIS IN NIGERIA

THE publication of another in a long and distinguished series of progress reports on the control of sleeping sickness in Nigeria (Thomson 1969) serves very well to introduce this and the next chapter. It focuses attention on the geography of persistent infection and raises more doubts about classical theories of the origins of epidemics. It draws attention to the recent apparent complete elimination of the infection from the Ndzorov clan of Tiv people by the use of pentamidine prophylaxis. There is still, in some hamlets, particularly close man–fly contact. The conclusion, surely a correct one, is drawn that it is extremely unlikely that in this area there is any important animal reservoir of *Trypanosoma brucei gambiense*. If there were an animal reservoir, either wild or domestic, such as the infected cattle described by Onyango, van Hoeve, and de Raadt (1966) in Alego (p. 278) then the withdrawal of prophylactic treatment of the people after three years (1956–8 inclusive) should have been the signal for reappearance of the disease. The whole programme of control of sleeping sickness in Nigeria, in the Congo basin, in West Africa generally, indeed wherever the disease has been obviously associated in its distribution with the presence of *palpalis*-group tsetses, has been based upon the hypothesis that man is the reservoir of the infective trypanosome; that the tsetse obtains its own infection from man which, when it has matured, it passes on to other people. The evidence for this appeared to be overwhelming, so much so that tsetse of the *morsitans* group have been almost completely ignored by medical entomologists while epidemiological relationships between the riverine tsetse and man have been very precisely observed. The classical account comes from Nash, whose work (Nash and Page 1953) on the climatic basis of *G. palpalis* concentration has been described briefly on p. 381.

Sambo is situated above a small stream which dries up after the rains. Exhaustive search along the stream bed for some miles on either side of the village failed to reveal the presence of a *single* tsetse or of any pools of water, but immediately below the hamlet there was a spot in the stream-bed where the sand was moist and where the villagers had scooped out a two-feet deep hole from which they obtained their meagre water supply. At this spot four *Glossina palpalis* were caught. The closeness of the man–fly contact presented ideal conditions for the spread of the disease. Each woman had to take her turn at sitting by the hole with a curved section of calabash with which she would scoop up a cupful of water and transfer it to the water pot. A pause would then be necessary to allow more water to seep into the hole. It took each woman about 15 minutes to fill her water pot. Thus for many hours each day this small tsetse population of probably less than a dozen flies could feed on the queue of women, without expending any energy in the search for food.

The case described is considered to afford a classical example of close man–fly contact. Annually, at the end of the dry season, man is forced to depend upon this one spot for his water supply. Annually the severity of the dry season climate compels the tsetse to evacuate the other parts of the stream as the pools dry up, and to concentrate at the village water hole where the damp sand produces conditions of lower temperature and higher humidity and where the presence of the water hole assures a steady food supply within the microclimate area.

In the writer's experience this is by no means an isolated case, but represents conditions commonly found in large areas of Northern Nigeria (Nash 1944).

Sambo was a hamlet with 43 inhabitants situated in the Zaria emirate; 70 per cent of these people were infected.

To variations upon this theme may be attributed most of the epidemics that have afflicted Nigeria in the last forty years. Nobody questions this, and all control schemes, without exception, have been based upon repeated observations that West African sleeping sickness is a disease transmitted by *Glossina* of the *palpalis* group. In these chapters, however, the argument will be developed in favour of a wild animal reservoir as the essential factor in maintaining the endemic state that has persisted in West Africa and the Congo basin over many centuries and perhaps two or three millennia.

The hypothesis is put forward that *brucei*-group trypanosomes, which include strains infective to man, are transmitted to his domestic animals by species of *Glossina* that readily bite wild and domestic Bovidae, but rarely man; and that from domestic animals they are transmitted to man by *palpalis*-group vectors that seldom feed on wild animals but avidly attack man and domestic livestock.

Strains of trypanosomes behaving in every way like the classical *Trypanosoma 'rhodesiense'* of eastern African have been isolated on various occasions in Nigeria, but to those who were concerned in controlling the epidemic that reached its peak in 1935 it was 'impossible to believe that more virulent strains are being derived directly from game' (Nigeria medical report 1938). Lester, who built up the Nigerian Sleeping Sickness Service, described a number of *rhodesiense* type strains collected from patients mostly, but not all, from the Chad basin (Lester 1933). He believed that '*Trypanosoma rhodesiense* is only a virulent type of *T. gambiense*' and that 'This more virulent type usually arises from the normal human trypanosome through idiosyncrasies in the human host' (Nigeria medical report 1934).

The suggestion that human trypanosomiasis, at least in the Chad basin, may originate as a zoonosis is due to Duggan (1962a) who, however, did not commit himself to this opinion and offered in addition an alternative theory to explain the epidemiological peculiarities of that region. Duggan's paper provides the foundation for much of the following account of Nigerian sleeping sickness.

Some few items of evidence about the presence of the disease in West Africa in ancient times have already been mentioned (Chapters 4 and 21). A review of this evidence suggested that 'Before 1900, the West African situation was fairly static; many endemic foci were present, but epidemics were unusual. . . . Major advances of the disease were probably rare, even on a tribal scale' (Duggan 1962a). Indeed, were there no historical evidence at all, this conclusion would still be forced upon one. It is hardly possible to conceive that epidemics of the magnitude of that which occurred in Nigeria in the 1930s could have happened frequently in West Africa. It was, in any event, not Nigeria alone that was involved (see, for example, Vaucel, Waddy, de Andrade e Silva, and Pons 1963, Neujean 1963, Hutchinson 1953, 1954, and Scott 1965). The long history of West African civilization is, in one respect, the history of the evolution of human societies along paths that enabled them to avoid frequent periodical decimation by trypanosomiasis.

In Northern Nigeria in 1935 about 90 000 cases were detected out of somewhat over 400 000 people examined. Between 1931, when the Sleeping Sickness Service was inaugurated, and 1946, 500 000 people had been given treatment (Fig. 23.1) in a campaign that involved the examination of over 3 million people in primary surveys and nearly million in re-surveys (McLetchie 1948).

A European forestry officer provided the first individually recorded Nigerian case of sleeping sickness in 1905. Probably he was infected somewhere in the Niger–Benue valley. The first African cases were among soldiers stationed at Akwatcha near the Benue river in 1906. The Colonial Office, alerted by the tragedy of the Uganda epidemic, had already issued a circular questionnaire regarding the distribution and incidence of the disease in the Colony in 1903. This produced evidence of earlier foci of infection, especially in the Chad basin, but none of persons known, at that time, to be infected. The Medical Service and, no doubt, the Administration, were certainly aware of the possibilities of the disease appearing and of its likely consequences. By 1912 sleeping sickness was being regularly reported and during the 1914–18 war a number of localized outbreaks were discovered. These reports were, perhaps, only a consequence of the build-up in the medical service. As more doctors came into the field, more infections were found. In 1921 a Tsetse Investigation Department was set up, with headquarters in the Chad river area.

Although it is probable that many thousands of people died before they could be reached by the Sleeping Sickness Survey teams during the great

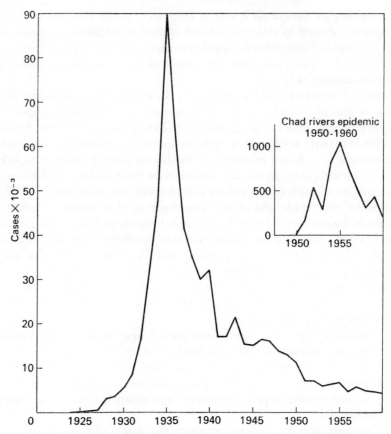

FIG. 23.1. Human trypanosomiasis (numbers of new cases yearly) in Nigeria, 1922–60 and (on a larger scale) the rise and fall of the 1954–7 Chad rivers epidemic.

epidemic period of the 1930s, there can be no reasonable doubt that the peak year, if not in fact 1935, was not very much earlier. The pandemic was developing during the 1920s but the timing indicated in Fig. 23.1 must be approximately correct. What is probably wrong is the slope of the curve before 1935: it should be far more gradual to accommodate the undetected cases, especially among so-called 'pagan' tribes who were severely afflicted and were more suspicious of Europeans than were the Muslims. Also it should not begin at zero.

The *Pax Britannica*

Subsequent studies have not greatly modified the conclusions derived from early data. There were two areas of endemic trypanosomiasis in Nigeria at the turn of the century. They were the Niger–Benue valley and the middle reaches of the Lake Chad rivers. 'This was the basic epidemiological situation from which all later events in Northern Nigeria developed'

(Duggan 1962a). The explanation usually offered for the development of the epidemic was the 'Pax Britannica'. How was it supposed to have worked?

There is no escape, indeed, from the conclusion that the epidemics of sleeping sickness that began in the Congo Independent State of King Leopold II and in Uganda at the end of the nineteenth century and continued well into the 1930s (if, indeed, they can yet be said to have ceased) were provoked by the colonial impact. In Nigeria the Atlantic slave trade was dying out by 1850 but from the Niger–Benue valley northwards slave raiding increased during the second half of the nineteenth century. A large part of the population lived in walled towns and had done so for centuries and, no doubt, in periods of formal war, as in the Jihad, the emirs had ensured that the walls were kept in repair. Later, when the new Fulani rulers of the Hausaland began their orgy of slave raiding, those people who were able to do so crowded into the towns and the walls were still maintained. The principal sufferers from the slave raids, the numerous small non-Muslim or pagan tribes, concealed themselves as best they might from the Fulani cavalry, especially in the rocky hills around the Bauchi Plateau. In the main Hausa area of the Sudan zone, 'The central plateau was so intensively cultivated that all tree growth was cut down over hundreds of square miles which are, to this day, entirely fly-free. Elsewhere in the countryside people were immobilized for fear of enslavement and large areas were depopulated by this remorseless trade. Undoubtedly this state of permanent defensiveness held sleeping sickness in check' (Duggan 1962a). Dense human settlement does not necessarily eliminate G. tachinoides. Nash (1948b) describes a tsetse-infested thicket in the moat of the town of Anchau where some 2500 people lived in only 0·118 mile².

In the last forty years, a steady movement of dispersal took much population from the relative safety of the old towns to new hamlets and homesteads which were too often sited near the most permanent pools of infested streams. The African's habits are no negligible factor in determining close and repeated contact.† He seeks shade and water, as do the tsetse, and often at time of day when the latter are most active. Conditions conducive to a persisting high degree of contact between man and the riverine tsetse are therefore common, especially in the Northern Provinces (McLetchie 1948).

One account of the operation of the Pax Britannica is of interest because it comes from an authoritative African source, the Emir of Zaria, within whose domains lie some of the most persistent foci of infection.

Before his country came under British authority, he stated, sleeping sickness was a problem of little importance. Owing to the existence of inter-tribal warfare,

---

† All people in hot dry climates seek shade and water. It is precisely this habit that accounts for the relatively high rate of infection among European holidaymakers in the Zambezi valley (see page 364).

the Hausas lived in walled towns, only daring to travel abroad in armed bands. The consumption of timber for building and as fuel produced a deep zone of clearance around the community. Farming was carried on intensively with the use of manure within the town walls and the farms were cropped almost annually, some of them for several generations. Sleeping sickness, when it occurred, was localised; it burnt itself out in the district and had little opportunity of spread. With the introduction of *Pax Britannica* it became safe to leave the towns, to travel, to develop farms in the bush, to open up trade with distant areas. Associated with these excellent results of peace were some serious disadvantages; the people became decentralised, freedom to travel brought contact with sleeping sickness, settling in the bush brought close contact between man and fly, and intensive farming gave place to a shifting cultivation. Sleeping sickness, which had only existed endemically and epidemically in small communities, became widespread as communications improved; and so was created the problem which now exists in Northern Nigeria (Davey 1948).

One difficulty in accepting the *Pax Britannica* as the cause of the epidemics of 1930–40 is that it avoids the issue of the origins of the causal trypanosomes. The depopulation by the slave trade can only have occurred where there were human communities to depopulate. There were wars, certainly, and always had been, but there is much to suggest that before the middle of the nineteenth century large areas were at peace and populated by prosperous communities. For example, the fourth volume of Denham (1831) describes how Captain Clapperton with his servant Richard Lander landed, in 1825, at Badagry 30 miles west of Lagos. For the first 70 miles of the journey Clapperton rode a horse. They passed through the Yoruba country where there were numerous Fulani-owned humped cattle and at the capital a cavalry regiment. In Borgu, at the town of Kaiama, which Clapperton thought had a population of 30 000 people, they also found horses and cattle. They travelled on to the town of Wawa (18 000–20 000 people) where they became acquainted with a widow who rode 'astraddle on a fine horse'. Richard Lander was given 'a beautiful mare' at Wawa and the Sultan of Kaiama also gave him 'a strong pony' (Denham 1831).

These references to a part of Nigeria which otherwise scarcely enters this story are made because the towns of Kaiama and Wawa now lie in the middle of the very extensive *G. morsitans* fly-belt of Borgu. The rivers are infested with *G. palpalis* and *G. tachinoides*. The depopulating agencies of the nineteenth century had operated here; the *Pax Britannica* had, in due course, intervened; people were free to move about the country and did so, but there was no sleeping sickness and there is none today. All the conditions needed for the '*Pax*' to lead to an epidemic were present, but nothing happened. If the theory of pacification and freedom of movement is sufficient to explain the development of the Nigerian epidemic it must also explain what were the conditions that confined the infection to certain parts of the country only.

The Ketare focus of infection

Ketare is a locality in the centre of Nigeria (Map 23.1) near the southern border of the emirate of Zaria. At the time of the great 1935 epidemic 10·8 per cent of the Ketare people were infected. In 1961 3 cases were found and more recently 19 people came in for treatment from some very remote villages (Thomson 1969). It is evident that the focus of infection persists.

A grave objection to the 'Pax' hypothesis is that the foci in which the great epidemic raged most actively are still in existence, except where they have been eliminated by entomological means. In 1911 J. J. Simpson went to Ketare at the request of the medical authorities because sleeping sickness was thought to be very prevalent.

Kateri . . . is a Kadara town situated in a small open clearing in the centre of a dense kurimi [*gallery forest*], which extends for several hundred yards all round. . . . The Kadaras are a very primitive and shy people; the women are devoid of clothing, and the children are supported on their backs by skins, chiefly those of a species of monkey and the harnessed antelope. The importance of this is seen when one remembers that the women are the water carriers, and that the water pools stand in thick bush swarming with tsetse, so that they have no protection from the attacks of these insects. One case of sleeping sickness was found in this village (Simpson 1912).

Kateri, or Ketare, lies between two rivers, the Dinya, a tributary of the Kaduna and the Gurara, both running into the Niger. Near Ketare they are only some 10 miles apart and it is not clear, on Simpson's map, into which river runs the stream whence the Kadara women drew their water. It is, perhaps, not important, for there is no doubt at all that they were infected through the bite of *G. palpalis* or *G. tachinoides*, both of which were present in 1911 as they still are today.

Simpson's most significant observation was that the harnessed antelope (*Tragelaphus scriptus*) was not uncommon. He did not observe *G. longipalpis* which in Nigeria takes 74·4 per cent of its blood meals from this antelope (Weitz 1963). However, infestations of *G. longipalpis* were found by Mahood (1955) on the Tapa river, a tributary of the Gurara, only some 25 miles south-west of Ketare. Glover (1965) summarizes Mahood's observations as well as collating most of the information available on this species in West Africa, and provides a map showing the known distribution of *G. longipalpis* in Nigeria in 1960.

G. longipalpis resembles the East African *G. pallidipes* so closely in its morphology that some systematists have suggested that they are races of the same species. Their habits are very similar. Wild pigs, buffaloes, and, in both cases, *Tragelaphus scriptus*, together form 90 per cent of their diet. The direction of the argument is apparent when comparison is made with Chapter 16. *G. longipalpis*, like *G. pallidipes*, on occasion attacks man, and

Morris (1934) thought it must be a vector of human trypanosomiasis in Ghana. There is a need to study the biting habits of *G. longipalpis* (as of *G. pallidipes* in East Africa). Near Koton Karifi, just north of the confluence of the Niger and Benue, recent surveys have found mixed aggregations of *G. longipalpis* and *G. tachinoides* in places where human population density is high and where the latter species takes most of its meals from man.

The Niger–Benue primordial focus of human trypanosomiasis

Duggan (1962a) believed that his tentative suggestion of a zoonotic origin for some epidemics in Nigeria could apply to the foci in the Chad basin. Here *G. morsitans* was present with the bushbuck and both might be associated in relatively small and compact areas with man and *G. tachinoides*. It is a situation yet to be described. Duggan did not suggest that it could apply elsewhere.

In the Niger–Benue primordial focus of human trypanosomiasis in Nigeria the disease is generally mild and very chronic. Its limits have been mapped by Duggan (1962a). Quite clearly *G. palpalis* and *G. tachinoides* are the vectors, and there is a long history of endemic trypanosomiasis in areas from which *G. morsitans* is absent. Nevertheless when Glover's (1965) map of the distribution of *G. longipalpis* is superimposed upon Duggan's map, the coincidence between the limits of endemic sleeping sickness and the distribution of this tsetse is remarkably close (Map 23.1). Perhaps even more remarkable are the places where the coincidence appears to fail. The principal failure lies in the centre of the Tiv country which occupies most of the eastern end of the Niger–Benue endemic area. The 'centrifugal expansion' of the Tiv people and their elimination of a belt of *G. morsitans* have been described in Chapter 22.

Duggan has illustrated the apparent movement of infection outwards from the Niger–Benue primordial focus. There were three eastern extensions. A movement of some 1500 Tiv up the Benue valley led to the appearance of infection among them and Jukun fishermen. It does not enter into the present account. It is presumed that the Tiv migrants took their infection with them. The eastern limit of the primordial focus is formed by the valley of the Donga river, a tributary of the Benue. The headwaters of this river are shown on the 1 : 1 750 000 map of Nigeria as the Kari, rising on the border of Cameroon. The disease apparently had spread along trade routes up the Donga–Kari valley to the district of Kentu where an epidemic developed. It was discovered in 1939 and successfully eliminated by mass survey and treatment and establishment of dispensaries.

Parallel to the Donga but some 40–50 miles further to the east is the Taraba river, with its main headwater, the Gasheka, also rising on the Cameroon border. In 1936 an extension from the endemic focus on the Donga reached the valley of the Taraba around the town of Bakundi. The disease began in epidemic form and survived in endemic form particularly

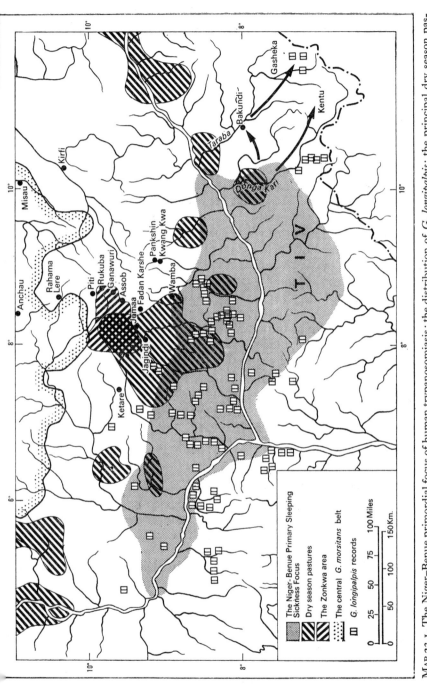

MAP 23.1. The Niger–Benue primordial focus of human trypanosomiasis; the distribution of *G. longipalpis*; the principal dry season pastures for migrant cattle; persistent foci of infection and two temporary epidemic extensions of sleeping sickness. (After Duggan 1962*a* Glover 1965, Thomson 1966, and with additional records supplied by D. A. T. Baldry 1969 *in litt.*)

at the town of Kungana-Kwossa. According to Thomson's (1969) map this area is now within the Tiv endemic area. It is noteworthy that Bakundi and Kungana-Kwossa lie in an area still infested by *G. morsitans*. The Bakundi focus apparently gave rise to a new extension southward into the Gasheka district. In 1957 hamlet infection rates of 3 per cent were found here. There were still very few people and it was possible easily to interrupt transmission and extinguish the epidemic.

In the headwater areas both of the Donga–Kari and Taraba–Gasheka rivers *G. longipalpis* has been discovered. The disease in both of these headwater areas was apparently successfully countered, because only relatively few people, on the outward fringe of peripheral expansion, were involved.

Duggan (1962a) also shows the distribution of sleeping sickness in Nigeria up to 1912. There is evidence for the antiquity of the infection and it is reasonable to suppose that where it was traditional or where information about it was obtained by doctors from older inhabitants, the disease must have appeared, at the places noted, in an unusually disruptive form. Of the eighteen early sites shown, all but two are in relatively close proximity to modern records of *G. longipalpis*. Many also are in areas in which *G. morsitans* is found today. The two sites not now in the area infested by these species of *Glossina* lie in the centre of the Tiv area where the endemic condition today is, undoubtedly, sustained by *G. tachinoides* and *G. palpalis*. So far a geographical correlation has been established between the area of persistent endemic sleeping sickness and the distribution of *G. longipalpis* and, hence, by implication, with the distribution of the bushbuck. The presence in the vicinity of *G. morsitans* shows that other possible wild hosts of *brucei*-group trypanosomes also live within the general area of the primordial focus.

The Lake Chad basin epidemics

All theories of the origin of epidemics of human trypanosomiasis begin with the observation of geographical and historical correlations that point to circumstances in which situations like those described in Ketare by Simpson (1912) or in Sambo by Nash (1944) may develop. The *Pax Britannica* encouraged people to leave their walled cities. The activities of the colonial authorities in promoting development determined the direction in which the epidemics thus supposed to have been engendered were spread. There were two movements. Infections spread north from the Niger–Benue valley and south or south-west from the Chad basin drainages. On the central watershed, where some of the worst epidemics occurred, it seemed possible that strains of trypanosomes from both of the persistent endemic areas were in circulation. The correlation between distribution of the Niger–Benue focus with the distribution of *G. longipalpis* has been noted.

The hypothesis that the disease on the Chad rivers is a zoonosis fits the general theme of this account.

Over long stretches of the Dingaiya and Gaya Rivers *G. tachinoides* co-exists with *G. morsitans*, and the harnessed antelope exists in Northern Nigeria. . . . it is conceivable that transmission of *rhodesiense*-like trypanosomes to man occurs through the agency of *G. morsitans*, this phenomenon being governed by cyclical conditions as yet unknown. Human infection, of course, would be perpetuated by *G. tachinoides*, perhaps until the trypanosome had been attenuated by continued passage through this species of tsetse (Duggan 1962a).

One is reminded of Busoga where transmission to man of trypanosomes probably from the same species of antelope also occurs, but where prolonged transmission involving only *G. fuscipes* as the vector may lead to a typical *gambiense*-like situation. One difficulty is that *G. morsitans* and *Tragelaphus scriptus* coexist with *G. tachinoides* and *G. palpalis* over large areas in other parts of Nigeria where epidemics of trypanosomiasis are unknown. What other correlations are detectable?

One has already been described. The Chad rivers runs through the frontier zone between the Fulani–Hausa emirates and the country of Bornu. The chain of buffer states were much involved in frontier disputes, but in times of peace served as staging posts of international trade. The situation emerges clearly from the writings of Barth (1857) already quoted in Chapter 22. He, as well as his predecessors, recorded other diseases but, as Duggan has noted:

Neither Park who died on the Niger in 1805, nor Clapperton who died in Sokoto twenty years later, nor Richard Lander who revealed the true course of the Niger in 1830, nor Barth, who covered tremendous distances in the 1850s, refer in their writings to sleeping sickness, which, in its later stages at least, is a sufficiently dramatic disease to inspire literary impressions (Duggan 1962a).

Why? In part because no epidemics were in progress. Lester, who had the task of dealing with the 1930–40 epidemic, was in a better position than any predecessor or successor to assess the effects of the disease. 'In dealing with a mild type of disease any infection rate of 1 per cent or less is of little importance. It would not be economical to reduce it further' (Lester 1939). This would not be an acceptable doctrine today. It was founded upon the belief that the classical chronic, mild disease, at a low level of incidence, did not interfere with the life of the community. Lester added that in these conditions, the majority of deaths in untreated cases would be due to lowered general resistance and intercurrent infection. 'My experience in West Africa and what I saw in six months touring in East Africa, led me to regard the text book story as representing a state of things that only happens occasionally. . . . We have places where people have kept on fifteen years or more with infection and are still alive.' Typical sleeping sickness cases comprised about 5 per cent of the whole. 'When the infection gets down to about 1 per cent you can find no real sign of the population being hit by it' (Lester 1939, discussion). The non-medical biologist who reads a large number of sleeping sickness reports inevitably forms the view that many so-called outbreaks of human trypanosomiasis owed their origin to the chance of a survey by a competent diagnostician and that not only was there no real sign of the community being hit by the disease, but people were often unaware of its presence among them. It was the epidemic condition, when produced by more virulent strains of trypanosome, that frightened people and led them to abandon their villages. The disease is now well known and the benefits of medical attention are widely appreciated, but even in 1967 voluntary patients in Northern Nigeria only formed 42 per cent of cases diagnosed (Thomson 1969).

The widespread endemic condition of mild disease is far more characteristic of the Niger–Benue valley than of the Chad river foci. Indeed, after their first investigation Lloyd, Johnson, and Rawson (1927) reported that the disease in the Chad basin appeared only periodically in its virulent form. The chronic form was unknown and there were no spontaneous cures. However, after the dying down of the 1927–38 epidemic in the area studied by Lloyd and his co-workers, Harding (1940) found a low endemicity with an incidence well under 1 per cent. The disease persisted among fishermen and others who frequented rivers and streams.

Duggan's alternative hypothesis for the Lake Chad epidemics was that in the intervals the disease remained in the condition described by Harding and behaved like a normal *gambiense* endemic condition. In these circumstances populations accumulate and the villages were restored only to break down again when their population density had reached a level at which man–fly contact was sufficiently frequent to precipitate another outbreak. In support of this argument Duggan produced evidence for a cycle of alternating epidemic and endemic phases. At Dizagore on the Jamaari river there was an epidemic in about 1859, after which the town was deserted for fifty years. Eleven years after its re-establishment around 1909 the disease broke out once more. In Babuwuri there was an outbreak in about 1886 and the town was deserted until 1905. The next outbreak was that studied by Lloyd and Johnson and began in about 1920. In the Bedde emirate there were histories of epidemics in 1846 and 1898, both with devastating consequences. The next came in 1930, forming part of the great epidemic spread in this region which seems to have begun in about 1920. Lloyd and Johnson took up their position at Sherifuri just as the third epidemic wave in sixty years broke about the place (Duggan 1962a).

It is difficult to see in these dates any synchronicity of epidemics in different villages before 1920. Perhaps beginning at about that time, but certainly developing very rapidly after 1926, a spread of infection took place throughout the Chad river basin and reached a peak in 1935. Carriage of trypanosomes by people in the earlier stages of the disease, who left their villages hoping to escape infection from those already dying, must have greatly assisted the spread of the epidemic. After 1935 the decline in numbers of cases was so spectacular that it could not be attributed to preventive measures but was due to a natural dying out of the infection. The quiescent endemic condition which followed began to break down in 1948. This time, however, the activities of the Sleeping Sickness Service over the next twelve years prevented any spread of the epidemic, while the numbers of cases were too few to affect the general shape of the curve of total infections for Nigeria as a whole. Duggan lists 38 towns or villages in the Chad basin, with the results of surveys in each between 1951 and 1960. Although the organization of surveys, by teams that can only deal with a limited number of local epidemics in one year, is such that complete accuracy for the peak year cannot be determined, it is evidence that it must have come between 1954 and 1957. It is also not possible to say what would have been the course of the epidemic without the work of the Sleeping Sickness Service. The available figures show two peaks twenty years apart (Fig. 23.1). Is there any correlation with other events which might suggest an explanation for these two epidemics other than that put forward by Duggan, namely the gradual build-up of man–fly contact frequency and its collapse when communities were overwhelmed or the disease extinguished by treatment? What arguments can be adduced in support of the hypothesis already applied to the situation in the north-east corner of Lake Victoria in Chapters 14–16, and earlier partly developed in respect of the Tanzanian epidemic spread which reached its peak in 1928 or thereabouts (Chapter 13 and Ford 1965)?

Environmental relationships of the Chad basin foci

Map 23.2 shows the present outlines of the more northerly *G. morsitans* fly-belts of Nigeria, including those that have now been eliminated (MacLennan 1963a, Davies 1964). It also shows, in the central belt only, evidence of its growth during the last twenty years from maps published by Nash (1948a), Nigeria Tsetse report (1956, 1964), Wilson (1958), and MacLennan (1963a). It is known that portions of the central fly-belt west of Kaduna were in existence in the early 1920s, although their precise limits were not defined (Johnson and Lloyd 1923).

Map 23.3 shows five groups of foci of infection of sleeping sickness taken from Duggan (1962a) and Thompson (1969). The first group, not shown individually, includes those sites for which there is historical evidence from the nineteenth century. All lie on the Chad rivers system, save one, on the Gongola, which Duggan thought to be of doubtful authenticity but which lies remarkably close to Thomson's Kirfi focus discovered in 1967. The second group are those places at which the disease was identified before 1920. The third group are those that appeared between 1920 and 1933 and

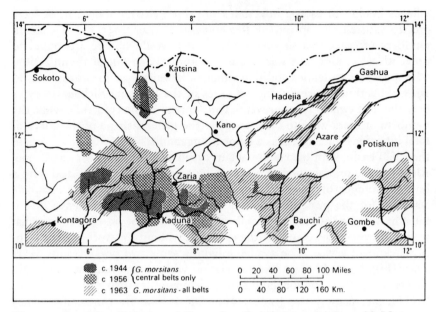

MAP 23.2. Expansion of the central *G. morsitans* fly-belt for comparison with Map 23.3.

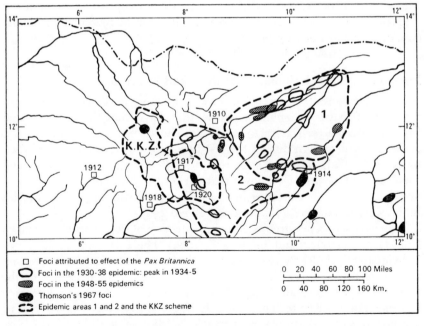

MAP 23.3. Northern foci of infection with epidemic areas (1) and (2) and limits of K.K.Z. scheme (after Duggan 1962 and Thomson 1969).

were involved in the major epidemic peak of 1934–5. The fourth group, also from Duggan (1962*a*), includes foci that became active during the suppressed epidemic period of 1948–55. Finally the fifth group is taken from Thomson (1969) and comprises those foci still known to be active.

The five groups of foci can be divided into two zones. Epidemic zone (1) includes foci located on the Chad rivers where they pass through the Hausaland–Bornu border emirates, in which both *G. tachinoides* and *G. morsitans* share the same riverine habitats. It is here that Duggan envisaged sporadic infection by *rhodesiense*-like trypanosomes, derived through *G. morsitans* from antelopes, as causing epidemics of zoonotic origin, but circulated among the people by *G. tachinoides*. This zone includes the historical foci with the exception of that on the Gongola.

Epidemic zone (2) includes no ancient foci and historical evidence is entirely negative. In the pre-1920 group that at Baserka, 1914, lies very close to or within the limits of the 1967 Misau focus. The epidemics at Gimi (1917),† Kaduna (1918), and Soba (1920) are regarded as having been initiated by the appearance at these places of infected persons who had come north, mostly as labourers on the new road and rail systems, and had brought with them trypanosomes derived from the Niger–Benue primordial focus. At this time there was a movement outwards from the walled cities and new villages sprang up in the bush where people came into close contact with riverine tsetses. Further south and on the Bauchi plateau recruitment of mining labour from communities living within the Niger–Benue primordial focus was another source for spreading infection. Evidence that sleeping sickness spread up the new lines of communication was well founded and is difficult to dispute. But it is possible to admit this spread of infection and at the same time to doubt that it was responsible for the devastation of the northern epidemic zones during the late 1920s and early 1930s.

It is difficult to use the events of 1910–30 to explain the persistence of foci of infection in virtually the same sites, some for as long as forty years, in the face of well-organized medical and, sometimes, entomological attacks on the disease and its vectors. In epidemic zone (1) it was possible to envisage sporadic zoonoses as the origins of periodical epidemics. But a particular feature of the foci in epidemic zone (2) is that they always appeared well outside the limits of *G. morsitans* distribution. Many of them later became engulfed in the spreading fly-belt, but when the epidemics began, only *G. tachinoides* and, in some parts *G. palpalis* as well, were the only possible vectors. There could have been no direct transmission by *G. morsitans* of antelope trypanosomes to man.

† On a modern map of Nigeria Gimi is shown on the railway between Zaria and Kano, some nine miles north of the Galma River, but it is clear from a map published by Johnson and Lloyd (1923) that at the time of the epidemic Gimi village lay within half a mile of the Galma.

Origins of epidemic zone (2)

In Chapter 5 it was recalled that at one time *Trypanosoma vivax* was regarded as the predominant trypanosome of cattle in West Africa. There tended to be a zonation in the geographical distribution of the cattle trypanosomiases and *T. congolense* became more frequent in veterinary diagnoses in more southerly regions. Two studies revealed the appearance of *T. vivax*, *T. brucei*, and *T. congolense*, in that order, in trade cattle moving from north to south. The *T. brucei* infections were transient in the peripheral circulation so that eventually only *T. vivax* and *T. congolense* were found in the bloodstreams of those animals that survived the journey.

Although veterinary staff regularly deplored the widespread infection of Nigerian cattle it was not until 1924 that the first note of anxiety about an increase in the disease was sounded. In 1930 the first treatment service was begun. In Chapter 15 it was shown that an epizootic among the cattle of Busoga nearly coincided with the first *rhodesiense* epidemic in that area. In Chapter 16 the demonstration that domestic cattle acted as a reservoir of the human trypanosome in a later epidemic in the region was described. Nobody seems to have been struck by the fact that Lester's Sleeping Sickness Service and the Veterinary Department's treatment service for trypanosomiasis in cattle both began in 1930. Severe trypanosome infection in cattle became increasingly evident during the 1920s. Over the same period the great sleeping sickness epidemic of the next decade gathered momentum. It would be remarkable if the concurrent development of trypanosomiasis in cattle and in man did not have the same ecological origin. The epidemic condition among the people and the epizootic condition among cattle appeared when the two conflicting ecosystems, in their recovery from the common affliction of the rinderpest some thirty to thirty-five years earlier, brought man and cattle once more into contact along relatively wide fronts with wildlife and its parasites. The latter, it may be inferred from what is known to have happened in other parts of Africa, had been reduced by the same disease which attacked, in particular, the natural hosts of the *morsitans* group tsetses, among them warthogs and bushbuck, called, in West Africa, the harnessed antelope.

When this correlation between recovery of the man–cattle–cultivation and the wildlife ecosystems and the appearance of the epidemic spread of rhodesian trypanosomiasis in Tanzania was first pointed out (Ford 1965), the work of Onyango, van Hoeve, and de Raadt (1966) at Alego had not yet appeared. If their work is considered in relation to the observations of Unsworth and Birkett (1952) and Godfrey, Killick-Kendrick, and Ferguson (1965) on the succession of parasitaemias in trade cattle, and these studies are, in turn, related to the increasing contact between cattle and *G. morsitans* which took place during the 1920s, it becomes clear that the great epidemic must have been preceded by a period in which the cattle provided a greatly expanded reservoir for the proliferation of *brucei*-group trypanosomes. In the course of the seasonal transhumance, cattle forming this reservoir of infection could now carry *brucei*-type infections, which included *rhodesiense*-type strains, into areas outside the *G. morsitans* belts where *G. tachinoides* lived very largely upon people and their domestic livestock.

In Chapter 22 it was pointed out that there had been a rapid rise in demand for tartar emetic from 1930 to 1933, and thereafter until 1937 the demand diminished. This period of reduced demand for treatment co-incided with the period of maximum incidence of the human infection. Indeed, Fulani examined during sleeping sickness surveys have shown high infection rates (Duggan 1962a). This is not surprising among people who live symbiotically with animals that periodically serve as reservoirs of human infection; but that they would keep away from villages where the inhabitants were dying of sleeping sickness is not unlikely. In doing so they removed their cattle from proximity to vector populations infected not only by *T. brucei* but also by *T. congolense* and *T. vivax*. This avoidance of infection foci was reflected in a diminished demand for drug treatment.

The 1948–57 epidemic period

One test of the probability for the hypothesis just developed is to observe if it is repeated when similar conditions arise again and, in particular, if in addition to the general correlation, detailed examples can be found.

Duggan's view that the collapse of the epidemic after 1935 could not have been entirely due to the activities of the newly formed Sleeping Sickness Service has been noted. The epidemic collapsed because the organisms involved, i.e. man, cattle, trypanosomes, wild reservoir animals, and tsetse, had adjusted themselves so that all could continue to live without mutual destruction. Such adjustments are essential in all successful parasitic re-lationships. They may be physiological, behavioural, or ecological and in trypanosomiasis they are still far from being understood. Very virulent and highly pathogenic strains of trypanosomes weed themselves out because they kill off cattle or people too quickly; alternatively highly susceptible hosts die, leaving the less susceptible still alive; people move their villages and stockmen choose new routes for their cattle; small residual populations of tsetse disappear because the women on whom they fed in the dry seasons are either dead or have migrated. These processes all contribute to the period of quiescence that follows the collapse of the epidemic. Such a period of quiescence would give way to a period of epidemics and epizootics if the population density relationships were to change. The rapid spread of *G. morsitans*, which began in the 1940s as the cattle population built up, outstripped the suppressive effects of the more slowly increasing human population. In particular, a very rapid acceleration, after the introduction of drugs had enabled cattle to form a more reliable blood supply for the tsetse, was observed from 1950 onwards. The spread of *G. morsitans*, which greatly exercised the veterinary service, was followed very shortly by the appearance of epidemic conditions among the people. Sleeping sickness in the Chad basin built up to a climax in 1955 (Fig. 23.1) before it was over-come by the surveys and treatment combined with an entomological attack on the vectors. Again, the authorities concerned did not perceive any connection, although veterinary and medical teams collaborated in controlling riverine tsetse infestations.

The best known of all trypanosomiasis control operations in Nigeria, perhaps in Africa, was the Anchau Rural Development and Settlement Scheme. In the Anchau district east of the town of Zaria about one third of the population had sleeping sickness and in some hamlets half the people were infected. The only tsetse present in the epidemic area were *G. tachinoides* and *G. palpalis*. The two nearest *G. morsitans* belts were 30 and 40 miles respectively from Anchau town in the centre of the scheme when it was begun in 1936 (Nash 1948*a*, *b*). So confident were the authors of this scheme that *G. morsitans* was of no significance in West African sleeping sickness, that this species is not mentioned in Nash's (1948*b*) most interest-ing account of the Anchau project. The scheme involved three principal operations. The first was the creation of the Anchau corridor from which all riverine tsetse were removed, and the second was the resettlement of people living near its edge into the centre of the corridor. Thirdly Anchau itself was enlarged by building a new suburb, Takalafya, to relieve the insanitary overcrowding in the old town. All this work was completed successfully.

The 30 per cent incidence of 1934 was reduced to 0·2 per cent in 1946. A few people still became infected on journeys that took them outside the corridor (McLetchie 1948). The Anchau Scheme later formed the most easterly portion of a large-scale bush-clearing project directed against the riverine *G. palpalis* and *G. tachinoides* only. This was the Katsina–Kano–Zaria (K.K.Z.) scheme (McLetchie 1948, 1953 and Duggan 1962*a*) in which, between 1950 and 1960, 3204 miles of river were cleared covering the western end of the epidemic zone (2) (Map 23.3). Although the benefits of this scheme were widespread numerous intractable endemic foci re-mained outside its area of influence. Some of these lie within the zone of recurrent epidemic foci that lies around the Bauchi plateau, particularly below its western and southern scarps. It will be dealt with separately. However, certain foci on the Chad basin rivers were believed, during the epidemic of the 1930s, to have received some of their infective strains from the Niger–Benue focus, carried north by people involved in the movements associated with the *Pax Britannica* and its accompanying projects for development such as rail and road building and mining. 'The hamlets of Tudun Wada District on the Kano River were involved in the Lake Chad basin epidemic of 1929 and an intermingling of trypanosome strains must have occurred there. Similarly, tributaries of the Galma (Niger system) and the Jare (Lake Chad basin) to the north, closely interdigitate and the ebb and flow of epidemic sleeping sickness in this area continued until well into the 1940s' (Duggan 1962a).

Tudun Wada was also involved in the epidemic resurgence of the 1950s. In 1956, 7 cases were found among 6000 people examined, and in 1957 another 22 cases in 46 000. These figures do not indicate a high incidence (0·1 and 0·05 per cent respectively) for the district as a whole, although no doubt they include hamlets with higher as well as lower incidences than these averages. What is of interest in this second Tudun Wada outbreak is its coincidence with the arrival of *G. morsitans* along cattle routes crossing the Anchau corridor.

Wilson's (1958) description of the invasion of the Anchau area by *G. morsitans* has already been mentioned in Chapter 22, and the role played in their movement by migrant cattle was illustrated by the spectacular rise in density of the tsetse along the Malamawa–Katini route between June 1955 and June 1957. Another route led north from Pambeguwa, where Nash had noted the fresh arrival of the tsetse in 1944, to Tudun Wada (Map 22.1). The route crossed the corridor in a northerly direction close to Anchau itself. *G. morsitans* was established in a small forest reserve just south of Tudun Wada village by 1955, the year before the reappearance of infection in this neighbourhood. Another route, between Hayin Kano and Burji, became infested in 1958. It lies parallel to and some 12 miles east of the Pambeguwa–Tudun Wada route. Both of these cattle tracks lead northward, the latter forking eatswards towards Gaya, another epidemic focus where *G. morsitans* was already present, in an extension of the Katagum river belt. Here epidemic conditions were located in 1952 and continued until 1956. Burji was a part of the Tudun Wada epidemic area in 1933. Between it and Gaya was another epidemic focus at Rano, which had been active in both the epidemic periods. It is difficult to escape the conclusion that the principal vehicles for carriage of *T. brucei* strains infective to man between these various centres are the cattle and that they have themselves received the infection from *G. morsitans* to which they are far more acceptable as hosts than is man.

Wilson (1958) also described the spread of *G. morsitans* eastwards in the direction of Ningi and noted that its invasion would involve the tsetse in establishing itself in the Sudan vegetation zone (or sub-Sudan zone according to Glover 1965). Wilson seems to have overlooked a small belt of *G. morsitans* shown on Nash's (1948a) map between Ningi and the advancing fly-front to the west. This must have been engulfed by the expanding main belt before it reached the limits of the Northern Guinea zone in about 1959. Tarry (1967) described the invasion of this sub-Sudan vegetation in 1959–60. Again, the tsetse used the migrating cattle as food supply although, in this lightly populated area, some wild animals, including warthog, were present (Tarry 1969). The people of Ningi were surveyed during the inter-epidemic period in 1938 when 159 cases were found among 11 000 examined, giving an incidence of 1·4 per cent. In 1953 three villages on the Bunga river showed infection rates of 2·6, 4·0, and 5·0 per cent. Accordingly tsetse control measures against *G. tachinoides* were undertaken. In 1959, the year in which *G. morsitans* invaded from the west, 65 cases were found among 16 000 people examined. Duggan's view is that in Ningi sleeping sickness is permanently endemic, with localized epidemics at hamlet level. One asks what maintains this endemism and again it is difficult to avoid the conclusion that the cattle are the vehicles by which the population of human trypanosomes is continually refreshed.

Residual epidemic foci around the Bauchi plateau

The adjustments to infection, both ecological and physiological, that lead to the establishment of an endemic condition can be upset in various ways. The movement of a new population into an area has three main effects. If numerous enough the newcomers may alter the social and geographical patterns that have developed between the human community and adjacent wildlife ecosystems. They may displace natural hosts and alter the feeding patterns of tsetse populations. They may introduce into local human society a substantial proportion of people who are not immunologically adjusted to local strains of trypanosomes. Severe epidemics may then develop among them. Thirdly, they may bring with them strains of trypanosomes to which they are partially adjusted, but against which indigenous people have no protection. Again, epidemics may develop and disruption of the community may spread disease further.

Are these various factors sufficient to explain the persistence of infection around the Bauchi plateau, especially on its southern and western edges? It is around this plateau that the *Pax Britannica* seems most obviously to have played an epidemiological role. Among the people who suffered most during the phase of Fulani aggressiveness that followed the Jihad were the so-called 'pagans' of the savannas north of the Benue–Niger valley. At first subjected to the proselytizing zeal of Usuman dan Fodio's followers, they later became ideal victims when this zeal was diverted to the commercial ends of slave raiding. Many pagan tribes took refuge in the inaccessible high forests of the scarps around the Bauchi plateau. The Ganawuri, a small tribe living in a district to which they gave their name, were afflicted by a severe epidemic of sleeping sickness first recognized among them in 1928. They numbered 5052 at a census taken a year earlier. Between November 1928 and December 1929 some 2600 cases were seen and treated, and between January and May 1930 a further 649 new cases were found. Taylor studied the epidemiological situation in 1929.

Endemic sleeping sickness of a very mild type with a low mortality has prevailed hitherto. The epidemic disease with a high mortality seems to be of recent origin and is probably due to the improved communications and unrestrained movement between different tribes and races throughout the Province, resulting in the introduction of new and virulent strains of *Trypanosoma gambiense*. The large labour camps at the tin mines are doubtless responsible for a good deal of this movement of population (Taylor 1930).

This is the classical statement. Nearly forty years later it is necessary to ask what is wrong with it. The tin mines labour have, for many years, been subject to special regulations to enforce their regular examination for trypanosome infection. Nevertheless, there have been numerous epidemics just west of the Bauchi plateau. The names of the villages where epidemics are observed change as control programmes follow one after the other. At Assob, less than 20 miles from Ganawuri, Thomson (1969) has reported that even the achievement of successful control of *G. palpalis* has not prevented the appearance of new cases. At Fadan Karshe, in the same locality, a survey in 1968 detected 154 cases (2·7 per cent incidence) with a maximum hamlet prevalence of 15·3 per cent (17 out of 111 people examined). For forty years, in this very small and circumscribed portion of Nigeria, the maintenance of dispensaries, the work of mobile survey and treatment teams, the control of labour movement, the use of pentamidine prophylaxis, the application of numerous schemes of tsetse control directed against *G. palpalis*, unquestionably the only vector between man and man, has failed to eliminate the infections that continually threaten to, and sometimes do, develop into serious epidemics. The presumption must be that circumstantial epidemiology is faulty and that therefore other correlations must be sought.

Other correlations were examined and rejected by Taylor. It is time to look at them afresh. The Ganawuri live near the northern tip of an island of forest–savanna mosaic on the western scarp of the Bauchi plateau. Nobody has yet found *G. longipalpis* here, although, apart from the riverine *G. palpalis* and *G. tachinoides*, this is what one might expect. But much forest vegetation still exists in which, according to Thomson (1969) 'tsetse control has generally been considered impracticable'. *G. longipalpis*, like its close relative *G. pallidipes*, has cryptic habits and it is doubtful if it has been sought in this inaccessible area by teams properly equipped for its discovery. It was also stated by Taylor that although the Ganawuri country was formerly well populated by game, the wild animals are now exterminated. This, he believed, perhaps correctly, was an important factor in the maintenance of the epidemic state. 'The absence of game and aquatic reptiles, the normal buffers between *G. palpalis* and man, has resulted in the fly obtaining a large proportion of its food from man.'

A possible source of trypanosomes from more distant areas is the Fulani cattle which yearly come south to find dry-season pasture either on the plateau itself or in the plains surrounding it. Taylor believed these animals were free of infection, but the evidence on which he based this belief would, today, be considered inadequate. More recent evidence shows that, whatever the parasitological condition of the area in 1929, twenty-five years later it was recognized as unusually dangerous for cattle.

The Kaduna river, which drains north-westwards into the central *G. morsitans* belt before turning south to the Niger, rises among the hills on either side of Ganawuri. Another river, the Mada, also rises close by and turns due south to the Benue. Between the two the Gurara rises, somewhat west of the plateau wall, and also turns south to join the Niger shortly before it meets the Benue. This watershed area was covered by the Zonkwa Veterinary Scheme started in 1958 in an attempt to eliminate *Glossina palpalis*, the only tsetse known to be present. Cattle became so heavily infected around Zonkwa that it could not be used for pasture throughout the year but had to be evacuated in the rains. Fifty miles to the south, however, in the neighbourhood of Keffi, although here *G. palpalis* also infested the rivers, cattle could be kept throughout the year without too much sickness (Maclennan 1963*b*). An account of the reclamation work is given by Glover (1965). Reinfestation took place from various points on the periphery of the scheme area and by 1964, after 1264 mile^2 of country had been given insecticide treatment, the economic benefits of the scheme were being weighed against its maintenance cost (*Nigeria Tsetse and Trypanosomiasis Unit* 1964).

In the search for geographical, ecological, and parasitological correlations with the distribution of human trypanosomiasis, the Zonkwa project is of singular interest. The majority of sites of local epidemics, which were supposed to have arisen because of the movement of infected persons between the Niger–Benue primordial focus and the Chad rivers focus, lie around the periphery of the Zonkwa area where enzootic cattle trypanosomiasis due to infection by *G. palpalis* is unusually serious (Map 23.1). In other examples the coincidence or near coincidence in time of epizootics and epidemics has been remarked; here the correlation is geographical. The foci of recurrent human epidemics that have defied a half-century of medical, entomological, and administrative effort to remove them, lie like a string of beads around the central area of heavy enzootic cattle infection.

The Ganawuri people gave a history of endemic typically *gambiense* type infection before they were hit by the epidemics of the 1920s. Less than 20 miles north of Ganawuri is the home of another 'pagan' tribe, the Rukuba. They too became involved in the spread of epidemic conditions, but not until some years after the Ganawuri. The epidemiological history of the Rukuba has been described in detail by Duggan (1962*b*). Sleeping sickness did not occur among them until after 1930. Like other 'pagan' tribes, they have survived the proselytizing zeal of Islam and they fought their last battle against the cavalry of the Emir of Zaria in 1892. At that time the Rukuba lived in hilltop villages.

Access was made difficult by cactus hedging which not only surrounded the villages and farms, but was planted at the sides of footpaths, making them easily barred. Not a single nook or cranny among the rocks was wasted. The compound type of house predominated. . . . Mud was, and is, used as a building material and the craft is so finely drawn that it is often impossible to put a hand between the walls of a granary and a sleeping hut. After the wars had ceased the Rukuba migrated down the hillsides from these packed and impenetrable domestic fortresses. The new environment on the edge of the escarpment contained more dense vegetation and less rock than previously and the old paths became overgrown and converted into tunnels of living cactus. The diet consists of the chief indigenous crops—millet, guinea-corn, coco-yams, yams and sweet potatoes, supplemented with meat and milk from the Fulani. A perennial water supply abounds from rocky streams (Duggan 1962b).

The Rukuba were hardly less suspicious of the new Christian rulers than they had been of the Muslim. When, in 1935, a second attempt was made to survey them for trypanosome infections the entire population fled into the hills as the team arrived and not a single examination was made. It appears that during this first epidemic period the tribe lost about 16 per cent of its strength as a result of sleeping sickness. A first partial survey in 1934 had indicated an infection incidence in one village of 18·3 per cent. Duggan's account of the prolonged and patient effort, culminating in success during the 1940s, to examine and treat these people gives an excellent idea of the complexities, social, religious, and economic that had to be understood before control was achieved. The Rukuba story puts the *Pax Britannica* in its proper context as an epidemiological agent. The Rukuba came down from their hilltop villages because Lugard's new administration put an end to the raids of the Emir of Zaria's cavalry. In so doing they put themselves epidemiologically in a vulnerable position. They did not have to move very far. Nash (1948a) who devised the entomological attack on *G. palpalis* which, together with mass treatment, brought the epidemic under control between 1942 and 1946, described the situations in which the people built their villages after their descent from the hilltops.

The Rukuba country lies at the western edge of the Plateau at an altitude of about 3200 feet. . . . The country between Jos [in the centre of the Plateau] and this area is fly-free, consisting of treeless grassland and rocky hills. Many streams flow westwards, but their banks are denuded of vegetation until they reach the edge of the escarpment, where they fall some 400 feet down rocky gorges, choked with evergreen vegetation which supports a large population of *G. palpalis*. On reaching the plain below, the stream banks are once more treeless, and the country tsetse-free; *G. palpalis* is confined to the edge and face of the escarpment. The villages consist of isolated groups of mud huts surrounded by cactus hedges and situated beside or just above these fly-infested gorges, from which they get their water. In the wet season tsetse are found inside the villages and frequent the sunken paths lined by cactus hedges. . . . Game is completely absent . . and there can be little doubt that the fly are dependent on man, his goats and his dogs. Man–fly contact was extremely close (Nash 1948a).

This situation and its consequences are illustrated by Nash in a somewhat grim map which he describes thus:

Following the map from east to west, it will be seen how the incidence of the disease steadily increases, as the edge of the escarpment and the tsetse-infested streams are approached. Thus Egbak 4 per cent., Agwaji 34 per cent., Buhuk 38 per cent., Ashirin 53 per cent., and Bunyu, Kago, Binchi Baku and Dutsen Abo 'all dead'. The 'all deads' follow the extreme edge of the escarpment, where tsetse were most numerous (Nash 1948a).

The Rukuba epidemic was a consequence of the creation of an appropriate biogeocoenosis. That this creation was, in one sense, an effect of the *Pax Britannica* is self-evident. The removal of the villages from the remote hilltop strongholds to the more convenient but much more dangerous escarpment sites was a sequel to Lugard's conquest of Zaria. This had taken place thirty years before the epidemic began and Duggan's account accepts local evidence that up to 1930 the Rukuba were free of infection. It follows that when they descended to the new locations and displaced the wild animals as hosts of *G. palpalis*, the latter were also free of trypanosomes infective to man. The Rukuba claimed that they had first become infected through their contacts with the neighbouring locality of Piti and they called the condition *ciwon Piti* meaning 'the Piti disease'. Piti is less than 10 miles away from the centre of Rukuba and the infection had been recognized there in the early 1920s (Duggan 1962b). The Piti infection had been derived from Lere, 25 miles to the north, and Lere had been earlier involved in an epidemic spread down the Galma river from the area just east of Zaria Town which included the districts of Soba and Anchau and the village of Gimi, also on the Galma, where the epidemic spread began in 1917.

Gimi had been established by the Emir of Kano to accommodate a local Christian community in 1915. Other, earlier, villages had been sited there, but survivors of the 1917 epidemic maintained that it had hitherto been 'fertile and salubrious' and that sleeping sickness was unknown in that part of Kano before 1917 (Duggan 1962a). Gimi is over 100 miles from Rukuba.

The Piti area continued as a dangerous focus of infection although the disease had seemed to have been eliminated by 1954. In 1958 a survey showed an infection incidence among some 2000 people of 0·8 per cent. By 1962 there were 200 cases among 2438 people examined, giving an incidence of 8·2 per cent. In that year Godfrey, Killick-Kendrick, and Leach (1962) published the result of a parasitological survey of cattle at Rahama, only about 5 miles from Lere town and situated between the headwaters of the Galma and the Karami rivers. Some 70 per cent were infected with *T. congolense*, suggesting close proximity to and infection from *G. morsitans* (cf. Chapters 9 and 18). The maps show that Rahama was then just on the edge of the salient of infestation by that tsetse which had been spreading south-eastwards through the country drained by the Karami and Kaduna rivers since Nash (1948a) had seen the first sign of it at Pambeguwa in 1944. The Rahama cattle also showed a 4·7 per cent infection of *brucei*-group trypanosomes.

This history of spread of infection up into the headwaters of the Kaduna river system has all the characteristic features of the spread of the disease that was described locally in the Anchau area, to Tudun Wada and to Ningi, and evidently was part of the same process. It involved the spread of *G. morsitans*, the growth of the cattle population and its use by the tsetse as a food supply and vehicle of spread, and the assumption of the role of reservoir of human trypanosomes by the migrant herds. It may well be that the Rukuba had never known infection before; but it was not the *Pax Britannica* which brought about the epidemic. The cessation of Fulani aggression allowed them to descend from their mountain fastnesses where they had retreated during the nineteenth century (this was, it is true, a sequel to the *Pax*), but the infection was derived from maladjustment of domestic animal and wildlife relationships brought about by the rinderpest and the subsequent processes of recovery. In particular it was brought into the Kaduna–Mada–Gurara watershed area, for which the name Zonkwa can be retained, by the migrant cattle on their annual transhumance. Again, the evidence is ready to hand in another map produced by the Veterinary Services, the significance of which, in the epidemiology of sleeping sickness, has not yet been considered. It was published by Glover (1965) and is reproduced in Map 23.4 to show the correlation between the various elements in the biogeocoenosis that has been described. This map was intended to indicate roughly, by means of the width of its arrows, the relative importance of the routes used in the annual transhumance. Four of them lead into the central dry-season grazing area of which Zonkwa forms the most northerly segment. One of the two more important routes runs south through the narrower portion of the central *G. morsitans* belt just east of Zaria; the second through the eastern extremity of this same belt. When these routes came into extensive use after the recovery of the cattle populations from the epizootic, the *G. morsitans* belts were fragmentary and the way south through Soba, Anchau, and other parts of the Galma and Kaduna valleys were probably free of this tsetse. Taylor (1930) may have been correct in thinking that the Fulani cattle near Ganawuri were not infected or, at any rate, were less heavily infected than they later became. But the boundaries of this central grazing area also abutted on the *G. longipalpis* belt and, indeed, overlapped it. It still does so, but now and for years past, its endemic infection has been annually reinforced by the contact made by cattle with the *G. morsitans* belts across the Kano, Galma and Kaduna valleys.

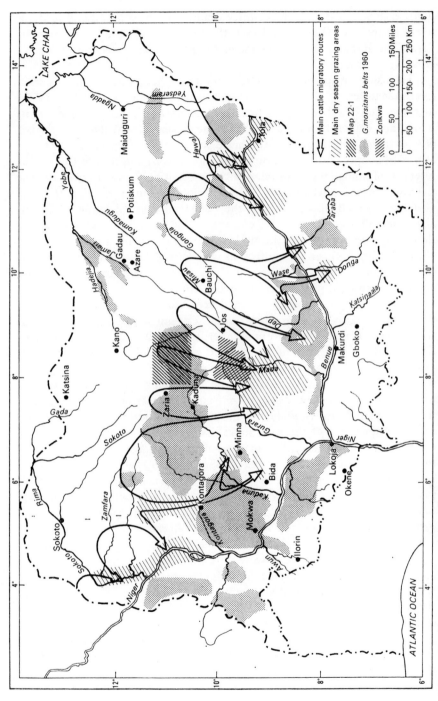

MAP 22.1. Map (from Glover 1965) to show the position of Map 22.1 and of the Zonkwa scheme in relation to major cattle transhumance routes.

Conclusion on epidemic zone (2)

In Chapter 22 it was suggested that the contrast between Heinrich Barth's estimate of 30–40 million for the population of Nigeria in 1854 and Lugard's 9 million in 1900 had, although much exaggerated, some foundation in fact. The depopulation brought about by Fulani aggression and intensified slave raiding after the death of Sultan Bello of Sokoto in 1840 continued into the early years of the colonial administration. The supposition that before this depopulation began the area of *G. morsitans* infestation was very much smaller than it became after 1930 is supported by the accounts of early travellers. In these circumstances the mechanism of spread and maintenance of infection through seasonally migrant cattle would not have been operative. Even if it were, and had been forgotten during the years of chaos, it must have been extinguished when the rinderpest panzootic killed off most of the cattle and most of the hosts of *G. morsitans* including, especially, *Tragelaphus scriptus*. A period followed in which the link provided by cattle between the game trypanosomes and the riverine vectors, if it had ever existed, must have been broken. This was not the case in epidemic zone (1), where *G. morsitans* and its wild hosts, *G. tachinoides*, man, and his cattle all shared the same dry-season water supplies and where infection persisted throughout the last century, but where, it is to be hoped, it has finally been eliminated by use of insecticides.

24

THE EPIDEMIOLOGY OF
WEST AFRICAN SLEEPING SICKNESS

Trypanosome strains and variations in the sleeping sickness syndrome

THE review of sleeping sickness given in the last chapter differs from that of Duggan (1962a), on which it is largely based, in maintaining that the pattern of epidemics was only in a minor degree a consequence of the *Pax Britannica*. It also suggested that gambian trypanosomiasis was caused by trypanosomes derived, at no very great interval of time, from wild animals as are those that cause the rhodesian and Zambezi varieties of the disease. Transmission is believed to occur through *morsitans*-group tsetses from the wild host to domestic animals (pigs and Muturu cattle) and thence, via the *palpalis*-group flies, to man. In the Niger–Benue primordial focus the principal agent in effecting the transfer of the trypanosome from the wildlife ecosystem to the human–domestic animal community is *Glossina longipalpis*. In the Chad river and Kaduna river headwaters foci, new strains of trypanosomes are periodically introduced into the Northern Guinea and Sudan zones by migrant Fulani cattle. The latter receive these infections either while in transit through the *morsitans* fly-belts or from *G. longipalpis* encountered in the southern dry-season pastures.

This hypothesis must be extended if it is to cover the whole range of epidemiological phenomena associated with West African sleeping sickness. The greatest obstacle to the understanding of trypanosomiasis has been and continues to be the fact that morphology, the image of the causal organism seen under the microscope, can only convey a very limited notion of its properties as a pathogen. A *brucei*-type trypanosome will probably kill dogs and horses easily and will usually produce an infection in cattle and pigs so mild that it may not be noticed. In man it either fails completely to infect or it may infect and kill. When a *brucei*-type trypanosome is recovered from a wild or domestic mammal or from a tsetse fly, its power to affect man can only be ascertained by inoculating it into a reasonably large sample of human volunteers. This is a method difficult to use and gives little scope for experimentation. In West Africa where chronic strains may take months to become patent, it may be useless and dangerous. It is still only possible to discuss the circumstantial epidemiology of human trypanosomiasis in a terminology invented many years ago, and it is not surprising that since Lester examined several strains of

Nigerian trypanosomes in the 1930s, little other comparative work has been done and little relevant advance beyond the position achieved by him has yet been made.

Lester recognized three disease categories:

(1) The commonest was the mild form which, in the 1930s, constituted more than 95 per cent of the cases at mass surveys. After initial fever and headache the patient reached a stage when the disease and his resistance to it seemed to have achieved a state of equilibrium. Symptoms included enlarged cervical glands, puffiness of face and limbs, some albuminuria. Patients were below par mentally and physically and might remain in this state for years. Some recovered but in general it was their lowered resistance to other diseases which was at the root of the very real depopulation that occurred.

(2) The second type was more rare and toxaemia was its salient feature. Oedema was more pronounced and certain patients became 'completely water-logged' and developed well-marked ascites. They died relatively quickly without showing signs of nervous involvement.

(3) In the third type, the disease followed the textbook description of 'gambiense' disease (see Chapter 4). The nervous system was affected and the patient commonly became a 'sleeper'. 'Varying degrees of mental aberration up to acute mania are common' (Lester 1938, 1945).

Some of the strains described by Lester (1933, 1939) were obtained from patients at Gadau, in the centre of the Chad rivers epidemic zone. Others came from Ayu, a focus of epidemic infection below the western scarp of the Bauchi plateau and associated perhaps with the Niger–Benue infestation of G. longipalpis, perhaps with the Zonkwa area around the Mada–Gurara–Kaduna watershed.

In both areas the strains could be grouped into two categories. Six from Gadau and five from Ayu could be regarded as variants of Trypanosoma 'gambiense'. But from both places strains were collected which in all respects save that they had been collected in West Africa from people who had almost certainly received them through the bite of palpalis-group tsetses behaved like T. 'rhodesiense'. These became famous as Gadau 6 and Ayu 6 and they were very similar to a strain collected some years before, from the Chad rivers area, and called 'Sherifuri K'.

Lester's general conclusion about the trypanosomes found in Nigerian patients was that not only do strains having all the characteristics ascribed to T. 'rhodesiense' occur, but there is a whole series of strains with characteristics intermediate between T. 'rhodesiense' and T. 'gambiense'. There was an implication that rapidly developing and disruptive epidemics were associated with an abundance of strains having 'rhodesiense' characteristics, and that 'gambiense' type strains were commoner where the disease was more chronic. But it is difficult to relate the variability characterizing different epidemic and endemic conditions with variability in strains classified by laboratory techniques. This difficulty has increased with time and is in part a consequence of the activities of medical services.

Sequels to mass treatment campaigns

Lester's successor in charge of the Nigerian Sleeping Sickness Service took a view of the disease somewhat different from that of his predecessor. He did not accept that the majority of cases were mild, chronic infections that were liable to collapse under the stress of intercurrent disease. To him the majority of patients that died did so from an acute toxaemia that was a direct consequence of the infection. 'A very considerable proportion of deaths, apart from advanced cases, arises from acute toxaemic exacerbation of the actual trypanosomiasis.' This was so even with people who had 'had the usual minor manifestations of the disease for months or even years' (McLetchie 1948).

It is possible that both doctors were correct. Lester's experience in the field had been built up by observing the effects on people of trypanosome populations hitherto subject to the natural environments provided by the blood and other tissues of a succession of various vertebrate and insect hosts. McLetchie, who joined Lester's team just at the peak of the epidemic of the 1930s, had seen the effects of trypanosome strains that, by the time he began his work, had been subjected to an entirely novel environment provided by the blood of some 200 000 people, flushed through with intravenously injected tryparsamide.

The spectacular effects of this drug in the Congo basin, as well as its failure to bring about the elimination of all infective trypanosome strains in the endemic areas of that country, were described by van Hoof (1947). The property of resistance to arsenical drugs was long regarded as a specific character of T. 'rhodesiense' (Chapter 4), but it is now clear, in part because of results seen in the field, that while normal arsenic-sensitive strains of T. 'gambiense' can be made resistant to arsenical drugs by underdosing, as happens when people fail to present themselves to complete a course of treatment, strains naturally resistant to arsenic do occur in areas where no medicaments have ever been used. Moreover, a high proportion of the milder, more chronic and near-symptomless cases are caused by strains very sensitive to tryparsamide. In short, a mass campaign using tryparsamide leaves behind a residual population of trypanosomes having properties different from those of the parent population from which they were derived. In particular it is now difficult to obtain information about the very mild forms of the disease. They were evidently far more common in the past than they have since become. It is not possible to understand the role of trypanosomiasis in West African communities before the colonial impact, especially before the vigorous application of the 'sterilization' principle of Koch took effect, without examining these mild forms of the disease at greater length.

The very mild chronic disease

At the height of the epidemic that Lester and his team were attempting to control in Northern Nigeria, medical officers in the south were concerned with a very widespread endemic condition. This had first been described by Scott Macfie (1913*b*) who had been so impressed by its apparent harmlessness that he thought it must have been caused by a trypanosome different from *T. 'gambiense'*. He therefore gave it a new name, *Trypanosoma nigeriense*. It was subsequently recognized as a form of *T. 'gambiense'*. Twenty years later the infection was still widespread. 'The "mild" areas in Southern Nigeria, where sleeping sickness may be so shy and modest in its manifestations that its presence often passes unnoticed' were described by Hope Gill (1935). 'In large areas where the disease has been long established and is endemic the actual percentage of infection may be very high, though the symptoms are slight or unrecognisable, the great majority of the infected being children whose only symptom complained of is enlarged glands.' That children displaying such swollen glands were likely to have a dramatically shortened life had for long been evident to residents of areas in which the condition occurred. 'It has been repeatedly observed in old-standing endemic areas that there are large numbers of comparatively healthy natives of all ages who show the scars of excision of neck glands, which is believed by them to be an effective cure and many of these operations have been performed in childhood' (Hope Gill 1935). This operation was studied by various colonial doctors with the verdict that it could not affect the course of the disease. It had to be concluded that in these areas a majority of cases either were symptomless and infection did not affect the patient's ability to perform his daily tasks or that many children threw off the disease completely. 'In the Eket area I can support Macfie's observation that the majority of young children have typically enlarged glands, whereas this condition is not nearly so common among the adults, and yet there is no sign of any abnormal diminution of the population which one would expect if each infected case proved fatal. The number of third stage cases [i.e. "sleepers"] is also remarkably small' (Hope Gill 1935).

Macfie (1913*b*) had described the environment of the people among whom these infections were found.

The country round Eket [*south-west, over the Cross River, from Calabar*] is an undulating plateau covered with dense bush, and intersected by numerous waterways. It includes a good deal of swampy land. The district is densely populated. The towns consist of scattered compounds standing some distance apart, and closely surrounded by farms and banana trees. They are usually very dirty, and some cattle, and a good many pigs, goats, and fowls are kept in them. The towns are generally some distance away from the waterside. Their water supply is obtained at two or three spots, which are closely surrounded by bush and trees, and approached along a narrow shaded path. The children and young adults are the water carriers, and Dr. Foran considers that this accounts for the majority of cases of sleeping sickness occurring in young people. Tsetse flies are prevalent all over the district. Dr. J. J. Simpson records *G. palpalis* and *G. caliginea* from Eket . . . but according to Dr. Foran, *G. tachinoides* is also a common species, at any rate during the months of September and October. He has shown that tsetse flies 'appear to follow pigs about more than any other animal, and it is generally easier to catch the flies where these animals are, than at the water'.

For the first time, the close association of *G. tachinoides* with pigs was observed. According to Simpson (1912) the southern half of the Eket district was at that time covered with virgin forest and practically uninhabited. The northern, inhabited portion was covered with low bush cut over every four years for cultivation.

Hope Gill (1930) had already compared 52 cases from an epidemic focus at Birnin Kudu on the Katagum river, in the Chad area, with a sample of the same size from Pankshin on the southern edge of the Bauchi plateau, on the northern boundary of the Niger–Benue primordial focus. Among the first group 35 showed symptoms of sleepiness and all had some complaint associated with the disease. Among Pankshin cases, who belonged to a 'pagan' tribe called Tof, 7 revealed no symptoms at all and were unaware that they were ill and none showed signs of becoming 'sleepers'. The majority of them were comparatively fit and only swollen glands gave a clue to diagnosis. The majority of the Birnin Kudu cases were of considerable severity.

The explanation adopted was that already applied to the Busitema and Namatala areas in Busoga by Van Hoof (see Chapter 16). 'Sleeping sickness varies in severity in proportion to the length of time a particular strain of trypanosome has been endemic in a population', and 'the virus becomes attenuated in an endemic area if no new elements, trypanosomes, flies, or men, are introduced' (Hope Gill 1935). To this statement the present account adds fourth and fifth elements. They are (1) reservoir mammals, whether wild or domestic, and (2) stress conditions that may arise from a variety of causes but include intercurrent infections. Further to this one may add that if the milder forms of the disease are looked upon as manifestations of the process of mutual adjustment of host and parasite, a sixth element tending to prevent adjustment, and so to maintain the severity of the disease, is the administration of drugs which preferentially select for elimination the milder strains. Support for this view comes from McLetchie's review of Hope Gill's (1930) work sixteen years later. 'Today sleeping sickness is rather more common and more deadly in the same area of Pankshin than it is in Birnin Kudu' (McLetchie 1948). This is not to say that treatment ought not to be undertaken. The problem was made explicit in a focus of infection studied in Sierra Leone. It is described here because it is is a comparatively recent example of what seems to have been the first appearance of a strain in mutual adjustment with its human hosts.

The Fuero strain

The Fuero strain was discovered by Harding and Hutchinson (1948) near the border of Sierra Leone and what is now the Republic of Guinea. The infection was not precisely similar to that described by Macfie and Hope Gill. A high proportion of cases were indeed symptomless but a few of them showed cervical gland enlargement. The disease was found by accident during the course of a survey of a much larger infected area which lay partly in Sierra Leone, partly in Guinea, and partly in Liberia. Later it became notorious as the Kissi focus, an excellent example of a modern *Grenzwildnis* situation (Hutchinson 1962, Bangoura-Alecaut 1962).

In the area as a whole the disease presented no outstanding peculiarities. Diagnosis was made by gland puncture and by blood-slide, and it was found that for every case diagnosed by positive blood another four were found with positive gland juice. Incidence of the disease varied from village to village, but was mostly between 6 and 14 per cent. The first peculiarity noted at Fuero was that a much higher proportion of people had trypanosomes visible in their blood. The ratio of gland to blood diagnoses was 1 : 2 instead of 4 : 1. Moreover, the trypanosomes when present in blood were often unusually abundant. One of these people with abundant trypanosomes in his circulation was examined a few days later and found to be negative. This suggested that cases were being missed with only a single examination. Re-survey was undertaken and more cases were found. Many of these people were without symptoms of disease and apparently quite healthy. The distribution of the infection was carefully plotted and found to be confined to an area, around Fuero, of only about 14 mile^2 in which about 900 people were living. Moreover, it seemed that it must have appeared between 1941 and 1942, for examination of the records of 1940 and 1941 surveys revealed no abnormality in the gland to blood positive ratios.

By 1944 the area in which the Fuero strain was dominant had greatly increased and at its centre, in Fuero itself, the strain characteristics had become more marked. The gland to blood positive ratio was now 1 : 10 (as against the normal 4 : 1); the proportion of symptomless cases was very high, and when trypanosomes were found in the blood they were often very numerous. This sort of situation presents considerable ethical problems to doctors. Harding and Hutchinson (1948) described the spread of the Fuero strain between 1942 and 1944 as 'very serious' with the implication that it was a dangerous condition, chiefly because so much more difficult to diagnose by routine procedures. On the other hand it was perfectly possible to see in it the emergence of physiological adjustment between the human host and the parasite which would have allowed the community to continue to live in comparatively good health without fear of the more dramatic forms of the disease making their appearance.

This was, of course, clear to Harding and Hutchinson. In 1944 they selected a number of cases for observation and left them untreated, but examined them weekly for two months. Fifty-one were symptomless at the beginning and only one developed symptoms. Twenty admitted intermittent headache at the initial diagnosis, but none of these showed any deterioration at the end of two months. Seventeen of these symptomless or very mild cases were followed for seven to nine months. All save 3 showed no change in condition and none showed any physical impairment.

The Fuero strain was very sensitive to tryparsamide, a typical *gambiense* character; but the low proportion of swollen and positive glands was atypical. A higher proportion than was usual with ordinary *T. gambiense* cases not only showed positive blood, but also an abnormal white cell count in the cerebro-spinal fluid. There were indications that a high proportion of infected people proceeded to spontaneous cure; although in some the disease developed normally and they would have died had no treatment been given.

The whole picture suggests that this particular race of man and this particular strain of *Trypanosoma gambiense* exist in a state of generally satisfactory adaptation to one another recalling the adaptation between game animals and their trypanosomes. Or to take another example, that between cattle and the less virulent strains of *T. congolense*. . . . It would, however, be entirely unsafe to assume that the Fuero epidemic, if left to itself, would not change its present comparatively harmless character. There are already some indications of a tendency towards reversal to the more normal type (Harding and Hutchinson 1948).

Adjustment of host and parasite

The 'normal' type was the type of sleeping sickness most characteristic of the Kissi area at the time. The Fuero strain differed in some respects from Scott Macfie's '*Trypanosoma nigeriense*' at Eket and the trypanosomes that infected Hope Gill's Tof villages near Pankshin in 1930. It is arguable that these very mild, nearly symptomless infections had been the true 'normal' for centuries. The possibility that those forms characterized by swollen glands might break down into the advanced form of the disease had long been recognized and dealt with by isolation and by gland excision (Hoeppli and Lucasse 1964). The former method kept infective persons out of range of tsetse inhabiting places where many people congregated. The second also had at least the value to the community, if not to the patients, that some must have died under the surgeon's knife and so ceased to exist as sources of infection. Both McLetchie's comment on the Pankshin cases and the observation by Harding and Hutchinson that the Fuero strain was reverting to the more 'normal' type suggest that mass treatment had the effect of selecting out the historically 'normal' strains and leaving as survivors the strains that more readily produced 'advanced' forms of the disease.

The second point is suggested by the comparison made between the effects of the Fuero strain in man and of a mild *T. congolense* strain in cattle. It is a comparison that could have been carried further for these mild, chronic strains of *T. brucei gambiense* were most commonly found in the two ecological zones in which had survived, over many centuries, two types of cattle distinguished by their ability to adjust themselves to trypanosome infection. The humpless longhorn or N'Dama cattle were first found on the Fouta Djallon highlands of Guinea and are essentially inhabitants of the high forest edge and Guinea zone of vegetation. The West African humpless shorthorn, known by a variety of local names, but most commonly called, in Nigeria, Muturu, belong to the forest-edge and forest–savanna mosaics. The geographical ranges of the two types met not far from Fuero, near the western frontier of Liberia. They are the two oldest cattle types in tropical Africa, having preceded the zebus by many centuries.

Calves of these cattle acquire from the dam's colostrum a temporary supply of antibody against trypanosome infection and, provided that they are themselves infected early in life, build up their own antibodies against local strains of trypanosomes. They do, much more efficiently, what zebu cattle can also do under favourable conditions. Like the zebus they are liable to collapse from the infection if subjected to stress conditions, such as are provided by intercurrent disease or, when they are moved into new areas, they encounter new strains of flagellates, or again, having been born outside tsetse-infested areas, are later introduced into them as adult animals (Desowitz 1959). In short, they reproduce, in respect of *T. congolense* and *T. vivax*, the condition postulated by Harding and Hutchinson for the people of Fuero—'this particular race of man and this particular strain' of *T. 'gambiense'* is duplicated by these particular races of cattle and these particular strains of *T. congolense* and *T. vivax*.

Trypanosoma brucei in domestic animals

In eastern Africa the picture of the association of the human trypanosome, *T. brucei rhodesiense*, with antelopes, domestic animals, and *Glossina* of both *morsitans* and *palpalis* groups is clear, at least in its broader outlines. The principal relevant studies are the Tinde experiment, the discovery of *T. brucei rhodesiense* in bushbuck by Heisch, McMahon, and Manson–Bahr (1958) and in domestic cattle by Onyango, van Hoeve, and de Raadt (1966; Chapters 4 and 16).

A partial replication of the Tinde experiment was carried out at Leopoldville (Kinshasa) by Van Hoof, Henrard, and Peel (1940). They infected a domestic pig with *T. brucei gambiense* from a patient and maintained the strain by cyclical transmission through *G. palpalis* from pig to pig over a period of four years during which time two volunteers were infected. At the end of the experiment the strain had ceased to be transmissible. The pigs showed no signs of disease and often no trypanosomes were visible in blood slides. However, until transmissibility was lost, flies could still be infected although the animals showed no patent parasitaemia. Especially in the early passages there was a striking contrast between the rarity of the flagellates circulating in the blood and the high degree of transmission. It was also observed that the reinfection of a pig which had been naturally cured could only be achieved with difficulty and that even when this was done successfully, the infection was of short duration. Thus it was thought that in looking for natural infections in pigs in endemic sleeping sickness areas, one should preferably examine young animals (Van Hoof 1947). One is reminded of the prevalence of patent infection in children observed by Macfie and Hope Gill in the 'mild' areas in Southern Nigeria.

Watson (1962) also infected a pig with *T. brucei gambiense*. It supported the infection for 70 days. During the first 41 days 10 out of 183 *G. palpalis* that were fed on it developed mature infections, but from the 42nd day onward the trypanosomes in infected flies did not develop beyond the 'gut' stage and failed to reach the salivary glands. Thus there is sound parasitological evidence that domestic pigs could act as a supplementary reservoir for *T. brucei gambiense* in addition to man himself in those parts of West Africa in which these animals are kept. These are the non-Muslim areas and include the Tiv country in the centre of the Niger–Benue primordial focus, many of the 'pagan' areas around the Bauchi plateau, and the Ibo country on the southern borders of which lay the former areas of 'mild' infection around Eket. These non-Muslim areas are, in general, the areas of persistent mild endemic disease.

In the Muslim north the foci of infection are markedly localized and characterized by alternating endemic and epidemic phases. The migrant cattle are not so much reservoirs of infection as carriers of infective strains along particular routes. The credit for demonstrating that this could happen with *T. brucei rhodesiense* belongs to Wilde and French (1945). They suggested that cattle could convey the parasites from endemic sleeping sickness areas to others where the disease was absent but the vector was present.

There is little specific evidence of the behaviour of *T. brucei gambiense* in cattle. Hornby (1952) recalls the few observations made and concludes that the infection is very mild as, indeed, is that of *T. brucei* in the sense of *brucei*-group trypanosomes not infective to man.

The evidence from trade cattle has already been mentioned (Chapters 5 and 22). Of the 28 animals examined by Godfrey, Killick-Kendrick, and Ferguson (1965) 12 became infected with *T. brucei* on their passage through the fly-belts north of the Niger. Of these infections 9 only became patent in the blood and 3 were discovered only by sub-inoculation into rats. Of the 9 patent infections it was observed that 'on most days after the initial patency it was difficult to find *T. brucei* in the blood'. All of these 9 were infective to rats at least one day before the trypanosomes were detectable in the blood. On the last day of the experiment, when only 9 animals were still alive, all were infected with *T. vivax*, 7 also had *T. congolense* infections, but *T. brucei* could only be detected in 4, by use of the sub-inoculation method. Cattle adjust themselves very easily and rapidly to infection by *T. brucei*, including the human infective strains. They are therefore particularly well adapted to serve as carriers of infection for limited periods of time.

The use of xenodiagnosis, that is the detection of infection in an animal yielding parasite-free blood slides by feeding tsetse flies on it and, in due course, showing that they have developed an infection, was particularly developed by Belgian workers. It is almost certain that the cattle on Nigerian trade routes that have acquired infection of *T. brucei* but have ceased to reveal it microscopically in the blood, would, for a time, continue to infect *Glossina*. Nevertheless, just as infected tsetse fail, at some meals, to inoculate an infective dose of metacyclic trypanosomes, so it may be supposed that the disappearance of the flagellates from blood slides must indicate a reduced opportunity for tsetse to imbibe them with its blood meal. It is reasonable to suppose that the short period in which *T. brucei* is patent in the peripheral blood of cattle that have traversed a fly-belt, is one in which its infectivity to *Glossina* is enhanced.

Biting rates, host choice, and infection rates in *Glossina*

Evidence from blood meals

Table 24.1 reproduces blood meal analyses for Nigerian species of *Glossina*, but omits data from meals identified as to host families only, save in the case of birds and reptiles. This is done so that blood meals obtained from man or domestic Bovidae can be shown precisely in relation to feeds from wild animals. The two *fusca*-group species showed no feeds from man, but both had taken a few meals from cattle. *G. tabaniformis* is predominantly a feeder on wild Suidae and *G. fusca* on wild Bovidae. Of its 74·9 per cent of meals from this family, 98·0 per cent were taken from the bushbuck, *Tragelaphus scriptus*. The third tsetse which may be grouped with the above as a forest or forest-edge dweller is *G. longipalpis*. It rarely attacks man or cattle, but lives predominantly on wild Bovidae among which the bushbuck supplies 81·0 per cent of its meals.

Table 24.1 indicates that in respect of biting attack on man the probability of transmission of infection to him is greatest in *G. tachinoides* and that the probability decreases through *G. palpalis* and *G. morsitans* to *G. longipalpis* and is nil in the two *fusca*-group species. With some reservations about the relative importance of the first two species this is the order in which most field workers would have placed the six species. If, however, the primary source of infection is the wild antelope reservoir (and this

TABLE 24.1

Summarized blood meal analysis of Nigerian tsetse†

Species	Number analysed	Wild Suidae (%)	Wild Bovidae (%)	Domestic Bovidae (%)	Other mammals (exc. man) (%)	Birds and reptiles (%)	Man (%)	Total (%)
Fusca group								
G. fusca . .	616	14·4	74·9	0·2	10·4	0	0	99·9
G. tabaniformis .	227	69·6	4·8	3·5	22·0	0	0	99·9
Morsitans group								
G. morsitans . .	1083	46·1	18·0	1·7	8·8	7·1	18·3	100·0
G. longipalpis . .	872	3·9	91·8	1·7	0·6	0·2	1·6	99·8
Palpalis group								
G. palpalis . .	298	4·0	13·1	5·7	4·7	36·9	35·6	100·0
G. tachinoides .	233	1·3	3·0	14·6	10·6	54·1	16·3	99·9

† From Weitz (1963).

might not be accepted by all field workers) then the species most important are *G. longipalpis* and *G. fusca*. Finally, if the hypothesis that trypanosomes derived from wild animals are first transmitted to domestic animals is acceptable, then it is necessary to combine the probabilities for feeding on wild and domestic bovids. The order of importance as agents for transmitting the parasite from a wild to a cattle reservoir emerges as:

G. longipalpis	$91{\cdot}8 \times 1{\cdot}7 =$	156·1
G. palpalis	$13{\cdot}1 \times 5{\cdot}7 =$	74·7
G. tachinoides	$3{\cdot}0 \times 14{\cdot}6 =$	43·8
G. morsitans	$18{\cdot}0 \times 1{\cdot}7 =$	30·6
G. tabaniformis	$4{\cdot}8 \times 3{\cdot}5 =$	16·8
G. fusca	$74{\cdot}9 \times 0{\cdot}2 =$	16·0.

From the same table and in the same way the order of probabilities for the six species transmitting infective trypanosomes from cattle to man is:

G. tachinoides	789·9
G. palpalis	202·9
G. morsitans	31·1
G. longipalpis	2·7
G. tabaniformis	Nil
G. fusca	Nil.

Using the same argument, the areas in which one would expect to find the most frequent double transmission, from wild to domestic Bovidae and from the latter to man, will be those in which one or the other or both of the two riverine tsetses, *G. tachinoides* and *G. palpalis*, occupy areas overlapping the habitat of *G. longipalpis*. Where the overlap of these species is with the *fusca*-group flies alone, then the transmission through cattle to man must be very rare, even discounting the fact that cattle themselves will be rare or absent in many *fusca* group habitats.

Similar arguments might be made in respect of the domestic pigs. It is usual for glossinologists to say that the *fusca*-group tsetse are of little economic importance and of none in respect of human health. This may be untrue. A pioneer family of forest dwellers moving to a new area and taking with them their domestic pigs (provided that the wild and domestic Suidae are equally acceptable as food for *Glossina*, and this is not known) would clearly be at greater risk of being inoculated with trypanosomes obtained at one remove in forest infested with *G. tabaniformis* than in the habitat of *G. fusca* (see also page 379).

The most notorious and long-standing focus of infection in the Central African Republic was at Nola on the Sangha river. Within 50 km of Nola five *palpalis* group and five *fusca*-group tsetse species have been found: *G. palpalis*, *G. fuscipes*, *G. caliginea*, *G. pallicera*, *G. newsteadi*, *G. fusca*, *G. nigrofusca*, *G. tabaniformis*, *G. haningtoni*, and *G. nashi*. Although only *G. palpalis* and *G. fuscipes* are regarded as of importance in transmitting infection from man to man, one knows of no other area in which there is evidence of so many and such varied transmission paths for trypanosomes parasitic in wild animals. At the same time it must be said that because of the horror with which Nola was regarded in the early years of this century and the difficulties encountered in bringing the infection there under control, it may have been the object of more intense entomological survey than other less recalcitrant centres. It should also be said that the persistence of Nola as an endemic focus with high infection incidence giving rise at intervals to epidemics is attributed, as are all other similar foci in the Congo basin and in the former French and British territories of West Africa, to a combination of topographical, hydrographical, demographical, and entomological circumstances particularly favouring the circulation of parasites from man to man through *G. palpalis*, *G. fuscipes*, and, perhaps, *G. caliginea*. The other seven species of tsetse and the wild and domestic animal hosts of trypanosomes have never been considered of any importance (Lotte 1952, Maillot 1961, 1962, Finelle, Itard, Yvore, and Lacotte 1963). It is an opinion that might profitably be revised.

The foregoing discussion of blood meal data would provide the basis for an epidemiological model if all hosts were equally available to all tsetses in an area or if the biting behaviour of a single species of tsetse were the same in all areas. Neither proposition is true.

Regional patterns of tsetse behaviour

Following the habitat studies on *G. palpalis* of Nash and Page (1953) and Page (1959*b*) in the Northern Guinea and forest zones respectively and

also the definitions of Nash (1944) of close personal and impersonal contact between man and tsetses, Page and McDonald (1959) compared the
recapture rates of marked flies to parties of men in these two ecological
zones in wet and dry seasons. They were chiefly concerned with those flies
that were recaptured at more than 17 days interval from marking, as this
was the time needed for an infection of *T. 'gambiense'* to mature. In the
more arid Northern Guinea zone the recapture rate in the dry season was
nine times and in the wet season seven times greater than in the more humid
forest region in the south. Their work gave a quantitative assessment of
'close personal man–fly contact' in the north as compared with the 'impersonal' contact characterizing the southern habitats. They suggested that
'the rarity of sleeping sickness in the south is believed to be due, in part at
least, to the absence of close man–fly contact' (Page and McDonald 1959).
Again taking a longer view it might, perhaps, be a more valid conclusion
that the former presence of a widespread, very mild, very chronic disease
in the south was associated with absence of close personal man–fly contact.

The same sort of geographical behaviour pattern in *G. tachinoides*,
studied by Baldry (1964, 1966, 1968), has been mentioned already and has
been shown by him to be associated with changes in feeding habit. In the
north it is a riverine fly, feeding readily on whatever host is available. In the
derived savanna or forest mosaics of the south it loses entirely its opportunist feeding habits, especially its readiness to feed on man, and becomes
a highly specific feeder on either domestic pigs or domestic cattle. The
situation is brought out clearly in Table 24.2 in which Baldry's results
(1968) are compared with the northern feeding pattern of *G. tachinoides*
given by Weitz (1963).

At Nsukka *G. tachinoides* is so dependent on pigs as hosts that its
populations decline almost to zero when these animals are removed from
the locality. The peri-domestic habit probably originated in the Benue
valley where *G. tachinoides* is essentially riverine, especially in the dry
season, but where, during the floods of the rainy season it moves to the new
water edge and finds temporary habitats in villages on higher ground where
man and his livestock are also concentrated. There is a 'transition from
northern riverine ecology to southern non-riverine ecology and the change
from feeding patterns that may be described as opportunist, but favouring man, to those that are specific and favour non-human hosts' (Baldry
1968).

These geographical distinctions of behaviour in two members of the
palpalis group are, perhaps, shared by *G. morsitans*. The differences observed in the responses of this species to an ox or to man at Yankari in the
Sudan zone and at Ilorin just south of the Niger–Benue primordial focus
have been described in Chapter 2. Man is far less acceptable as a food host
in this southern area, unless to teneral flies, which are of necessity still free
of trypanosomes. Although, therefore, as Unsworth and Birkett (1952) and

TABLE 24.2

Feeding patterns of G. tachinoides *at various localities south of the Niger–Benue valley compared with the pattern in the Sudan zone*†

Locality	Man	Domestic Bovidae	Domestic Suidae	Wild animals	Unidentified
Ilorin . .	1·0	99·0	0	0	0
Awka . .	0	97·3	1·3	0	0
Nsukka . .	1·8	5·6	76·0	0	16·6
Sudan zone .	54·1	14·6	0	31·3	0

% of meals derived from:

† After Baldry (1968), and Weitz (1963).

Godfrey, Killick-Kendrick, and Ferguson (1965) showed, cattle that had come through the Kontagora *G. morsitans* belt displayed, for a few days, abundant *brucei*-type trypanosomes in their circulations, *G. morsitans* would be far less likely to act as a direct zoonotic agent than in the northern Sudan zone (Ford 1969*b*).

Accompanying the change in the disease as one moves from north to south, that is, from an endemo-epidemic situation where the periodical epidemics are seriously disruptive and relatively frequent to the essentially endemic zone where the disease is milder, more chronic, and, at least in the past, often symptomless, there is a change in the responses of *Glossina* to man.

Personal and impersonal man–fly contact and the development of immunity

Nash's (1944) concept of close personal contact implied that the same group of people was being constantly bitten by the same small population of tsetses. The idea of *impersonal* contact did not in any way imply that people living in or visiting tsetse habitats were less frequently bitten by tsetses, nor should this notion be read into the results of Page and Mc-Donald, although it is implied by observation on peri-domestic *G. tachinoides* and the difference of intensity of attack on man and ox at different places by *G. morsitans*.

In Scott Macfie's (1912*b*) account of the biting attack by *G. palpalis* on children and adolescents visiting their village water holes there need be no implication that the same flies bit the same group of people every time they fed. In the forest there is no climatic barrier to movement by *G. palpalis*. In this environment more or less wide dispersal is possible throughout the year and as the recapture experiments showed, individual flies do not come back frequently to the same place.

In these conditions, provided there is a sufficiently dense and evenly distributed population of vertebrate hosts, i.e. of men, pigs, and Muturu cattle, the same strain of trypanosome would be widely and variously distributed throughout a community, two components of which, pigs and cattle, would serve as temporary reservoirs unaffected by the pathogenic properties of the parasite. Among the people adjustment to infection is effected by the operation of social practices already described and by physiological change.

In Chapter 4 it was shown that in the series of blood meals that it takes throughout its life, the infected tsetse may, in some of them, inoculate sufficient metacyclic trypanosomes to set up an infection in its host, but in other meals it may inoculate metacyclics that are too few to establish themselves and in yet other meals it may fail to inoculate any trypanosomes.

During the course of an infection trypanosomes multiply until they are visible in the blood and the patient feels the effects of the parasite when suffering fever and headache. He responds to the growth of the trypanosome population by producing antibodies which are in some degree protective and bring about a reduction of the parasite population; but not completely, for the trypanosomes again multiply and are no longer responsive to the first set of antibodies. Their antigenic properties have changed and the host must now make a new antibody response. He may overcome the infection. This is, perhaps, the least common result. He may reach a state of adjustment and, after an illness, continue to support a population of parasites which is controlled at a level at which its toxic properties do not seriously inconvenience him. This was the commonest condition in areas of endemic mild disease. This state of balance between parasite and host may represent a condition of premunity (Chapter 4). Thirdly, the patient may be unable to respond to the succession of antigens produced by the trypanosomes which continue to multiply, invade other organs, and kill him, either by an overwhelming toxaemia produced by the abundant parasite population or through damage to the central nervous system.

In the conditions of close personal contact described by Nash (1944) at the water-hole at Sambo, it is possible to imagine that some individuals may receive, from a single bite, a fully infective dose of metacyclic trypanosomes. Another may receive too small a dose of trypanosomes to overcome the antibody response they invoke and, as a result of this interaction the individual may be protected for a time against subsequent infection because his or her bloodstream contains protective antibodies induced by the first sub-infective bite. Yet again, a third individual might receive two bites more or less simultaneously, neither large enough to establish an infection, but both together adding up to a fully infective dose of metacyclic trypanosomes. Thus even if the vector population at the pool is originally only infected with a single strain of *T. brucei gambiense* the situation already includes the means for providing antigenic situations of considerable complexity among people visiting the pool. Included in these variant conditions may be some which offer the persons affected a chance of coming to terms with the infection. At the same time the substrains derived by inoculation into a number of people and, from them, the infection of hitherto uninfected tsetses might provide a mechanism for the sorting out of different antigenic variants, some of which might be linked with variation in pathogenicity. People who react unfavourably to infection and become ill more rapidly and suffer more severely will stay at home, perhaps to die, but in any case to remove from circulation the more dangerous substrains of trypanosomes they carry in their bloodstreams. This process will lead to community adjustment to infection, for all at risk of new infection will, increasingly, encounter strains to which the individual is able to produce a favourable immune response. Also involved in this process, it may be supposed, will be idiosyncratic differences between persons, some better able to develop protective antibody than others. Selection will take place in favour of persons better endowed than others to give adequate protective antibody response.

In the view of doctors concerned with the earlier outbreaks of sleeping sickness, strains that gave rise to very mild chronic infections were more easily transmissible than those having *rhodesiense*-like properties. The process envisaged above would therefore lead to the spread among susceptible populations of a mild easily propagated disease.

The chances that all these processes would together lead to the production of strains like the Fuero strain of Harding and Hutchinson (1948) or the '*Trypanosoma nigeriense*' of Scott Macfie (1913b) would be minimal in two sorts of situation. The first occurs where the actual focus of infection is small and the number of vectors is also small, as in Nash's Sambo example. Here an infective trypanosome will be quickly circulated among a small, select population (of water-drawers, washerwomen, etc.) who, when they become ill, withdraw from the scene and are replaced by other members of their families. There will be the minimum of opportunity for selection either for survival of milder substrains of trypanosomes or of persons giving a favourable response to infection. A high rate of infection in the hamlet will lead to its evacuation.

The second situation in which the effects of infection on a community will be exacerbated is that in which the vector population is liable to intermittent infection with new or heterologous strains of trypanosomes. In the foregoing account of trypanosomiasis in Nigeria the migrant herds of cattle have been seen as the vehicle by which a large population of *brucei*-type trypanosomes are annually concentrated along routes which bring them into the proximity of numerous hamlets like Sambo.

Human carriers of infection

Infective trypanosomes may be introduced into new communities by travellers who bring them with them in their bloodstreams. Sporadic outbreaks of sleeping sickness among people normally free of the disease may be explained in this way. A community lives in proximity to a river infested with *G. palpalis* or *G. tachinoides*, close personal contact is maintained, and all that is lacking is an appropriate trypanosome. An infected visitor arrives and all the elements needed to produce an epidemic are brought together. Much work has been done and much ingenuity used to prove that this is the way in which most epidemics of sleeping sickness have developed. It has been, perhaps even frequently, a way in which infection is spread; but that it was thus that the great devastating epidemics arose seems so improbable as to be impossible.

Movement of susceptible communities into endemic areas

The appearance and spread throughout a community of a chronic, mild disease has been seen as a process in which both the parasite and its hosts become more or less, though seldom completely, adjusted. There is some evidence that the properties of a trypanosome strain can change in response to its environment. In the course of twenty-two years at Tinde a gradual decline took place in the virulence of the strain of *T. brucei rhodesiense* in use. The vectors used were *G. morsitans* and the hosts sheep and men. A similar change, but a more rapid one, has been described in van Hoof's *T. brucei gambiense* in pigs. On the other hand Sandground (1947) enhanced the virulence, by repeated passage in rats, of *T. brucei gambiense* until it behaved, in those animals, like *T. brucei rhodesiense*. Such work suggests that the arrival in an endemic area of persons who had had no previous contact with infective trypanosomes might, because themselves unadjusted to infection, change the properties of the local trypanosomes so that even among the indigenous and already adjusted community an epidemic ensues that affects them as well as the newcomers. This could have been the cause of epidemics in areas where mine labour had been imported. The men did not bring the parasites with them, but in the places where they worked they provided a new physiological environment for local trypanosomes.

Serology and epidemiology

Serological research has been directed chiefly towards the problem of diagnosis of infection especially in West Africa where a high proportion of cases show negative blood and gland juice. Surveys using recently devised techniques for measuring change in the proportion of immunoglobulins in sera of persons at risk of infection soon began to show results of epidemiological significance. The development of these tests was due chiefly to

French workers at Dakar under the leadership of Mattern. They first showed, by use of electrophoresis, that the sera of 39 out of 41 patients, taken before treatment, contained a significantly high proportion of β-2-macroglobulin. After treatment the amount of this protein reverted to normal (Mattern, Masseyeff, Michel, and Peretti 1961). They suggested that their technique might be used as a means of diagnosis and they also noted that the β-2-macroglobulins possessed properties that suggested they were antibodies against trypanosomes. Enhanced immunoglobulins (IgM) may be found in other diseases, but in general other diagnostic information permits these to be excluded.

The entire population of an Ivory Coast village in an endemic area was surveyed by IgM estimation in blood sera in 1962. None of these 380 people had ever been given prophylactic treatment against infection. One of them was diagnosed as a new case in the first stage of the disease by conventional tests (blood slide, gland puncture). Sera from this one case as well as from 330 of his fellows was analysed by immuno-electrophoresis. Thirty-five, including the one new case, showed a significantly raised IgM level. Of these, 3 were old cases. The remaining 31, all apparently well, were taken into hospital for further tests. From 6 of them trypanosomes were isolated by triple centrifugation of blood. This left 25 people symptomless and all negative by the usual diagnostic tests. The only other likely source of enhanced IgM was chronic hepatitis and this was excluded (Bentz and Macario 1963, Macario and Bentz 1963).

All those shown to be positive by the IgM test, whether or not any other test had confirmed the diagnosis, were treated with pentamidine, and in all but two the IgM level fell to normal. One interpretation of this result is that the 25 entirely symptomless persons were, in fact, infected and therefore were trypanosome carriers, from whom, presumably, in favourable circumstances, the local *Glossina* might acquire an infection. The existence of such persons in a community would explain why mass survey and treatment might fail to eliminate the disease, as they would be missed by conventional diagnostic routines. That they were infected was suggested by the fact that although nearly all of them had previously declared themselves symptomless, after treatment many remarked upon the disappearance of headaches, muscular pains, and other symptoms which they recalled having suffered, usually at night.

On the other hand, there was no proof that they were a source of danger to their fellows. Trypanosomes could not be found. If they were present in other organs and only circulated in the bloodstream spasmodically it is possible that, like the strains in van Hoof's pigs, they would no longer infect *G. palpalis*. The third conclusion is that treatment with pentamidine, while relieving them of minor aches and pains, had also deprived them of antibodies which might have saved them from reinfection with more virulent and more highly pathogenic strains. These studies confirm accounts of early endemic situations in Nigeria. In times of comparative social stability, populations, particularly in the southern forest and forest–savanna areas, were able to achieve a considerable degree of physiological adjustment to infection.

Recapitulation: sequence of events and their epidemiological and epizootiological significance

How do the various factors postulated above fit into the historical sequence of events preceding and following the epidemic peak of 1935? As with other narratives, it is useful to finish with a timetable of these events and their epidemiological and epizootiological consequences.

1809–37   End of Jihad and consolidation and extension of the Fulani rule over Hausaland. Eastern limit provided by line of small buffer emirates between Hausaland and the Empire of Bornu.

1837–1900   Death of Sultan Bello of Sokoto in 1837. The Fulani spread southwards becomes involved with the Atlantic slave trade, as well as the traditional trans-Saharan and internal trade. Disintegration of Sokoto hegemony. Concentration of population in walled cities intensifies. 'Pagan' tribes hide in remote and inaccessible areas. Population decline.

Disruptive epidemics of sleeping sickness in the Chad river emirates along the *Grenzwildnis* between Hausaland and Bornu are said to have occurred at intervals during the second half of the nineteenth century. These were possibly provoked by the disturbed condition of the emirates during this period.

Indications of a reduction in the size of the horse population in the Southern Guinea and forest–savanna mosaic zones suggest that the human population decline since 1840 had permitted expansion of the *G. morsitans* fly-belts.

1887–91   Severe epizootic of contagious bovine pleuro-pneumonia followed by rinderpest panzootic. Periodically severe epizootics of rinderpest continue until mid 1920s when vaccination campaigns begin to bring disease under control.

The main effects of the rinderpest panzootic were:

(1) The cattle population was greatly reduced.

(2) Similar devastation affected the hosts of *morsitans*-group tsetses. Reduction of warthog and bushbuck populations were of especial epidemiological importance.

(3) This destruction of tsetse hosts caused a widespread shrinkage of the *G. morsitans* and perhaps *G. longipalpis* fly-belts.

(4) A secondary effect of the reduction of the cattle population and of the size of the fly-belts was the enlargement of available pasture.

(5) The recovery of the cattle population was very rapid although interrupted by further severe epizootics of rinderpest.

1889   Severe smallpox epidemic.

1900–6   Lugard's conquest of Hausaland.

1904   Famine.

1900–20   The human population first continues to decline and not until after 1920 is there evidence of the beginnings of recovery.

1905   First case of sleeping sickness diagnosed in the Niger–Benue area. Thereafter sporadic cases begin to appear throughout the country. This, in part, reflects the growth of the Medical Service.

1911   Simpson describes Kadara women at Ketare, where sleeping sickness has been identified, getting water from *G. palpalis*-infested streams and carrying their babies slung in bushbuck skins. Widespread, mild chronic or near symptomless sleeping sickness west of Calabar (Macfie's '*T. nigeriense*').

1914   Famine; rinderpest.

1918   Influenza pandemic.

1919   Rinderpest. The first severe local epidemic of trypanosomiasis is encountered on the Galma river at Gimi, having begun there in 1917.

1920–30   The disease is located at numerous foci, but particularly along the routes leading through the centre of the country into Hausaland and also among the 'pagan' tribe areas west and south of the Bauchi plateau. Many of these foci appear to be associated with the introduction of labour for gold and tin mining. Trypanosomiasis in the south and among 'pagans' around Bauchi plateau tends to be mild and chronic, but in the north on the Chad rivers and Kaduna system headwaters it is an acute infection.

Epidemics among mine labourers may be attributed either to importation of new strains in themselves or to the effects of local trypanosomes on people who had either not encountered trypanosome infections earlier in life or who, in their homes, had become accustomed to strains different from those they were now meeting.

1921   Johnson and Lloyd start tsetse-fly investigation.

1923–5   References to northward spread of cattle trypanosomiasis.

1927   Famine.

1930   Lester establishes the Sleeping Sickness Service based upon principles developed by the French Dr. Jamot. Veterinary services organize centres for administration of tartar emetic for cattle trypanosomiasis.

1931–41   Major epidemic period. Peak of 89 597 cases treated in 1935.

1941–51   Continuing decline in incidence of human trypanosomiasis. 17 202 cases treated in 1941, 7220 in 1951.

1944   First indication of spread of central G. morsitans fly-belt.

1930–58   Cattle trypanosomiasis treatments rise from 2313 in 1930 to 34 225 in 1949 using tartar emetic, and from 45 445 in 1950 to 771 438 in 1957 using new organic drugs.

1945–56   The Wukari G. morsitans belt, at its greatest extent covering some 2000 mile², disappeared under pressure of Tiv population growth.

1956–65   By contrast, the central fly-belt stretching east and west of Zaria expanded from about 7760 mile² in 1956 to 16 666 mile² in 1961 and 18 600 mile² in 1965.

1948–57   Second epidemic period. The epidemic fails to develop because adequately countered by the Sleeping Sickness Service, including large-scale entomological counter-measures, but some old foci are reactivated and this reactivation is associated with the spread of G. morsitans along cattle migration routes.

This correlation supports the view that the epidemic peak of 1935 was a sequel to the recovery of domestic and wild animal populations from the effects of the rinderpest panzootic.

1967   Thomson (1969) shows that foci identified over half a century ago are still active.

Thomson's paper demonstrates that endemic human trypanosomiasis is maintained over large areas by transmission from man to man by *palpalis*-group tsetses. In this it is in line with classical views of *T. brucei gambiense* as a purely human trypanosome. At the same time its evidence for the antiquity of certain foci of infection is best explained by the hypothesis that domestic animals serve as reservoirs of trypanosomes derived from wild hosts by transmission through tsetses of the *morsitans* or *fusca* groups. From the domestic animals the flagellates are conveyed to man by *G. palpalis* or *G. tachinoides*. The virulence of local strains is thus refreshed and, where this happens, there is repeated immunological failure by the population involved to overcome infection, even when assisted by medical treatment. This repeated introduction of new strains can only happen where appropriate biogeocoenoses favour their rapid circulation among local people and their domestic livestock. The residual foci of infection so created are persistent or, if they are extinguished, are easily reinfected because all the elements in the system are present except the one or two which nature or the control services have, for the time being, temporarily eliminated.

Parallels in Ghana

Nigeria was taken as an example for West Africa as a whole. It is necessary to ask if the same situations that have been described there have been met elsewhere. The history of sleeping sickness in Ghana has been reviewed by Scott (1965).

From 1901 to 1927 incidence of human trypanosomiasis in the country as a whole was low. In 1907 there were 34 cases and in 1926 37. The highest incidence had been observed in 1912 when there were 104 cases. In 1922 there were only 3. Numbers increased significantly in 1930 and reached a peak with 6826 cases in 1939. The epidemic subsided, but there was a reappearance of epidemic conditions between 1955 and 1959. As in Nigeria at about the same time this second epidemic phase was kept in control. The parallels are close, except that the major epidemic reached a peak four years later than that in Nigeria but having started between five and ten years later, in 1930 as against 1921–5.

Scott has pointed out that epidemic human trypanosomiasis spread across West Africa, beginning in Cameroon in the early 1920s, reaching Ghana and Haute Volta in 1930, and finally appearing in border areas of Guinea, Sierra Leone, and Liberia in 1939. He believes that the Cameroon epidemic was a spread from the Congo basin where, he suggests, an epidemic developed in 1912. This I find difficult to accept, for the Congo basin epidemic was already long-lived by that time; rather it is that Belgian and French medical services had, in 1912, begun to assess the magnitude of their problem. Maillot (1962) has mapped foci north and west of the Congo river in the former French Equatorial Africa that were active as early as 1887. The Congo epidemics had their origin in the social disruption produced on the one hand by Arab slave traders in the eastern Congo and by the brutalities of *concessionaires* of the Congo Independent State of Leopold II and, eventually, the conflict between the Europeans and the Arabs (Slade 1962). The westward progress of the epidemic from Cameroon is well established.

Two maps show that during the first and second epidemic periods the principal areas of infection lay in the north of Ghana, one overlapping the territory of Haute Volta in the Black Volta basin, the other, in the east, lying partly in Togo. In these areas transmission of the disease was through *G. tachinoides* and *G. palpalis* and both abut upon belts of *G. morsitans*. The vegetation map (Keay, Aubréville, Duvigneaud, Hoyle, Mendonca, and Pichi-Sermolli 1958) shows that the northern areas of persistent infection lie on or near the junction of the Sudan and Northern Guinea zones. Their ecological situation resembles that of the Chad–Kaduna river watershed foci of Northern Nigeria. In the more recent epidemic period these northern areas contained five residual foci defined as places where 'the disease is most prevalent in endemic periods and where epidemics first appear'. There is one other persistent focus. This, named Kpembe South, lies just north of a salient of 'transitional' vegetation, between the southern forest and the savanna zone. Keay *et al.* (1958) show this salient as composed of lowland moist forest. The focus is associated with the Daka and Oti rivers, tributaries of the Volta. Within 50 miles of it *G. palpalis, G. tachinoides, G. morsitans, G. longipalpis, G. fusca,* and *G. medicorum* have been recorded (Potts 1953–4). Entomologically it has, therefore, the characteristics of forest edge or forest–savanna mosaic foci seen in Nigeria and territories further east.

The geographical contexts are similar. Is there any similarity in historical antecedents, particularly with the parasitological upheaval attributed to the rinderpest panzootic and later disruptive epizootics? Can the westward movement of the rinderpest account for the later westward movement of the spread of sleeping sickness? According to Curasson (1932) the Fulani expected waves of rinderpest every twenty-five to thirty years. They always spread from the east. The French West African colonies were all infected, in the great panzootic, by 1892. The epizootic that appeared in Nigeria in 1914 reached Niger in 1915, Mali and Haute Volta in 1916, and thence to Senegal. Guinea and the Ivory Coast were invaded in 1917 and Togoland and neighbouring British territories were the last to be infected. It has been noted that there was an epizootic of some severity in Nigeria in 1919.

This sequence is of interest. The virus spread most rapidly through the areas of dense cattle populations. In Nigeria these are found in the Sudan and Sahel regions whence, in the dry seasons, the herds supplement their fodder by migration into the tsetse-infested regions of the Guinea zones. Every year large numbers move into territory that also supports the hosts of the *morsitans*-group tsetses. North of Ghana, however, this pattern is altered. The main areas of cattle concentration (especially the Fulani-owned cattle) are based upon the Niger. In the wet weather when grass and surface water are more readily available they spread throughout the Sahel, but in the dry weather, instead of moving south into the *Glossina* zone, they concentrate upon the Niger on the great bend between Niamey and Mopti (Stenning 1959). Here they are some 100–150 miles north of the tsetse line. Nomadic cattle between 2°E. and 5°W. are out of contact with the wild hosts of tsetse. Spread of the virus was westward from the Niger bend to the cattle based upon the basin of the Senegal river. Thence it moved eastwards again, but now it left the immunized survivors of the nomadic herds of the Sahel and travelled through the more sparsely distributed populations of N'Dama, Ghana shorthorn, and Muturu of the forest–savanna mosaics. The two cattle zones are clearly shown in Ady (1965). This return spread of rinderpest came through the *Glossina* zone and, though there are no data available, again it is to be supposed that the wild Suidae, the bushbuck, and other host animals of *morsitans*- and *fusca*-group tsetses were affected.

Scott remarks that the epidemic spread across West Africa must have had a cause shared in succession by each of the countries involved. This he takes, rightly it would seem, to be an argument against the *Pax Britannica* theory. He was unable to suggest the cause for the spread. The passage of the rinderpest provides a possible cause that would repay further historical and epidemiological study.

It was suggested that the cause of the minor epidemic peak observed in Nigeria in 1955 might be the rapid growth of the cattle population, assisted by the new drugs, which enlarged the size of the bovine reservoir for *brucei* group trypanosomes. The drugs came into use at about the same time throughout Africa. Vaucel, Waddy, de Andrade Silva, and Pons (1963) produce evidence of augmentation of the incidence of human infection in Sierra Leone, 1955–8; Mali, 1951–61; Ivory Coast, 1950–9; and Togo, 1958–60. Richet (1962) shows graphs of new cases and of the incidence of infection in a number of francophone countries of West Africa since 1940. The overall incidence throughout these countries in 1950 had been reduced to 0·2 per cent, so that evidence of what Vaucel *et al.* (1963) spoke of as '*poussées épidemiques locales*' as making up this increase in the 1950s are not very obvious compared to the rapid fall in incidence since 1940. Richet's data show that both Senegal, in 1957, and Dahomey, in 1956, also showed slight but distinct increases. Again, the proliferation of cattle, providing an enlarged reservoir for trypanosomes, suggests a cause in common throughout West Africa.

25

TSETSE-BORNE TRYPANOSOMIASIS:
A CONTINENTAL DISEASE

Peculiarities of African trypanosomiasis

THE presence of tsetses in Africa has often seemed to give a unique character to the tropical zone of that continent. Over a vast area, somewhat larger than the United States, the trypanosomes conveyed by these insects to man and to his domestic animals seem to offer hazards to health of a kind not encountered elsewhere. The distinction is apparent rather than real. Other large areas of the world present similar hazards. Numerous viral, bacterial, or protozoal infections are transmitted from their natural hosts by insects and other arthropods to man and his domestic livestock. There are many diseases of this kind in tropical Africa as well as the trypanosomiases. There is also at least one dangerous trypanosomiasis outside Africa. Chagas' disease, in Central and South America, is a distressing and often fatal infection caused by *Trypanosoma* (*Schizotrypanum*) *cruzi* which is transmitted by the reduviid bug, *Triatoma*. Among many reviews of the zoonoses those of Burnet (1953), Cockburn (1963), and Fiennes (1964), as well as reports of various symposia such as those edited by Horton-Smith (1957) and, recently, by McDiarmid (1969), illustrate, in one way or another, the features held in common by the African tsetse-borne trypanosomiases and other vector-borne diseases.

What was peculiar about African trypanosomiasis was its spectacular effect in eastern and southern Africa and the fact that, from the earliest times, this effect was obviously associated with one conspicuous insect. Cattle and horses died if their owners tried to take them into the valley of the Limpopo river, and it was quite clear that these deaths were a consequence of fly-bite. Many African cattle-owning tribes had long been aware of the connection and it seems difficult to avoid the conclusion that it was also known to the prophet Isaiah (Isaiah 7: 18–25).† Austen's (1903) monograph is still the best introduction to this aspect of the problem. The outer world was made aware of the human infection in an equally spec-

---

† See Westwood (1850). Verse 18 is well known to students of *Glossina*, but few have bothered to read to the end of Chapter 7. The late Professor Saul Adler was kind enough to look at this chapter in its original Hebrew and agreed that Verse 19 might well imply that the fly in the uttermost parts of the rivers of Egypt lived, as do the tsetses of the drier savanna areas, in land covered with thorns and bushes. It is in this drier sort of country that 'holes of the rocks' are most commonly used for larviposition. The most convincing verses, however, are Verses 23 and 25, for they describe, respectively, the apparent effects of tsetse 'advances' and the conditions in which tsetse are excluded by cultivation. An interesting speculative paper is that of Townshend (1923).

tacular manner. The role of tsetse in its transmission had remained as obscure as that of *Anopheles* in the transmission of malaria and until about the same date. Almost certainly if Europeans became infected with sleeping sickness before 1900, then their deaths must have been attributed to the same 'fevers' that made the west coast a 'white man's grave'. But hardly had the European powers assumed their various imperial roles when the Uganda epidemic, soon recognized as being identical with that already afflicting the Congo, was shown to be tsetse-borne. The discovery struck with alarm the imagination of those looking forward either to the commercial exploitation of the continent or to the spiritual reclamation of its inhabitants.

Essentially there is no fundamental difference between the epidemiologies of the African trypanosomiases and the numerous other infections that man and his livestock acquire through contacts with arthropods that normally live by sucking the blood of wild animals. In the next chapter some comparisons will be made between factors controlling the development of epidemics of trypanosomiasis and of malaria.

It has been a principal object of this study to show that notions of the circumstantial epidemiology of trypanosomiasis put forward in the first quarter of the century, even in its first decade, are long out of date. One consequence of their persistence is that much basic field work has not been done. The intention of these two concluding chapters is to suggest some ways in which a new outlook on control policies for African trypanosomiasis may be developed.

Measurement of ecosystems replacement

An aspect of the development of both human and animal trypanosomiasis, shared, indeed, with other diseases, is made clear in the foregoing narratives. It is usually neglected, except in the most general terms, in formal epidemiology and epizootiology. It is the aspect of the origin of zoonotic disease that has been referred to, from time to time in the preceding pages, as the conflict or confrontation of ecosystems. In the sense in which it has been used, it can be described quantitatively.

The effects of the decline and growth of Sukumaland upon the nature of the contacts between man and his cattle on the one hand and the tsetse belts on the other were described in Chapter 13. During the phase of growth or recovery of that area between 1938 and 1947 the *G. morsitans* belt west of Sukumaland receded by about 1000 mile[2] and at the same time, on its eastern boundaries, the *G. swynnertoni* belt also shrank by about 2500 mile[2]. It was possible to estimate roughly that this change resulted in the reduction of the total population of the former tsetse by about 21 million and of the latter by about 225 million individual insects. It was also possible to say that these events followed and, indirectly, were caused by, the growth of the Sukuma tribe by about 300 000 and of their

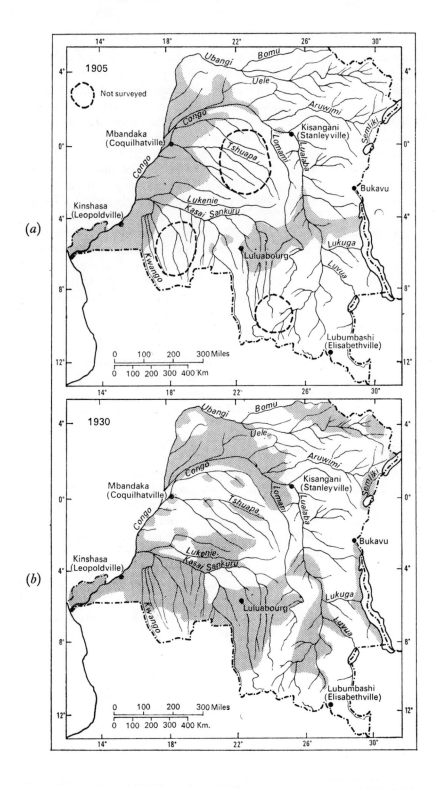

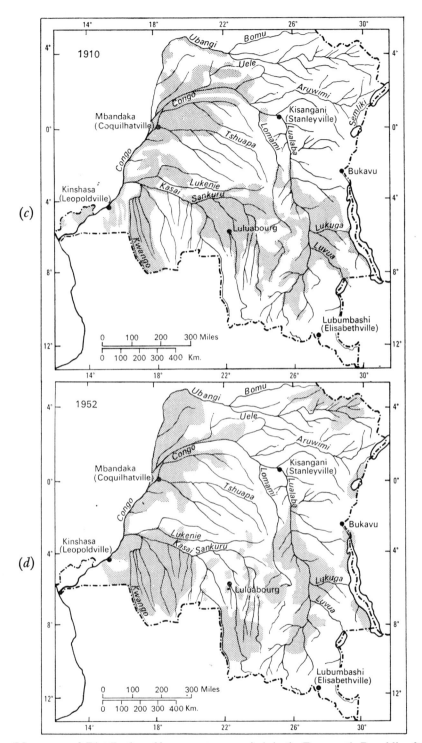

MAPS 25.1a–d. Distribution of human trypanosomiasis in the Democratic Republic of the Congo. 1905 from Dutton and Todd (1906); 1910 from Stohr (1912); 1930 and 1952 from Neujean and Evens (1958).

domestic cattle and small stock (sheep and goats) each by about 750 000 (Ford 1968). These are not the sort of statistics that usually interest entomologists or epidemiologists; but in underdeveloped countries they provide measurements of factors that are of the first importance in understanding the conditions in which diseases get out of control. One reason for this lack of interest among those directly responsible for the control of disease is that there is no possibility of interfering with an event that took place in the comparatively distant past. The present task is to diagnose infection and administer treatment or, perhaps, to locate the resting sites of tsetse and spray them with insecticide. These operations are not greatly assisted by a knowledge that a focus of infection is currently active because of the demographical consequence of a different infection twenty years earlier. Nevertheless once this kind of relationship is understood then it should be possible to define the ecological situations in which they are likely to occur. Conversely, where it can be shown that peasant farmers practising a subsistence type of agriculture are capable, above certain critical densities of population, of extinguishing the sources of infection, then it should be possible to define the conditions in which progress in development can continue without risk of severe epidemics or epizootics.

The Congo situation

Another approach to these wider aspects of epidemiology may be made by defining, in the first place geographically, the nature of those areas in which infection is persistent and where outbreaks are most likely to arise. This will not, at once, reveal the cause of localization of infection, but will lead to a more comprehensive view of its environmental contexts.

Maps 25.1a–d reproduce, in a somewhat simplified form, four maps of the distribution of human trypanosomiasis in the Democratic Republic of the Congo, formerly Congo Belge (Dutton and Todd 1906, Stohr 1912, Neujean and Evens 1958). Throughout the country the rivers are infested with tsetse of the *palpalis* group. As regards the principal vectors, all areas are equally dangerous. The centre of the country, that is, the basin of the Tshuapa river, the middle reaches of the Lomami and Lualaba rivers, and, in general, south, east, and north of Kisangani (Stanleyville) for some 150–300 miles and including most of the Aruwimi and the central Uele rivers, is free of infection. Except for very occasional localized outbreaks, this always has been so. Although this central portion is less heavily populated than the peripheral endemic areas, it is not devoid of people and its inhabitants are, for the most part, riverine dwellers. More is needed than the mere contiguity of people and *G. fuscipes*.

A minimum density of human population is a fundamental requirement for the maintenance of the endemic condition if, as is certainly the case, the overwhelming majority of transmissions are, via *G. fuscipes*, from man to man. There is nothing in this observation to provoke any doubts that gambian sleeping sickness is a purely human disease.

The campaign against the infection was begun in the first decade of the century. By the time of independence it seemed, at least on paper, that the task was nearing its completion. The campaign had passed through three main phases. During the first quarter of the century, when drug treatment was largely experimental and certainly inadequate, the main effort was directed towards locating infected people and isolating them in special hospitals (lazarets), thus interrupting the circulation of the parasite among people still uninfected. It was also a period of development of the field services and of training of personnel

During the first phase, in the middle of which, around 1912, the epidemic condition was extremely grave, it is only possible to obtain figures from village and other localized population surveys. A history of sleeping sickness in the Kwango district (Gabba 1938) shows: at Pondo, 21 per cent infected; at Bagata 17 per cent; at Leverville 17 per cent; at Kikwit 29 per cent; at Kimbinja 44 per cent. In the same area in 1918, after the medical services had been depleted by military needs for some three years, figures of 10, 13 and 20 per cent were still being obtained. Meanwhile the efficiency of the service greatly improved and in 1926, of 2 145 177 people examined in the endemic areas of the Congo as a whole, there were only 24 982 new cases (1·20 per cent) plus 50 775 old cases. These figures disguise local incidences much greater than the average, but they provide a base-line from which to examine the next two phases.

The first of these runs from 1926 to 1947. During this time the system of mass survey was developed with follow-up treatment with the drug tryparsamide. It is now evident that use of this drug had achieved its maximum effect by about 1942. During the next five years the incidence of appearance of new cases continued to fluctuate at about the same level, although the coverage of the population under survey continued to increase. In 1946, at the end of this phase, described in some detail by van Hoof (1947), the incidence of new infections was 0·23 per cent, a reduction of over 80 per cent of that observed at the opening of the tryparsamide campaign.

Failure, between 1942 and 1947, to improve on this figure could be attributed to two factors: failure to locate and diagnose a proportion of new cases, and an increase in the proportion of strains resistant to the drug.

In 1947 a new drug, pentamidine, was introduced, not containing arsenic and possessing marked prophylactic properties. This was administered periodically to all persons living in endemic areas. It gave spectacular results and by 1956 had lowered the new case incidence to 0·012, a reduction of 95 per cent from the 1946 figure and of 99 per cent on the 1926 figure. But already there were signs that the rate of progress in reducing incidence was slackening. At this time 50 per cent of the population of the whole country was subjected to examination twice a year. During the next three years the programme was extended to cover 70 per cent of the population and the incidence of new cases was reduced by 1959 to 0·006 per cent. In the next year the Democratic Republic of the Congo achieved its independence. Neujean (1963) who had conducted the last phase of the campaign felt able, with some justification, to report that 'the methods used by the former Belgium administration have proved their worth. The campaign against sleeping sickness, thanks to the latest developments in chemotherapy, presents more an executive problem than one of research.' For success to be sustained two conditions had to be fulfilled.

(1) There must be available a well-educated, trained and disciplined staff at all levels.

(2) The people must be induced, through their traditional or administrative leaders, to accept periodic examination and movement control in endemic zones and the areas surrounding them (passport or medical visa) and to accept treatment and prophylactic injections. The medical services should, in turn, reduce to a minimum the need for people to travel to case-finding and chemoprophylaxis centres and motor transport should be used as much as possible in the interests of speed and efficiency (Neujean 1963).

It is easy to say that the drop in proportion of the population surveyed from 70 per cent in 1958 to about 2 per cent in 1960 was to be expected after independence, even without the political disorders that attracted so much attention. Yet it is doubtful if the populations of the most advanced European countries would voluntarily submit to prophylactic injections twice a year, in the buttocks, for the prevention of a disease of which often only their parents and grandparents had any vivid memories. The number of new cases reported in the Congo in 1967 was 2438, almost the same as that found in 1955, viz 2117. But the latter were discovered after the examination of some 6 million persons and the former after examination of less than 500 000. It is difficult, in fact, to make a comparison, for although, in some areas, medical auxiliaries remaining after the termination of the Belgian rule endeavoured to maintain services, it is still only in limited areas that data are again becoming available. These have shown a very rapid rise in infection incidence (Fig. 25.1).

The situation has been described by Burke (1964) and Janssens and Burke (1968) who gave evidence of the rapid resurgence of the disease and stated that many of the cases now displayed the rapid involvement of the central nervous system characteristic of rhodesian type infection. A second observation has been that while the major foci of infection may themselves be suppressed by mass prophylaxis, yet the sources of infection still seem to persist as evidenced by the appearance of cases around the periphery of the original focus, even when it remains itself still suppressed and inactive.

Human trypanosomiasis in the Democratic Republic of the Congo after

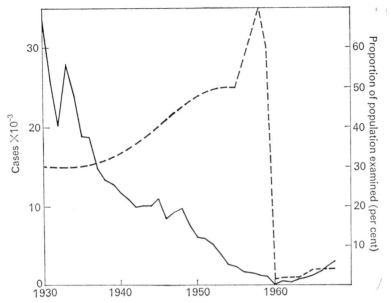

FIG. 25.1. New cases of sleeping sickness diagnosed in the Democratic Republic of the Congo, 1930–68, and the percentage of the whole population examined (after Janssens and Burke 1968).

———— no. of cases;
– – – – % of population examined.

independence shows features that characterize the epidemiology of the disease elsewhere.

(1) The infections persist in residual foci that were not eliminated by twenty years of mass treatment followed by over a decade of compulsory prophylaxis.

(2) The recrudescence of infection after control was allowed to lapse indicated a change in properties of the parasite suggesting the emergence of 'rhodesian' strains.

(3) Although the system of mass prophylaxis used by the Belgians was admirably organized and very effective in protecting people at risk, it did not affect the fundamental ecology of the parasites.

The conclusion that seems most likely to emerge from studies now being directed towards problems of this sort is that the effect of massive drug treatment of the human population is to protect the adventitious host of the parasite, man, from infection, while leaving the natural host undiscovered and untouched. A secondary result is that mass prophylaxis removes from populations of the adventitious host, man, the store of antibody built up and sustained by constant contact with the parasite.

To make these assertions is not to affirm that the campaign against sleeping sickness in the Congo was misdirected. Its results, in terms of the freedom from infection that it conferred upon the inhabitants of that vast country, were admirable. There is every reason to suppose that had the Belgian regime persisted the further development of the country would have accelerated the replacement of the natural ecosystems by others that were more fully managed by human activity. In these circumstances the habitat of *Glossina* and of its natural hosts would have become more and more restricted and more and more easily managed. In due course medical prophylaxis would have been replaced by '*le prophylaxie agronomique*'.

Now it is necessary to begin again. It is worth recalling a report on human trypanosomiasis in the Katanga in 1910–12 carried out by Dr. Stohr. Here the disease was particularly acute. He discussed the situation with a resident of some long experience and wrote as follows: 'La virulence de la maladie s'écroit-elle avec le temps? J'ai entendu affirmer par un homme influent— qui n'était pas médecin—que la meilleure façon de s'y prendre avec la trypanosomiase était de faire rien, que la prochaine génération aurait acquis l'immunité et que dans vingt ans tout serait comme autrefois' (Stohr 1912). This suggested an approach to the problem that was biologically and ecologically more desirable than those that were later devised; but in every other respect it was obviously impossible.

One further point is to be noted from this report on Katanga. 'Je crois que sans doute la maladie du sommeil sur la côte ouest est d'un type moins aigu que la maladie dans les localités où elle vient d'éclater' (Stohr 1912). Much of Katanga is infested by *G. morsitans*, *G. pallidipes*, and *G. brevi-palpis* as well as the riverine *G. fuscipes*. Some years later Bourguignon (1937), working on the upper Lualaba around Bukama, isolated a strain which had all the characteristics of *T. 'rhodesiense'*. At about the same time Lester, in Nigeria, was examining *rhodesiense*-like strains found in analogous ecological environments (Chapter 24). Bourguignon advanced a theory, similar to Lester's, that *T. 'rhodesiense'* had been derived from *T. 'gambiense'* by transmission through a tsetse of the *morsitans* group, in this case *G. pallidipes*, and that some of the Katanga infections were of rhodesian trypanosomiasis. In the next year van Hoof, Henrard, and Peel (1938) undertook an investigation to determine whether or not rhodesian sleeping sickness existed in the Congo. Although they found a number of charac-teristically rhodesian strains, they concluded that only *T. 'gambiense'* was present because the infection was only found among people living in areas where *Glossina* of the *palpalis* group infested the rivers. The distinction is no longer valid and where, as in Busoga (Chapter 16), such strains are first transitted by *G. pallidipes*, they are soon transferred to a *palpalis* group transmission cycle.

The observations of Stohr (1912) and of Bourguignon (1937), the first made before and the second during the first great treatment campaign, suggest that in spite of its very different geographical context, the pattern of infection in the Congo is ecologically similar to that in Nigeria. There are, however, no areas of contact between the *Brachystegia–Julbernardia* woodlands (*miombo*) and more arid *Acacia*-dominated savanna. There are therefore no infection foci corresponding to those located, in Nigeria, on or near the junction of the Northern Guinea and Sudan vegetations.

The major environmental contexts of human infection in West and Central Africa

Within the limits of *palpalis* group infestation in West and Central Africa, the location of the major centres of human infection can be related to vegetation (used as an indicator of distribution of natural ecosystems), to tsetse distribution, and to the pattern of distribution of mankind. When this is done it is clear that residual foci of persistent infection tend to be located adjacent to three biotic interzones. They are:

(1) The interzone between the central closed or moist forest and the savanna–forest mosaic and/or the relatively moist savanna and savanna woodland (South Guinea zone in Nigeria). Here the pattern of biting by the principal vectors (impersonal man–fly contact) leads to the development of the typical gambian disease—easily transmissible, chronic, and often exhibiting a high degree of mutual adjustment with the human host. Domestic animals (pigs and/or dwarf cattle) may act as temporary reservoirs of infection. The principal contact with the wild reservoir of trypanosomes is through these animals and the *fusca*- and *morsitans*-group tsetses of the forest edge. There is little direct contact between man and the latter two groups and infection in man is maintained solely by *palpalis*-group flies. In nature (i.e. under stable social conditions and without intervention of mass therapy and prophylaxis) adjustment between man and trypanosome has allowed numerous major African societies to develop on the moist forest periphery.

(2) The interzone between the forest–savanna mosaic and/or moist savanna and the *miombo* (*Brachystegia–Julbernardia* or *Isoberlinia* woodland and associated vegetations). The vectors concerned in transmission of trypanosomes between people are of the *palpalis*-group. Introduction of heterologous strains, causing epidemics and, especially, leading to formation of highly stable foci of infection, is chiefly due to *G. pallidipes* and/or *G. longipalpis*. Again the spread of infection from man via the riverine flies leads to adjustment to infection and the prevalence of typical gambian strains.

(3) The interzone between the *miombo* and savanna vegetations in which acacias and other thorny and spinose trees adapted to a semi-arid environment are prevalent. In Nigeria this is the interzone between the Northern Guinea and Sudan zones. Here, because of the stringencies of climate, the riverine tsetses are seasonally restricted to habitats which are also vital to the survival of human communities. Close personal man–fly contact develops seasonally with small selected elements of the human populations.

There is a minimum of opportunity for adjustment between man and trypanosome to develop. New strains of trypanosomes causing epidemics are periodically introduced from the *G. morsitans* belts of the *miombo*, either through the agency of cattle or directly to man himself. Epidemics are most frequent during periods of expansion of the fly-belts.

Along these three interzones, where infection risk has been highest, human activity has been vigorous. In Nigeria the earliest of the great West African art cultures, that of Nok, developed in the area in which, today, are situated the foci of infection just west of the Bauchi plateau. The Nok people must have been in part responsible for the maintenance, if not the creation, of the forest–savanna mosaic of central Nigeria.†

Starting on the south of the Congo basin and moving eastwards were Kongo itself, the Luba and Lunda states, and, just south of them, the Lozi kingdom (Fage 1958, Vansina 1966, Balandier 1968). East of the Congo, in the same ecological zone, were the interlake kingdoms, the empire of Kitara and the kingdom of Buganda. Through here also came the great southward movement of nilotes in which, on the north-east corner of Lake Victoria, the Luo became involved in the epidemics described in Chapters 14–16. In West Africa, in the same situation, one can name Benin as well as the long-lived Oyo empire in Nigeria, and the Asante, Fante, and Akan states in the region of modern Ghana. On the other hand the Hausa states, the empire of Bornu, as well as, one may suppose, the Songhay, Mali, and old Ghana empires, abutted upon and to some extent, although not fully, overcame the infection risks associated with the *G. tachinoides–G. palpalis–G. morsitans* association of trypanosome vectors on their southern borders.

Infection foci in absence of tsetse of the *palpalis* group

In those parts of East and southern Africa where *Glossina* of the *palpalis* group are not found the incidence of the human infection is trivial when compared with that of the West and Central African countries. From 1922–46 the total of cases observed in Tanzania was 23 955 (Fairbairn 1948), little more than a quarter of the total diagnosed in Nigeria in 1935. The two countries are comparable in area.

Widespread epidemic conditions were observed in Tanzania between 1925 and 1937, with peak years in 1929 and 1932. Two authors (Fairbairn 1948, Ormerod 1961) have seen this as the spread of human infective trypanosomes northward from the Zambezi valley. It has, on the other hand, been argued (Ford 1965) that the cause of the Tanzanian epidemic was, as described in Chapters 11–13, the re-invasion by tsetse of land from which they had disappeared following the destruction of their natural hosts by rinderpest. This took place in a period when the human population still had

---

† Mr. Bernard Fagg has informed me that the Nok sites yield abundant seeds of *Canarium schweinfurthii*. This tree is a conspicuous indicator of the forest–savanna mosaic as far east as Busoga, where its seeds are still cooked and eaten (Eggeling and Dale 1951).

not recovered from the disorders of the colonial onset, and were too sparsely distributed in marginal areas to prevent the recovery of pig and antelope populations with their attendant tsetses and trypanosomes. Later when people were multiplying and the areas of human occupation were expanding at the expense of *Glossina*, ephemeral epidemics occurred as pioneer families penetrated the fly-bush. This was followed by a period (still in progress) of spread of an endemic state in which local epidemics begin by the sporadic infection of individuals by bite of *G. morsitans*, *G. swynnertoni*, or *G. pallidipes*. In natural, pre-colonial conditions, many such sporadic single infections must have failed to start local epidemics and their sole result was the death of the individual concerned. The epidemic spread in Tanzania in the 1925–37 period was confined to communities within or, in most cases, on the edge of the western *G. morsitans* fly-belt (*G. morsitans centralis*). Around or within the eastern fly-belt there have never been any large-scale disruptive epidemics. In the period examined by Fairbairn (1948) the eastern fly-belt (*G. morsitans morsitans*) only produced 4·8 per cent of cases observed, while the western belt produced 78·8 per cent. The remainder were associated with a number of smaller central fly-belts, including the *G. swynnertoni* belt which was the source of the Maswa outbreak described in Chapter 13.

Human trypanosomiasis was discovered in southern Tanzania very soon after the rhodesian type of infection was first recognized. Its presence in the Rovuma valley, where the border between Mozambique and German East Africa divided the eastern *G. morsitans* belt into two, was investigated by Drs. Beck and Weck (1913, also Beck 1914, Weck 1914). Like their contemporaries all over Africa their main concern was to get evidence that the infection had been brought in from a neighbouring territory. It was not difficult, on the northern banks of the Rovuma, to find a few infected persons who had visited the Portuguese territory to the south.

TABLE 25.1

Human population densities per mile² within the Tanzanian fly-belts

Year	Western belt	Central belt	Eastern belt	All belts	Fly-belt population as % of territorial population
1934–5†	3·5	1·3	8·1	5·7	20·8
1945–6‡	6·6	8·5	12·1	9·1	23·9
1948–55§	6·2	9·5	9·8	8·1	22·0

† Gillman (1936).
‡ East Africa Royal Commission (1955).
§ *Tanganyika atlas* (1956).

The contrast between the endemic condition of the disease in the eastern fly-belt and its spreading, epidemic state in the western belt may be attributed to a number of factors. In the eastern belt *G. pallidipes* and *G. brevipalpis* are widely distributed; in the western belt these two species are rare except in the north and have still not been recorded in the parts of the fly-belt where the epidemic spread was most in evidence. A second distinction lies in the density of population of people living within the fly-belts. This is set out in Table 25.1. People living within the eastern belt tend to be about twice as thick on the ground as those living in the western belt. The classical paper on human trypanosomiasis in the eastern fly-belt is that of Dye (1927) who concluded that the disease was endemic and that in village outbreaks transmission via *G. morsitans* proceeded from man to man.

A new interpretation of the Tanzanian epidemic of 1925–37

In an earlier examination of the Tanzania situation the supposed endemic condition of the disease in the eastern fly-belt and its absence in the western was used in part explanation for the rapid epidemic spread around the latter and its non-occurrence where people had achieved some degree of adjustment to infection (Ford 1965). It was not an entirely satisfactory explanation, even when linked to somewhat tenuous evidence for a higher infection rate among *Glossina* and their natural hosts in the southern portions of that belt. No account was taken of the evidence of Wilde and French (1945) that cattle might act as reservoirs of *T. brucei rhodesiense* infection, while the confirmation of this in the Alego epidemic, by Onyango, van Hoeve, and de Raadt (1966) had yet to be made. The interactions between East coast fever and trypanosomiasis as controlling agents of cattle population density and distribution had also not become clear. Applying these notions to the Tanzanian epidemic spread it is now possible to see more clearly why it was confined to the periphery of the western *G. morsitans* belt and the *G. swynnertoni* belts and missed the people living in and around the eastern belt.

The eastern, *G. morsitans morsitans*, subspecies lives for the most part below the main African plateau, at altitudes under 4000 ft above sea level. The flies of the western belt, *G. morsitans centralis*, live above this altitude. In Tanzania the low-level, eastern fly-belt is sharply demarcated on its western boundary by the highlands that run from Mbeya and Njombe at the northern end of Lake Nyassa north-west through Iringa to Kilosa and beyond. These highlands, under a somewhat more humid climate than the rest of central Tanzania, support a major focus of endemic East coast fever. In 1957, the last year in which full cattle counts were published by the government of Tanganyika Territory, 83 per cent of the cattle of the territory lived in the higher plateau country, west of the highlands. Not only were they separated from the eastern *morsitans* belt by the scarp bounding the highland zone, but they were also separated from it by the zone of endemic theileriosis.

In 1921, when the first cattle count was published by the British administration, the disproportion between cattle numbers west and east of the highlands was even greater. The western area then contained 93 per cent of the whole cattle population. An examination of three maps, topography, tsetse, and cattle population, in the *Tanganyika atlas* (1956) shows that the cattle which occupy the tsetse-free country of Central Tanzania are pushed, as it were, westwards and northwards so that the limits are sharply outlined by the boundaries of the western *G. morsitans centralis* belt and the north-central *G. swynnertoni* belts. In their eastern pasture, however, they are not sharply confined by tsetse, but diminish in density as they impinge upon the East coast fever belt of the central highlands.

The reasons already advanced for the appearance of the epidemic spread of sleeping sickness in Tanzania in the 1920s, still seem valid.

The slowing down of growth of the cattle population and of the rate of expansion of the fly-belts were both consequences of the collision of two mutually exclusive biotic communities, the woodland/savanna–game animal–tsetse and the cultivation–man–cattle ecosystems. These had been separated for 25 to 30 years because of their reduction by rinderpest acting on cattle as well as on the wild fauna and aided by severe local collapses, from various causes, of the human population. The period 1920 to 1930, in which the collision made its widest impact, was also that in which the first rapid epidemic spread of *rhodesiense* sleeping sickness took place (Ford 1965).

To this explanation may be added the notion, already developed in Chapters 16, 23, and 24, that cattle brought in large numbers into contact with *Glossina* may act, temporarily, as an enormously expanded reservoir for *T. brucei rhodesiense*. In Tanzania it explains not only why the epidemic peak developed during the 1920s but also why it was only observed around the western and central, but not the eastern, fly-belts.

The epidemics of rhodesian trypanosomiasis in Western Tanzania in the 1920s were, in respect of their comparatively large scale, a new phenomenon. Lester's opinion that, in Nigeria, an infection incidence of 1 per cent was tolerable has been noted. From data given in Ford (1965) it is possible to calculate very crude incidence rates for populations living in the *morsitans* infested areas of Tanzania. Between 1950 and 1960 the overall rate in the western fly-belt was of the order of 0·07–0·15 per cent. In the same period the rate in the eastern fly-belt was about 0·01 per cent. These figures, of course, mask much higher rates shown in local outbreaks and endemic foci. In about 1930, at the peak of epidemic spread, the western belt showed an incidence rate of about 0·9 per cent, but incidence in the eastern belt was, if anything, less than the 0·01 per cent rate of later years. In periods of ecological stability, incidence of rhodesian trypanosomiasis throughout very large areas of eastern Africa was so low that it was scarcely recognized.

Where *G. pallidipes* in the Zambezi valley and, probably, the eastern belt of Tanzania, sets up permanent foci of infection associated with small localized populations of host animals particularly suited to become reservoirs of *brucei*-type trypanosomes, then constant exposure to infection in adjacent communities allowed the sort of adjustment described in Rhodesia by Blair, Burnett Smith, and Gelfand (1968) to develop (Chapter 20). This adjustment probably also involved the movement of hamlet and village populations away from localized foci when deaths or sickness became too frequent.

Trypanosomiasis and the continental distribution of cattle

The pattern of distribution of domestic cattle throughout the African continent was studied in the 1930s at the Onderstepoort Laboratory in South Africa and the main conclusions were discussed by Curson and Thornton (1936). Among other papers from the same establishment were those of Epstein (1933, 1934) and of Bisschop (1937). One outcome of this work was a conception of African cattle as derived from four parent stocks, none of which was indigenous in the African tropics. A second result was the compilation of a map showing the approximate routes by which these animals achieved their present pattern of distribution. The map, with slight modifications, has been reproduced more recently by Faulkner and Epstein (1957) and by Payne (1964). Mason and Maule (1960) do not entirely agree with Faulkner and Epstein, still less with Curson and Thornton, regarding the four parent stocks and the ancestry of a fifth type, the Sanga, supposed to be descendants of crosses between zebus and the earliest of African cattle, the hamitic longhorns. There is no need to discuss these problems, but it remains to note that Joshi, McLaughlin, and Phillips (1957) adopted a classification that was chiefly geographical. In the following account the classification of Epstein (Faulkner and Epstein 1957) is followed.

(1) Longhorn humpless cattle are now represented only by (a) the Kuri cattle which live out of range of tsetse in the Lake Chad swamps, and (b) the N'Dama which are West African cattle living especially in and around the Republic of Guinea, particularly the Fouta Djallon highlands.

(2) Shorthorn humpless or *Brachyceros* cattle are represented by a number of West African types of dwarf cattle (Muturu, Lagunes, West African shorthorn) and the Nuba cattle of the Koalib hills in the Sudan.

(3) The neck-humped zebus survive in the Afrikander cattle of South Africa.

(4) The chest-humped zebus include many types, among which are the East African zebus and the Sokoto Gudali of Nigeria. They are believed to have been introduced by Arab and Indian traders since the Arab invasion of the East African coast in A.D. 669.

(5) The Sangas which may be neck- or chest-humped zebu crosses with

the original longhorn humpless cattle now include the Ankole cattle, the White Fulani, and Rahaji of the Fulani, and the Shona, Ndebele, and Barotse cattle.

In the royal cemeteries of Cush, in decorated chapels below the pyramids at Meroe and Barkal, in the Nile valley some 150–200 miles north of Khartoum, the wall decorations depict both longhorn and shorthorn humpless cattle. As well as these, in a small relief reproduced by Chapman (1952), there are the outlines of four humped animals. Meroe flourished between 590 B.C. and A.D. 325 and these latter must have been neck-humped zebus according to Epstein's classification, for zebus are to be seen in Egyptian reliefs as far back as the Eighteenth and Nineteenth Dynasties. Epstein believes the Sangas to have originated in the highlands of Ethiopia. The meroitic remains show that there was ample genetic material at the right latitude and at the right time. (See also Lucas in Tothill 1948, Arkell 1961.)

Two problems require attention. How did the first two types in Epstein's classification become adapted to withstand constant infection by trypanosomes, and how did the many varieties of the remaining three types disperse themselves throughout much of the African tropics and, in particular, how did they traverse the continental fly-belt from 14°N. to 20°S. to reach and populate the tsetse-free regions of South Africa?

Throughout this study it has been emphasized that adjustment to infection takes two forms: one is physiological through the development of partially protective immunities or premunities; the other is ecological and is expressed in various activities which isolate the potential adventitious host from the vectors. In Chapter 1 it was remarked that colonial scientists had generally failed to study the achievements of African peoples in overcoming the hazards presented by the presence of tsetses and trypanosomes. Many of these achievements were evidently empirical and success followed upon much trial and error. Curson (1924) described how white South African farmers, in country surrounding the forest that now survives in the game reserves of Mkuzi, Hluhluwe, and Umfulozi, found that, unlike the Zulus whom they had supplanted, they could not keep cattle. Following their European traditions they had divided up the area into separate farms and those of them with low-lying ground found their cattle seriously infected with *nagana* in the summer months. The Zulus who had occupied the area as a community had practised a form of transhumance that took them into the high veld in the wet summer and into the low veld in the dry winter. It was supposed that the infections acquired during the summers were a consequence of the wandering habit of the tsetses (*G. pallidipes*) in wet weather and their restriction to dense thicket in the dry. It is more likely that at the latitude of Zululand tsetse in the cold winter months were relatively free of infection and that only in the warm summers did they transmit trypanosomes. Flexibility in the use of pasture by the community as a whole allowed infection to be avoided, in a way not possible when the land was divided up into individually owned farms. Similar development of patterns of behaviour in grazing have been noted elsewhere. Foci of infection in the *Grenzwildnisse* of the interlake region were known and avoided. The seasonal migrations of the Fulani were caused chiefly by the need to find dry-season pasture and water, but their pattern over the face of the land was also determined by distribution of areas of high infection risk. The habit of the Sukuma and Masai, in years of very severe drought, of driving their cattle into tsetse-infested bush where they know that many will die of trypanosomiasis, while outside all will die of starvation, is, perhaps, the first stage in achieving that physiological adjustment to infection that now seems to be so much better developed in West than in East and southern Africa.

As in so much else in African rural life, the chaos of the rinderpest makes it difficult to be entirely confident of conditions before 1890. Jeffreys (1953) makes the interesting point that cattle owned by African cultivators tend to be small or dwarf animals, while those owned by the semi-nomadic pastoralists like the Masai, Boran, Hima, Tusi, and Fulani are much bigger. Zeuner (1963) has suggested that dwarf cattle may have been bred deliberately or had a selective advantage in adverse conditions. The small size would be favoured as making the animals more manageable. Since the rinderpest, and also as a consequence of trade and of breeding policies deliberately fostered for one reason or another, many of the older cattle types have disappeared or become very rare.

The origins and uses of pasture

The conquest of African trypanosomiasis began with the 'neolithic revolution', that is with cultivation and domestication of animals. Whether this revolution began in various parts of the Old World, including Africa, as Murdock (1959) thinks, or whether it was brought to the African tropics by people who came from or had had contacts with Mediterranean cultures, is not important. Its effect was to create relatively large settled communities whose activities profoundly altered their environment and displaced the natural vegetation and its wildlife (including small nomadic groups of hunting and gathering predecessors) with cultivation and domestic livestock. These early agricultural communities flourished most vigorously on the interzones between the major natural ecosystems—on the edge of the forest where it abutted upon woodland or upon the contact zone between woodland and the drier savanna. Their successors have continued to expand from these areas, occupying different soil types and destroying different vegetations as new crop plants became available and new techniques were learnt or invented for their propagation. The interzones favoured such developments because they offered, within relatively small areas, the widest variety of ecological situations for agricultural experiment.

They also were easy to exploit. Rain forest is easier to destroy on its edge, where it encounters a climate more favourable to woodland, than it is where it enjoys optimum conditions of climate. Change in the direction of increased dryness in the continental climate, or over large parts of the continent, must have produced conditions of instability in forest–woodland or woodland–savanna interzones which endured for very long periods. Moreau (1967), who has reviewed our knowledge of Pleistocene climates in some detail, concludes that the Mega-Chad lake lasted from 22 000 to 8000 years ago. During this period there may have been a northward shift of the central rain forest; but later the rain belt moved southward, and the extreme desert conditions of the modern Sahara began to develop about 5000 years ago. The 'neolithic revolution' in Africa profited by the instability of the forest edge created by this movement. Tree felling, burning of fire-sensitive species, the invasion of grasses, and the development of grass burning as a definite land-management technique all progressed more rapidly on the interzones.

In 1939, Michelmore suggested that natural climax grasslands, with the possible exceptions of some flood plain areas, did not occur in tropical Africa. It is a view now generally accepted. Cattle are grazing animals and it is therefore to be supposed that they did not begin to penetrate the savannas, woodlands, and forests until agricultural communities had not only expanded sufficiently to destroy enough of the wildlife ecosystems to create a profound reduction of the risk of trypanosome infection, but also to produce enough secondary grassland to maintain cattle populations. However, before this happened one may suppose cattle-owning peoples first moved latitudinally along the tsetse-free steppe between the expanding desert and the retreating savannas and wooded grasslands in much the same way as the Fulani and Baggara Arabs and other cattle nomads do today.

At some point in their history cattle owners, searching for more pastures, must have encountered the cultivation of people living within the *Glossina* zone and discovered that here were other relatively infection-free pastures. Once this contact had been made the various mechanisms of ecological and physiological adjustment began to operate. While this was happening other people, with other types of cattle, were circumventing or traversing the desert barrier of the Sahara and creating pressures that drove their forerunners into taking increasing risks of infection.

The N'Dama of the Guinea and Sierre Leone derived savannas are descendants of the first wave of cattle, the humpless hamitic longhorns that have become adjusted to a life of constant exposure to infection, as have the descendants of the next wave of humpless shorthorns. The arrival in the tropics of zebu stocks led, according to Epstein, to the appearance of Sanga crossbreeds from which many distinctive types have developed. Probably the crucial circumstances favouring the spread of Sangas was that

they began to proliferate at a time when agricultural activity, assisted perhaps among some peoples by their possession of earlier cattle types, had
converted enough land into relatively fly-free pasture to permit of nomadism.
Iron Age nomad pastoralists were able to move down the infection-free
corridors along the cultivated interzones or to develop systems of transhumance, like the Fulani and Zulus, into and out of the infected areas
where the need for more pasture and water coincided seasonally with
intervals of lower infection risk.

It seems likely that an essential factor in the regular development of
transhumance systems that involve penetration into tsetse-infested zones is
exposure to a more or less continuous but low infection risk. In Zululand
this was associated with cold (Ford and Leggate 1961) and in West Africa
with exposure to the bites of the riverine tsetses, *G. tachinoides* and *G. palpalis*. Partly owing to their diet but also because of a specific inability to
develop a high infection incidence, they present both man and his livestock with a challenge to which their imperfect powers of physiological
adjustment to infection can often successfully respond.

The cattle routes and their penetration

The occupation of the pastures created by the efforts of the cultivators
was at first a peaceful process and cattle grazed the fallows with the agreement or at the invitation of cultivators. Only later did the pastoralists
assume a dominant role, again, perhaps, because of a need to control the
use of pasture for their multiplying herds.

This process was studied by a Belgian ecologist in Rwanda. Like most
biologists of his time in Africa he was less interested in the creation of
pasture than, as he saw it, the bad effects of forest destruction. He described how the Tusi cattle aristocrats drove the agricultural Hutu deeper
into the forest areas and took over from them the pastures they had made
by forest felling, cultivation, and grass burning. 'Nous assistons de nos
jours à un déplacement en masse de populations Bahutu vers l'ouest, à une
véritable vague d'assaut contre les zones humifères de haute montagne. . . .
Devant cette poussée, la forêt rétrocède constamment d'une façon im-
pressionante. Le recul est valué de l'ordre d'un kilomètre par an sur tout le
front du Nord au Sud' (Scaetta 1932). The distance from the Lake Victoria
shore to the eastern slopes of the Rwanda volcanoes where this retreat of the
forest was said to be in progress is about 250 km. The Tusi and Hima
arrived in the interlake region in about A.D. 1400 and must have found
infection-free pastures awaiting them. It follows that the destruction of
forest by the Hutu cannot possibly have taken place as rapidly as Scaetta
imagined.

There is a tradition in Karagwe that the Nyambo, before the arrival of the
Hima with their longhorned Ankole type of Sangas, had owned shorthorn
humpless cattle (Ford and Hall 1947). Stuhlmann (1894), travelling north

in 1891 through what is now the western part of modern Ankole, saw a herd of shorthorned humpless cattle. Similar animals were to be seen in Kigezi district, south-west of Ankole, at the time of the present writer's first visit there in 1934. Whoever, long before the Tusi and Hima arrived, had introduced the ancestors of these shorthorned animals must also have come in in the wake of cultivating predecessors who had destroyed the forest edge to make an unstable, if enduring, zone of tsetse-free pasture.

The instability of these routes is important. The collapse of part of the most westerly route to the south in the interlake zone was described in Chapters 7–10. At some earlier date it had forked eastwards around the south of Lake Victoria as well as continuing down the east coast of Lake Tanganyika, but these movements were extinguished from causes unknown, but including perhaps competition with the East African zebus as well as with tsetses. Today a few small herds with Ankole characteristics are still to be found in islands of tsetse-free land in the Tanzanian western *G. morsitans* belt. In Chapter 19 it was noted that former inhabitants of the Rhodesian plateau carved longhorn Sangas on their soapstone bowls and that they appear to have had cultural connections with the rulers of the interlake kingdoms.

An earlier movement down this route, formed by the forest–savanna mosaic around the Congo basin, was followed by the first of the two zebu stocks, the neck-humped zebus which, in recent times, have been developed into the Afrikander breed of South Africa. These had moved around the forest-edge route to the Atlantic coast and continued their journey southwards and, eventually, with their Hottentot owners, penetrated the Cape region of South Africa from the west (Faulkner and Epstein 1957). In recent years, because of their size, hardiness as work oxen, and their good beef qualities, they have moved north from the Cape into Rhodesia, Zambia, and the Tanzania highlands as well as rejoining the peripheral Congo route with Belgian settlers in the pre-independence Katanga.

In Chapter 20 Selous's observation that the Shona cattle of the 1870s were 'small but beautiful' was linked with a very recent observation that control of trypanosomiasis in the Sabi valley was likely to lead to overstocking and that this in turn would reduce the size and quality of the cattle. Shona cattle are Sangas. They are still, sometimes, called Kalanga, a name that links them to the Karanga rulers of Mutapa. Faulkner and Epstein (1957) say they are 'a small to medium size breed, cows weighing 600–800 lbs'.

Jeffreys (1953) was so much impressed by the smallness of Shona cattle according to nineteenth-century pre-rinderpest accounts that he argued that they were dwarf humpless shorthorns or *Brachyceros*. He quoted Bent (1896) who described the Mtoko area of Rhodesia as having 'more cattle than we had seen elsewhere, but all of the same calibre', that is, dwarf. Jeffreys also quoted Nobbs (1927) who gave weights of Shona cattle at

300–400 lb, about half that given thirty years later by Faulkner and Epstein. The modern Shona cattle are often much interbred with exotic stock, but it is possible that they gained much in weight after the rinderpest when grazing was virtually unlimited and that they will, when free of disease but limited to available pasture, return to the small size of earlier times. Dwarfism may characterize the cattle of cultivators, as Jeffreys suggested, and certainly many of the zebus of the trypanosome-free pastures of Sukumaland might be so classified. Faulkner and Epstein (1957) give 482 lb for an average Sukuma cow, but this is a figure from animals reared on a veterinary stock farm; many locally owned animals might fall below this and so below the weight of mature, well-cared-for, Nigerian Muturus, which are undoubted dwarfs. The dwarfism of the Muturu (448 lb for an average cow, again at a veterinary livestock centre) is associated with adjustment to continuous trypanosome infection. This property is shared by the only obviously dwarf cattle in Rhodesia today, those descendants of the Tonga cattle seen by Livingstone. It is possible that they are, in fact, merely Shona cattle of the pre-rinderpest type that, in the harsh environment of the Zambezi valley and subjected to continual infection but still out of contact with larger exotic breeds, have retained their ancient characteristics.† It is difficult, as witness the disagreement of veterinary anatomists, to classify African cattle by their morphological characteristics. Evidently the whole subject of their systematic relationships as well as their physiological responses to infection and the stresses of tropical life awaits genetic exploration of such indicator factors as blood groups and serum protein composition. Meanwhile the best explanation for the small size of the Shona cattle seen by Selous and Bent is that it represented a response to conditions of high population density in a land heavily populated by agricultural people and limited, ultimately, by harsher conditions of the *Grenzwildnisse* of the Limpopo and Zambezi. The condition of Sukuma zebus today is similar, except that they still have room there for further expansion.

There were three routes through eastern Africa (Ford 1960b). One has been described as following the forest–savanna mosaic around the borders of the rain forests of the Congo basin. The second is essentially provided by the secondary grasslands that developed from cultivation along the interzones bordering the lower montane forests of the highlands running south through Kenya and Tanzania to Malawi. Some of these grasslands, today, lie above the altitude limits of *Glossina*, but it is wrong to suppose, like Clark (1959), that penetration of the African tropics was accomplished by nomads who guided their animals along the high ground above the levels to which tsetse belts might rise. The process was much more complex. It

† Payne (1964) publishes a photograph of one of these dwarf Tonga cattle and attributes it to me. It was taken by my colleague D. F. Lovemore. Payne takes the view that these animals may be dwarfed hamitic longhorns with some Sanga characteristics.

involved first the use by cultivators of instability zones along the edges of Pleistocene sub-montane forests which, under an early climatic regime, had grown up over areas far larger than would be achieved in the climate of today. Secondly, it involved the creation of a man–cultivation ecosystem in which neither the forest tsetses nor those of the savanna could survive. Thirdly, it involved the political take-over of fallow lands by pastoralists and the development of fire as a means of control of tree growth. This in turn led to changes in the species composition of the larger wild vertebrate fauna. In some areas, where circumstances were favourable, both men and cattle also adjusted themselves to infection, presumably by selection of individuals better endowed than others with the capacity to produce immunoglobulins. Such events did not always take place in sequence. Reverses were initiated by epidemics and epizootics or by political or administrative decisions, as when Gungunyana in Gazaland said of the wildlife, *azi-zale*, 'let them multiply' or, in recent times, where colonial governments controlled grass fires in the interests of forest regeneration or wildlife preservation and so assisted the spread of *Glossina* and trypano-somiasis. (See, for example, Kenya Ministry of Agriculture 1956: 'The prohibition of grass fires by the British Government . . . led probably to the advance of tsetse fly in several regions.')

The third route had been opened, or at least was kept open, by Arab colonizers of the East African coast. It collapsed, as Napier Bax (1943) has shown, when suppression of slavery led to the disappearance of Arab coast agriculture. It was used only by the latest arrivals, the chest-humped zebus.

26

A NEW APPROACH TO
THE TRYPANOSOMIASIS PROBLEM

The need for a new approach

IN this book much attention has been paid to demolishing what has been called the *Pax Britannica* theory of the epidemiology of trypanosomiasis. To some this may have seemed an unnecessary task. Colonial empires in tropical Africa are dead; but knowledge of tsetse-borne infections in nature is largely confined to a dwindling group of ex-colonial civil servants, who tend to look upon each new epidemic as a consequence of the too hasty granting of political freedom and the collapse of the control services they had themselves helped to build up. At the same time research on some aspects of the problem is being vigorously pursued in the laboratories of Europe and North America and to a lesser degree in some Asiatic countries by a new generation of scientists, many of whom have not yet visited Africa. A third group is formed by Africans themselves who are slowly building a cadre of research and field workers with the object of taking the task of solving their own problems out of the hands of foreigners.

One source of confusion and misplaced effort comes from the uncritical acceptance by the two latter groups of the ideas about the role of trypanosomiasis in African ecology propounded by the first group. Entomologists dream of a great project in which expert teams will move across the continent exterminating *Glossina*. Immunologists are inspired by the thought of vaccines that will be injected into millions of people and millions of cattle so that they may move at will through the bush unaffected by the bites of tsetses which will continue to feed on the wild animals, while all will live together in idyllic harmony. Such ideas betray a complete ignorance of the logistics of rural population growth and industrial expansion in under-developed countries.

A fourth group of people interested in a solution to the trypanosomiasis problem is formed by staffs of international bodies such as the World Health Organization and the Food and Agricultural Organization, the overseas aid departments of some richer countries, as well as the great private research financing agencies. At present these tend to find themselves either preoccupied with emergencies or else, lacking any policy but impelled by the notion that any idea may, by a lucky chance, turn up a solution, sponsoring a host of uncoordinated research projects.

The practical problem

A number of lessons may be drawn from the narratives related in the foregoing chapters. Throughout tropical Africa the epidemics, epizootics, and famines that characterized the early years of this century and, in turn, set off the epidemics and epizootics of trypanosomiasis during the 1920s and 1930s, were a consequence of ecological, political, and parasitological disharmony caused by the unforeseen events that accompanied the colonial impact. Lugard in the despatch quoted on p. 140 had been aware of this, although in his *Dual Mandate* (Lugard 1922), written thirty years later, he outlined the foundations of *Pax Britannica* epidemiology. His first assessment was right. It was not *Pax* but *bellum*, an outbreak of biological warfare on a vast scale none the less terrible to its sufferers because they only vaguely perceived its cause while most colonial civil servants were quite unaware of the events that accompanied their advent.

The disappearance of the colonial empires may well be followed by epidemiological disorders as profound and as devastating as those that accompanied its inception. High incidences of the human infection in the Congo basin were soon measurable after 1960, at least in those limited portions of that vast territory in which the inadequate medical service operated. The present position in the southern Sudan can only be guessed from the numbers of infected refugees moving down the Nile valley into the north-west corner of Uganda. It is a reasonable assumption that Biafra, the Eastern region of the old colonial Nigeria, will, sooner or later, be similarly affected; the only real doubt lies in when the epidemic will appear. It is unlikely that it will take the form of the old, classical gambian disease such as Scott Macfie (1913b) described. It will be an acute infection, killing in a few months. In western Ethiopia cattle have recently fled from the valleys to the tsetse-free highlands and the human infection has been diagnosed for the first time in history. The information available suggests that the spread of *Glossina* which has brought about these happenings must itself be a consequence of earlier population movement, possibly associated with the campaigns of 1940–1. Elsewhere there are large areas of tropical Africa in which it is quite possible that severe epidemics are now in progress, unknown to anyone save those who are the victims.

It is one of the inevitable features of countries in course of development that persons with valuable technical skills—and these include doctors and veterinarians as well as those who are less highly educated but still relatively sophisticated—confine their activities to the larger towns where profit is to be made and life is comfortable. Here also the doctor can find most patients as well as hospitals and other facilities that allow him to offer to the greatest number of people the benefits of his skill. The diseases that are associated with the confrontation between the wildlife ecosystems and those artificial systems created by peasant cultivators and pastoralists pass unseen for there are few, and sometimes none, to see them. For example, Thomson (1967*b*) has described an epidemic of unknown origin only discovered, in Nigeria, after all its victims were dead. The exceptions are those outbreaks, such as recently occurred in the Serengeti park in Tanzania, where tourism may be affected. They are soon noticed, but in the vast areas away from the roads and air strips the peasant who is and has always been the principal contestant against zoonotic infection works on alone.

In some countries, however, control services have survived in full or even greater vigour the end of colonialism. In them the application of tsetse elimination techniques at very high cost creates situations which promise to be even more dangerous than the almost total lack of services to be seen elsewhere. In the latter case the mechanisms for natural re-adjustment to infection, both ecological and physiological, still exist. Where a policy of extensive elimination of *Glossina* or of the trypanosomes is pursued, often with the use of external financial aid on a scale unrelated to the potential of the country for economic growth, both these mechanisms cease to operate. A rapid expansion of the cattle population is the first consequence of successful, large-scale, 'tsetse reclamation' in savanna vegetations. But human beings, even when relieved of the burden of many of their parasites, multiply far more slowly. Under a natural system of human community growth, such as took place in Sukumaland, the area of tsetse-free land available to cattle is controlled by the rate of human population expansion. Where *Glossina* is artificially eliminated over thousands of square miles there is, of necessity, no human activity to destroy the habitat of the insects or to suppress their natural hosts. Indeed, to the latter is added an abundant population of domestic trypanosome hosts. In Uganda, where tsetse elimination programmes have been particularly successful, attempts have been made to attract settlers from neighbouring territories to occupy 'defence lines' (Turner and Baker 1968). Another disadvantage of over-rapid elimination of *Glossina* is that, sooner or later, sections of the surviving *Grenzwildnis* too are freed of infection and the activities of the applied entomologist must stop at a line, usually one drawn about 1900, on the other side of which thousands of square miles of bush, owned by another government, perhaps wiser in adopting a policy of relating its disease control to its rate of economic growth or, on the other hand, as in the Southern Sudan, completely ineffectual.

The illusion that large-scale tsetse elimination can free a country of the burden of its trypanosomiasis still persists. The relief obtained by very heavy expenditure on tsetse control is only temporary, and reduction of expenditure or relaxation of effort must be followed by catastrophic losses of cattle. The lesson was clear in Rhodesia, where an efficient system of control had been used for many years. The attempt to abandon it, as in the Urungwe reserve in 1944–52, or to change it, as in the Gwaai river area in 1961, was followed by a very rapid development of epizootic conditions.

Since 1960 insecticides have provided an easily used means of tsetse destruction. Their effects are even less durable than are those of wildlife control. In Uganda, in 1949, a development plan to last ten years made available £1 million sterling to rid the country of its *Glossina* belts (Worthington and Harris 1949). From the completion of that plan, near to the time of independence, to the present day, expenditure has continued to increase, mostly in the effort to prevent reinfestation and is now said to exceed a quarter million pounds a year. But with some small exceptions, the main foci of tsetse infestation and of endemic human trypanosomiasis have not been eliminated and the limits to which the indigenous people of the country had reduced them before 1890 are still not reached. Moreover, the populations which, at that time, controlled and confined the spread of tsetse no longer exist. Indeed they cannot do so, for their former habitats are now occupied by game parks which preserve both the faunas which provide the reservoirs for the trypanosomes as well as the tsetses which transmit them. What then are the needs of sound policy? They are two:

(1) An assessment of the nature and rate of development expected in each ecological area, regardless of the presence of tsetse and trypanosomiasis.

(2) A much more profound understanding than exists at present, of the causes of epidemics and epizootics of tsetse-borne disease.

Development potentials and trypanosomiasis control

Comprehensive continent-wide reviews of the development potentials of African countries are not lacking (e.g. F.A.O. 1962, Phillips 1959), and most, if not all countries, at one time or another have been surveyed by teams of experts who have suggested a variety of development plans. Often much has been done to implement them, with corresponding benefits in disease control. In general, development potentials are known within the limitations of modern technical expertise. There are large areas where development potential is very low and which are infested with *Glossina*. Elsewhere valuable land still lies empty because the populations required to work it are as yet unborn. Some aspects of the problem of development potential and tsetse infestation were discussed in Chapter 20. Using as bases the maps already produced by meteorologists, pedologists, agronomists, agriculturists, and others, and in consultation with such experts, those responsible for trypanosomiasis control should produce maps to show those areas of tsetse infestation which are (1) not capable of development because of inherent poverty of resources, (2) capable of productive development by peasant agriculture but which remain unused because of insufficient demand, and (3) capable of productive development by injection of new techniques. In the latter category would be included at one extreme national parks and at the other large-scale irrigation works. For each land category assessments should be made of appropriate techniques already available for control both of the infections and of the vectors. There are large areas of Africa in which it is possible to list, for any given type of land development, a number of methods of control which could be effectively applied and their approximate cost. What is more immediately important is once more to build upon and maintain predictive surveillance services which can give advance warning of the likelihood of outbreaks appearing.

Field investigational teams ought to include in their assessment of local trypanosomiasis situations not only the obstacles to development that the presence of the tsetse-borne diseases will provide and how to deal with them, but should also consider what ill-effects might result from removal of infection. These ill-effects would embrace not only pasture impoverishment, erosion, and stock control by starvation, but also the removal of the partial immunities enjoyed by cattle and human populations living in the presence of *Glossina* in areas where control services are likely to prove inadequate. At present this embraces nearly all tropical Africa. What ought to be avoided are all forms of mass treatment, whether by mass injection of curative or prophylactic drugs, or by blanket spraying with insecticides, or by large-scale felling of vegetation, or destruction of wildlife. All sorts of biological as well as mechanical bulldozing may, on occasion, control the spread of disease but at a cost to future generations that cannot be fully assessed. Equally undesirable, on the other hand, are the activities of conservationists who have often succeeded in the past in invoking the law to preserve inviolate as natural parks and wildlife reserves known major foci of human trypanosomiasis. It is not so much that these places endanger the health of tourists, or that game parks, when controlled and isolated from intimate contact with relatively large populations, are likely to give rise to epidemics. The real danger lies in their preservation not of wildlife as such, but of populations of pathogenic trypanosomes. This is not to advocate abolition of game parks. Apart from other considerations their present value to the economy of some tropical African countries is so great that governments would not contemplate their closure. What is needed is the development of methods of wildlife management that take into account not only the preservation of the fauna but also the elimination of its more dangerous parasites. Indeed, until this aspect of wildlife preservation is studied and understood, the role of the game animals as reservoirs of fatal infections ultimately endangers their own survival.

The need for an integrated approach to these problems has been well appreciated by field biologists for at least two decades. This appreciation is reflected today in the composition of teams sent to emergency areas. These teams include doctors, veterinarians, and entomologists, and have access to whatever laboratory services they may need. So far as they are able they collaborate not only among themselves but with administrators, agronomists, foresters, game wardens, and others concerned with rural development. But in an emergency, even if a sound theoretical basis existed for integration of data (which it does not), there is no time to adopt an approach to the local situation that will not only save people's lives, but will also ensure minimal destruction of natural resources.

Towards a formal epidemiology of trypanosomiasis

Much effort and expense might be spared if it were borne in mind that Africans, centuries ago, found solutions to the problems created by the presence of tsetses and trypanosomes. They were interrupted in the work of converting bush to cultivation and pasture by the European impact. The problem that now confronts scientists concerned with trypanosomiasis is how best to use their knowledge to facilitate and accelerate the Africans' task of reducing and managing the wildlife ecosystems of the continent. Clearly the first need is to improve existing services for the prevention of suffering and death in those who become infected while engaged upon that task. Such services can only operate to the best advantage if their work and deployment is founded on a proper understanding of the prevalence of infection and of the causes of epidemics and epizootics. This involves the development of a sound epidemiology of tsetse-borne disease. A superficial study of the epidemiology of malaria shows that this will not be easily done; but it also shows that the deliberate attempt to classify and measure the factors responsible for the presence of disease can assist significantly in the planning of research programmes and control campaigns.

The malaria parasite was discovered by Laveran in 1880. Its cyclical transmission through mosquitoes was demonstrated by a number of workers during the last five years of the nineteenth century. Prominent among them was Sir Ronald Ross, the founder of mathematical epidemiology. His attempts to formulate equations that would express the quantitative relationships between the various factors that control the incidence of the disease were not, in fact, successful. The main reason for this lack of success was that the biology of the interactions of the organisms involved—mosquitoes, plasmodia, man—were not yet fully understood. Macdonald (1957) revised the Ross equations and his book has many points of interest for the student of trypanosomiasis. The object of mathematical model making is to show 'how the various factors concerned in transmission interact with each other to build up a composite picture of endemic or epidemic conditions resembling that seen in nature'. The model obviously must include all known factors thought to be relevant. Its chief value emerges from its failures, for each failure indicates a gap in knowledge and a new field for investigation. Its success confirms the completeness of research.

Macdonald showed that the mathematical phase forms a third stage in epidemiological study. The first is the growth of circumstantial epidemiology, which describes in essentially historical, geographical, and sociological terms the conditions in which disease occurs. The second is provided by aetiological epidemiology which defines the causal organism and describes its transmission from man to man. Without these preliminary studies the mathematical approach cannot begin; moreover, in so far as the premises derived from circumstantial and aetiological epidemiology are wrong, so will the logical approach of the applied mathematician fail through misdirection.

It may be useful briefly to review some aspects of the epidemiology of trypanosomiasis in the light of Macdonald's ideas. A major object in writing this book has been to show that because of preconceived notions about Africa and Africans held by colonial research workers, basic circumstantial epidemiology has often been wrongly described. Its main assumption was that the succession of violent epidemics that beset the African peoples in the first forty years of this century were results of barbarism and lack of 'law and order'. In fact they were a consequence of quantitative changes in the relationships of three of the five populations involved— man, his domestic livestocks, and the wild fauna—and the effects of these changes upon the remaining two populations, the trypanosomes and the tsetses. The quantitative data are of poor quality, but they are not entirely lacking. If predictive surveillance is to be efficient, the first need is to continue and improve census taking of man and his domestic livestock and to use the data collected to assess population growth and decline and distribution change. In some countries censuses are completely lacking. In others their political connotations have led to them being rigged. Elsewhere the conservatism of pastoralists and their suspicions that cattle counts are a prelude to increased taxation lead to evasion and concealment. These are difficulties to be overcome.

In the list of parameters used in his equations Macdonald puts first 'the anopheline density in relation to man' and second, 'the average number of men bitten by one mosquito in one day'. Clearly analogous factors would be of the first importance in the epidemiology of any vector-borne disease. Because of the illusion that persisted among British workers that they could eliminate tsetses, and among French and Belgians that they could eliminate trypanosomes, their measurement in trypanosomiasis has barely yet begun. Moreover, the malaria equations dealt with transmission of the blood parasites from man to man. Although it is likely that human trypanosomiasis takes an epidemic form only when transmission is from man to man, some epidemics at least begin by transmission to man from a wild host, perhaps via a different tsetse or, perhaps, not only through a different tsetse, but also through the intermediary of other adventitious hosts, the domestic animals.

The third of Macdonald's parameters, if translated to the language of trypanosomiasis, would run, 'the proportion of those tsetses with meta-cyclic trypanosomes in the glands or mouth parts which are actually infective'. The fifth and sixth parameters similarly transformed are, respectively, 'the time taken for completion of the cycle of development of the trypanosome in the tsetse' and 'the proportion of tsetses infected with mature infections'. The time taken for the completion of the cycle of development of single strain infections of some species of trypanosomes has been known for many years (Kleine 1909, Robertson 1913). Measurements of the third and sixth parameters have been the subject of recently renewed research (Chapters 4 and 5); but the problem is complicated in nature by multiple infection with various strains of *brucei-*, *vivax-*, and *congolense*-group trypanosomes. The interactions of the three species in the infected tsetse have not been studied. The consequences of multiple infection in domestic animals also await detailed investigation. An ox can support an infection of *T. 'rhodesiense'* for several months. Will it continue to do so if it is also infected with, but does not die from, *T. congolense* and *T. vivax*?

Only one of Macdonald's parameters, applied to *Glossina*, has had detailed intensive study by entomologists. This is the fourth, 'the probability of a tsetse surviving through one day'. Work done on this subject, during the colonial period, was summarized by Glasgow (1963a). It is far from complete.

Macdonald's equations employ fifteen parameters. The mere setting down of the first six has been sufficient to outline a programme of research on *Glossina* as a vector, most of which remains to be done.

One further point may be taken from Macdonald's preliminary discussion of his subject. 'The disease to be analysed must first be established by criteria of recognition.' Macdonald used as his criterion the presence in the peripheral blood of parasites demonstrable by normal techniques. In trypanosomiasis failure to demonstrate trypanosomes in the bloodstream by normal techniques, whether in the human or the animal infection, is not sufficient evidence that they are absent. Nevertheless techniques are available to detect the trypanosomes in sites other than the bloodstream. But the identification of the human trypanosome in the insect vector or in the naturally infected animal host is impossible save by one method. This is to inoculate the flagellates into a number of human beings, a method that is unsatisfactory because of its danger and because it is difficult, perhaps impossible, to muster a sufficiently large sample of volunteers. A great deal of current research is directed towards the problem of identifying the human-infective trypanosomes and of separating them from those strains of *T. brucei* which are harmless. It is a problem being approached from many directions, though not necessarily yet from one that will provide the answer.

A main reason for the failure of Ross's mathematics was that one of his major premises was wrong. He supposed that 'an individual infected with malaria could not be again infected until after complete recovery from the initial infection. This is certainly untrue' (Macdonald 1957). It is perhaps not possible to make a parallel statement about the trypanosomiases, whether animal or human. It may be that geographical variation in patterns of sleeping sickness and their social and entomological relationships can be explained by varying frequency of inoculation of sub-infective doses of trypanosomes, or, indeed, of inoculation by trypanosomes specifically incapable of infecting man, but nevertheless provoking in him an immune response. Here again current research uses several avenues of approach.

It is in the field, however, that the study of factors that will lead to measurement of essential parameters in a formal epidemiology of trypanosomiasis are conspicuously lacking. It is matched on the control side by inadequate surveillance services. One can foresee a situation—indeed it already exists—where there is knowledge of how to control infection, but no knowledge of the habits and circumstances of the populations among which it needs to be applied. Entomologists in the past neglected, with a few notable exceptions, to study the people and livestock that were being bitten. In this respect, at least, political freedom offers a better prospect of progress than did colonial rule. Whatever may be the contributions made or yet to be made by research in the laboratories of the temperate regions, the solution to the problem of tropical African trypanosomiasis lies, as it has always done, in the hands of Africans themselves.

BIBLIOGRAPHY

ABRAHAM, D. P. (1964) Ethno-history of the empire of Mutapa. Problems and methods. In *The historian in tropical Africa*. International African Institute, London.

—— (1966) 'Chaminuka' and the Mhondoro cults. In *The Zambesian past* (ed. E. STOKES and R. BROWN). University Press, Manchester.

ABRAHAMS, R. G. (1967) The peoples of Greater Unyamwezi, Tanzania. *Ethnographic survey of Africa: East Central Africa*, Pt. 17. International African Institute, London.

ADAMANTIDIS, DR. (1956) Monographie pastorale du Ruanda-Urundi. *Bull. agric. Congo Belge*. **47,** 585.

ADAMSON, G. (1965) Learning to live free. *The Times*, London, 7 July, p. 12.

ADY, P. H. (ed.) (1965) *Regional economic atlas: Africa*. Oxford University Press, London.

ALLEN, W. and THOMSON, T. R. H. (1848). *A narrative of the expedition sent by Her Majesty's Government to the River Niger in 1841 under the command of Captain H. D. Trotter, R.N.*, 2 vols. Bentley, London.

ALPERS, E. (1968) The Mutapa and Malawi. In *Aspects of Central African history* (ed. T. O. RANGER). Heinemann, London.

Ankole district book Records kept in the District Commissioner's Office, Mbarara, Uganda.

ANSORGE, W. J. (1899) *Under the African sun. A description of native races in Uganda, sporting adventures and other experiences*. Heinemann, London.

APTED, F. I. C., ORMEROD, W. E., SMYLY, D. P., STRONACH, B. W., and SZLAMP, E. L. (1963) A comparative study of the epidemiology of endemic Rhodesian sleeping sickness in different parts of Africa. *J. trop. Med. Hyg.* **66,** 1.

ARKELL, A. J. (1961) *A history of the Sudan from the earliest times to 1821*. Athlone Press, London.

ASHCROFT, M. T. (1958) An attempt to isolate *Trypanosoma rhodesiense* from wild animals. *Trans. R. Soc. trop. Med. Hyg.* **52,** 276.

—— (1959*a*) A critical review of the epidemiology of human trypanosomiasis in Africa. *Trop. Dis. Bull.* **56,** 1073.

—— (1959*b*) The importance of African wild animals as reservoirs of trypanosomiasis. *E. Afr. med. J.* **36,** 289.

—— (1959*c*) The Tinde experiment. A further study of the long-term cyclical transmission of *Trypanosoma rhodesiense*. *Ann. trop. Med. Parasit.* **53,** 137.

—— BURTT, E., and FAIRBAIRN, H. (1959) The experimental infection of some African wild animals with *Trypanosoma rhodesiense*, *T. brucei*, and *T. congolense*. *Ann. trop. Med. Parasit.* **53,** 147.

AUBRÉVILLE, A. (1949) *Climats, forêts, et désertification de l'Afrique tropicale*. Société d'Éditions Géographiques, Maritimes et Coloniales, Paris.

AUSTEN, E. E. (1903) *A monograph of the tsetse-flies genus* Glossina, *Westwood based on the collection in the British Museum*. British Museum (Natural History), London.

AXELSON, E. (1960) *Portuguese in south-east Africa, 1600–1700.* Witwatersrand University Press, Johannesburg.

BAIKIE, W. B. (1856) *Narrative of an exploring voyage up the rivers Kwo'ra and Bi'nue (commonly known as the Niger and Tsadda) in 1848.* John Murray, London.

BAILEY, N. M. and BOREHAM, P. F. L. (1969) The number of *Trypanosoma rhodesiense* required to establish infection in man. *Ann. trop. Med. Parasit.,* **63,** 201.

—— DE RAADT, P., and KRAMPITZ, H. E. (1967) The investigation of an epidemic of human trypanosomiasis in Yimbo, Central Nyanza, Kenya. *East African Trypanosomiasis Research Organization report 1966,* p. 65. Government Printer, Entebbe.

BAKER, J. R. (1960) The influence of the number of trypanosomes inoculated on the prepatent period of the subsequent trypanosomiasis in laboratory rodents. *Ann. trop. Med. Parasit.* **54,** 71.

—— (1963) Speculations on the evolutions of the family Trypanosomidae Doflein, 1901. *Expl Parasit.* **13,** 219.

—— (1969a) *Parasitic Protozoa.* Hutchinson, London.

—— (1969b) Trypanosomes of wild mammals in the neighbourhood of the Serengeti national park. In MCDIARMID (1969) (*q.v.*).

—— SACHS, R., and LAUFER, I. (1967) Trypanosomes of wild mammals in an area northwest of the Serengeti national park, Tanzania. *Z. Tropenmed. Parasit.* **18,** 280.

BALANDIER, G. (1968) *Daily Life in the Kingdom of the Kongo.* Allen and Unwin, London.

BALDRY, D. A. T. (1964) Observations on a close association between *Glossina tachinoides* and domestic pigs near Nsukka, Eastern Nigeria. II Ecology and trypanosome infection rates of the fly. *Ann. trop. Med. Parasit.* **58,** 32.

—— (1966) On the distribution of *Glossina tachinoides* in West Africa, Pts. 1 and 2. *Proc. 11th Meet. int. scient. Comm. Trypanosom. (Nairobi), O.A.U./ S.T.R.C. Publ.* No. 100, pp. 95 and 103.

—— (1967) A species list of the Nigerian tsetse flies, genus *Glossina* (Diptera: Muscidae) in Nigeria. *Niger. ent. Mag.* **1,** 44.

—— (1968) The epidemiological significance of recent observations in Nigeria on the ecology of *Glossina tachinoides.* Paper presented to 8th International Congresses of Tropical Medicine and Malaria, Teheran, September 1968.

—— (1969) Distribution and trypanosome infection rates of *Glossina morsitans submorsitans* Newst. along a trade cattle route in south-western Nigeria. *Bull. ent. Res.* **58,** 537.

BALIS, J. and BERGEON, P. (1968) Étude de la repartition de glossines en Ethiopie. *Bull. Wld Hlth Org.* **38,** 809.

BANGOURA-ALECAUT, A. (1962) Contribution à la lutte concertée contre la trypanosomiase dans le territoire des Kissis. *Proc. 9th Meet. int. scient. Comm. Trypanosom. (Conakry), C.C.T.A. Publ.* No. 88, p. 311.

BARNES, J. A. (1951) The Fort Jameson Ngoni, i. In *Seven tribes of British Central Africa* (ed. E. COLSON and M. GLUCKMAN). Oxford University Press, London.

BARNES, O. (1958) North Maswa Survey. Report to Director of Tsetse Survey and Reclamation, Tanyanyika Territory. (Typescript.)

BARTH, H. (1857) *Travels and discoveries in north and central Africa being a journal of an expedition undertaken under the auspices of H.B.M.'s Government in the years 1849–1855*, 3 vols. Harper Brothers, New York.

BAUMANN, O. (1894) *Durch Massailand zur Nilquelle. Reisen und Forschungen des deutschen Anti-Sklaverei Komitee in den Jahren 1891–1893.* Dietrich Reimer, Berlin.

BEATON, W. G. (1968) Trypanosomiasis in African wild animals. Summary of paper by M. P. CUNNINGHAM in *Symposium on wildlife and land use.* Nairobi, Kenya, 1967. *Bull. epizoot. Dis. Afr.* **16**, 247.

BECK, M. (1914) Untersuchungen über ein um Rovuma (Deutsch-Ostafrika) vorkommendes *Trypanosoma* beim Menschen. *Arch. Schiffs- u. Tropenhyg.* **18**, 97.

—— and WECK, S. (1913) Die menschliche Trypanosomen Krankheit an Rovuma im Deutsch-Ostafrika. *Arch. Schiffs- u. Tropenhyg.* **17**, 145.

BEDFORD, G. A. H. (1927) Report on the transmission of nagana in the Ntalanama and Mhlatuze settlements, Zululand. 11th and 12th reports of the Director of Veterinary Education and Research, Pretoria Pt. 1, p. 275.

BEGUIN, H. (1960) La mise en valeur agricole du sud-est du Kasai. Essai de géographie agricole et de géographie agraire et ses possibilités d'application pratiques. *Publs. Inst. National pour l'étude agronomique du Congo (I.N.E.A.C.) Série scient.* **88**, Bruxelles.

BELL, H. HESKETH (1909) Report on the measures adopted for the suppression of sleeping sickness in Uganda. *Colonial reports—Miscellaneous* No. 65, Uganda. Cd. 4990, H.M.S.O., London.

BENT, T. (1896) *The ruined cities of Mashonaland.* Longmans, London.

BENTZ, M. and MACARIO, C. (1963) Le traitement systématique des individus porteurs d'hyper-béta-2-macroglobinemies (A.I.E. qualitatives) en zone d'endémie trypanique. *Bull. Soc. Path. exot.* **56**, 416.

BERNACCA, J. P. (1963) *Uganda Protectorate annual report of the Department of Veterinary Services and Animal Industry* Pt. 6, Tsetse control, p. 43. Government Printer, Entebbe.

BISSCHOP, J. H. R. (1937) Parent stock and derived types of African cattle, with particular reference to the importance of conformational characteristics in the study of their origin. *S. Afr. J. Sci.* **33**, 852.

BLAIR, D. (1939) Human trypanosomiasis in Southern Rhodesia 1911–1938. *Trans. R. Soc. trop. Med. Hyg.* **32**, 729.

—— BURNETT SMITH, E., and GELFAND, M. (1968) Human trypanosomiasis in Rhodesia—A new hypothesis suggested for the rarity of human trypanosomiasis. *Cent. Afr. J. Med.* **14**, supplement.

BOHANNAN, L. and BOHANNAN, P. (1953) The Tiv of Central Nigeria. *Ethnographic Survey of Africa: Western Africa* Pt. 8. International African Institute, London.

BOHANNAN, P. (1954a) Tiv farm and settlement. *Colonial research studies* No. 15. H.M.S.O., London.

—— (1954b) Expansion and migration of the Tiv. *Africa* Jan. 1954, p. 2.

BOUGHEY, A. S. (1957) *The origin of the African flora.* Inaugural lecture, University College of Rhodesia and Nyasaland. Oxford University Press, London.

BOURGUIGNON, G. C. (1937) Notes épidémiologiques sur la trypanosomiase humaine dans le Sud-Est du Congo Belge. *Bull. méd. Katanga* **14**, 3, 11, 21, 31.

BOYT, W. P., LOVEMORE, D. F., PILSON, R. D., and SMITH, I. D. (1962) A preliminary report on the maintenance of cattle by various drugs in a mixed *G. morsitans* and *G. pallidipes* fly-belt. *Proc. 9th Meet. int. scient. Comm. Trypanosom. (Conakry)*, *C.C.T.A. Publ.* No. 88, p. 71.

BRITISH SOUTH AFRICA COMPANY (1896, 1898) Reports on the Company's proceedings and the condition of the territories within the sphere of its operations, 1894–1895 and 1896–1897. London.

BROOKS, A. C. and BUSS, I. O. (1962) Past and present status of the elephant in Uganda. *J. Wildl. Mgmt* **27**, 36.

BROWN, K. N. (1963) The antigenic character of the *brucei* trypanosomes. In *Immunity to Protozoa*. A symposium of the British Society for Immunology, 1961. Oxford University Press, London.

BRUCE, D. (1915) *Rep. sleep. Sick. Commn. R. Soc.* No. 16, p. 18.

—— HARVEY, D., HAMERTON, A. E., DAVEY, J. B., and BRUCE, LADY (1913) The trypanosomes found in the blood of wild animals in the sleeping sickness area. *Rep. sleep. Sick. Commn. R. Soc.* No. 15, p. 16.

—— NABARRO, D., and GREIG, E. D. W. (1903) Further report on sleeping sickness in Uganda. *Rep. sleep. Sick. Commn. R. Soc.* No. 4, p. 3.

BUECHNER, H. K. and DAWKINS, H. C. (1961) Vegetation change induced by elephants and fire in Murchison Falls national park, Uganda. *Ecology* **42**, 752.

Bukoba District Book. Records kept in the District Commissioner's office, Bukoba, Tanzania.

BURKE, J. A. M. E. (1964) Considérations épidémiologiques sur la trypanosomiase à *T. gambiense* dans la République Démocratique du Congo. *Proc. 10th Meet. int. scient. Comm. Trypanosom. (Kampala)*, *C.C.T.A. Publ.* No. 97, p. 187.

BURNET, MACFARLANE (1953) *Natural history of infectious disease*. Cambridge University Press, London.

BURSELL, E. (1958) The water–balance of tsetse pupae. *Phil. Trans. R. Soc.* (B) **241**, 179.

—— (1959) The water balance of tsetse flies. *Trans. R. ent. Soc. Lond.* III, 205.

—— (1960) The effect of temperature on the consumption of fat during pupal development in *Glossina*, *Bull. ent. Res.* **51**, 583.

—— (1961) The behaviour of tsetse flies (*Glossina swynnertoni* Austen) in relation to problems of sampling. *Proc. R. ent. Soc. Lond.* (A) **36**, 8.

—— (1963) Aspects of the metabolism of amino acids in the tsetse-fly, *Glossina* (Diptera). *J. Insect Physiol.* **9**, 439.

—— (1965) Nitrogenous waste products of the tsetse-fly *Glossina morsitans*. *J. Insect. Physiol.* **11**, 993.

—— (1966) The nutritional state of tsetse-flies from different vegetation types in Rhodesia. *Bull. ent. Res.* **57**, 171.

—— (1969) Theoretical aspects of the control of *Glossina morsitans* by game destruction. *Zoologica Africana*, Capetown. (In press.)

—— and SLACK, E. (1968) Indications concerning the flight activity of tsetse flies (*Glossina morsitans* Westw.) in the field. *Bull. ent. Res.* **58**, 575.

BURTON, RICHARD (1860) *The Lake Regions of Central Africa*, 2 vols. Longmans, London.

BURTT, B. D. (1937) A report by the tsetse botanist on a preliminary ecological survey of north-western Uzinza with special reference to the population, soils, vegetation and the tsetse fly *Glossina morsitans*. E.A.T.R.O. Archives, Uganda. (Typescript.)

—— (1942) Some East African vegetation communities. *J. Ecol.* **30,** 67.

BURTT, E. (1946a) Incubation of tsetse pupae: increased transmission rate of *Trypanosoma rhodesiense* in *Glossina morsitans*. *Ann. trop. Med. Parasit.* **40,** 18.

—— (1946b) Salivation by *Glossina morsitans* on to glass slides: a technique for isolating infected flies. *Ann. trop. Med. Parasit.* **40,** 141.

BUSS, I. O. (1961) Some observations on food habits and behaviour of the African elephant. *J. Wildl. Mgmt* **25,** 131.

BUXTON, P. A. (1955) *The natural history of tsetse flies*. H. K. Lewis, London.

—— and LEWIS, D. J. (1934) Climate and tsetse-flies. Laboratory studies upon *Glossina submorsitans* and *tachinoides*. *Phil Trans. R. Soc.* (B) **224,** 175.

BUYCKX, E.-J.-E. (1964) Note préliminaire sur la biologie de *Glossina morsitans* Westw. au Bugesera (Rwanda). *Acad. roy. Sci. Outre-Mer. Bull. Séanc.* **805.**

CAGNOLO, C. (1933) *The Akikuyu. Their customs, traditions and folklore*. Nyeri, Kenya.

CARMICHAEL, J. (1938) Rinderpest in African game. *J. comp. Path.* **51,** 264.

CARPENTER, G. D. H. (1916) Dr. G. D. H. Carpenter's notes on South West Uganda and on late German East Africa west of Victoria Nyanza. *Proc. R. ent. Soc. Lond.* **68.**

—— (1920) *A naturalist on Lake Victoria with an account of sleeping sickness and the tsetse fly*. Fisher Unwin, London.

—— (1924) Report on an investigation into the epidemiology of sleeping sickness in Central Kavirondo, Kenya Colony. *Bull. ent. Res.* **15,** 187.

—— (1925) Manuscript notes. Library of Hope Department of Entomology, Oxford.

CARTER, R. M. (1906) Tsetse fly in Arabia. *Brit. med. J.* **2,** 1393.

CASEWELL, J. J. (1968) The control of tsetse and trypanosomiasis in the north-eastern districts of Rhodesia. Paper presented to 8th Congresses of Tropical Medicine and Malaria, Teheran, September 1968.

CHALLIER, A. (1965) Amélioration de la méthode de détermination de l'âge physiologique des Glossines. *Bull. Soc. Path. exot.* **58,** 250.

CHAPMAN, R. F. (1960) A note on *Glossina medicorum* Aust. (Diptera) in Ghana. *Bull. ent. Res.* **51,** 435.

—— (1961) Some experiments used to determine the methods used in host-finding by the tsetse fly, *Glossina medicorum* Austen. *Bull. ent. Res.* **52,** 83.

CHAPMAN, S. E., with text by DOWS DUNHAM (1952) *The royal cemeteries at Kush. Vol. 3. Decorated chapels of the Meroitic pyramids at Meroe and Barkal*. Museum of Fine Arts, Boston.

CHEVALIER, A. (1900) Les zones et les provinces botanique de l'A.O.F. *C. r. Acad. Sci.* **130,** 1205.

CHIEF NATIVE COMMISSIONER (1914) *Southern Rhodesia: Annual report of the Chief Native Commissioner*. Government Printer, Salisbury.

CHILD, G. and WILSON, V. J. (1964) Delayed effects of tsetse control hunting on a duiker population. *J. Wildl. Mgmt* **28**, 866.

CHORLEY, J. K. (1943) Tsetse fly operations, 1942. Short survey of the operations by districts for the year ending December 1942. *Rhodesia agric. J.* **40**, 174.

—— (1944) Tsetse fly operations. Short survey of the operations by districts for the year ending December 1943. *Rhodesia agric. J.* **41**, 412.

—— (1945) Tsetse fly operations. Short survey of the operations by districts for the year ending December 1944. *Rhodesia agric. J.* **42**, 493.

—— (1947a) Distribution of tsetse in Southern Rhodesia. *Conferencia inter-colonial sobre Tripanossomiases, Lourenco Marques, August, 1946*, vol. 1, p. 63.

—— (1947b) Tsetse fly operations in Southern Rhodesia. Short survey of the situation in the year ended December 1946. *Rhodesian agric. J.* **44**, 520.

—— (1954) Annual report of the Director of Tsetse Fly Operations for the year October 1st 1951 to September 30th 1952. *Rhodesia agric. J.* **51**, 197.

—— (1956) La lutte contre la mouche tsé-tsé en Rhodesie du Sud. *Proc. 6th Meet. int. scient. Comm. Trypansom. (Salisbury), C.C.T.A. Publ.*, p. 123.

CHORLEY, T. W. (1944) *Glossina palpalis fuscipes* breeding away from water (Diptera). *Proc. R. ent. Soc. Lond.* (A) **19**, 1.

CHRISTY, C. (1903) The epidemiology and etiology of the sleeping sickness in East Equatorial Africa with clinical observations. *Rep. sleep. Sick. Commn. R. Soc.* No. 3, p. 3.

CLARK, C. (1967) *Population growth and land use*. Macmillan, London.

CLARK, J. D. (1959) *The prehistory of Southern Africa*. Penguin Books, London.

COCKBILL, G. F. (1958a) Report of the Acting Director of Tsetse and Trypano-somiasis Control and Reclamation. *Report of the Secretary to the Federal Ministry of Agriculture for the year ended 30th September 1957*, Salisbury, p. 152.

—— (1958b) The use of records from traffic control points in Southern Rhodesia. *Proc. 7th Meet. int. Scient. Comm. Trypanosom. (Brussels), C.C.T.A. Publ.* No. 41, p. 231.

—— (1960a) District Reports, D. Other Areas. *Report of the Secretary to the Federal Ministry of Agriculture for the year ended 30th September 1959*, Salisbury, p. 206.

—— (1960b) The control of tsetse and trypanosomiasis in Southern Rhodesia. *Proc. Trans. Rhod. scient. Ass.* **47**, 1.

—— (1964) Report of the Assistant Director of Veterinary Services (Tsetse and Trypanosomiasis Control) for the year ended 30th September 1964, Salisbury. (Typescript.)

—— (1965) Report of the Assistant Director of Veterinary Services (Tsetse and Trypanosomiasis Control) for the year ended 30th September 1965, Salisbury. (Typescript.)

—— (1966) Report of the Assistant Director of Veterinary Services (Tsetse and Trypanosomiasis Control) for the year ended 30th September 1966, Salisbury. (Typescript.)

—— (1967) Recent developments in tsetse and trypanosomiasis control. The history and significance of trypanosomiasis problems in Rhodesia. *Proc. Trans. Rhod. scient. Ass.* **52**, 7.

COCKBURN, A. (1963) *The evolution and eradication of infectious diseases.* Johns Hopkins Press, Baltimore.

COCKERELL, T. D. A. (1918) New species of North American fossil beetles, cockroaches and tsetse flies. *Proc. U.S. natn. Mus.* **54,** 301.

COLBACK, H. R. F. (1952) Note au sujet de la carte des trypanosomes animales au Congo belge et au Ruanda-Urundi. *Proc. 4th Meet. int. scient. Comm. Trypanosom. (Lourenco Marques), C.C.T.A. Publ.,* No. 52, p. 26.

COLE, S. (1964) *The Prehistory of East Africa.* Weidenfeld and Nicolson, London.

COOK, A. R. (1945) *Uganda Memories (1897–1940).* Uganda Society. Kampala.

CORNEVIN, R. (1963) *Histoire des peuples de l'Afrique noire.* Berger-Levrault, Paris.

CORSON, J. F. (1935) Experimental transmission of *Trypanosoma rhodesiense* through antelopes and *Glossina morsitans* to man. *J. trop. Med. Hyg.* **38,** 9.

CRAZZOLARA, J. P. (1950, 1951) *The Lwoo. Pt. 1, Lwoo migrations; Pt. 2, Lwoo traditions,* 2 vols. Missioni Africane, Verona.

CROWDER, M. (1962) *The story of Nigeria.* Faber and Faber, London.

CULWICK, A. T., FAIRBAIRN, H., and CULWICK, R. E. (1951). The genetic relationship of the polymorphic trypanosomes and its practical implications. *Ann. trop. Med. Parasit.* **45,** 11.

CUNNINGHAM. M. P. and HARLEY, J. B. M. (1962) Preservation of living metacyclic forms of the *Trypanosoma brucei* sub-group. *Nature, Lond.* **149,** 1186.

—— and VAN HOEVE, K. (1965) Diagnosis of trypanosomiasis in cattle. *Proc. 10th Meet. int. scient. Comm. Trypanosom. (Kampala),* 1964, *C.C.T.A. Publ.* No. 97, p. 51.

CURASSON, A. (1932) *La peste bovine.* Vigot Frères, Paris.

CURD, F. H. and DAVEY, D. G. (1949) 'Antrycide': a new trypanocidal drug. *Nature, Lond.* **163,** 89.

CURSON, H. H. (1924) Notes on *Glossina pallidipes* in Zululand. *Bull. ent. Res.* **14,** 445.

—— (1932) Distribution of *Glossina* in Bechuanaland Protectorate. 18th Report of the Director of Veterinary Services and Animal Industry, Onderstepoort, August 1932, Pretoria.

—— and THORNTON, R. W. (1936) A contribution to the study of African native cattle. *Onderstepoort J. vet. Sci.* **7,** 613.

DARBY, H. C. (1956) The clearing of woodland in Europe. In *Man's role in changing the face of the earth* (ed. W. L. THOMAS). University of Chicago Press, Chicago.

—— (1957) The face of Europe on the eve of the great discoveries. *The new Cambridge modern history,* vol. 1, ch. 2. Cambridge University Press, London.

DAVEY, T. H. (1948) *Trypanosomiasis in British West Africa.* H.M.S.O., London.

DAVIDSON, B. (1965) *The growth of African civilisation. A history of West Africa, 1000–1800.* Longmans, London.

DAVIDSON, G. (1945) Report to the Chief Field Zoologist, Department of Veterinary Services, Kabete, Kenya. (See WIJERS, 1969.)

DAVIES, H. (1962) *Tsetse flies in Northern Nigeria. A handbook for junior control staff.* The Gaskiya Corporation, Zaria.

DAVIES, H. (1964) The eradication of tsetse in the Chad river system of Northern Nigeria. *J. appl. Ecol.* **1**, 387.

DAVISON, E. (1967) *Wankie: the story of a great game reserve.* Books of Africa, Capetown.

DAWE, M. J. (1906) *Report on a botanical mission through the forest districts of Buddu and the Western and Nile provinces of the Uganda Protectorate,* Cd. 2904, H.M.S.O., London.

DELMÉ-RADCLIFFE, C. (1947) Extracts from Lt. Col. C. Delmé-Radcliffe's diary report on the delimitation of the Anglo-German boundary, Uganda, 1902–1904. *Uganda J.* **11**, 9.

DENHAM, MAJOR (1831) *Travels and discoveries in Northern and Central Africa in 1822, 1823, and 1824 by Major Denham, F.R.S., Captain Clapperton, and the late Doctor Oudney, with a short account of Clapperton's and Lander's second journey in 1825, 1826, and 1827 in four volumes.* John Murray, London.

DEOM, J. (1949) La méthode du réveil provoqué dans le diagnostic des trypano-somiases bovines au Congo Belge. Communication préliminaire. *Annls Soc. belge Méd. trop.* **29**, 1.

DESART, THE EARL OF (Chairman) (1914) *Report of the Interdepartmental Committee on Sleeping Sickness,* Cd. 7349, and *Minutes of Evidence.* Cd. 7350, H.M.S.O., London.

DESOWITZ, R. S. (1959) Studies on immunity and host–parasite relationships. I. The immunological response of resistant and susceptible breeds of cattle to trypanosomal challenge. *Ann. trop. Med. Parasit.* **53**, 293.

—— (1960) Studies on immunity and host–parasite relationships. II. The immune response of antelope to trypanosomal challenge. *Ann. trop. Med. Parasit.* **54**, 281.

DOBBS, C. M. (1914) The Kisingiri and Gwasi districts of South Kavirondo, Nyanza province. *Jl E. Africa Uganda nat. Hist. Soc.* **4**, 129.

DUGGAN, A. J. (1962a) A survey of sleeping sickness in Northern Nigeria from the earliest times to the present day. *Trans. R. Soc. trop. Med. Hyg.* **56**, 439.

—— (1962b) The occurrence of human trypanosomiasis among the Rukuba tribe of Northern Nigeria. *J. trop. Med. Hyg.* **65**, 151.

DUKE, H. L. (1913) Some trypanosomes from wild game in Western Uganda. *Rep. sleep. Sick. Commn. R. Soc.* No. 14, p. 37.

—— (1919) Some observations on the bionomics of *Glossina palpalis* on the islands of Victoria Nyanza. *Bull. ent. Res.* **9**, 263.

—— (1923) An enquiry into an outbreak of human trypanosomiasis in a '*Glossina morsitans*' belt to the east of Mwanza, Tanganyika Territory. *Proc. R. Soc.* (B) **94**, 250.

—— (1928) Studies on the bionomics of the polymorphic trypanosomes of man and ruminants. *Final Report of the League of Nations International Commission on Human Trypanosomiasis.* C.H. 629, p. 21. Geneva.

—— (1930) The discovery of *T. rhodesiense* in man in Uganda Protectorate. *Trans. R. Soc. trop. Med. Hyg.* **24**, 201.

—— (1944) Rhodesian sleeping sickness. *Trans. R. Soc. trop. Med. Hyg.* **38**, 163.

DUNBAR, A. R. (1965) *A History of Bunyoro.* Oxford University Press, London.

DU TOIT, R. M. (1959) The eradication of the tsetse fly (*Glossina pallidipes*) from Zululand, Union of South Africa. *Advances in Veterinary Science* **5**, 227.

DUTTON, J. E. and TODD, J. L. (1906) Distribution and spread of sleeping sickness in the Congo Free State. Reports of the Expedition to the Congo, 1903–5. *Liverpool School of Tropical Medicine Memoir* 18, p. 23.

DYE, W. H. (1927) The relative importance of man and beast in human trypanosomiasis. *Trans. R. Soc. trop. Med. Hyg.* **21,** 187.

EAST AFRICA ROYAL COMMISSION (1955) *East Africa Royal Commission 1953–1955 report.* Cmd. 9475, H.M.S.O., London.

EAST AFRICAN TRYPANOSOMIASIS (1956 onwards) East African Trypanosomiasis Research Organization Annual Reports. East African High Commission and East African Common Services Organization, Nairobi.

EDNEY, E. B. and BARRASS, R. (1962) The body temperature of the tsetse fly, *Glossina morsitans* Westwood (Diptera, Muscidae). *J. Insect Physiol.* **8,** 469.

EGGELING, W. J. and DALE, I. R. (1951) *The indigenous trees of the Uganda Protectorate.* Crown Agents, London.

EMINSON, R. A. F. (1915) Observations on *Glossina morsitans* in Northern Rhodesia. *Bull. ent. Res.* **5,** 381.

ENGLEDOW, F. (1958) Agricultural policy in the Federation of Rhodesia and Nyasaland. *Report to the Federal Ministry of Agriculture by the Federal Standing Committee on Agricultural Production* in collaboration with Professor Sir Frank Engledow, C.M.G., F.R.S. C. Fed. 77, Government Printer, Salisbury.

EPSTEIN, H. (1933) Descent and origin of Afrikander cattle. *J. Hered.* **24,** 449.

—— (1934) Studies in Native Animal Husbandry. No. 9 The West African Shorthorn. *Jl S. Afr. vet. med. Ass.* **5,** 187.

—— (1955) The Zebu cattle of East Africa. *E. Afr. agric. J.* **21,** 83.

EVENS, F. M.-J.-C. (1953) Dispersion géographique des glossines au Congo Belge. *Mém. Inst. r. Sci. nat. Belg.* 2nd ser. fasc. 48.

FAGE, J. D. (1958) *An Atlas of African history.* Edward Arnold, London.

FAIRBAIRN, H. (1948) Sleeping Sickness in Tanganyika Territory, 1922–1946. *Trop. Dis. Bull.* **45,** 1.

—— (1954) The animal reservoirs of *Trypanosoma rhodesiense* and *Trypanosoma gambiense. Annls. Soc. belge Méd. trop.* **34,** 663.

—— (1956) The infectivity to man of syringe-passaged strains of *Trypanosoma rhodesiense* and *T. gambiense. Ann. trop. Med. Parasit.* **50,** 167.

—— and BURTT, E. (1946) The infectivity to man of a strain of *Trypanosoma rhodesiense* transmitted cyclically by *Glossina morsitans* through sheep and antelope: evidence that man requires a minimum infective dose of metacyclic trypanosomes. *Ann. trop. Med. Parasit.* **40,** 270.

—— and CULWICK, A. T. (1950) The transmission of the polymorphic trypanosomes. *Acta trop.* **7,** 19.

—— and WATSON, H. J. C. (1955) The transmission of *Trypanosoma vivax* by *Glossina palpalis. Ann. trop. Med. Parasit.* **43,** 250.

FALLERS, L. A. (1965) *Bantu bureaucracy.* University of Chicago Press, Chicago.

FARRELL, J. A. K. (1961) Maps to illustrate departmental reports on the vegetation of the Sabi river valley. Department of Tsetse and Trypanosomiasis Control and Reclamation, Federation of Rhodesia and Nyasaland, Salisbury, Rhodesia.

FAULKNER, D. E. and EPSTEIN, H. (1957) *The indigenous cattle of the British dependent territories in Africa.* H.M.S.O., London.

FEDERAL MINISTRY OF AGRICULTURE (1960) Tsetse and Trypanosomiasis Control and Reclamation: C. Sabi–Lundi area. *Report of the Secretary to the Federal Ministry of Agriculture* for the year ended 30 September 1960, Salisbury, p. 201.

—— (1962) Department of Veterinary Services, Tsetse and Trypanosomiasis Control. *Report of the Secretary to the Federal Ministry of Agriculture* for the year ended 30 September 1961, Salisbury, p. 216.

—— (1963) Department of Veterinary Services, Tsetse and Trypanosomiasis Control. *Report of the Secretary to the Federal Ministry of Agriculture* for the year ended 30 September 1962, Salisbury, p. 200.

FIENNES, R. N. T.-W. (1950) The cattle trypanosomiases. Cryptic trypanosomiases. *Ann. trop. Med. Parasit.* **44,** 222.

—— (1953) The therapeutic and prophylactic properties of antrycide in trypanosomiasis of cattle. *Br. vet. J.* **109,** 280.

—— (1964) *Man, nature and disease.* Weidenfeld and Nicolson, London.

FINELLE, P., DESROTOUR, J., YVORE, P., and RENNER, R. (1962) Essai de lutte contre *Glossina fusca,* par pulvérisation de dieldrin, en République Centrafricaine. *Revue Élev. Med. vét. Pays trop.* **15,** 247.

—— ITARD, J., YVORE, P., and LACOTTE, R. (1963) Répartition des glossines en République Centrafricaine. État actuel des connaissances. *Revue Élev. Med. vét. Pays trop.* **16,** 337.

FISKE, W. F. (1920) Investigations into the bionomics of *Glossina palpalis. Bull. ent. Res.* **10,** 247.

FLEMING, A. M. (1913) Trypanosomiasis in Southern Rhodesia. *Trans. R. Soc. trop. Med. Hyg.,* **6,** 298.

F.A.O. (1962) *Africa Survey.* Report on the possibilities of African rural development in relation to economic and social growth. F.A.O., Rome.

FORD, J. (1944a) A survey of the wet season limits of *G. pallidipes* in South Busoga, May 1944. E.A.T.R.O. archives, Tororo. (Typescript.)

—— (1944b) Busoga defence line: Igwe sector. E.A.T.R.O. archives, Tororo. (Typescript.)

—— (1948) *A safari to Uzinza, December 1947.* Report to Chief Entomologist, E. African Tsetse Research Organization, Shinyanga, dated 20.1.48. (Typescript.)

—— (1950) Early anti-trypanosomiasis measures treated as ecological field experiments. *Proc. 2nd Meet. int. scient. Comm. Trypanosom. (Antwerp). Publs. Bur. perm. interafr. Tsé-tsé* No. 112/0.

—— (1953) Tsetse fly in Ankole: A Hima song. *Uganda J.* **17,** 186.

—— (1958a) A note on the location of *Glossina morsitans* Westw. on transect fly-rounds. *Proc. 7th Meet. int. scient. Comm. Trypanosom. (Bruxelles), C.C.T.A. Publ.* No. 41, p. 237.

—— (1958b) Tsetse reclamation and development in eastern Africa. *Proc. 6th Int. Congr. trop. Med. Malaria* No. 3, p. 223.

—— (1960a) The advance of *Glossina morsitans* and *Glossina pallidipes* into the Sabi and Lundi River basins, Southern Rhodesia. *Proc. 8th Meet. int. scient. Comm. Trypanosom. (Jos), C.C.T.A. Publ.* No. 62, p. 219.

—— (1960b) The influence of tsetse flies on the distribution of African cattle. *Proceedings of the 1st Federal Science Congress*, Salisbury, p. 357.

—— (1962) Microclimates of tsetse fly resting sites in the Zambezi Valley, Southern Rhodesia. *Proc. 9th Meet. int. scient. Comm. Trypanosom. (Conakry). C.C.T.A. Publ.* No. 88, p. 165.

—— (1963) The distribution of the vectors of African pathogenic trypanosomes. *Bull. Wld Hlth Org.* **28**, 653.

—— (1964) The geographical distribution of trypanosome infections in African cattle populations. *Bull. epizoot. Dis. Afr.* **12**, 307.

—— (1965) Distributions of *Glossina* and epidemiological patterns in the African trypanosomiases. *J. trop. Med. Hyg.* **68**, 211.

—— (1966) The role of elephants in controlling the distribution of tsetse flies. *Bull. int. Un. Conserv. Nat.*, N.S. **19**, 6.

—— (1968) The control of populations through limitation of habitat distribution as exemplified by tsetse flies. *R. ent. Soc. Lond. Symposium on Insect Abundance* (ed. T. R. E. SOUTHWOOD). Blackwell, Oxford.

—— (1969a) Age groups in feeding and following *Glossina morsitans* males. 9th Seminar on Trypanosomiasis. *Trans R. Soc. trop. Med. Hyg.* **63**, 126.

—— (1969b) Feeding and other responses of tsetse flies to man and ox and their epidemiological significance. *Acta trop.* **26**, 249.

—— (1969c) The control of the African trypanosomiases with special reference to land use. *Bull. Wld Hlth Org.* **40**, 879.

—— and CLIFFORD, H. R. (1968) Changes in the distribution of cattle and of bovine trypanosomiasis associated with the spread of tsetse-flies (*Glossina*) in south-west Uganda. *J. appl. Ecol.* **5**, 301.

—— GLASGOW, J. P., JOHNS, D. L., and WELCH, J. R. (1959) Transect fly rounds in field studies of *Glossina. Bull. ent. Res.* **50**, 275.

—— and HALL, R. DE Z. (1947) The history of Karagwe, Bukoba district. *Tanganyika Notes Rec.* **24**, 3.

—— and LEGGATE, B. M. (1961). The geographical and climatic distribution of trypanosome infection rates in *G. morsitans* group of tsetse flies. *Trans. R. Soc. trop. Med. Hyg.* **55**, 383.

FOSTER, R. (1963) Contributions to the epidemiology of human sleeping sickness in Liberia. *Trans. R. Soc. trop. Med. Hyg.* **57**, 465.

FRIES, R. E. (1921) *Wissenschaftliche Ergebnisse der Schwedischen Rhodesia-Congo Expedition 1911–1912 inter leitung von Eric Graf von Rosen.* Bd. 1. Botanische Untersuchungen, Stockholm.

FULLER, C. (1923) Tsetse in the Transvaal and surrounding territories. An historical review. *9th and 10th reports of the Director of Veterinary Education and Research*, Pretoria.

FURON, R. (1963) *The geology of Africa.* Oliver and Boyd, Edinburgh.

GABBA, DR. (1938) *La maladie du sommeil dans le district de Kwango avant l'occupation de ce district par* Foreami *jusqu'à fin 1934.* Foreami, Bruxelles.

GANN, L. H. (1965) *A history of Southern Rhodesia. Early days to 1934.* Chatto and Windus, London.

GARSTIN, W. (1904) *Despatch from His Majesty's Agent and Consul-General at Cairo inclosing a report by Sir William Garstin, K.C.M.G., Under-Secretary.*

of State for Public Works in Egypt, upon the basin of the Upper Nile. Cd. 2165, H.M.S.O. London.

GELFAND, M. (1961) *Northern Rhodesia in the days of the Charter.* Blackwell, Oxford.

—— (1966) The early clinical features of rhodesian trypanosomiasis with special reference to the 'chancre' (local reaction). *Trans. R. Soc. trop. Med. Hyg.* **60,** 376.

GILLMAN, C. (1936) A population map of Tanganyika Territory. *Geogr. Rev.* **26,** 353.

GLASGOW, J. P. (1947) Notes on the history of *G. pallidipes* in Samia. Report in E.A.T.R.O. Archives, Uganda. (Typescript.)

—— (1954) *Glossina palpalis fuscipes* Newst. in lake-side and riverine forest. *Bull. ent. Res.* **45,** 563.

—— (1960) Shinyanga: a review of the work of the Tsetse Research Laboratory. *E. Afr. agric. For. J.* **26,** 22.

—— (1961a) The feeding habits of *Glossina swynnertoni* Austen. *J. Anim. Ecol.* **30,** 77.

—— (1961b) Ecological effects of tsetse fly control in particular as a consequence of bush clearing. *International Union for the Conservation of Nature Symposium,* Warsaw 1960, p. 85, Leiden.

—— (1963a) *Distribution and abundance of tsetse.* Pergamon, Oxford.

—— (1963b) Tsetse in the environment of ancient man in Southern Rhodesia. *Nature, Lond.* **197,** 414.

—— (1967) Recent fundamental work on tsetse flies. *Ann. Rev. Ent.* **12,** 421.

—— ISHERWOOD, F., LEE-JONES, F., and WEITZ, B. (1958) Factors influencing the staple food of tsetse flies. *J. Anim. Ecol.* **27,** 59.

—— and WILSON, F. (1953) A census of the tsetse fly *Glossina pallidipes* Austen and of its host animals. *J. Anim. Ecol.* **22,** 47.

GLOVER, P. E. (1965) *The tsetse problem in Northern Nigeria* (2nd edn.). Patwa News Agency, Nairobi.

GODFREY, D. G. (1960) Types of *Trypanosoma congolense.* I. Morphological differences. *Ann. trop. Med. Parasit.* **54,** 428.

—— and KILLICK-KENDRICK, R. (1961) Bovine trypanosomiasis in Nigeria. I. The inoculation of blood into rats as a method of survey in the Donga valley, Benue province. *Ann. trop. Med. Parasit.* **55,** 287.

—— —— and FERGUSON, W. (1965) Bovine trypanosomiasis in Nigeria. IV: Observations on cattle trekked along a trade cattle route through areas infested with tsetse fly. *Ann. trop. Med. Parasit.* **59,** 255.

—— —— and LEACH, T. M. (1962) Recent findings on the incidence of bovine trypanosomiasis in Nigeria. *9th Meet. int. scient. Comm. Trypanosom. (Conakry), C.C.T.A. Publ.* No. 88, p. 111.

GOLDTHORPE, J. E. (1955) The African population of East Africa: A summary of its past and present trends. Appendix 7 to EAST AFRICA ROYAL COMMISSION (*q.v.*).

GOODIER, R. (1958) Some effects of bush clearing in Southern Rhodesia. *Proc. 7th Meet. int. scient. Comm. Trypanosom. (Brussels). C.C.T.A. Publ.* No. 41, p. 241.

—— (1961a) The Sabi–Lundi tsetse fly front. *Report of the Secretary to the*

Federal Ministry of Agriculture for the year ended 30 September 1960, Salisbury, p. 238.

—— (1961b) *A note on the use of biting fly traverses to detect tsetse.* Report to Director, Tsetse and Trypanosomiasis Control Department, Salisbury, Rhodesia, dated 25.3.61. (Typescript.)

—— (1962) Blood feeding by *Philoliche (Dorcaloemus) silverlocki* Austen (Diptera, Tabanidae). *Nature, Lond.* **193,** 1003.

GORDON, R. M., CREWE, W., and WILLETT, K. C. (1956) Studies on the deposition, migration, and development to the blood forms of trypanosomes belonging to the *Trypanosoma brucei* group. I. An account of the process of feeding adopted by the tsetse-fly when obtaining a blood meal from the mammalian host, with special reference to the ejection of saliva and the relationship of the feeding process to the deposition of metacyclic trypanosomes. *Ann. trop. Med. Parasit.* **50,** 426.

—— and WILLETT, K. C. (1958) Studies on the deposition, migration, and development of the blood forms of trypanosomes belonging to the *Trypanosoma brucei* group. III. The development of *Trypanosoma rhodesiense* from the metacyclic forms as observed in mammalian tissue and in culture. *Ann. trop. Med. Parasit.* **52,** 346.

GORJU, PÈRE J. (1920) *Entre le Victoria, l'Albert, et l'Edouard.* Imprimeries Oberthür, Rennes.

GRANT, J. A. (1864) *A walk across Africa.* Blackwood, Edinburgh.

GRAY, A. C. H. (1908) Report on the Sleeping Sickness camps, Uganda, from December 1906–November 1907. *Rep. sleep. Sick. Commn. R. Soc.* No. 9, p. 62.

GRAY, A. R. (1962) The influence of antibody on serological variation in *Trypanosoma brucei. Ann. trop. Med. Parasit.* **56,** 4.

—— (1965) Antigenic variation in a strain of *Trypanosoma brucei* transmitted by *Glossina morsitans* and *G. palpalis. J. gen. Microbiol.* **41,** 195.

—— (1966) Immunological studies on the epizootiology of *Trypanosoma brucei* in Nigeria. *Proc. 11th Meet. int. scient. Comm. Trypanosom. (Nairobi). O.A.U./S.T.R.C. Publ.* No. 100, p. 57.

—— (1967) Some principles of the immunology of trypanosomiasis. *Bull. Wld Hlth Org.* **37,** 177.

GRIFFITHS, J. A. (1937) *Trypanosomiasis of the horse in Nigeria.* Reprinted from the Veterinary Report for Nigeria for the year 1936. Government Printer, Kaduna.

GROGAN, E. S., and SHARP, A. H. (1900) *From Cape to Cairo.* Hurst and Blackett, London.

GROVE, A. T. (1961) *Population densities and agriculture in Northern Nigeria.* In *Essays on African Population* (ed. K. M. BARBOUR and R. M. PROTHERO). Routledge and Kegan Paul, London.

GRUVEL, J. (1966) Les glossines vectrices des trypanosomiases au Tchad. *Revue Élev. Med. vét. Pays trop.* **19,** 169.

HALL, P. E. (1910) Notes on the movements of *Glossina morsitans* in the Lundazi district, north-eastern Rhodesia. *Bull. ent. Res.* **1,** 183.

HALL, S. A. (1962) The cattle plague of 1865. *Med. Hist.* **6,** 45.

HARDING, R. D. (1940) A trial with 4:4'-diamidino-stilbene in the treatment of sleeping sickness at Gadau, Northern Nigeria. *Ann. trop. Med. Parasit.* **34,** 101.

HARDING, R. D. and HUTCHINSON, M. P. (1948) Sleeping sickness of an unusual type in Sierra Leone and its attempted control. *Trans. R. Soc. trop. Med. Hyg.* **41,** 481.

HARKER, K. W. (1959) An *Acacia* weed of Uganda grasslands. *Trop. Agric., Trin.* **36,** 45.

HARLEY, J. M. B. (1966a) Seasonal and diurnal variation in physiological age and trypanosome infection rate of females of *Glossina pallidipes* Aust., *G. palpalis fuscipes* Newst., and *G. brevipalpis* Newst. *Bull. ent. Res.* **56,** 595.

—— (1966b) Studies on age and trypanosome infection rates in *Glossina pallidipes* Aust., *Glossina palpalis fuscipes* Newst., and *G. brevipalpis* Newst. in Uganda. *Bull. ent. Res.* **57,** 23.

—— (1967a) Further studies on age and trypanosome infection rates in *Glossina pallidipes* Aust., *G. palpalis fuscipes* Newst., and *G. brevipalpis* Newst. in Uganda. *Bull. ent. Res.* **57,** 459.

—— (1967b) A population of *G. fuscipes* without trypanosome infections. *E. Afr. Tryp. Res. Org. Report. 1966,* p. 52. Government Printer, Entebbe.

—— CUNNINGHAM, M. P., and VAN HOEVE, K. (1966) The numbers of infective *Trypanosoma rhodesiense* extruded by *Glossina morsitans* during feeding. *Ann. trop. Med. Parasit.* **60,** 455.

—— and WILSON, A. J. (1968) Comparison between *Glossina morsitans, G. pallidipes,* and *G. fuscipes* as vectors of the *Trypanosoma congolense* group: the proportions infected experimentally and the number of infective organisms extruded during feeding. *Ann. trop. Med. Parasit.* **62,** 178.

HARROY, J. P. (1949) *Afrique, terre qui meurt.* Marcel Hayez, Brussels.

HEINZ, H. J. (1968). Trypanosomiasis in Ngamiland: an ethnoparasitological investigation. *S. Afr. geogr. J.* **50,** 93.

HEISCH, R. B., McMAHON, J. P., and MANSON-BAHR, P. E. C. (1958) The isolation of *Trypanosoma rhodesiense* from a bushbuck. *Br. med. J.* **2,** 1203.

HENNING, M. W. (1956) *Animal diseases in South Africa* (3rd edn.). Central News Agency, Johannesburg.

HERRMANN, HAUPTMANN (1894) Die Wasiba und ihr Land. *Mitt.dt.Schutzgeb.* **7,** 46.

—— (1899) Aufnahmen zwischen dem Victoria Nyanza und dem Kagera. *Mitt. dt. Schutzgeb.* **12,** 105, 168.

D'HERTEFELT, M., TROUWBORST, A., and SCHERER, J. (1962) Les anciens royaumes de la zone interlacustre méridionale (Rwanda, Burundi, Buha). *Ethnographic Survey of Africa,* International African Institute, London.

HILL, J. F. R., and MOFFETT, J. P. (1955) *Tanganyika: A review of its resources and their development.* Government of Tanganyika, Dar-es-salaam.

HOARE, C. A. (1931) Studies on *Trypanosoma grayi.* III. Life cycle in the tsetse fly and in the crocodile. *Parasitology* **23,** 449.

—— (1949) *Handbook of medical protozoology.* Baillière, Tindall, and Cox, London.

—— (1964) Morphological and taxonomic studies on mammalian trypanosomes. X. Revision of systematics. *J. Protozool.* **11,** 200.

—— (1965) Discussion on K. C. Willett (1965). *Trans. R. Soc. trop. Med. Hyg.* **59,** 390.

HODGES, A. D. P. (1908) Report on sleeping sickness in Uganda from 4 January to 30 June 1906. *Rep. sleep. Sick. Commn. R. Soc.* No. 9, p. 3.

HOEPPLI, R. (1969) *Parasitic diseases in Africa and the western hemisphere: early documentation and transmission by the slave trade. Acta trop.* Supplement 10, Verlag für Recht und Gesellschaft AG, Basel.

—— and LUCASSE, C. (1964) Old ideas regarding cause and treatment of sleeping sickness held in West Africa. *J. trop. Med. Hyg.* **67,** 60.

HOGBEN, S. J., and KIRKE-GREEN, A. H. M. (1966) *The emirates of Northern Nigeria.* Oxford University Press, London.

HOLTZ, W. (1911) Der Minsirowald in Deutsch-Buddu, seine Beschaffenheit, sein Wert und seine wirtschaftliche Bedeutung. *Ber. ü. Land- und Forstwirtschaft in Deutsch-Ost-Afrika* **3,** 223.

HOPE-GILL, C. W. (1930) A comparative study of human trypanosomiasis in Kano and the Plateau provinces (Northern provinces of Nigeria). *W. Afr. Med. J.* **3,** 53.

—— (1935) The problem of *T. gambiense* sleeping sickness in Southern Nigeria. *W. Afr. med. J.* **8,** 10.

HOPEN, C. E. (1958) *The pastoral Fulbe family in Gwandu.* Oxford University Press, London.

HORNBY, H. E. (1930) Control of Animal Trypanosomiasis. *11th International Veterinary Congress.* Bale, Sons and Danielson, London.

—— (1938) in *Annual Report of the Department of Veterinary Science and Animal Husbandry, 1937.* Government Printer, Dar-es-salaam.

—— (1947) Report on the tsetse fly problem of Maputo. *An. Inst. Med. trop. Lisbon* **4,** 313.

—— (1948) Tsetse problems in relation to those of soil conservation. Communication No. 84, Conférence africaine des sols, Goma. *Bull. agric. Congo belge.* **40,** Fasc. 3–4, 2189.

—— (1952) *Animal trypanosomiasis in eastern Africa, 1949.* H.M.S.O., London.

HORTON-SMITH, C. (ed.) (1957) *Biological aspects of the transmission of disease.* Oliver and Boyd, Edinburgh.

HOWARD, L. O. and FISKE, W. F. (1911) The importation into the United States of the parasites of the gypsy moth and the crown-tail moth. *U.S. Dept. Agriculture, Bureau of Entomology, Bull.* No. 91.

HUTCHINSON, M. P. (1953, 1954) The epidemiology of human trypanosomiasis in British West Africa. Pts I, II, and III. *Ann. trop. Med. Parasit.* **47,** 156 and **48,** 75.

—— (1962) Northern Liberia—Human trypanosomiasis 1959–60. *Proc. 9th Meet. int. scient. Comm. Trypanosom. (Conakry), C.C.T.A. Publ.* No. 88, p. 301.

INTERNATIONAL BANK (1955) *The economic development of Nigeria. A report of a mission organized by the International Bank for Reconstruction and Development.* Johns Hopkins Press, Baltimore.

JACK, R. W. (1914) Tsetse fly and big game in Southern Rhodesia. *Bull. ent. Res.* **5,** 97.

—— (1927) Some environmental factors relating to the distribution of *Glossina morsitans* Westw. in Southern Rhodesia. *S. Afr. J. Sci.* **24,** 457.

—— (1933) The tsetse fly problem in Southern Rhodesia. *Rhodesia agric. J.* **30,** 365.

JACK, R. W. (1939) Studies in the physiology and behaviour of *Glossina morsitans* Westw. *Mem. Dept. Agriculture, Southern Rhodesia* No. 1, Salisbury.

—— (1941) Further studies in the physiology and behaviour of *Glossina morsitans* Westw. *Mem. Dept. Agriculture, Southern Rhodesia* No. 3, Salisbury.

—— and WILLIAMS, W. L. (1937) The effect of temperature on the reaction of *Glossina morsitans* Westwood to light. A preliminary note. *Bull. ent. Res.* **28,** 499.

JACKSON, C. H. N. (1930) Contributions to the bionomics of *Glossina morsitans*. *Bull. ent. Res.* **21,** 491.

—— (1933) The causes and implications of hunger in tsetse flies. *Bull. ent. Res.* **24,** 443.

—— (1937) Some new methods in the study of *Glossina morsitans*. *Proc. zool. Soc. Lond. 1936,* 811.

—— (1940) The analysis of a tsetse fly population. *Ann. Eugen.* **10,** 332.

—— (1943) Interim report on sleeping sickness epidemic in Busoga. Dept. of Tsetse Research, Tanganyika Territory. E.A.T.R.O. archives. (Typescript.).

—— (1945) Comparative studies of the habitat requirements of tsetse fly species. *J. Anim. Ecol.* **14,** 46.

—— (1946) An artificially isolated generation of tsetse flies (Diptera). *Bull. ent. Res.* **37,** 291.

—— (1949) The biology of tsetse flies. *Biol Rev.* **24,** 174.

—— (1954) The hunger cycles of *Glossina morsitans* Westw. and *G. swynnertoni* Aust. *J. Anim. Ecol.* **23,** 368.

—— (1955) The pattern of *Glossina morsitans* communities. *Bull. ent. Res.* **46,** 517.

JACKSON, P. J. and PHELPS, R. J. (1967) Temperature regimes in pupation sites of *Glossina morsitans orientalis* Vanderplank (Diptera). *Rhod. Zamb. Malawi J. agric. Res.* **5,** 249.

JANSSENS, P. G. and BURKE, J. A. M. E. (1968) Situation actuelle de la trypanosomiase humaine en République démocratique du Congo. Personal communication of data presented to FAO/WHO Expert committee, Geneva.

JEANNEL, R. (1942) *La genése des faunes terrestres. Éléments de biogéographie.* Presses Universitaires de France, Paris.

JEFFREYS, M. D. W. (1953) *Bos brachyceros* or dwarf cattle. *Vet. Rec.* **65,** 393, 410.

JOHNSON, W. B. and LLOYD, LL. (1923) First report of the tsetse fly investigation in the Northern provinces of Nigeria. *Bull. ent. Res.* **13,** 373.

JOHNSTON, H. (1900) *Preliminary report by Her Majesty's Special Commissioner on the Protectorate of Uganda.* Cd. 256, H.M.S.O., London.

—— (1901) *Report of His Majesty's Special Commissioner on the Protectorate of Uganda.* Cd. 671, H.M.S.O., London.

JORDAN, A. M. (1961) An assessment of the economic importance of the tsetse species of Southern Nigeria and the Southern Cameroons based on their trypanosome infection rates and ecology. *Bull. ent. Res.* **52,** 431.

—— (1963) The distribution of the *Fusca* group of tsetse flies (*Glossina*) in Nigeria and West Cameroon. *Bull. ent. Res.* **54,** 307.

—— (1964) Trypanosome infection rates in *Glossina morsitans submorsitans* Newst. in Northern Nigeria. *Bull. ent. Res.* **55,** 219.

—— (1965a) The hosts of *Glossina* as the main factor affecting trypanosome infection rates of tsetse flies in Nigeria. *Trans. R. Soc. trop. Med. Hyg.* **59**, 423.

—— (1965b) Observations on the ecology of *Glossina morsitans submorsitans* Newst. in the Northern Guinea savannah of Northern Nigeria. *Bull. ent. Res.* **56**, 1.

—— (1965c) Bovine trypanosomiasis in Nigeria. V. The tsetse fly challenge to a herd of cattle trekked along a trade-route. *Ann. trop. Med. Parasit.* **59**, 270.

—— (1965d) The status of *Glossina fusca* Walker (Diptera, Muscidae) in West Africa. *Ann. trop. Med. Parasit.* **59**, 219.

—— LEE-JONES, F., and WEITZ, B. (1961) The natural hosts of tsetse flies in the forest belt of Nigeria and the Southern Cameroons. *Ann. trop. Med. Parasit.* **55**, 167.

—— —— —— (1962) The natural hosts of tsetse flies in Northern Nigeria. *Ann. trop. Med. Parasit.* **56**, 430.

JOSHI, N. R., McLAUGHLIN, E. A., and PHILLIPS, R. W. (1957) *Types and breeds of African cattle.* F.A.O., Rome.

KAMUGUNGUNU, L. (1946) Personal communication on movements of cattle from Ankole to Karagwe in 1917.

KEAY, R. W. J. (1949) *An outline of Nigerian vegetation.* Government Printer, Lagos.

—— (1953) *An outline of Nigerian vegetation* (2nd edn.). Government Printer, Lagos.

—— (1959) Derived savanna—derived from what? *Bulletin de l'IFAN* **21**, A, 427.

—— AUBRÉVILLE, A., DUVIGNEAUD, P., HOYLE, A. C., MENDONCA, F. A., and PICHI-SERMOLLI, R. E. G. (1958) *Vegetation map of Africa south of the Tropic of Cancer.* Oxford University Press, London.

KENYA MINISTRY OF AGRICULTURE (1956) *African land development in Kenya 1946–55.* Ministry of Agriculture, Animal Husbandry, and Water Resources, Nairobi.

KENYA (various dates) *Veterinary Department annual reports.* Government Printer, Nairobi.

KILLICK-KENDRICK, R. and GODFREY, D. G. (1963) Bovine trypanosomiasis in Nigeria. II. The incidence among some migrating cattle with observations on the examination of wet blood preparations as a method of survey. *Ann. trop. Med. Parasit.* **57**, 117.

KINGHORN, A., YORKE, W., and LLOYD, Ll. (1913) Final report of the Luangwa Sleeping Sickness Commission of the British South Africa Company, 1911–12. *Ann. trop. Med. Parasit.* **7**, 183.

KLEINE, F. K. (1909) Positive infektionsversuche mit *Trypanosoma brucei* durch *Glossina palpalis. Deutsch. med. Wschr.* **35**, 469.

—— (1928) Report of the new sleeping sickness focus at Ikoma. *Final report of the League of Nations International Commission on Human Trypanosomiasis,* Geneva, C.H. 629, p. 7.

—— and FISCHER, W. (1912) Schlafkrankheit und Tsetsefliegen. *Zeitschr. f. Hyg. u. Infektionskrankheiten* **23**, 253 (in *Trop. Dis. Bull.* **1**, 270).

KOCH, R. (1907) in *Deutsch. med. Wschr.* **333**, 1889; quoted in Diagnosis of human trypanosomiasis, *Bull. Sleep. Sickn. Bur.* December 1908, 58.

KOLLMAN, P. (1899) *The Victoria Nyanza.* Swann, Sonnenschein, London.

KUCZYNSKI, R. R. (1937) *Colonial population.* Oxford University Press, London.

—— (1948) *Demographic survey of the British colonial empire. Vol. 1, West Africa.* Oxford University Press, London.

LAMBORN, W. A. (1915) Second report on *Glossina* investigations in Nyasaland. *Bull. ent. Res.* **6**, 249.

LAMBRECHT, F. (1955) Contribution à l'étude de la répartition des tsétsés dans les territoires du Ruanda-Urundi. *Annls Soc. belge Méd. trop.* **35**, 427.

—— (1964) Aspects of evolution and ecology of tsetse flies and trypanosomiasis in prehistoric African environment. *Jl Afr. Hist.* **5**, 1.

LANGDALE-BROWN, I., OSMASTON, H. A., and WILSON, J. G. (1964) *The vegetation of Uganda and its bearing on land use.* The Government Printer, Entebbe.

LANGHELD, W. (1909) *Zwanzig Jahre in deutschen Kolonien.* Wilhelm Weicher, Berlin.

LANGLEY, P. A. (1968) The effect of feeding the tsetse fly *Glossina morsitans* Westw. on impala blood. *Bull. ent. Res.* **58**, 295.

LAURIE, W., BRASS, M. A., and TRANT, H. (n.d.) A health survey in Kwimba district Tanganyika. East African Medical Survey Monograph No. 3. East African Medical Research Organisation, Mwanza. (Mimeograph.)

LAVERAN, A. and MESNIL, F. (trans. NABARRO, D.) (1907) *Trypanosomes and trypanosomiasis.* Baillière, Tindall, and Cox, London.

LAVIER, G. (1928) A morphological study of iolated strains at Entebbe Laboratory by the International Sleeping Sickness Commission. *Final report of the League of Nations International Commission on human trypanosomiasis,* Geneva, C.H. 629, p. 122.

LAWRENCE, D. A. and BRYSON, R. W. (1958) Trypanosomiasis in Southern Rhodesia. *Symposium on animal trypanosomiasis, Luanda, Angola. C.C.T.A. Publ.* No. 45.

LE BERRE, R. and ITARD, J. (1960) Validité des sous-espèces *Glossina fusca fusca* Walker 1849 et *Glossina fusca congolensis* Newstead and Evans 1921, Diptera, Muscidae. *Bull. Soc. Path. exot.* **53**, 542.

LEGGATE, B. M. (1962) Trypanosome infections in *Glossina morsitans* Westw. and *G. pallidipes* Aust. under natural conditions. *Proc. 9th Meet. int. scient. Comm. Trypanosom. (Conakry), C.C.T.A. Publ.* No. 88, p. 213.

LESTER, H. M. O. (1930) Annual Report, Tsetse Investigation 1929, Appendix B to Nigeria Annual Medical and Sanitary Report for the year 1929. Government Printer, Lagos.

—— (1933) The characteristics of some Nigerian strains of polymorphic trypanosomes. *Ann. trop. Med. Parasit.* **27**, 361.

—— (1938) The progress of sleeping sickness work in Northern Nigeria. *W. Afr. med. J.* **10**, 2.

—— (1939) The results of sleeping sickness work in Northern Nigeria. *Trans. R. Soc. trop. Med. Hyg.* **32**, 615.

—— (1945) Further progress in the control of sleeping sickness on Nigeria. *Trans. R. Soc. trop. Med. Hyg.* **38**, 425.

LEWIS, E. A. (1934) Tsetse-flies in the Masai Reserve, Kenya colony. *Bull. ent. Res.* **25**, 439.

—— (1937) Tsetse-flies in the Ol Orukuti area of the Masai reserve, Kenya colony. *Bull. ent. Res.* **28,** 395.

—— (1939 Observations on *Glossina fuscipleuris* and other tsetses in the Oyani valley, Kenya colony. *Bull. ent. Res.* **30,** 345.

—— (n.d.) Report of experiments on the control of *Glossina pallidipes* in Kenya colony. Tsetse flies in the Lambwe valley, Kenya colony. Veterinary Research Laboratory, Kabete, Kenya. (Mimeograph.)

LEWIS, I. J. (1963) See WILSON, S. G., MORRIS, K. R. S., LEWIS, I. J., and KROG, E. (1965).

LIVINGSTONE, D. (1857) *Missionary travels and researches in South Africa.* John Murray, London.

—— (ed. WALLIS, J. P. R.) (1956) *The Zambezi expedition of David Livingstone 1858–63,* 2 vols. Chatto and Windus, London.

—— and LIVINGSTONE, C. (1865) *Narrative of an expedition to the Zambezi and its tributaries; and of the discovery of the Lakes Shirwa and Nyassa.* London.

LLOYD, LL. (1912) Notes on *Glossina morsitans* Westw. in the Luangwa valley, Northern Rhodesia. *Bull. ent. Res.* **3,** 233.

—— and JOHNSON, W. B. (1924) Trypanosome infections of tsetse flies in Northern Nigeria and a new method of estimation. *Bull. ent. Res.* **14,** 265.

—— —— and RAWSON, P. H. (1927) Experiments in the control of tsetse fly. *Bull. ent. Res.* **17,** 423.

—— —— YOUNG, W. A., and MORRISON, H (1924). Second report of the tsetse fly investigation in the Northern provinces of Nigeria. *Bull. ent. Res.* **15,** 1.

LOTTE, A. J. (1952) Historique du foyer de trypanosomiase de Nola. *Publs. Bur. perm. interafr. Tsé-tsé* No. 194/0.

LOURIE, E. M. and O'CONNOR, R. J. (1937) A study of *Trypanosoma rhodesiense* relapse strains *in vitro. Ann. trop. Med. Parasit.* **31,** 319.

LOVEMORE, D. F. (1958) *Glossina pallidipes* Austen in Southern Rhodesia's northern tsetse belt. *Proc. 7th Meet. int. sci. Comm. Trypanosom. (Brussels),* C.C.T.A. Publ. No. 41, p. 235.

—— (1963) The effects of anti-tsetse shooting operations on the game populations as observed in the Sebungwe district, Southern Rhodesia. *Symposium on Conservation of Natural Resources in Modern African States, 1961* I.U.C.N. Publ. N.S. No. 1., p. 232.

—— (1967) Annual report of the Branch of Tsetse and Trypanosomiasis Control Department of Veterinary Services, Ministry of Agriculture, Rhodesia, for the year ending 30 September 1967. Salisbury. (Mimeograph.)

LUCAS, A. (1948) Some Egyptian connections with Sudan agriculture. In TOTHILL, J. D. (1948) *Agriculture in the Sudan.* Oxford University Press, London.

LUGARD, F. D. (1891) F. D. Lugard to Administrator General, Imperial British East Africa Company, Fort Edward, Toro, Unyoro, 13 August 1891. Enclosure 3 in No. 2 of Africa No. 4 (1892) *Papers relating to the Mombasa railway survey and Uganda.* Cd. 6555, H.M.S.O., London.

—— (1893) *The rise of our East African Empire,* 2 vols. Blackwood, Edinburgh.

—— (1922) *The Dual Mandate in British tropical Africa.* Blackwood, Edinburgh.

LUKYN WILLIAMS, F. (1935) Early explorers in Ankole. *Uganda J.* **2,** 196.

LUMSDEN, W. H. R. (1962) Trypanosomiasis in African wildlife. *Proc. 1st int. Conf. Wildl. Disease*, New York, p. 68.

—— (1963) Quantitative methods in the study of trypanosomes and their applications, with special reference to diagnosis. *Bull. Wld Hlth Org.* **28**, 745.

—— (1965) Biological aspects of trypanosome research. *Advanc. Parasit.* **3**, 1.

—— (1967) Trends in research on the immunology of trypanosomiasis. *Bull. Wld Hlth Org.* **37**, 167.

—— and HARDY, C. J. C. (1965) Nomenclature of living parasite material. *Nature, Lond.* **205**, 1032.

MACARIO, C. and BENTZ, M. (1963) Données épidémiologiques nouvelles sur la trypanosomiases humaine africaine à *T. gambiense. Bull. Soc. Path. exot.* **56**, 422.

MACAULAY, J. W. (1942) *A tsetse fly and trypanosomiasis survey in Bechuanaland, 1940–2.* Bechuanaland Protectorate Veterinary Department, Mafeking.

McCULLOCH, B. (1967) Trypanosomes of the *brucei* sub-group as a probable cause of disease in wild zebra (*Equus burchelli*). *Ann. trop. Med. Parasit.* **61**, 261.

—— SUDA, B'Q. J., TUNGARAZA, R., and KALAYE, W. J. (1968) A study of East coast fever, drought and social obligations, in relation to the need for the economic development of the livestock industry in Sukumaland and Tanzania. *Bull. epizoot. Dis. Afr.* **16**, 303.

McDIARMID, A. (ed.) (1969) Diseases in free-living wild animals. *Symposia of the Zoological Society of London* No. 24. Academic Press, London.

MACDONALD, G. (1957) *The epidemiology and control of malaria.* Oxford University Press, London.

MACDONALD, J. R. L. (1897) *Soldiering and surveying in East Africa.* Edward Arnold, London.

MACFIE, J. W. SCOTT (1913a) Trypanosomiasis of domestic animals in Northern Nigeria. *Ann. trop. Med. Parasit.* **7**, 1.

—— (1913b) On the morphology of the trypanosome (*T. nigeriense* n. sp.) from a case of sleeping sickness from Eket, Southern Nigeria. *Ann. trop. Med. Parasit.* **7**, 339.

MACHADO, A. DE BARROS (1954) Revision systématique des Glossines du groupe *palpalis* (Diptera). *Publcoes cult. Co. Diam., Angola* No. 22.

—— (1959) Nouvelles contributions à l'étude systématique et biogéographique de Glossines (Diptera). *Publcoes cult. Do. Diam., Angola* No. 46.

—— (1970 Les races géographiques de *Glossina morsitans. Criacao da mosca tsétsé no laboratorio e sua aplicacao pratica, I° Symposium Internacional de 1969,* Junta de Investigacoes do Ultramar (Publ. nao numerada), Lisbon (in press).

MACKICHAN, I. W. (1944) Rhodesian sleeping sickness in Eastern Uganda. *Trans. R. Soc. trop. Med. Hyg.* **38**, 49.

MACLEAN, G. (1935) Report on Karagwe. Report to Director of Medical Services, Tanganyika Territory, 15 June 1935. (Typescript.)

MACLENNAN, K. J. R. (1958) The distribution and significance of *Glossina morsitans submorsitans* in Northern Nigeria. *Proc. 7th Meet. int. scient. Comm. Trypanosom. (Brussels), C.C.T.A. Publ.* No. 41, p. 357.

—— (1963a) Cattle trypanosomiasis in Northern Nigeria. The problem in the field. *Bull. epizoot. Dis. Afr.* **11,** 381.

—— (1963b and 1969). Personal communications.

McLETCHIE, J. L. (1948) The control of sleeping sickness in Nigeria. *Trans. R. Soc. trop. Med. Hyg.* **41,** 445.

—— (1953) Sleeping sickness activities in Nigeria, 1931–52. Pts. I and II. *W. Afr. med. J.* **2** (n.s.), 70, 138.

MAHOOD, A. R. (1955) Map of tsetse distribution in Abuja area, Northern Nigeria. In *Veterinary Department Tsetse and Trypanosomiasis Unit 2nd annual report, April 1955–March 1956.* Kaduna.

MAILLOT, L. (1961) Répartition des Glossines et maladie du sommeil. Les races géographiques. *Bull. Soc. Path. exot.* **54,** 856.

—— (1962) Notice pour la carte chronologique des principaux foyers de la maladie du sommeil dans les états de l'ancienne fédération d'Afrique Équatoriale Française. *Bull. Inst. Rech. Scient. Congo* **1,** 45.

MALCOLM, D. W. (1953) *Sukumaland. An African people and their country.* Oxford University Press, London.

MANSON-BAHR, P. H. (1966) *Manson's tropical diseases* (16th edn.). Baillière, Tindall, and Cassell, London.

MARTIN, C. J. (1961) In *Essays on African population* (ed. K. M. BARBOUR and R. M. PROTHERO). Routledge and Kegan Paul, London.

MARTIN, G. and LEBŒUF, A. (1908) Diagnostic microscopique de la trypanosomiase humaine. Valeur comparée des divers procédés. *Bull. Soc. Path. exot.* **1,** 126.

MASON, I. L. and MAULE, J. P. (1960) The indigenous livestock of Eastern and Southern Africa. *Commonwealth Agricultural Bureaux, Technical Communication No. 14 of the Commonwealth Bureau of Animal Breeding and Genetics,* Edinburgh.

MATTERN, P., MASSEYEFF, R., MICHEL, R., and PERETTI, P. (1961) Étude immunologique de la macroglobuline des serums de malades atteints de trypanosomiase africain à *T. gambiense. Annls Inst. Pasteur, Paris* **101,** 382.

MECKLENBERG, THE DUKE OF (1910) *In the Heart of Africa.* Cassell & Co., London.

MELDON, J. A. (1907) Notes on the Bahima of Ankole, I and II. *Jl R. Afr. Soc.* **6,** 136, 234.

MELLANBY, K. (1936) Experimental work with the tsetse fly *Glossina palpalis* in Uganda. *Bull. ent. Res.* **27,** 611.

MEYER, H. (1913) Ergebnisse einer Reise durch das Zwischenseengebiet Ostafrikas 1911. *Mitt. dt. Schutzgeb.* Erganzungsheft No. 6.

MICHELMORE, A. P. G. (1939) Observations on tropical African grasslands. *J. Ecol.* **27,** 282.

MILBRAED, J. (1914) *Wissenschaftliche Ergebnisse der Deutschen Zentral-Afrika-Expedition 1907–8 unter Fuhrung Adolf Friedrich, Herzog zu Mecklenberg, Vol. 2, Botanik.* Leipzig.

MITTENDORF, H. J. and WILSON, S. G. (1961) *Livestock and meat marketing in Africa.* F.A.O., Rome. Quoted in WILSON, MORRIS, LEWIS, and KROG (1963).

MOFFETT, J. P. (ed.) (1958) *Handbook of Tanganyika* (2nd edn.). Government Printer, Dar-es-Salaam.

518   BIBLIOGRAPHY

MONTAGUE, F. A. (1926) *On distribution of fly and thicket areas in Simiyu River sleeping sickness area.* Typescript report dated Kizumbe, 23.12.26. E.A.T.R.O. Archives, Uganda.

MONTGOMERY, E. (1923) The stock industry in Uganda. *Uganda Protectorate Annual report of the Veterinary Department, year ended 31 December 1921,* p. 19. Government Printer, Entebbe.

MOORE, M. S. (1922) Report on investigation of tsetse fly on the mainland west and south of the Island of Juma. Report to Director of Game Preservation, Tanganyika Territory. (Typescript.)

MOREAU, R. E. (1967) *The bird faunas of Africa and its islands.* Academic Press, London and New York.

MORNET, P. (1954) The pathogenic trypanosomes of French West Africa. *Proc. 5th Meet. int. scient. Comm. Trypanosom. (Pretoria), Publs. Bur. perm. interafr. Tsé-tsé.* No. 206, p. 37.

—— and MOREL, P. (1956) Further observations on the distribution of pathogenic trypanosomes in domestic animals in French West Africa. *Proc. 6th Meet. int. scient. Comm. Trypanosom. (Salisbury), C.C.T.A. Publ.* p. 173.

MORRIS, H. F. (1960) The murder of H. St. G. Galt. *Uganda J.* **24,** 1.

—— (1962) *A History of Ankole.* East African Literature Bureau, Nairobi.

—— (1964) *The heroic recitations of the Bahima of Ankole.* The Clarendon Press, Oxford.

MORRIS, K. R. S. (1934) The bionomics and importance of *Glossina longipalpis* Wied. in the Gold Coast. *Bull. ent. Res.* **25,** 309.

—— (1958) Studies of *G. pallidipes* in Busoga, Uganda. *E. Afr. Tryp. Res. Org., July 1956–December 1957.* Government Printer, Nairobi, p. 63.

—— (1960a) The epidemiology of sleeping sickness in East Africa. III. The endemic area of Lakes Edward and George in Uganda. *Trans. R. Soc. trop. Med. Hyg.* **54,** 212.

—— (1960b) The epidemiology of sleeping sickness in East Africa. II. Sleeping sickness in Kenya. *Trans. R. Soc. trop. Med. Hyg.* **54,** 71.

—— (1963) The movement of sleeping sickness across Africa. *J. trop. Med. Hyg.* **66,** 57.

MORRIS, R. M. (1956) Incidence de la trypanosomiase humaine en Rhodésie. *Proc. 6th Meet. int. scient. Comm. Trypanosom. (Salisbury), C.C.T.A. Publ.* p. 5.

MOSSOP, M. C. (1948) Report of the Division of Entomology, 31 December 1947. *Rhodesia agric. J.* **45,** 230.

MOUCHET, J., GARIOU, J., and RATEAU, J. (1958) Distribution géographique et écologique de *Glossina palpalis palpalis* Rob.-Desv. et *Glossina fuscipes fuscipes* Newst. au Cameroun. *Bull. Soc. Path. exot.* **51,** 652.

MUHLPFORDT, H. (1964) Generationsdauer verschniedener Trypanosomenarten. *Z. Tropenmed. Parasit.* **15,** 145.

/ MULLIGAN, H. W. (ed.) (1970) *The African trypanosomiases.* Allen and Unwin, London (in press).

MURDOCK, G. P. (1959) *Africa. Its peoples and their culture history.* McGraw-Hill Book Company Inc., New York.

MWAMBU, P. M. (1966) The incidence of cattle trypanosomiasis in areas adjoining the South Busoga fly-belt. *E. Afr. Trypanosom. Res. Org. report* 1965, p. 48.

—— (1967) Cattle trypanosomiasis in the area adjoining the South Busoga fly-belt: (a) the incidence and (b) the effect of block treatment of the cattle in the area with ethidium bromide. *11th Meet. int. scient. Comm. Trypanosom.* (*Bangui*), 1966, p. 25.

—— and ODHIAMBO, J. O. (1967) Cattle trypanosomiasis in the area adjoining the South Busoga fly-belt. *E. Afr. Trypanosom. Res. Org. report* 1966, p. 56.

NAPIER BAX, S. (1937) The senses of smell and sight in *Glossina swynnertoni. Bull. ent. Res.* **28**, 539.

—— (1940) *Tsetse research report 1935–8.* Government Printer, Dar-es-salaam.

—— (1943) Notes on the presence of tsetse fly, between 1857 and 1915, in the Dar-es-Salaam area. *Tanganyika Notes Rec.* **16**, 1.

—— (1944) A practical policy for tsetse reclamation and field experiment. Reprinted from *E. Afr. agric. J.* **9**.

NASH, T. A. M. (1930) A contribution to our knowledge of the bionomics of *Glossina morsitans. Bull. ent. Res.* **21**, 201.

—— (1933) The ecology of *Glossina morsitans* Westwood and two possible methods for its destruction. *Bull. ent. Res.* **24**, 107, 163.

—— (1939) The ecology of the puparium of *Glossina* in Northern Nigeria. *Bull. ent. Res.* **30**, 259.

—— (1942) A study of the causes leading to the seasonal evacuation of a tsetse breeding ground. *Bull. ent. Res.* **32**, 327.

—— (1944) A low density of tsetse flies associated with a high incidence of sleeping sickness. *Bull. ent. Res.* **35**, 51.

—— (1948a) *Tsetse flies in British West Africa.* H.M.S.O., London.

—— (1948b) *The Anchau rural development and settlement scheme.* H.M.S.O., London.

—— (1952) Some observations on resting tsetse fly populations and evidence that *Glossina medicorum* is a carrier of trypanosomes. *Bull. ent. Res.* **43**, 33.

—— (1968) Personal communication.

—— and DAVEY, J. T. (1950) The resting habits of *Glossina medicorum, G. fusca,* and *G. longipalpis. Bull. ent. Res.* **41**, 153.

—— and PAGE, W. A. (1953) The ecology of *Glossina palpalis* in Northern Nigeria. *Trans. R. ent. Soc. Lond.* **104**, 71.

NEAVE, S. A. (1911) Report on a journey to the Luangwa valley, north-eastern Rhodesia, from July to September 1910. *Bull. ent. Res.* **1**, 303.

—— (1912) Notes on bloodsucking insects in eastern tropical Africa. *Bull. ent. Res.* **3**, 275.

NELSON, G. S. (1965) Discussion on K. C. WILLETT (1965) *Trans. R. Soc. trop. Med. Hyg.* **59**, 391.

NEUJEAN, G. (1963) Aspects pratiques de la lutte contre la trypanosomiase humaine dans la République du Congo (Léopoldville). *Bull. Wld Hlth Org.* **28**, 797.

—— and EVENS, F. (1958) Diagnostic et traitement de la maladie du sommeil à *T. gambiense. Mém. Acad. r. Sci. colon.* **7**.

NEWLANDS, H. (1956) Personal communication.

NEWSTEAD, R. and EVANS, A. M. (1921) New tsetse-flies (*Glossina*) from the Belgian Congo. *Ann. trop. Med. Parasit.,* **15**, 95.

NEWSTEAD, R., EVANS, A. M., and POTTS, W. H. (1924) *Guide to the study of tsetse flies. Liverpool School of Tropical Medicine, Mem. (New Series) No. 1.* Hodder and Stoughton, London.

NIGERIA MEDICAL REPORT (1934, 1938) *Annual medical and sanitary reports.* Government Printer, Lagos.

NIGERIA TSETSE AND TRYPANOSOMIASIS UNIT (1956, 1964) Northern Nigeria: Ministry of Animal and Forest Resources: Tsetse and Trypanosomiasis Division, Kaduna.

NIGERIA VETERINARY SERVICE (1925, 1928, 1940, 1945, 1947) *Colony and Protectorate of Nigeria. Annual Reports of the Veterinary Department.* Government Printer, Lagos.

NOBBS, E. A. (1927) Native cattle of Southern Rhodesia. *S. Afr. J. Sci.* **24,** 328.

NORTHERN NIGERIA REGION (1955) *This is Northern Nigeria.* Northern Region Government, Kaduna.

OKONJO, C (1968) A preliminary medium estimate of the 1962 mid-year population of Nigeria. In *The population of tropical Africa* (ed. J. C. CALDWELL and C. OKONJO). Longmans, Green and Co., London.

OLIVER, R. and MATTHEW, G. (eds.) (1963) *History of East Africa,* 2 vols. The Clarendon Press, Oxford.

OMER COOPER, J. D. (1966) *The Zulu aftermath. A nineteenth century revolution in Bantu Africa.* Longmans, Green and Co., London.

ONYANGO, R. J., SOUTHON, H. A. W., DE RAADT, P., CUNNINGHAM, M. P., VAN HOEVE, K., AKOLO, A. M., GRAINGE, E. B., and KIMBER, C. D. (1965) Epidemiological studies on an outbreak of sleeping sickness in Alego Location in Central Nyanza, Kenya. *East African Trypanosomiasis Research Organization report* July 1963–December 1964, Nairobi, p. 54.

—— VAN HOEVE, K. and DE RAADT, P. (1966) The epidemiology of *T. rhodesiense* sleeping sickness in Alego Location, Central Nyanza, Kenya. *Trans. R. Soc. trop. Med. Hyg.* **60,** 175.

ORCHARDSON, I. Q. (1932) Religious beliefs and practices of the Kipsigis. *Jl E. Africa Uganda nat. Hist. Soc.* **47–48,** 154.

ORMEROD, W. E. (1960) Cell inclusions and the epidemiology of Rhodesian sleeping sickness. *Trans. R. Soc. trop. Med. Hyg.* **54,** 299.

—— (1961) The epidemic spread of Rhodesian sleeping sickness 1908–60. *Trans. R. Soc. trop. Med. Hyg.* **55,** 525.

—— (1963) A comparative study of growth and morphology of strains of *Trypanosoma rhodesiense. Expl Parasit.* **13,** 374.

—— (1967) Taxonomy of the sleeping sickness trypanosomes. *J. Parasit.* **53,** 824.

ORMSBY-GORE, W. (chairman) (1925) Report of the East African Commission. Cmd. 2387, H.M.S.O., London.

OVAZZA, M. (1956) Contribution à l'étude du diptères vulnérants de l'Empire d'Éthiopie. IV. *Glossina. Bull. Soc. Path. exot.* **49,** 204.

OWEN, W. E. (1932) The Bantu of Kavirondo. *Jl E. Africa Uganda nat. Hist. Soc.* **45,** 67.

OYENUGA, V. A. (1967) *Agriculture in Nigeria.* F.A.O., Rome.

PAGE, W. A. (1959a) Some observations on the *fusca* group of tsetse flies (*Glossina*) in the South of Nigeria. *Bull. ent. Res.* **50,** 633.

—— (1959b) The ecology of *Glossina palpalis* (R.-D.) in Southern Nigeria. *Bull. ent. Res.* **50,** 617.

—— (1959c) The ecology of *Glossina longipalpis* Wied. in Southern Nigeria. *Bull. ent. Res.* **50,** 595.

—— and MACDONALD, W. A. (1959) An assessment of the degree of man–fly contact exhibited by *Glossina palpalis* at water holes in Northern and Southern Nigeria. *Ann. trop. Med. Parasit.* **53,** 162.

PARKE, T. H. (1891) *My personal experiences in equatorial Africa.* Sampson Low, London.

PATTERSON, J. H. (1907) *The man-eaters of Tsavo and other East African adventures.* Macmillan, London.

PAVER, B. G. (1957) *Zimbabwe cavalcade: Rhodesia's romance.* Cassell, London.

PAVLOWSKY, Y. N. (ed.) (D. ROTTENBURG trans.) (1964) *Human diseases with natural foci.* Foreign Languages Publishing House, Moscow.

PAYNE, W. J. A. (1964) The origin of domestic cattle in East Africa. *Emp. J. exp. Agric.* **32,** 97.

PEEL, E. and CHARDOME, M. (1954) *Trypanosoma suis* (Ochmann 1905) trypanosome monomorphe pathogène de mammifères, évoluant dans les glandes salivaires de *Glossina brevipalpis* Newst., Mosso, (Urundi). *Annls Soc. belge Méd. trop.* **34,** 277.

PERCIVAL, A. BLAYNEY (1918) Game and disease. *Jl E. Africa Uganda nat. Hist. Soc.* **13,** 302.

PHELPS, J. R. (1959) Sabi-Lundi area. *Report of the Secretary to the Federal Ministry of Agriculture for the year ending 30 September 1958.* Salisbury, p. 209.

PHILLIPS, J. (1959) *Agriculture and ecology in Africa.* Faber and Faber, London.

—— HAMMOND, J., SAMUELS, L. H., and SWYNNERTON, R. J. M. (1962) *The development of the economic resources of Southern Rhodesia with particular reference to the role of African agriculture. Report of the Advisory Committee.* Government Printer, Salisbury.

PIGAFETTA, P. (trans. CAHUN, L.) (1883) *Le Congo. La véridique description du royaume Africain appelé, tant par les indigènes que par les Portugais, le Congo, telle quelle a été tirée récemment des explorations d'Édouard Lopez, par Phillipe Pigafetta, qui l'a mise en langue italienne.* J.-J. Gay, Brussels.

PILSON, R. D. (1961) The crossing of the Sebungwe game-free barrier by *G. morsitans. Report of the Secretary to the Federal Ministry of Agriculture for the year ended 30 September, 1960.* Salisbury, p. 235.

—— and LEGGATE, B. M. (1962a) A diurnal and seasonal study of the resting behaviour of *Glossina pallidipes* Aust. *Bull. ent. Res.* **53,** 551.

—— —— (1962b) A diurnal and seasonal study of the feeding activity of *Glossina pallidipes* Aust. *Bull ent. Res.* **53,** 541.

—— and PILSON, B. M. (1967) Behaviour studies of *Glossina morsitans* Westw. in the field. *Bull. ent. Res.* **57,** 227.

PIRES, F. A., MARQUES DA SILVA, J., and TELES E CUNHA, E. G. (1950) Posicao actual da tsetse na area da Sitatonga circonscricao do Mossurize. Mocambique, Lourenco Marques, No. 62, p. 1.

PITMAN, C. R. S. (1931) *A game warden among his charges.* Nisbet, London.

POLLARD, J. (1912) Notes on the tsetse flies of Muri province, Northern Nigeria. *Bull. ent. Res.* **3**, 219.

POTTS, W. H. (1926) Report on safari to Nindo and Salawe districts. Department of Game Preservation, Tanganyika Territory. (Typescript.)

—— (1930) A contribution to the study of numbers of tsetse fly (*Glossina morsitans* Westw.) by quantitative methods. *S. Afr. J. Sci.* **27**, 491.

—— (1951) The distribution of tsetse flies in Africa. Proc. 3rd. Meet. int. scient. Comm. Trypanosom. (Bobo-Dioulassou), Publs. Bur. perm. interafr. tsé-tsé. (Mimeograph.)

—— (1953–4) The distribution of tsetse species in Africa, Map sheets 1, 2, and 3. D.C.S. (Misc.) 48*a*, *b*, and *c*. Directorate of Colonial Surveys, London.

—— (1955) A new tsetse fly from the British Cameroons. *Ann. trop. Med. Parasit.* **49**, 218.

—— and JACKSON, C. H. N. (1952) The Shinyanga game destruction experiment. *Bull. ent. Res.* **43**, 365.

POULTON, W. F. (1938) Anti-*Glossina* measures: South Ankole. Unpublished report to the Uganda Protectorate government, Entebbe.

PRATES, M. N. (1928) Posterior nuclear forms of polymorphic trypanosomes (*brucei, gambiense,* and *rhodesiense*). *Final report of the League of Nations International Commission on human trypanosomiasis*, C.H. 629, p. 154, Geneva.

PULLAN, R. A. (1962) The concept of the middle belt in Nigeria—an attempt at a climatic definition. *J. geogr. Assoc. Nigeria* **5**, 39.

QUINTON, H. J. (chairman) (1960) *Southern Rhodesia Legislative Assembly. Second report of the Select Committee on resettlement of natives*, L.A.S.C. 3, Government Printer, Salisbury.

RAJAGOPAL, P. K. and BURSELL, E. (1965) The effect of temperature on the oxygen consumption of tsetse pupae. *Bull. ent. Res.* **56**, 219.

—— —— (1966) The respiratory metabolism of resting tsetse flies. *J. Insect Physiol.* **12**, 287.

RANDALL, J. B. (1944) *Report on livestock production in Uganda.* Government Printer, Entebbe.

—— (1958) Animal trypanosomiasis in Uganda. *Symposium on animal trypanosomiasis, Luanda, Angola.* C.C.T.A., Publ. No. 45.

RANGER, T. O. (1967) *Revolt in Southern Rhodesia 1896–7. A study in African resistance.* Heinemann, London.

—— (ed.) (1968) *Aspects of Central African history.* Heinemann, London.

REHSE, H. (1910) *Kiziba, Land und Leute.* Strecker und Schröder, Stuttgart.

RENNIE, J. K. (1966) The Ngoni states and the European intrusion. In *The Zambezian past* (eds. E. STOKES and R. BROWN). Manchester University Press, Manchester.

RICHARDS, P. W. (1952) *The tropical rain forest.* Cambridge University Press, London.

RICHARDSON, J. F. and KENDALL, S. B. (1963) *Veterinary Protozoology* (3rd edn.). Oliver and Boyd, Edinburgh.

RICHET, P. (1962) La trypanosomiase residuelle. *Proc. 9th Meet. int. scient. Comm. Trypanosom. (Conakry),* C.C.T.A. Publ. No. 88, p. 283.

RICHTER, OBERLEUTNANT (1899) Der Bezirk Bukoba. *Mitt. dt. Schutzgeb.* **12**, 67

RITZ, H. (1916) Über Rezidive bei experimenteller Trypanosomiasis. II Mitteilung. *Arch. Schiffs- u. Tropenhyg.* **20**, 397.

ROBERTSON, A. G. (1957) *Uganda Protectorate: annual report of the Tsetse Control Department for the year ended 31 December 1956.* Government Printer, Entebbe.

—— (1968) The Nagupande experiment. Tsetse and Trypanosomiasis Control Branch, Salisbury. (Mimeograph.)

—— and KLUGE, E. B. (1968) The use of insecticide in arresting an advance of *Glossina morsitans* Westwood in the south-east lowveld of Rhodesia. *Proc. Trans. Rhod. scient. Ass.* **53**, 17.

ROBERTSON, D. H. H. (1963) Human trypanosomiasis in south-eastern Uganda. A further study of the disease among fishermen and peasant cultivators. *Bull. Wld Hlth Org.* **28**, 627.

—— and BAKER, J. R. (1958) Human trypanosomiasis in south-east Uganda. I. A study of the epidemiology and present virulence of the disease. *Trans. R. Soc. trop. Med. Hyg.* **52**, 336.

ROBERTSON, M. (1913) Notes on the life history of *Trypanosoma gambiense*, with brief reference to the cycles of *Trypanosoma nanum* and *Trypanosoma* in *Glossina palpalis*. *Phil. Trans. R. Soc.* (B) **203**, 161.

ROBSON, J. and HOPE-CAWDERY, M. J. H. (1958) Prophylaxis against trypanosomiasis in Zebu cattle. A comparison of prothidium, the suraminate of ethidium and RD 2902 and antrycide prosalt. *Vet. Rec.* **70**, 870.

RODHAIN, J. (1919) Observations médicales recueillies parmi les troupes coloniales belges pendant leur campagne en Afrique Orientale, 1914–17. *Bull. Soc. Path. exot.* **12**, 137.

—— PONS, C., VANDENBRANDEN, F., and BEQUAERT, J. (1912) Contribution au mécanisme de la transmission des trypanosomes par les glossines. *Arch. Schiffs- u. Tropenhyg.* **16**, 732.

ROSCOE, J. (1923) *The Bagesu and other tribes of the Uganda Protectorate.* Cambridge University Press, London.

ROSS, G. R. and BLAIR, D. M. (1956) Cas de 'porteurs en bonne santé' de trypanosomiase humaine en Rhodésie du Sud. *6th Meet. int. scient. Comm. Trypanosom.* (*Salisbury*), *C.C.T.A., Publ.* p. 9.

ROUBAUD, E. and MAILLOT, L. (1952) Les modalités de l'infection cyclique trypanosomienne observées chez les *Glossinea caliginea* des gîtes à palétuviers de Douala. *Bull. Soc. Path. exot.* **45**, 228.

—— —— and RAGEAU, J. (1951) Infection naturelle de *Glossina caliginea* dans les gîtes à palétuviers de Douala (Cameroun français). *Bull. Soc. Path. exot.* **45**, 206.

ROUGET, J. (1896) *Annls Inst. Pasteur, Paris* **10**, 716, quoted by M. A. SOLTYS (1963).

ROUNCE, N. V. (1949) *The agriculture of the cultivation steppe of the Lake, Western, and Central provinces.* Department of Agriculture, Tanganyika Territory. Longmans, Green and Co., Capetown.

RUTHENBERG, H. (1964) *Agricultural development in Tanganyika.* Springer-Verlag, Berlin.

—— (ed.) (1967) *Smallholder farming and smallholder development in Tanzania. Ten case studies.* Hurst, London.

RUTTLEDGE, W. (1928) Tsetse-fly (*Glossina morsitans*) in the Koalib hills, Nuba Mountains province, Sudan. *Bull. ent. Res.* **19**, 309.

SACHS, R., SCHALLER, G. B., and BAKER, J. R. (1967) Isolation of trypanosomes of the *T. brucei* group from lion. *Acta trop.* **24**, 109.

ST. CROIX, F. W. DE (1945). *The Fulani of Northern Nigeria*. Government Printer, Lagos.

SALEM, I. F. (1930) *Cattle plague in Egypt*. Government Printer, Cairo.

SANDGROUND, J. H. (1947) Experimental studies of an old strain of *Trypanosoma gambiense*. I. The enhancement of virulence and the relationship of this phenomenon to the species of the polymorphic trypanosomes of Africa. *Ann. trop. Med. Parasit.* **41**, 293.

SANTOS DIAS, J. TRAVASSOS (1961) Resultado de um reconhecimento glossinico em algumas circonscricaos do distrito de Cabo Delgado. *Anais Servs Vet. Ind. anim. Moçamb.* **7**, 167.

—— (1962) The status of the tsetse fly in Mozambique before 1896. *S. Afr. J. Sci.* **58**, 243.

SAUNDERS, D. S. (1960) The ovulation cycle in *Glossina morsitans* Westwood (Diptera; Muscidae) and a possible method of age determination for female tsetse flies by examination of their ovaries. *Trans. R. ent. Soc. Lond.* **112**, 221.

—— (1967) Survival and reproduction in a natural population of tsetse fly, *Glossina palpalis palpalis* (Robineau-Desvoidy). *Proc. R. ent. Soc. Lond.* (A) **42**, 129.

SCAËTTA, H. (1932) Les famines périodiques dans le Ruanda. *Mém. Inst. r. colon. belge Sect. Sci. nat. méd.* **1**, Fasc. 4.

SCOTT, D. (1965) *Epidemic disease in Ghana*. Oxford University Press, London.

SCOTT, G. M. (1962) The soils of East Africa. In *The Natural Resources of East Africa* (ed. E. W. RUSSELL). East African Literature Bureau, Nairobi.

SCOTT ELLIOT, G. F. (1896) *A naturalist in mid-Africa*. Innes & Co., London.

SCUDDER, T. (1962) *The ecology of the Gwembe Tonga*. Manchester University Press, Manchester.

SHAW, G. D. (1958) Animal trypanosomiasis in Northern Rhodesia (A detailed survey of the problem). *Symposium on Animal Trypanosomiasis, Luanda, Angola, Publs. C.C.T.A.* No. 45, 124.

SHAW, T. and COLVILLE, G. (1950) *Report of Nigerian Livestock Commission*. H.M.S.O., London.

SIMMONS, R. J. (1929) Notes on a tsetse belt in Western Uganda. *Bull. ent. Res.* **19**, 421.

—— and CARMICHAEL, J. (1940) *Rinderpest control and research*. Government Printer, Entebbe.

SIMON, N. (1962) *Between the sunlight and the thunder. The wildlife of Kenya*. Collins, London.

SIMPSON, G. G. (1950) *The meaning of evolution*. Oxford University Press, London.

SIMPSON, J. J. (1912) Entomological research in British West Africa. II. Northern Nigeria. *Bull. ent. Res.* **2**, 301.

SLADE, R. (1962) *King Leopold's Congo*. Oxford University Press, London.

SLEEPING SICKNESS BUREAU (1909a) Sleeping sickness news: Uganda. *Bull. Sleep. Sickn. Bur.* **1**, 315.

—— (1909*b*) Sleeping sickness news: East Africa. *Bull. Sleep, Sickn. Bur.* **1**, 394.

—— (1911) Sleeping sickness news: Uganda. *Bull. Sleep. Sickn. Bur.* **3**, 426.

SOLTYS, M. A. (1955) Studies of resistance to *Trypanosoma congolense* developed by zebu cattle treated prophylactically with antrycide prosalt in an enzootic area of East Africa. *Ann. trop. Med. Parasit.* **49**, 1.

—— (1963) Immunity in African trypanosomiasis. *Bull. Wld Hlth Org.* **28**, 753.

SOUSA, A. E. DE (1960) The advances of *Glossina* in Southern Mozambique. *Proc. 8th Meet. int. scient. Comm. Trypanosom. (Jos), C.C.T.A. Publ.* No. 62, p. 203.

SOUSA, J. DE (1947) Carta da distribuicao dos casos de tripanossomiases humana encontrados nos ultimos vinte anos. *Conferencia intercolonial sobre tripanossomiases,* Lourenco Marques, 26–31 August 1946, vol. 1, p. 198.

SOUTHERN RHODESIA (1912) *Report on the public health for the year ended 31 December 1911.* Government Printer, Salisbury.

SOUTHON, H. A. W. (1960) Ecology of *T. rhodesiense* sleeping sickness in Busoga, Uganda. *E. Afr. Tryp. Res. Org. Report, January–December 1959,* p. 29. Government Printer, Nairobi.

—— CUNNINGHAM, M. P. and GRAINGE, E. B. (1965) The infectivity of trypanosomes derived from individual *Glossina morsitans. E. Afr. Tryp. Res. Org. Report, July 1963–December 1964,* p. 33. E. A. Common Services, Nairobi.

—— and ROBERTSON, D. H. H. (1961) Isolation of *Trypanosoma rhodesiense* from wild *Glossina palpalis. Nature, Lond.* **189**, 411.

SPEKE, J. H. (1863) *Journal of the discovery of the source of the Nile.* Blackwood, Edinburgh.

—— (1864) *What led to the discovery of the source of the Nile.* Blackwood, Edinburgh.

STANLEY, H. M. (1878) *Through the dark continent,* 2 vols. Sampson Low, London.

—— (1890) *In darkest Africa,* 2 vols. Sampson Low, London.

STENNING, D. J. (1959) *Savannah nomads.* Oxford University Press, London.

STEPHENS, J. W. W. and FANTHAM, H. B. (1910) On the peculiar morphology of a trypanosome from a case of sleeping sickness and the possibility of its being a new species (*T. rhodesiense). Proc. R. Soc.* (B) **561**, 28.

STEUDEL, GENERALOBERARZT (1912) Der Kampf gegen die Schlafkrankheit. *Deutsch. Kolonialblatt* **22**, 434 (Summary in *Bull. Sleep. Sickn. Bur.* **4**, 244).

STEVENSON-HAMILTON, J. (1912) *Animal life in Africa.* Heinemann, London.

STEWART, D. R. M. and STEWART, J. (1963) The distribution of some large mammals in Kenya. *Jl E. Afr. nat. Hist. Soc. & Coryndon Mus.* **24**, 1.

STOHR, F. O. (1912) *La maladie du sommeil en Katanga.* Constable, London.

STUHLMANN, F. (1894) *Mit Emin Pascha ins Herz von Afrika.* Dietrich Reimer, Berlin.

—— (1916–27) *Die Tagebücher von Dr. Emin Pascha,* 6 vols. Westermann, Brunswick.

SUMMERS, R. (1958) *Inyanga. Prehistoric settlements in Southern Rhodesia.* Cambridge University Press, London.

—— (1960) Environment and culture in Southern Rhodesia: A study in the 'personality' of a land-locked country. *Proc. Am. phil. Soc.* **104**, 266.

SUMMERS, R. (1963) *Zimbabwe. A Rhodesian mystery*. Nelson, Capetown.

SURVEYOR GENERAL, SALISBURY (1963) Southern Rhodesia: Land apportionment map, 1 : 1 000 000. Federal Government Printer, Salisbury, Rhodesia.

SWYNNERTON, C. F. M. (1921) An examination of the tsetse problem in North Mossurisse, Portuguese East Africa. *Bull. ent. Res.* **11,** 315.

—— (1923a) The entomological aspects of an outbreak of sleeping sickness near Mwanza, Tanganyika Territory. *Bull. ent. Res.* **13,** 317.

—— (1923b) Tsetse flies breeding in open ground. *Bull. ent. Res.* **14,** 119.

—— (1923c) Report on elephants to the Uganda Protectorate government. E.A.T.R.O. Archives, Tororo, Uganda. (Typed draft.)

—— (1925a) An experiment in control of tsetse flies at Shinyanga, Tanganyika Territory. *Bull. ent. Res.* **15,** 313.

—— (1925b) The tsetse fly problem in the Nzega sub-district, Tanganyika Territory. *Bull. ent. Res.* **16,** 99.

—— (1936) The tsetse flies of East Africa. *Trans. R. ent. Soc. Lond.* vol. **84,** 579 pp.

TABLER, E. C. (1955) *The far interior: chronicles of pioneering in the Matabele and Mashona countries, 1847–1879*. A. A. Balkema, Capetown.

TANGANYIKA ATLAS (1956) *Atlas of Tanganyika* (3rd edn.). Department of Lands and Surveys, Dar-es-salaam.

TANGANYIKA CENSUS (1963) *African census report 1957*. Government Printer, Dar-es-salaam.

TANGANYIKA TSETSE (1948 onwards) *Annual reports of the Tsetse Survey and Reclamation Department*. Government Printer, Dar-es-salaam.

TANGANYIKA VETERINARY (1921 onwards) *Annual reports of the Department of Veterinary Science and Animal Husbandry*. Government Printer, Dar-es-salaam.

TANSLEY, A. G. (1949) *The British Islands and their vegetation*, 2 vols. Cambridge University Press, London.

TARRY, D. W. (1967) Observations on the ecology of *Glossina morsitans sub-morsitans* Newst., in the Guinea–Sudan transition savanna of Northern Nigeria. *Ann. trop. Med. Parasit.* **61,** 457.

—— (1969) Personal communication.

TAUTE, M. and HUBER, F. (1919) Die Unterscheidung des *Trypanosoma rhodesi-ense* vom *Trypanosoma brucei*: Beobachtungen und Experimente aus dem Kriege in Ostafrika. *Arch. Schiffs- u. Tropenhyg.* **23,** 211.

TAYLOR, A. W. (1930) *Glossina palpalis* and sleeping sickness at Ganawuri, Plateau province, Northern Nigeria. *Bull. ent. Res.* **21,** 333.

TAYLOR, B. K. (1962) *The western lacustrine Bantu. Ethnographic Survey of Africa*. International African Institute, London.

TERNAN, T. (1930) *Some experiences of an Old Bromsgrovian*. Cornish Brothers, Birmingham.

THOMAS, H. B. and SCOTT, R. (1935) *Uganda*. Oxford University Press, London.

THOMAS, W. E., DAVEY, T. H., and POTTS, W. H. (1955) *Report of the Commission of Enquiry on human and animal trypanosomiasis in Southern Rhodesia*. Federation of Rhodesia and Nyasaland, C. Fed. 24, Salisbury.

THOMÉ, M. (1964) Peste bovine: Historique. *Rapport annuel 1964, Ministère de l'Agriculture et de la Production Animale, République de Tchad: Direction d'Élévage*, Fasc. 7, p. 5. Fort Lamy.

THOMSON, K. D. B. (1967a) *Trypanosomiasis in Northern Nigeria: rural health report, 1965*. Government Printer, Kaduna.

—— (1967b) Rural health in Northern Nigeria: Some recent developments and problems. *Trans. R. Soc. trop. Med. Hyg.* **61,** 277.

—— (1969) The present sleeping sickness situation in the northern states of Nigeria. *J. trop. Med. Hyg.* **72,** 27.

TOWNSHEND, C. H. T. (1923) The tsetse problem. *S. Afr. J. nat. Hist.* **4,** 36, 139.

TRYPANOSOMIASIS COMMITTEE (1945) The scientific basis of the control of *Glossina morsitans* by game destruction. *Rhodesia agric. J.* **42,** 124.

TURNER, B. J. and BAKER, P. R. (1968) Tsetse control and livestock development: a case study from Uganda. *Geography* **53,** 249.

TURNER, R. D. (1967) Personal communication.

UDO, R. K. (1968) Population and politics in Nigeria. In *The population of tropical Africa* (ed. J. C. CALDWELL and C. OKONJO). Longmans, London.

UGANDA ATLAS (1962) *Atlas of Uganda* (2nd edn.). Department of Lands and Surveys, Kampala.

UGANDA BLUE BOOKS (1909 to 1921) *Uganda Protectorate Government blue books*. Government Printer, Entebbe.

UGANDA MEDICAL (1927) *Annual medical and sanitary report, 1926*. Government Printer, Entebbe.

UGANDA TSETSE (1949 onwards) *Annual reports of the Department or Division of Tsetse Control*. Government Printer, Entebbe.

UGANDA VETERINARY (1921 onwards) *Annual reports of the Department of Veterinary Services and Animal Industry*. Government Printer, Entebbe.

UNSWORTH, K. (1953) Studies on *Trypanosoma vivax*. VIII. Observations on the incidence and pathogenicity of *T. vivax* in Zebu cattle in Nigeria. *Ann. trop. Med. Parasit.* **47,** 361.

—— and BIRKETT, J. D. (1952) The use of antrycide prosalt in protecting cattle against trypanosomiasis when in transit through tsetse areas. *Vet. Rec.* **64,** 351.

VAN DEN BERGHE, L., CHARDOME, M., and PEEL, E. (1963) Sur l'extrême variation de virulence des souches de trypanosomes du groupe *brucei* isolées de *Glossina morsitans* au Mutara (Rwanda). *Annls Soc. belge Méd. trop.* **2,** 169.

—— and LAMBRECHT, F. L. (1954) Notes on the discovery and biology of *Glossina brevipalpis* Newst. in the Mosso Region (Urundi). *Bull. ent. Res.* **45,** 501.

—— —— (1956) Notes écologiques et biologiques sur *G. pallidipes* dans le Mutara (Ruanda). *Annls Soc. belge Méd. trop.* **36,** 205.

—— —— (1962) Étude biologique et écologique de *Glossina morsitans* Westw. dans le région du Bugesera (Ruanda). *Mém. Acad. r. Sci. d'outre-mer Cl. Sci. nat. méd.* 8° **13.**

—— —— and CHRISTIAENSEN, A. R. (1956) Étude biologique des glossines dans la région du Mutara (Ruanda). *Mém. Acad. r. Sci. colon. Cl. Sci. nat. méd.* 8° **4.**

VANDERPLANK, F. L. (1947a) Experiments in the hybridization of tsetse flies (*Glossina*, Diptera) and the possibility of a new method of control. *Trans. R. ent. Soc. Lond.* **98,** 1.

VANDERPLANK, F. L. (1947b) Seasonal and annual variation in the incidence of trypanosomiasis in game. *Ann. trop. Med. Parasit.* **41,** 365.

—— (1949a) The classification of *Glossina morsitans* Westwood (Diptera, Muscidae) including a description of a new sub-species, varieties and hybrids. *Proc. R. ent. Soc. Lond.* (B) **18,** 56.

—— (1949b) The classification of *Glossina palpalis* including the description of new sub-species and hybrids. *Proc. R. ent. Soc. Lond.* (B) **18,** 69.

VAN HOOF, L. (1928a) Sleeping sickness in the Semliki valley, Belgian Congo. *Final report of the League of Nations International Commission on human trypanosomiasis.* Geneva, C.H. 629, p. 329.

—— (1928b) Epidemiology of sleeping sickness in Budama and Kavirondo. *Final report of the League of Nations International Commission on human trypanosomiasis.* Geneva, C.H. 629, p. 363.

—— (1947) Observations on trypanosomiasis in the Belgian Congo. *Trans. R. Soc. trop. Med. Hyg.* **40,** 728.

—— HENRARD, C. and PEEL, E. (1937) Influences modificatives de la transmissibilité cyclique des *Trypanosoma gambiense* par *Glossina palpalis. Annls Soc. belge Méd. trop.* **17,** 249.

—— —— —— (1938) Contribution à l'epidémiologies de la maladie du sommeil au Congo Belge. *Annls Soc. belge Méd. trop.* **18,** 143.

—— —— —— (1940) Recherches sur le comportement du '*Trypanosoma gambiense*' chez le porc. *Annls Soc. belge Méd. trop.* **20,** 203.

VANSINA, J. (1966) *Kingdoms of the savanna.* University of Wisconsin Press, Madison.

VARLEY, G. C. (1957) Ecology as an experimental science. *J. Anim. Ecol.* **26,** 251.

VAUCEL, M. and FROMENTIN, H. (1958) Nouvelles observations au cours d'infections expérimentales par mélange de souches de trypanosomes polymorphes. *Proc. 7th Meet. int. Comm. scient. Trypanosom. (Brussels), C.C.T.A.,* Publ. No. 41, p. 187.

—— and JONCHERE, H. (1954) Observations made during the course of hybridization trials with different 'species' of polymorphic trypanosomes. *Proc. 5th Meet. int. scient. Comm. Trypanosom. (Pretoria), Publs. Bur. perm. interafr. Tsé-tsé* No. 206, p. 126.

—— WADDY, B. B., DE ANDRADE E SILVA, M. A., and PONS, V. E. (1963) The geographical distribution of trypanosomiasis in man and animal in Africa. *Bull. Wld Hlth Org.* **28,** 545.

VESEY-FITZGERALD, D. F. (1960) Grazing succession among East African game animals. *J. Mammal.* **41,** 161.

VINCENT, V., THOMAS, R. G., ANDERSON, R., and STAPLES, R. R. (n.d.) *An agricultural survey of Southern Rhodesia.* Pts. I and II. Government Printer, Salisbury.

VON GÖTZEN, GRAF (1895) *Durch Afrika von Ost nach West.* Dietrich Reimer, Berlin.

VON STUEMER (1904) Bezirk Bukoba in Auszuge aus dem Berichte der Bezirksämter, Militärstationen und andere Dienstellen über die wirtschaftlichen Entwicklung im Berichtsjähre vom 1 April 1902 bis 31 Marz 1903. *Ber. Land- u. Forstw. Dt.-Ostafr.* **2,** 37.

WALKER, E. A. (1957) *A history of Southern Africa.* Longmans, Green, London.

WALLIS, H. R. (1920) *The handbook of Uganda* (2nd edn.). Crown Agents for the Colonies, London.

WALTON, J. (1957) Some features of the Monomotapa culture, In *Third pan-African congress on prehistory* (eds. J. D. CLARK and S. COLE). Chatto and Windus, London.

WATSON, H. J. C. (1962) The domestic pig as a reservoir of *T. gambiense. Proc. 9th Meet. int. scient. Comm. Trypanosom. (Conakry), C.C.T.A., Publ.* No. 88, p. 327.

WATSON, T. Y. (chairman) (1954) *Report of the Agricultural Productivity Committee, Uganda Protectorate.* Government Printer, Entebbe.

WECK, STABSARZT (1914) Beobachtungen über Trypanosomen des Menschen und der Tiere an Rovuma Flusse. *Arch. Schiffs- u. Tropenhyg.* **18**, 113.

WEINMAN, D. (1963) Problems of diagnosis of trypanosomiasis. *Bull. Wld Hlth Org.* **28**, 711.

WEIR, J. and DAVISON, E. (1965) Daily occurrence of African game animals at water holes during dry weather. *Zoologica africana* **1**, 353.

WEITZ, B. (1958) The immunological approach to problems relating to trypanosomiasis. *Proc. 7th Meet. int. scient. Comm. Trypanosom. (Brussels), C.C.T.A. Publ.* No. 41, p. 71.

—— (1963) The feeding habits of *Glossina. Bull. Wld Hlth Org.* **28**, 711.

—— (1964) The reaction of trypanosomes to their environment. *Symp. Soc. Gen. Microbiol.* No. 14, p. 112.

—— and JACKSON, C. H. N. (1955) The host animals of *Glossina morsitans* at Daga-Iloi. *Bull. ent. Res.* **46**, 531.

WERTHER, C. W. (1894) *Zum Victoria Nyanza.* Hermann Paetel, Berlin.

WESTWOOD, J. O. (1850) Observations on the destructive species of dipterous insects known in Africa under the names of tsetse, zimb, and tsaltsalya and on their supposed connection with the fourth plague of Egypt. *Proc. zool. Soc. Lond.* **18**, 258.

WHELLAN, J. A. (1949) A review of the tsetse fly situation in S. Rhodesia, 1948. *Rhodesia agric. J.* **46**, 316.

—— (1950) Tsetse fly in S. Rhodesia, 1949. *Rhodesia agric. J.* **47**, 416.

WHITE, F. (1962) Geographic variation and speciation in Africa with particular reference to *Diospyros.* In *Symposium on Taxonomy and Geography* (ed. D. NICHOLS). *The Systematics Association Publ.* No. 4, p. 71.

WHITESIDE, E. F. (1949) An experiment in control of tsetse with DDT-treated oxen. *Bull. ent. Res.* **40**, 123.

—— (1953) Kenya. *East Africa Tsetse and Trypanosomiasis Research and Reclamation Organization, annual report 1952,* p. 31. East African High Commission, Nairobi.

WIGGINS, C. A. (1960–1) Early days in British East Africa and Uganda. *E. Afr. med. J.* **37**, 699, 780.

WIJERS, D. J. B. (1958) Factors that may influence the infection rate of *Glossina palpalis* with *Trypanosoma gambiense. Ann. trop. Med. Parasit.* **52**, 385.

—— (1969) The history of sleeping sickness in Yimbo location (Central Nyanza, Kenya). *Trop. geogr. Med.* **21**, 323.

WILDE, J. K. H. and FRENCH, M. H. (1945) An experimental study of *Trypanosoma rhodesiense* infection in zebu cattle. *J. comp. Path.* **55**, 206.

WILLETT, K. C. (1955) Trypanosomiasis Research. *East Africa Tsetse and Trypanosomiasis Research and Reclamation Organization, annual report 1954–5*, p. 31. East African High Commission, Nairobi.

—— (1956) An experiment on dosage in human trypanosomiasis. *Ann. trop. Med. Parasit.* **50,** 75.

—— (1965) Some observations on the recent epidemiology of sleeping sickness in Nyanza Region, Kenya, and its relation to the general epidemiology of Gambian and Rhodesian sleeping sickness in Africa. *Trans. R. Soc. trop. Med. Hyg.* **59,** 374.

—— and FAIRBAIRN, H. (1955) The Tinde experiment: a study of *Trypanosoma rhodesiense* during eighteen years of cyclical transmission. *Ann. trop. Med. Parasit.* **49,** 278.

WILLS, A. J. (1964) *An introduction to the history of Central Africa.* Oxford University Press, London.

WILSON, S. G. (1958) Recent advances of *Glossina morsitans submorsitans* in Northern Nigeria. *Proc. 7th Meet. int. scient. Comm. Trypanosom. (Brussels), C.C.T.A. Publ.* No. 41, p. 367.

—— MORRIS, K. R. S., LEWIS, E. A., and KROG, E. (1963) The effects of trypanosomiasis on rural economy with special reference to the Sudan, Bechuanaland, and West Africa. *Bull. Wld Hlth Org.* **28,** 595.

WILSON, V. J. and ROTH, H. H. (1967) The effects of tsetse control operations on common duiker in Eastern Zambia. *E. Afr. Wildl. J.* **5,** 53.

WOLLASTON, A. F. R. (1908) *From Ruwenzori to the Congo.* John Murray, London.

WOODALL, J. P. (1968) Some problems of virus ecology in the Amazon forest. Tropical Group, British Ecological Society. *J. Ecol.* **56,** 1 P.

WOOFF, W. R. (1964) The eradication of *G. morsitans morsitans* Westw. in Ankole, Western Uganda, by dieldrin application. *Proc. 10th Meet. int. scient. Comm. Trypanosom. (Kampala), C.C.T.A. Publ.* No. 97, p. 157.

—— (1968) Map: Distribution of tsetse species. *Atlas of Uganda* (2nd edn.). Department of Lands and Surveys, Kampala.

WOOSNAM, R. B. (1914) Report on a search for *Glossina* on the Amala (Engabei) river, Southern Masai reserve, East Africa Protectorate. *Bull. ent. Res.* **4,** 271.

WORTHINGTON, E. B. and HARRIS, D. (1949) *A development plan for Uganda,* and the 1948 revision of the plan. Government Printer, Entebbe.

YEOMAN, G. (1966) Field vector studies of epizootic East coast fever. Parts I, II, and III. *Bull. epizoot. Dis. Afr.* **14,** 5, 115, **15,** 89.

—— (1967) Field vector studies of epizootic East coast fever. Part IV. The occurrence of *R. evertsi, R. pravus, R. simus,* and *R. sanguineus* in the East coast fever zones. *Bull. epizoot. Dis. Afr.* **15,** 189.

ZEUNER, F. E. (1963) *A history of domesticated animals.* Hutchinson, London.

AUTHOR INDEX

SUBJECT INDEX